EMILY'S BIRTH BOOK

YOUR GUIDE TO A CONSCIENTIOUS BIRTH

[Original cover]

A 16-week interactive course in pregnancy and birth preparation

Learn to participate in your medical care and build agency in your birth process.

Nourish your pregnancy with evidence-based information, art, and meditations.

Learn practical skills for birth and parenting with a partner or solo. Define your birth values and navigate your maternity care accordingly.

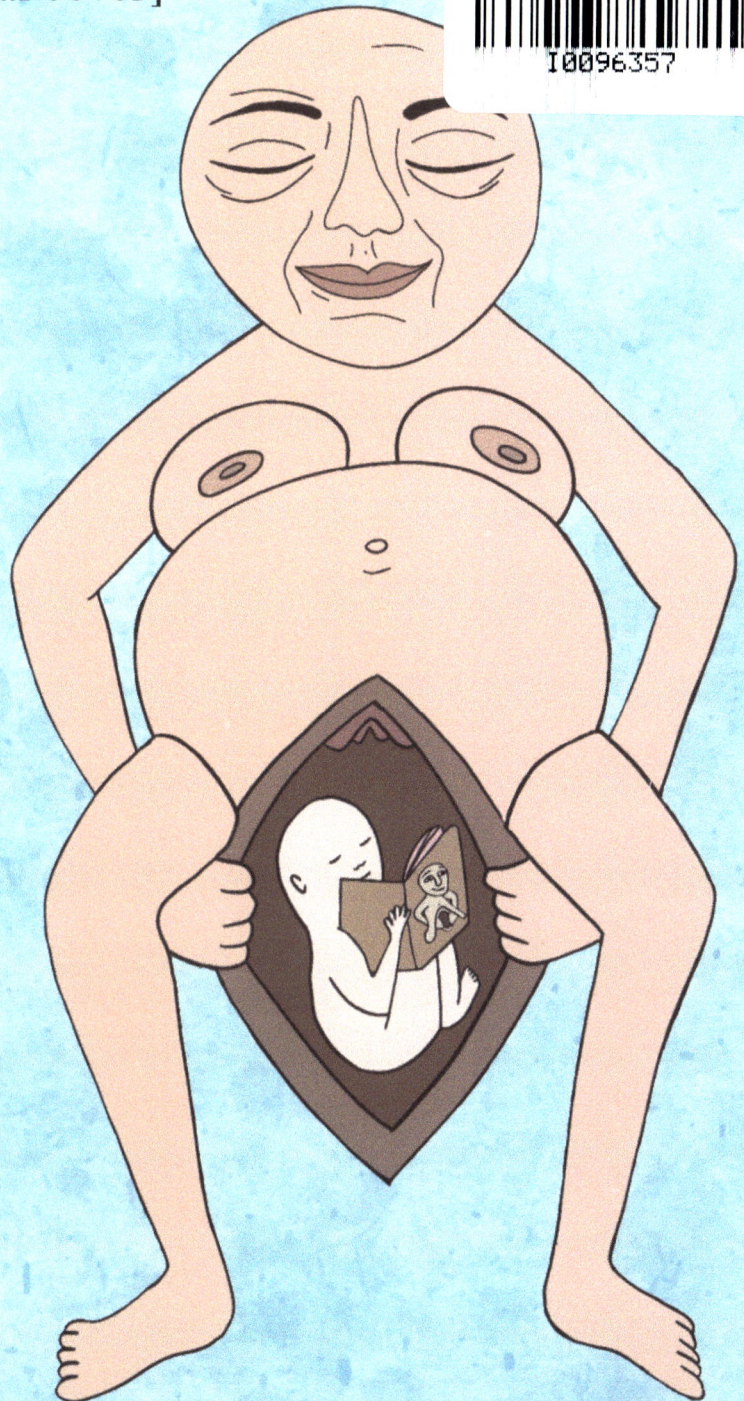

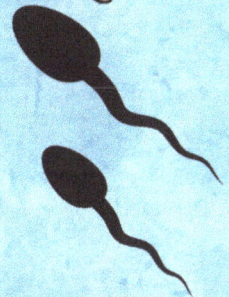

Emily Sherman Marynczak

ART BY Anna Schupack

EMILY'S BIRTH BOOK

YOUR GUIDE TO A CONSCIENTIOUS BIRTH

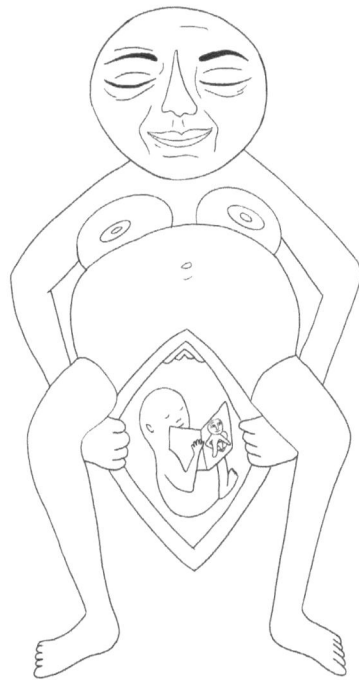

Emily Sherman Marynczak

ART BY Anna Schupack

Disclaimer

The information included in this book is not intended to take the place of medical/midwifery care. It is a presentation of opinions and ideas bolstered by experience and research. All medical and exercise decisions should be made by individuals in consultation with their healthcare providers. I am an affiliated instructor of the Bradley Method®, developed by The American Academy of Husband-Coached Childbirth®, but have no further connections or associations with the organization. As the author, I specifically disclaim all responsibility for any risk or loss incurred directly or indirectly related to the material in this book.

Critical resources

- In a mental health emergency call or text the national crisis hotline: **988**
- If you are actively bleeding get immediate medical attention, call: **911**
- If you are pregnant or lactating and need assistance with food, you may be eligible through the government program WIC (Women, Infant and Children): https://www.fns.usda.gov/wic/wic-how-apply

Author's note on the illustrations

It was a special honor to work with the artist Anna Schupack. I brought her my ideas and then she used her intuition and talent to help me realize my visions. It was important to me to bring both humor and beauty to the seriousness of this topic. It is my hope that the art brings some respite and inspiration from all the heavy weight of birthing and becoming a parent. Having babies and raising families is at its core a creative process. I wanted learning about birth to be creative, too. Thank you also to photographers Kyle Avery and Sable Trappenburg, who took photographs that were used as labor position references, and to Nana Adusei-Poku, Nic Kornegay, Shannon Hatfield, Willis Hatfield, Kendall Ross, and Khloe who were our fabulous reference models. (Some drawings were made from an amalgamation of various sources.)

Emily's Birth Book: Your Guide to a Conscientious Birth
Copyright © 2023 by Emily Sherman Marynczak

Book design by The Troy Book Makers
The Troy Book Makers • Troy, New York • thetroybookmakers.com

Printed in the United States of America

ISBN: 979-8-21830-748-6

CONTENTS

Dedication

Emily's Birth Book is dedicated to Julian,
Jasper, Arlo, and Sadie, our sweet family dog.
May her memory forever be a blessing.

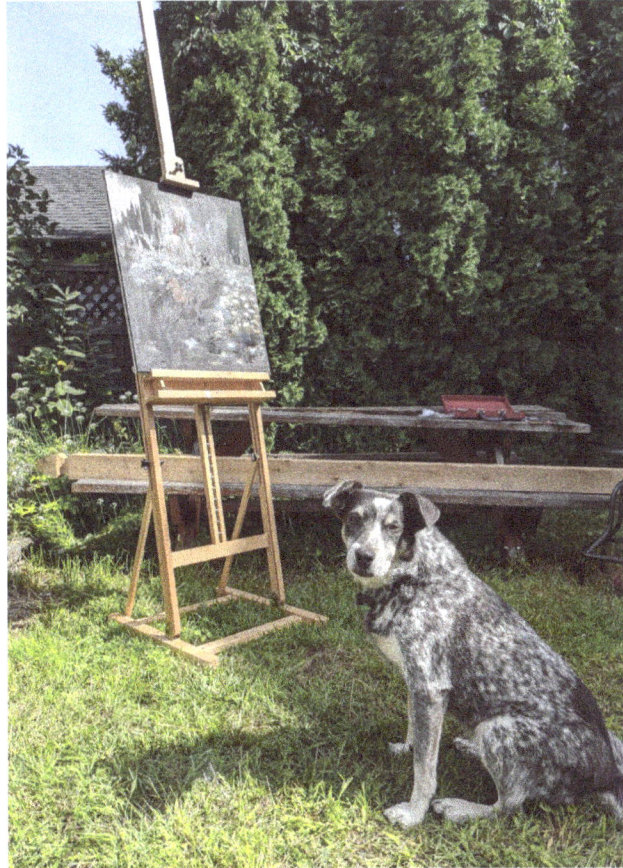

PHOTOGRAPH BY JASPER MARYNCZAK

SHEELA NA GIG

Sheela Na Gig[1] is an architectural adornment that has been found scattered around Europe, primarily in Ireland. The sculptures date back to at least the 11th Century. There is much speculation as to what their purpose was. One view is that they were used to ward off evil spirits. Another idea is that these sculptures were used to demark buildings where birth support and education took place. Regardless of their original intent, *Sheela Na Gig* is an excellent visual guide for contemporary people preparing to birth. If we can see ourselves getting big and open, we can better work to attain that opening.

PREFACE

I come to the writing of this book not as a scientist or a journalist, but as a mom, and a scholar of birth. I am also a childbirth educator, birth activist, and doula. I have been studying, instructing, nurturing, advocating for, and learning from families through their pregnancies, births, and postpartum adjustments for nearly three decades. I understand birth to be a creative and healthy human function, with a tremendous capacity for parental growth and empowerment. I believe that a birth partner, the support person (or persons) of the gestational parent's choosing, likely wants to be truly excellent at providing support. And yet, practical support tools are generally hard to come by, and many support people feel afraid of the birth and what exactly their role is to be. I have empathy. I am courageous and steadfast in my belief that birth is a reliable bodily function, and yet I respect how real our mortality is. My calm comes from knowing that our shared history of human birth has worked well over time, and that the safer and more empowered a gestational parent feels the safer the birth process will be. I understand that when you are pregnant it feels like an infinite number of things can go wrong suddenly and without warning. But for those without significant complicating medical conditions, who made it through the first trimester, the list of what can go wrong becomes finite. Moreover, many of the complications that can occur give us warning signs with time to redirect their trajectory.

Think of *Emily's Birth Book* as a portable mentor, "your guide to a conscientious birth." I wrote it to help you develop practical skills for being pregnant and to provide extended insight into how best to support someone pregnant through birth and into postpartum life. My goals for your pregnancy, birth, and beyond are quite simple: eat well, love well, and stay safe by making informed decisions that include realistic and physiologically sound plans for birth, breastfeeding, and postpartum adjustment. This book can help you be proactive in your maternity care and in your preparation for family life.

To help you make your own best choices, I have synthesized what I understand about working within our current maternity care system, including its political and economically focused dysfunction, with what I know about birth and family-life preparation:

○ Well-informed choices in maternity care will help ease you into parenthood through a more empowered birth experience.

○ Learning about your birth will help you to build confidence.

○ Realizing your legal rights and how to select and work with your care providers will help you to stay safe and get the care you want.

○ Cultivating your confidence will help you to trust your instincts, which will in turn help you to make better decisions as you work with your care providers and, later, with your children.

○ Learning to navigate the healthcare system effectively will be a useful skill throughout your life as you take responsibility for your family.

The childbirth course I teach is called the Bradley Method of Natural Childbirth Education®, a 12-week course taught by instructors trained and certified by The American Academy of Husband Coached Childbirth®. The organization's title comes from the title of Dr. Bradley's book: *Husband Coached Childbirth*. The inherent bias in this title is not upheld in my book. It is this bias, in part, that helped motivate the writing of my book because all kinds of people can make great support partners and parents! The Bradley® curriculum acts as a safety net for childbearing that stresses taking responsibility for self-education and focuses on the application of evidence-based, scientifically sound labor practices and the integration of the birth partner into the pregnancy, birth, and family life. A Bradley® class covers consumer (healthcare) rights and legal issues, prenatal nutrition, prenatal exercise, anatomy, birth physiology, labor positions and coping techniques, labor complications, interventions, pain management, unexpected birth (when you have to catch the baby yourself), postpartum preparation, postpartum adjustment, and breastfeeding education. This book covers these things, too, contextualized through my personal and professional experiences. Using the Bradley Method® as a framework, I present you with what to expect during your pregnancy. I also expose the politics informing birth and the dangers of the capitalistic, biased, and overmedicalized system of maternity care in the United States.

There are many books out there that already cover this information, but they almost never combine the biology and healthcare of birth with its sociopolitical challenges. Likewise, there are books available that are directed specifically at the mother's experience, while other books are directed at the father's experience—and with no acknowledgement of same-sex partnerships or gender-neutral identities, etc. By contrast, I wanted to present a book that honored both the gestational parent and the support person(s), regardless of where they are on the gender spectrum, their race, class, age, religion, or political leaning. Moreover, I wanted to create a shared experience for all involved. In short, I envision this book as a bridge builder, constructed with anecdotes (personal and professional), strung with empirical evidence and data, and bolstered with ample room for you, dear reader(s), to add your own voice(s). *Emily's Birth Book* aims to wrap your pregnancy journey in strength, knowledge, creativity, mindfulness, and experience—giving you agency over your own process.

I did not come to the profession of childbirth education and support through my academic career (that was based on the arts); I came to it through my life experience as a mother. And I stay in this profession due to the couples and clients that I have the honor to teach and privilege to assist through their pregnancy journey. With this book, I can now support you, too, in your remarkable journey of family life, as a couple, a single parent, gay, straight, transgendered, or nonbinary, and regardless of age, class, race, or religion. I acknowledge the gender bias that often accompanies discussions of gestational parents and their partners, and I recognize and work to interrupt the systemic bias and racism inherent in maternity care throughout the United States and across the globe. In addition, if you are a single parent-to-be, I encourage you to adapt this book's information on the partner's role to better understand your own needs and what support-blanks you will want to fill in—be it for and by yourself or with the help of friends, family, neighbors, etc. It does take a village to raise a child, and you can create your village with or without a primary partner. I believe family is created out of love, support, and commitment. It doesn't have to be tied to bloodlines.

To be clear, this book has been written for all. I use gender neutral pronouns when possible and purposefully avoid using "woman" or "female" or "mother" in favor of "pregnant person" or "gestational parent" (as you read above). Nevertheless, it is important to mention here that I do use female pronouns (she/her) when I refer to the baby in various scenarios. This is a conscious choice on my part. I have two beautiful, now full-grown boys, so you will forgive me the enactment of my dream here to theorize my own girl baby!

Maybe my language choices feel shocking. Perhaps they mirror any shock you may have felt encountering this book's unabashed cover art. Well, having a baby is shocking! And the road ahead in parenting is paved with all kinds of feelings, some known and experienced already and some that will come as complete surprises. This book works to reflect the full spectrum of feelings coupled to my effort to be honest and inclusive and transparent as I guide you through its contents. This being said, it is also important to testify that I, as an individual, am unapologetically pro-vagina. What I mean by this is that I am adamant in my personal identification as "mother." However, while I embrace and feel empowered by my own female biology, I also believe that the patriarchy and gender norms harm everybody. And thus, to chip away at this prevailing power structure, everybody has to bend. For my part, and in this book, language plays a powerful role in this. I wrote this book so that you—all of you—can have a safe space to get real about the intimate and amazing circumstances of your transformation through pregnancy. I trust you to define yourself.

Ultimately, this book is an interactive meditation and workbook for pregnant people and their partners. It will guide you through health optimization, birth physiology education, and skill development and confidence building for making medical decisions and managing the sensations of birth. It utilizes personal stories from my own (Emily's) birth experiences plus anecdotes and testimony from clients in my birthing classes to frame guided exercises. And it is all grounded by empirical research, wit, wisdom, humor, and art. As you read, I hope to engage many, if not all of your senses, intellectual thoughts and emotional responses. So please do your homework! You'll see this and other important recommendations repeated often and on purpose throughout this book. As another example, I will mention often that you'll want to align yourself with care providers who will work with you, respectfully engaging in a process of shared decision-making. These providers, those who support physiologically sound practices, are out there. I will provide you the tools to use in your quest to find them. Sadly, not everyone is able to find or access best care; don't panic. With the following information on birth, you will also be able to extract the best care possible from the circumstances and providers you face. Once again, this book is meant to help you and those supporting you to cultivate confidence in your voice and your decisions, to give you greater agency throughout your pregnancy and beyond. With its workbook format, this book will also transform into a memento of your pregnancy journey, a keepsake to treasure and revisit—for renewed strength and insight whenever you need it.

Before setting off together on your pregnancy journey, there is one more thing I need to mention about how this book came into existence: This book and I have grown up together over the last 15 years of its writing. During these years, in between raising my children, caring for my aging parents and educating expectant families, I wrote with the assumption that people had, or at least were supposed to have, agency over their own healthcare decisions. And then, just as this book was nearly ready for publication (Fall 2022), the U.S. Supreme Court overturned Roe v. Wade—and gone were the medical decision-making protections it afforded. Therefore, dear reader, please keep in mind that the question and issue of choice and control remain fraught with uncertainty. As you will learn in the pages ahead, my ultimate advice will always be to "do your homework/research," ask questions, and gather all the information you can, so that you can make *your own* best-informed healthcare decisions with the options available to you.

Now... *thank you* for bringing me into your pregnancy journey. I tend to love people easily and honestly. I care deeply and I care about you. My experiences and expertise have taught me that how other people feel after their births will inform their parenting and thus impact our shared potential for a happier, more socially connected, and more peaceful world. Conscientious birth is therefore as much an informed practice as a state of mind. Let's work together to open up this experience!

TRIGGER WARNING

Mostly, I am not a fan of trigger warnings. We must ultimately learn new things and confront our responses to difficult material. Facing our fears, feeling our grief, and expressing our emotions head on is a healthy way to process the big stuff—and having a baby is big stuff. In fact, crying is common in a Bradley® class. However, in class and in person we can comfort each other and help each other heal and find courage. As I write this book, I don't know what circumstances you will be in when you read it. I want you to be able to take care of your feelings. Each of you brings your own hurt spots and vulnerabilities, and many of us have considerable scarring—emotional and physical—to contend with during pregnancy. And let's face it, some days are better than others.

In various parts of this book I introduce some frightening facts on medical racism and maternal and infant mortality. I am sorry to deliver this material, but it is imperative to be honest about the risks that face birthing people in America. This will be unsettling and difficult to read for many. However, I believe that it is of the utmost importance that you understand how serious the consequences of birth-ignorance can be. When triggering material is presented, you will see this image at the start ⚠️. When this material has concluded, you will see this image at the end ✅. The following Introduction to this book, for example, includes a trigger warning because of its focus on the effects of medical racism.

This book will take time and dedication to read. My belief is that if you understand how serious the stakes of American maternity care are at the start, then you will increase your motivation to complete this book and further your education toward an empowered birth experience. I can assure you that if you do the work to learn how to best support your pregnancy, then you will significantly improve your chances for excellent outcomes. But if reading about medical racism or loss is too much for today, consider skipping the parts you need to. Then maybe, on another day, you can go back and face the information you skipped, under different circumstances and with renewed courage. To each of us in our own time...

INTRODUCTION

⚠ One night in 1995 (the same year I completed my certification to become a Bradley Method® childbirth educator and doula), a staff member called me from the group home I volunteered with. She was concerned about a young mother I hadn't yet met. She was in labor, and she was alone. Could I go help? I raced out the door.

I was told to go to the second largest hospital in my city, and I was grateful for the opportunity. My heart was pounding as I navigated the city streets. What will it be like to meet this woman for the first time, and while she is in labor? How will she react to me as her doula? How will the hospital staff react to me as her doula? How will my own toddler manage without me? How long will I be gone? I had many questions, but one singular plan: get to the hospital, find this young woman, and love her. I would love her baby and love their birth, as completely and genuinely as I could, with my heart open.

When I arrived at the hospital and found the laboring mother's room, I took a few deep breaths then walked in the door. "Hi, my name is Emily, and I am here to help support you through your birth, if you would like that. I got a phone call that you were here, alone, and I thought you might appreciate some company. How's it all going? Is there anything I can get you or help you with?" She was timid and uncertain about all the words I had just poured out and what they actually meant for her. But she didn't have long to contemplate my arrival before the next, very powerful contraction graced her body. I bolted to her side and began, with as soothing a tone as I could manifest, to guide her to exhale fully and breathe deeply into her body and through what was happening. I made gentle suggestions about relaxing her facial muscles and trying to soften in other parts of her body. I told her she and her baby were safe during these big sensations, and she was very responsive to my words. When the contraction was over, she smiled at me and said thank you. I took a few breaths of my own and settled contently into the work of loving this brave young woman. Over the course of the next few hours, in between contractions and sips of water and changes in position, I learned that she was 17 years old, very in love with her baby's father, and so in love with her baby and the idea of becoming a mother. I thought of my own mother who had had her first baby at age 18.

The nurse hadn't been in the room when I first arrived. When she did come in, she was fairly disinterested in my client and in me. I remember that she looked me up and down before saying, "Who are you?" I introduced myself and explained that I was the doula. "Oh. I didn't know she had a doula," was her only response. Then she did some charting and left the room. She continued to appear occasionally over the hours that followed, saying few words and making almost no eye contact with my client or myself. All the while, my client—or, as I quickly came to think of her, my "new love"—was working away beautifully in birth. She was so receptive to my soothing tone and guided relaxation and breath work. I helped her change positions and told her I believed in her completely. She was doing amazingly well, and we were working together like a team that had been close for years. The nurse was in the room when my new love started to make really clear grunting sounds for the first time. (Note that the sounds are quite different between first and second stage labor, as I'll discuss in this book). It was clear to the nurse and to me that the second, or expulsive phase of labor had begun. The nurse went to get the doctor.

A White male doctor in his early 50s, along with a White male resident in his late 20s, walked into the room. The doctor looked very uneasy when he saw me and questioned, "You're with her?" "Yes, I am," I answered calmly.

"And she's doing an amazing job, laboring so beautifully." He responded with a sour face and an abrupt, "Step aside. We need to examine her."

This doctor never introduced himself to his patient or to me. And the resident remained silent and avoided eye contact. Meanwhile, they both placed their bodies around the bed, which took up any room for me to be near the laboring parent. Consequently, the young woman and I did our best to look at each other over and around them. I would smile and breathe in a slightly exaggerated manner so that she could see me clearly. She and I were dialed in; she was making fantastic progress. And then, suddenly, the nurse pulls over a rolling tray table with tools on it. The doctor grabs the surgical scissors and, with no discussion, no informed consent, and no words whatsoever to anyone in the room, cuts an episiotomy. (An episiotomy is a surgical incision made into the vagina and perineum ostensibly to aid in delivery.) I knew, deep down, that I had just witnessed an assault.

I could visually see the baby had been making good progress down the birth canal (a euphemism for vagina). What the doctor did is something called a "pressure episiotomy"; this incision can be made at the height of a contraction, without anesthesia, so that a birthing person likely won't feel it (and, thankfully, my new love, the laboring mother, didn't). An episiotomy can speed up the delivery, but not by more than 5 – 10 minutes, maybe. This surgical procedure should only be used if there is a clear medical indication, which there was not, and should never be used without informed consent, and there was none. It seemed so clear to me that this woman was going to birth her baby without this cut. There was no indication that her baby was having trouble moving down. And throughout the birth there had not been a single questionable heart rate recording.

Once the baby was out, she appeared robust, even if small—a bit less than six pounds. I remember thinking: I bet no one told this young mom how important eating protein is and that this could be why her baby was small. Nevertheless, here was a healthy baby! But I also knew in my heart that the doctor had not been thinking about her or her baby when he performed what, in my opinion, was an unnecessary surgical procedure—after which he spent nearly one whole hour teaching the White male resident how to suture the incision (thus proving, at least to me, that the procedure was less about his patient and more about his own agenda). Generally, suturing an episiotomy is a 10- to 15-minute procedure at most, and often, from what I have since seen, much shorter than that.

Beyond having successfully given birth to her baby, my client didn't appear to understand what had happened to her or why. She assumed the whole procedure of the episiotomy was a normal and reasonable part of birth. By contrast, I was witnessing—experiencing, even—a trauma. I felt terrified and helpless, horrified and consumed with guilt that I hadn't been able to protect the new mother. I knew she was now at risk for potential healing complications that could be lifelong. But, in the moment, there was no time for such "me things." We have a baby!

Mama was jubilant and falling wildly in love with her baby right in front of my eyes. Her baby began to nurse with gusto. Mama and I both sat there gushing with love. This new parent was overcome with pride and amazement in her accomplishment, and she expressed deep gratitude for my companionship and support. (Of course, I had to correct her gently when she said that she could not have gotten through the birth without me. She was strong and capable; her body knew what to do.) We were now bonded indeed. I set out to love her and I was able to rise to that occasion. She set out to birth her baby, and she did—wondrously. I believed and still believe that love is the most important labor tool there is.

My new bestie was leaving town shortly after her discharge; she would go to her father's home with her new baby. And two quick months later, I moved across the country. I still love her to this day, and I know that I have a little spot inside her heart as well. Although she and I moved on in our worlds, I had to admit that the trauma I experienced did not. I knew that doctor would not have been so egregious had I been the patient. I am a White female. My client is a Black woman and was broke and unwed at the time. I also knew that the situation would have been especially different if my White adult male partner had been there, too. I was sickened that I could not have stopped him from cutting her, and I was certain that I had witnessed an act of medical racism, ageism, and classism. It felt like violence. It was violence. And I carry that sadness and those scars still. At the same time, I also knew I had made a positive impact on an individual's birth experience, and that the confidence and joy she grew through her labor would serve her well in her life ahead. I also felt my confidence grow in the labor techniques I had been studying—my labor of love now rooted. The whole experience, including the caregiving and professional support, the joy, the love between strangers, and the darkness of unrealized trauma, affirmed my dedication to a profession I have now held for 30 years and counting.

✅ There are many challenges facing a pregnant person: body changes, emotional changes, eating right, and most crushingly racism, genderism, poverty, and the politics of power and money that infiltrate birth in America.[2] Once the baby is out the challenges continue: raising the baby, paying the bills, doing the laundry, and for those of you coupled, there is also trying to keep a spousal relationship together... it's all a lot of hard work. Although I can't help with the laundry (and I really wish I could!), I can help by encouraging you to take some time now to prepare for this massive life transformation. By reading this book, working through its exercises and searching for local resources (including independent, evidence-based birth classes and respectful and competent doulas, midwives, and doctors), you really can set sail into parenthood with important navigation skills and, if you want, a well informed and fully participating co-pilot.

In the pages ahead, I will discuss ways to create plans for a labor that reduce risk to the gestational person and baby, increase empowerment and birth satisfaction, and help ease a family into and through the postpartum adjustment. Good risk-reducing birth plans include creating a calm environment filled with encouragement and birth knowledge. The people on your team should be gentle, patient, skilled, and not overly stressed or fearful themselves—all skills that can be coached into existence. Within a sphere of intimate and birth-wise support you can, more optimally, yield to the forces of nature that will pass through you as you open yourself for birth. In a loving and knowledgeable environment, you can find the courage to let go of inhibitions and allow your process to take over. Unfortunately, this ideal environment is not the typical hospital experience. Many nurses and providers are themselves tired or otherwise stressed from their own workload, and all of them are vulnerable to implicit biases regarding race, gender, class, religion, age, and size. Many partners are especially fearful from a lack of birth education and then further marginalized by staff and hospital protocols. Additionally, many routine hospital practices create stress and complicate the birth process.[3]

My role through this book is to encourage detailed planning for birth that emphasizes not a solid plan, but a *flexible action plan*. While planning helps you to have options, you really cannot plan a birth. The work is more like planning for an improvisational dance performance. Dancers plan by preparing their bodies; they plan their wardrobe; plan for their environment; they plan to have a technical support crew; and, importantly, they discuss ways to make decisions and contingency plans for performance. Planning for birth means much the same thing: caring for and preparing your body and mind; planning for your environment; planning your support crew; planning ways to actively cope with labor; and planning by learning how to make medical decisions as they arise. In short, planning to adapt.

To make your medical decisions, you need to learn what questions to ask and how to ask them. Once you know how to ask the right questions, you will get useful answers, which you will then need to balance with what you are feeling and what you want and need. That is how you make medical decisions. Spoiler alert: medical decisions are yours to make, not your provider's. It is an awesome burden of responsibility. Life is full of unpredicted obstacles, some are of biological origin and others are from human interference. Sadly, many of the common curve balls thrown at birthing parents in the United States do not come from nature; they come from our current protocols and medical routines.[4] In other words, they emerge from our basic model of hospital maternity care. However, with an educated, flexible action plan, and a good grasp on what questions to ask and how to ask them, you will become empowered to navigate your own, unique childbirth experience. You will have a conscientious birth!

What is a conscientious birth?

A conscientious birth is attained after you use your pregnancy to take responsibility to optimize your outcomes, learn to trust your instincts, and make plans for coping with what you cannot control. In preparation for a conscientious birth you learn about how your body works, what the common routines and interventions are that are used by the care providers to which you have access, and how each of these routines and interventions relate to your personal health history, your culture, and your preferences. Once you have learned about what choices will need to be made, and what choices might need to be made, you will have to do the often-hard work of accessing what you really think and feel about each decision. What are your instincts telling you about your options? What kind of science is there on this topic? Is there a difference between what the midwifery model and the obstetric model present? Once you have figured out what you think, you will need to make your preferences clear to your providers; this takes courage in addition to information. In other words, you want to have a strong, informed voice. A conscientious birth is one in which you use your pregnancy for advance preparation, empowerment building for yourself and a dedicated support partner(s), and you apply critical thinking skills to make informed decisions out of whatever your birth journey brings.

How do you work toward a conscientious birth?

The short answer: you use your pregnancy to create time for and pay attention to your health and education. You open and hold space for yourself and your baby. The longer answer is that having a baby is inherently creative work; you are creating a human. Tuning into, or reframing, your pregnancy as a creative process can help you to build vital empowerment, to explore your feelings (through joy, sadness, and everything in between), to truly understand your biology as a pregnant person, and to trust your instincts. Knowing your feelings and your body and trusting your instincts will help you to clarify your values, which in turn helps you to make decisions for your maternity care and birth. To approach all of this creatively is to welcome and embrace flexibility/adaptability. To do this tuning in, or reframing, you study the physiology of how your magnificent body works; you learn how best to support these incredible processes.

Pregnancy also puts you face to face with the for-profit healthcare system in the United States, your own mortality, and the mortality of your loved ones, including your baby. Many choices you will need to make will not have certain outcomes. Your self-care, fetal-care, healthcare, birth-care, and baby-care are all areas in which there are choices of care to be made. Many of these decision points are complicated by the fact that there are a variety of birth professionals who don't agree with each other about best practices. Some of your choices will have data to help drive answers, while for other choices the data may be non-existent or less clear or skewed by economics (who paid for the study?), politics (maternal rights vs. fetal rights), or bias (some pregnant people receive over-treatment and some under-treatment; some receive compassion while others do not). The medical choices available to you are impacted by the training, values, and experiences of your practitioners. There are also variations that differ regionally, and/or are culturally influenced. Still other choices will be affected by emotions: yours, your family's, your healthcare provider's, your co-workers', the media, etc. In order to make your own, best-informed decisions you first have to figure out what your pregnant body needs to thrive in pregnancy and how the birth process can be best supported. Then you need to learn about what the pros and cons of common birth practices are in the United States, particularly as they directly apply to you. It is also helpful to learn about the law as it pertains to your rights as a patient depending on the region in which you live.

This is a lot! And this where I come in.

By you reading and working through this book, I can help guide you to:

- Optimize your health through attention to nutrition
- Employ techniques for stress reduction
- Discover ways to be physically active
- Build empowerment in your patient/provider relationship
- Gain tips for building social support
- Learn ways to utilize your history
- Receive information about how your body works during birth

I will guide you to ask questions so that the answers you receive in return can help you to fully participate in your healthcare. By using this book and the guided exercises within, you will gain a variety of labor coping and support techniques that will allow you to use your creative powers to "dance" through the improvisation of your birth process. This guide will help you to tune into your instincts. It will help you to face your fears. Connecting to the specifics of your unique fears will in turn help you to build strategies for handling what you cannot control and to take responsibility where you can. Striving for a conscientious birth will strengthen your own agency in the process. It will help to empower you, to trust your instincts. It will illuminate the birth process and give you the tools to work with your support partner(s) and providers toward the goal of attaining your safest and most joyful experience.

Why work toward a conscientious birth?

Because it is protective to work toward a conscientious birth. The United States ranks quite low in the world when it comes to maternity care, so following the status quo may not be in your best interest. Out of the top 10 industrialized countries in the world, gestational parents are, at a minimum, nearly twice as likely to die in the United States. Out of 100,000 live births we lose 17.4 gestational parents compared to France at 8.7 deaths and Canada at 8.6. And the US fares even worse compared to the other top countries: United Kingdom, Australia, Switzerland, Sweden, Germany, The Netherlands, Norway, and New Zealand. In these other countries the deaths per 100,000 live births range from 6.5 to 1.7.[5] Here in the United States we also spend more money on these heartbreaking outcomes. Our system of healthcare is rigged toward making money while access to care remains inequitable. Like so many social systems, it is impacted by bias. Race, income, gender expression, sexual orientation, education levels, and more can all affect the care you receive. For example, while maternity care outcomes are worse for people who are not White and people who are under-resourced and under-represented, these same outcomes can often be found to be unfavorable for White people with money, too. Working toward a conscientious birth can help you to steer away from these systemic obstacles and statistics. Additionally, the empowerment you build on your path to a conscientious birth will inform your parenting and the medical decisions that your family will face over your lifetime.

When you work toward a conscientious birth, you help lay the foundation for your birth memories to fill you with pride. Birth is a wild ride that is ultimately beyond our control. But when you learn how best to support your process, and to take an active role in the decisions that abound, you are much more likely to have memories filled with joy and a sense of accomplishment. Likewise, should you experience less-than-optimal care from your providers, you will have a much better chance of understanding that your body did not fail you; your healthcare system failed you. Placing blame where it is deserved will help prevent you from turning your negatives in toward yourself, and this will help you to heal.

What to expect in this book

Week 1: Open and Breathe

- O Breath awareness
- O Diet assessment

Week 2: Eat and Relax

- O Wholistic prenatal health assessment
- O Diet development
- O Relaxation/meditation/breath awareness

Week 3: Move Your Body

- O Prenatal general fitness
- O Prenatal specific exercises for comfort in pregnancy and birth

Week 4: Take Responsibility

- O Maternity care choices
- O Interview skills for hiring maternity care providers
- O Prenatal screening and ultrasound

Week 5: Your Pregnant Body

- O Explore basic anatomy
- O Understand common pregnancy discomforts
- O Explore basic physiology

Week 6: Love and Service
- Confidence building
- Support skill development

Week 7: Waiting Wondering Working
- Explore waiting for birth and how it might begin
- Develop your mental approach and make coping plans for when labor arrives
- Explore fetal positioning and back labor

Week 8: First Stage Birth
- Develop your physical approach for first stage labor
- Explore time-tested labor positions

Week 9: Second and Third Stages of Birth
- Explore the baby's journey out
- Develop your physical approach for second stage labor
- Explore second stage positions
- Third stage labor decisions and safety considerations

Week 10: Expressions of Birth
- The emotions and physical feelings of birth
- Labor interruptions
- The vaginal exam in labor

Week 11: Inquire and Decide
- Build skills for making medical decisions
- Dig into your feelings around anticipated decision points

Week 12: Science and Your Nature
- Explore pain medications
- Explore inductions and labor augmentation

Week 13: Fear and Fortitude

○ Explore when cesarean sections are indicated and how to cope with the procedure

○ Explore the reality of stillbirth

Week 14: Yes, You Can!

○ Further development of birth tools

○ When to transport in a planned hospital birth

○ How to catch your baby if you get caught by surprise

○ Tips on sibling and pet birth-preparation

Week 15: Plan and Prepare

○ Explore doula care

○ Get real about your transition to family life

○ Learn about postpartum emotions and adjustment challenges

Week 16: Eat Sleep Repeat

○ Develop your breastfeeding skills

○ Explore introducing bottle-feeding to a breast-fed baby

○ Tips on picking a pediatrician

○ Explore issues in infant and family sleep

I encourage you to read this book in order, one chapter (one lesson) at a time, and to read through each lesson once a week. This schedule will help you to mimic an actual class experience, giving you time to practice the exercises and let the information digest. Before you begin each week, make yourself comfortable. Use the bathroom, pour yourself some water, get a snack if you need one. As you work through each week's lesson, please keep a pen nearby so you can jot down your answers to my questions and keep track of your own questions, comments, and reflections. You may also want to use some colored pencils, pens, crayons, etc. to write or draw in color. I have made room directly in this book for you to take notes, do some coloring, draw, preserve your responses to the exercises, and generally ruminate on your pregnancy process. Writing down or drawing your fears, dreams, and needs will help to propel your emotional growth. I encourage you to take time and make space to ponder the questions, fears, joys, and thoughts that arise.

If you have a partner, I suspect that the ideal way for you to read this is in bed, taking turns reading aloud to each other and offering up space for your partner to also take notes and make written and drawn comments. I also happen to believe that the intimacy of this subject matter can be greatly enhanced by the connection of shared nakedness. So please consider taking your clothes off and cuddling naked in bed together as you read. Pregnancy is a time of great power, but also a time of tremendous vulnerability. Learning about your journey together, in a mutual state of openness, can enhance your intimacy and increase your abilities to share. In addition to this, pregnancy can be so wonderfully sexy! There is no reason not to enjoy the sexiness of this miracle. Skin-to-skin contact is an important part of baby-care and breastfeeding, so maybe you can start to practice some skin-to-skin skills now to warm up!

Some of my most enjoyable times with my partner of more than 30 years are when we read a book out loud together. But regardless of where you are, who you are with, what your reading schedule is, and what you are wearing or not wearing, I sincerely hope you will have fun and celebrate your own courage, your own love, and your own powers to create and nurture life.

Congratulations on your pregnancy and your commitment to being a great parent!

Introducing Sadie the Super Bitch!

Sadie is a beloved family pet by day, but by night she is a Super-Shero-Power-Dog! Her super powers are that she has been alive forever, she can fly, and she telepathically communicates with midwives all over the Globe. She transmits a wealth of midwifery support and education throughout time and all around the world. As you see images of Sadie throughout this book, consider that she just might bring opening wide-wisdom from Sheela Na Gig.

Back in the 11th century, Sheela and Sadie were close pals.

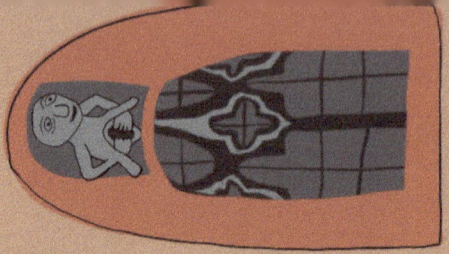

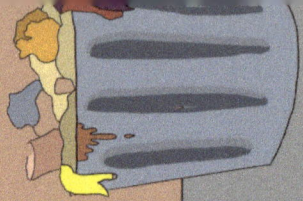

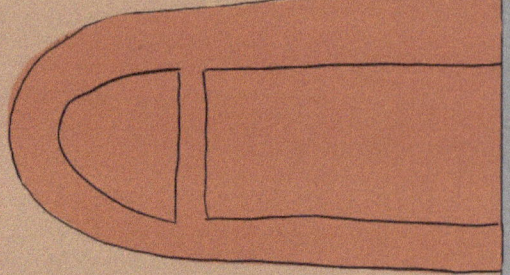

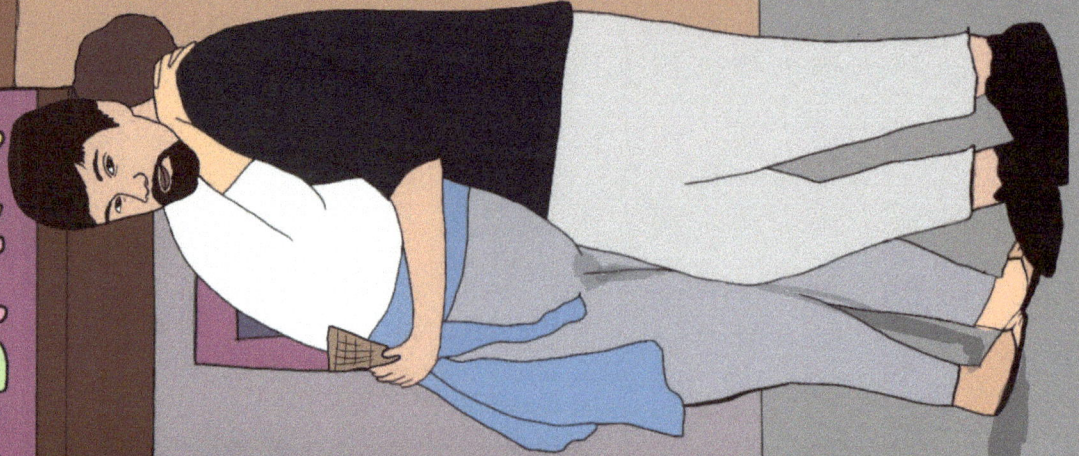

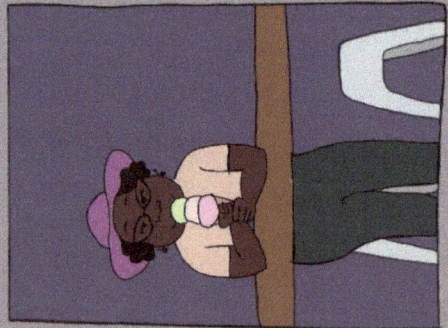

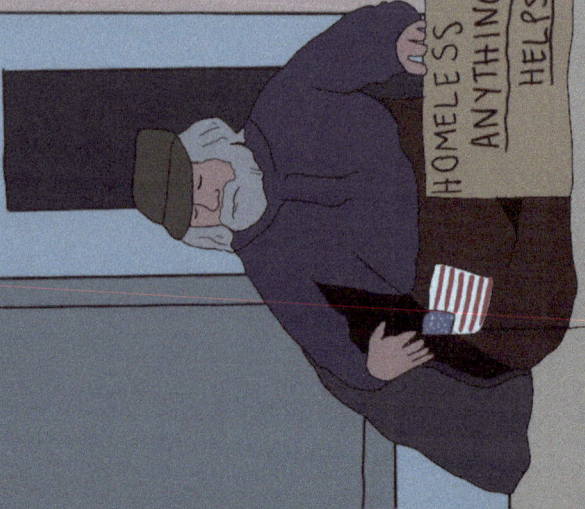

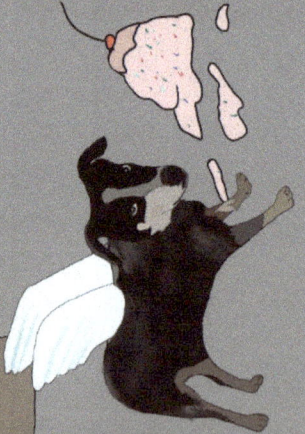

WEEK 1

Chapter contents:

- O *Introductions*
- O *Breath awareness*
- O *Diet assessment*

THIS SPACE IS FOR YOUR NOTES AND DRAWINGS

Welcome to class and congratulations again on your pregnancy! In a live class I enjoy and learn from the social connections I develop with my clients. Through this book I am excited to bring these years of experience directly to you, where you are, to create a sense of dialogue between us, and to introduce you to me through my own stories of pregnancy and birth. I want you to understand what I bring to this work and how I came to do it, so that you can open yourself up fully to the experience and the lessons presented here. So let's get started!

I have two biological children, though they are already men.

My personal birth education began on a night in my mid 20's, sitting around my apartment with a few girl-friends. I was single. Babies weren't even on my radar. I was a dancer/artist by degree. To make ends meet, I worked a combination of jobs—tying together early education, film production (as a script supervisor), and waiting tables. Beyond simply living in a woman's body, I had no experience related to women's health.

That night in my 20's, as we were all sitting around chatting, I mused: "I can't imagine how a baby actually comes out! But I guess that if I think about my dance training, I imagine it must require such complete and extreme relaxation. There must be some way to just... dissolve myself open. How else could these muscles and soft tissues stretch to such a phenomenal degree? How does this work when it just seems so impossible?" I have since learned that blood flow to the genitals helps them to expand, and deep relaxation helps everything. But let's not get ahead of ourselves yet.

One of the women at the table, my beautiful friend Angela, said:

"Do you know about the Bradley Method®? That is what Laurie used, and she said that relaxation is the premise of what they teach and that it really helped her."

Well no, I hadn't heard of the Bradley Method®. Reflecting back, I truly knew very little about birth and my body as a twentysomething adult. Luckily for me, my friend was a good and open resource. Her information settled into my head and a couple of years later when I was pregnant with my first child, I was excited to remember that there was this technique out there based on relaxation. Nevertheless, in the moment of my first pregnancy, medical care was my initial target, all but ignoring education as an empowering context. I often wonder what might have happened had I focused more immediately on education and relaxation. My hindsight is now your foresight!

My first pregnancy

When I found out I was pregnant, my first logical step was to find an obstetrician through my insurance office. They gave me the name of someone in my neighborhood and I set up an intake visit. It never occurred to me to research *all* of my possible options—or even determine what all these options were. What's more, I was ignorant of how to evaluate a medical relationship.

The practice I contacted had one obstetrician and one midwife. My first appointment was with the midwife. The office looked nice and the midwife was very friendly. She even smelled good. It all seemed so lovely. I thought, "This is great, I found an office." I also thought it was cool that there was a midwife, though I didn't really understand what that meant at the time. It just seemed groovy to say I was going to a midwife. I liked that. I thought of birth as a natural event that didn't need to be medicalized, even if society was now seeming to convince me otherwise. When I was in graduate school, I lived in The Netherlands and someone I knew there used a midwife for her home birth.

Beyond the obvious, I didn't know exactly what that meant, but I thought it intriguing, if also messy. But unlike this Dutch midwife, my new midwife worked in hospitals. So maybe less messy? I left my first appointment feeling good, happy to have medical providers.

I was really excited about the whole baby making experience. I loved trying to get pregnant and I loved being pregnant. I was amazed at what was happening in my body; I was joyful, trusting, and excited. I thought it was just about the sexiest and most romantic adventure I could be on. And I was eager to experience what came next.

And then at one of my early prenatal appointments the midwife handed me a couple of brochures, flimsy little things, on prenatal testing. She informed me that I would have to let her know which tests I would like to schedule.

I was stopped cold in my tracks, stunned and perplexed. How was *I* going to make these decisions? I didn't have a clue. I asked, "Didn't *you* go to school for this? Don't *you* know what I am supposed to do?" I really believed that when I got pregnant I would go to the doctor/midwife and she would tell me what I needed to do, and then I would do it. I thought, of course, the doctor or midwife would know what I needed. I was stumped. I believed in natural things. I believed in my body, and I figured my care provider would too. I expected their experience and knowledge to be helpful to me. It was mind boggling that I would have to take responsibility for decisions I knew nothing about.

I also mistakenly thought that this prenatal medical testing was all about *safety*. I thought that picking the right tests would somehow improve my odds at a healthy pregnancy and a healthy baby, and that my midwife or doctor would be guiding me through the safest route possible. But that, as I learned, is not how the medical system is designed. Medical testing/screening is not always a path to steering safely through the mortal journey we're on as a patient.

I didn't inherently have a lot of fears about pregnancy or birth. I easily imagined myself as a happy mommy with a happy, healthy baby. I had an intuition that everything would be fine biologically. People all around me were having babies, and many of these people were less healthy or health conscious than I was. And I hadn't wanted to do any invasive tests that would have obvious risks. I felt by instinct that I didn't want to have an amniocentesis or ultrasound scan. To my own mind, I have never understood why we don't call ultrasound an invasive procedure. During an ultrasound, a targeted concentration of sound waves go *into* your body, then bounce off of your baby, the placenta, or whatever else they are aimed at, in order to examine the fetus. That seems as "*in*vasive" to me now as it did back in 1992 when I first learned about it. There was also another test offered, the *alpha fetoprotein test,* which screens for neural tube defects and Down syndrome.[6] In 2013 this test was bundled into a group of tests called "quad screen." According to the Mayo Clinic, this screens for "Down syndrome, trisomy 18, neural tube defects, and abdominal wall defects."[7] When I was pregnant (in 1993) I was offered only the alpha fetoprotein test. Now a variety of prenatal screening tests exist, with more being developed every day. "Harmony" is one such newer blood test: "The Harmony test analyzes cell free DNA in maternal blood and gives a strong indication of whether the fetus is at high or low risk of having trisomy 21 (Down syndrome), trisomy 18 (Edwards syndrome) or trisomy 13 (Patau syndrome).[8]

When I read my little brochure from the midwife, I learned that they would take some blood from me, as a sample to analyze, which didn't sound like it would do anything to the baby. And while I did not receive any information—or more brochures—on neural tube defects or Down syndrome, I knew that they were both serious. (I had some basic familiarity with what Down syndrome looked like, but no real understanding of the wide spectrum of symptoms and level of functioning the anomaly could produce.) I believed that in either scenario there might be things to learn ahead of the birth. What I understand now, so many years later, is that I was really counting on the test results being normal. Would I have terminated my pregnancy based on any of the tests I was offered? That is a fundamentally important question, and only one of the many important things I hadn't considered ahead of time. I merely wanted some extra assurance that everything was going to be fine. And sure, there was an extremely low probable chance that we'd receive bad news. I now also understand that looking for prenatal anomalies can bring inconclusive and stressful results with frequent regularity.

As of today, where are you in your feelings toward—and knowledge and decisions about—prenatal screening tests? Please write or draw your answers here:

I had no idea what my rights and responsibilities were with regard to medical decision making. I did not understand that agreeing to take one test meant there was a high probability of "needing" more tests. And I didn't know that there were so few medical fixes if an anomaly was actually detected. There are now experimental surgeries that some doctors are performing in utero, which involve opening the womb surgically, working on the baby, and then sewing up all the parts to put the womb back together. There are some success stories to be read; there are also many losses. Finding a doctor who would tackle these surgeries in 2022 (forget about 1993) is not easy to do. It's also possible that many health insurance plans would not cover such surgery. With fetal surgery there is considerable fetal risk for prematurity, injury, and death. In hindsight, I wish I had been counseled ahead of time about the actionability of results, inconclusive test results, and false-positive results—that there could be lab errors, misinterpretations, and possible decisions about experimental surgeries and termination. I didn't understand ahead of time how the fears can so rapidly escalate, both mine and my provider's, and that I could be in for a long, costly, stressful cycle of uncertainty.

Beyond the emotional toll, which can be enormous, consider that each new test ordered is also another billable procedure. Uncertainty and fear become profitable. Fear from the patient and/or provider can lead to economic gain for providers, hospitals and the broader medical industry. I do not mean to accuse my provider of a greedy motive; it's the nature of the beast. Our current healthcare system rests upon the slippery ethics of profiting from healthcare. In the United States, we currently live in a fee-for-service, profit-driven medical system. Healthy people having healthy physiological births do not boost the medical economy.

At my next routine prenatal visit, I consented to the alpha fetoprotein blood test, and blood was drawn right then. Once I left the office, I put it out of my mind. Then, about a week later, the phone rang: my midwife had the test results. She said I was not within the normal values. She said they wanted me to have an ultrasound, and that they went ahead and scheduled one for the next morning. She hoped I would keep the appointment. She also said I needed to schedule an appointment for an amniocentesis and make an appointment to see a genetic counselor. (Cue the scary music.)

I did not see any of that coming! It seemed like the end of the world was speeding towards me. I had been so relaxed and in love with my baby and my body. Now, all of a sudden, I was crying and it sure seemed like my midwife was worried something was really wrong.

She said they wanted the ultrasound test to confirm my dates. That sometimes when a person's dates are wrong, it can throw off the interpretation of the test results. (In 1993 ultrasound screening was not yet as prevalent as it is today.) I was convinced my dates were accurate. We had been *trying* to conceive. I had been aware of my own fertility. I highly doubted that confirming my fetus' age would explain away my test results. I believed trouble must be lurking within. It never occurred to me that the lab could have screwed up—that maybe the test results that were read to me weren't even mine! And I knew nothing about the concept of false positives, and that this test might just be wrong. Experience has taught me since then: shit happens.

The next day I went in for the ultrasound, as recommended, and they said, "Your due date aligns with the baby's measurements." They also said they saw none of the bone length markers that suggest Down syndrome, such as a shortened femur, or a missing nasal bone, nor anything else remarkable. But this was only somewhat reassuring, because it wasn't convincing enough for my providers to rule out the "need" for further testing. Next step: amniocentesis and genetic counseling. Bad news might still be forthcoming. No one explained that the decision to do further testing should be thoroughly considered before consent, and that that consent was mine to give. Simply scheduling the amniocentesis and genetic counseling didn't erase the possibility to re-evaluate the decision to do further testing. But it felt like it did, and I didn't know any better.

I don't know if you are familiar with genetic counseling. I wasn't. It was a crazy experience for me. The counselor sat us down and asked us a lot of questions about the physical and mental health of our family members. She then proceeded to throw a seemingly unending stream of numbers at us. The probability of this vs. the probability of that. If you get this number, then that number has a such and such number of chances to mean that this other number will cause an increased incidence of blah blah blah... By the end of the appointment my head was spinning. I lived in Manhattan at the time, and I asked myself, "What are the chances that a cab might jump the curb and kill me? How am I supposed to process this information? What do I do now?" I didn't understand the numbers and now I was even more scared.

So onward we trudged towards the amniocentesis. It took time to get in for these appointments; everything was spread out over days and weeks. We couldn't get anything done as quickly as we felt it should be done. The waiting was hard and consuming.

During an amniocentesis they insert a very long needle through the abdomen and into the uterus to extract some of the amniotic fluid. They use ultrasound as a guide to help them avoid the baby, placenta, and umbilical cord. Then they send your sample off to the lab to grow the extracted cells in a culture medium so they can examine and count the chromosomes. They look for abnormalities. Amniocentesis has risks, including miscarriage, puncturing something unintentionally (like the baby), infection, or problems with the amniotic sac needle-hole.[9]

After my procedure the obstetrician said I should go home, get into bed and rest. He told me to contact them immediately if I leaked any fluid or had any spotting or cramping during the next 24 hours.

Ok, I thought, *I'll just go home and relax and rest... and what? What symptoms? Whoa, this sounds serious. Cramping, bleeding, and leaking fluid!?*

My stress at that moment was largely because I had been ill-prepared and not educated about the risks associated with the procedure ahead of time. I don't remember the little pamphlet that the midwife handed me containing any of these warnings. I hadn't originally wanted an amniocentesis, so I had not researched it (this was the dawn of owning a personal computer and the internet was itself a baby). Now I was to go home and rest while being on high alert for complications we may have just caused!

Okay, freak out! How will I know if I am leaking amniotic fluid? Would it really be obvious? If it's just a little bit, isn't it possible that I might miss it? I did have increased vaginal discharge, which is normal during pregnancy. Would I know for sure that it wasn't amniotic fluid? What if I sneezed hard or got caught by a laugh and I leaked some urine?

"Oh, and by the way," the nurse said, "because of your insurance company, the lab we need to use is going to take 10 days, maybe two weeks to get you the results. If we could have used this other lab, then we would receive the results much sooner. Sorry."

Because I had been born healthy, economically privileged, and White, I had the ignorant assumption that the healthcare system in the United States worked well and had my best interests as a priority. Now, all I could think about was *what is going on with our healthcare system!?* My experience felt as dizzying and disorienting as it was disappointing. I had no idea what I was up against, or how deeply racial bias and other injustices are interwoven into America's health-care system, or just how many other countries fare far better in maternity care outcomes than we do.[10]

After the amniocentesis, my partner Julian and I went to the video rental store (that surely dates us, I miss those stores!) and returned home with a stack of movies to wait out our post-procedural recovery period. One movie later, no problems. Two movies later, no problems. Six movies later, no problems... I can't even remember how many movies we actually watched while we waited. Thankfully, no problems ever arose related to my amniocentesis.

Two agonizing weeks later, the results arrived. My baby was deemed healthy, "everything looks normal" revealed the results. But the care providers were also quick to point out that "of course, there are still no guarantees." The testing avalanche was over, at least for the moment, and with a parting gift of continued uncertainty.

Now it was time to emotionally recover and settle back into my pregnancy. The testing ordeal had gobbled up more than a month. During that time, I had felt disconnected from my baby and my body. I was afraid for my baby and afraid *of* my baby. I wasn't eating or exercising as well as I had been, and I certainly wasn't sleeping as well. I understand now that my midwife's "urgency" was likely little more than "efficient" office management, an automatic protocol: if this happens, then do that. All along, she repeated, "oh this might be nothing." But at the time this struck me only as her way of trying to calm me down.

Thankfully, we had already registered for our Bradley® class and it was just about to begin. I was now on a mission to learn everything I could about the rest of my pregnancy and my birth, including information like this from the family physicians at Wayne State University:

> "The test [alpha-fetoprotein] is not completely accurate. A baby may have a birth defect even with AFP levels that are normal. Or a baby may be quite normal even though AFP levels are abnormal. ... For every 1000 pregnant women tested, about 50 have abnormal test results. Of

these 50, just 1 or 2 with high AFP levels have babies with problems. The test finds 90% of babies with anencephaly and 75% with spina bifida."[11]

That information definitely wasn't in the little brochure. My Bradley® class was giving me the confidence and the information I needed to help me understand when to ask medical questions and how to work with my providers.

As my first pregnancy continued, I considered changing providers. I did some research and found a midwife that I wanted to switch to, but she wouldn't take me on so late in my pregnancy. (There are providers who will take on clients late in pregnancy.) I ended my search and decided to stay put with the midwife/doctor combo I had. I began to focus instead on how well my body would work in labor and the fact that it was my work to birth, not my providers'. Plus, I mostly liked my midwife. I just felt a little mistrusting as I wished she had given me better counsel on prenatal screening. In the end I made peace with my plans by thinking, "How do I really know who will be with me or where I'll even be when my baby arrives? What if I deliver on a train or in a taxi? Well, wherever I am, it will always be my work to do."

My first birth, Jasper's arrival

A day and a half before my due date, in the middle of the day, I sat down on the toilet to urinate. I felt and heard a POP! I was confused, "A water balloon just popped?" It took me a moment or two to realize that the water balloon was me! It was my amniotic sac. Yes, it was *my* water balloon. I had to call Julian! We had the new, cutting-edge technology of the times: a pager. I paged him but he didn't respond. It turned out that he was just a couple of blocks away and didn't want to stop, get off the bus, and call... from a pay phone. (Cell phones were still the stuff of science fiction.) My contractions started within about 20 minutes of my water breaking.

We started off happy and in good shape with the early contractions. We knew that we had a lot of work in front of us, so we went out for an important last-minute supply: ice cream! But there was something I didn't know ahead of time: once your water breaks, each time you have a contraction you are going to leak some fluid. I learned this lesson well and quickly that day, on West 23rd Street in mid-town Manhattan. We were walking down the block, and I had to ask Julian for his jacket; I needed to tie it around my waist to cover my wet pants. Wet pants were not going to stop *me* from getting ice cream. I was a little embarrassed, but also pretty excited. With ice cream in hand we came home and I put on dry clothes. We ate ice cream, had contractions, and watched TV until TV got instantly annoying during a very strong contraction. It felt like the people on the screen were somehow in the room. I started to need the positions, techniques, and approaches we had learned in our Bradley® class. And thankfully, it was all working really well for us.

Several hours into labor I looked up and asked Julian how we were going to get to the hospital. I couldn't seem to remember our plan, and I really couldn't imagine going out in public. Disorientation can be an emotional signpost for the phase of labor birth-workers often call "transition." The hospital was across town; we had planned to take a taxi.

Riding in a New York City cab in labor was a surreal experience. I kept wondering if I was in a movie. The cabbie seemed consumed with angst that I might pop at any second. Thankfully I wasn't contracting too insanely for our short ride. (Stress hormones, which distort the process of labor, are often released during the emotional and physical rigors of traveling during labor.[12])

When we got to the hospital and settled into a room, my midwife checked my progress by inserting her gloved hand into my vagina; I was on my back on the bed with my legs splayed. She reached her first two fingers deep into me to feel for my cervix. She said, "You are four, almost five centimeters dilated already." My midwife's report was good news, yet I wished she had said 10 centimeters (when the cervix is completely open). But, hey, 4-5 is just about halfway. I took it as very good news.

The nurse then hooked me up to the electronic fetal monitor. The equipment consisted of an electronic box that sat on a cart. The box had a medium-sized screen on it and several knobs and buttons, a paper spool that looks almost like a cashier's receipt only wider, and two long wires coming out of it, each with a circular sensor on the end; they looked like hockey pucks about 3 inches around and black. The nurse helped me put a stretchy cloth band over my enormous abdomen and then she took the first sensor, squirted a transducer gel on the end of it to help the soundwaves get into the body, and moved that around on my belly until she heard the baby's heartbeat from a speaker on the box. We could also see a squiggly line on the screen that correlated to the heart tones. She then added gel to the second sensor and put that on the other side of my belly, also under the stretchy band. The second sensor measures the strength of the contractions, and we could see this represented on the screen in concert with the heart tones line. The electronic box can be made to print a paper readout of the two squiggly lines that represent the fetal heart tones in relation to the contractions. The nurse had wanted me to get in bed and lay on my back. But I wasn't happy on my back and asked her to monitor me while I stood up and leaned over the bed rail, which she did. When I was released from the monitor I got into the shower, and out of the shower, and back into the shower again. I was working hard and using everything I had learned in our Bradley® class. After a couple of hours, the midwife came back (she had not stayed with us, as expected) to do another vaginal exam. She wanted to check my progress.

Once again, she put her gloved hand into my vagina to feel for my cervix, but this time she had a funny look on her face. She pulled her fingers out and said that she thought there might be something going on with the baby's position. She wanted to bring the ultrasound machine in again to take a quick look. Her funny look translated to me as concern, which definitely scared me. I consented to more ultrasound hoping for nothing more than a brief exposure. And because the doctor happened to be nearby, she wanted to bring him in for a consultation as well.

Most babies come out head first, a *vertex* position (97% of babies are head down-vertex position at term)[13]. But when they turned on the ultrasound machine, my very athletic son was now butt down and head up: *breech* position. I knew enough at that point to know that my doctor didn't have any experience delivering breech babies vaginally. Although it used to be common practice, vaginal breech delivery techniques are no longer routinely taught in medical schools. And this has created a serious information gap. Today, medical doctors with the know-how for breech birth are few and far between. Historically, midwives have successfully managed the risks of breech delivery. Today, however, many have no experience at all.

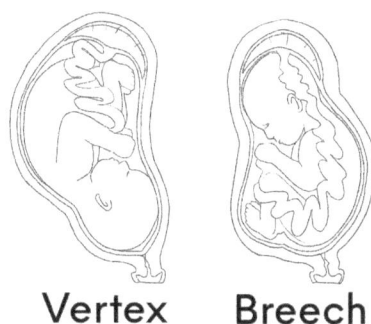

Vertex   Breech

My doctor's only recourse was to perform a cesarean section. Reflecting back, I wonder why it never occurred to me to ask if my certified nurse midwife (CNM) was trained to catch breech babies. She was a hospital midwife. Midwives that work in hospitals sometimes have little autonomy compared to their home birth colleagues, regardless of the training they actually have. For some CNM's, their practices are heavily controlled by doctors. In these cases, the midwives act more like physician assistants than midwives. Some of these doctor-extending midwives have been sarcastically named "med-wives" by several of my colleagues, friends, and relations. By the same token, there are also good examples of hospital midwives with ample autonomy and extensive training. These midwives practice a midwifery model of care and only call the doctors when they need them for consultation and advanced procedures, such as surgery. My midwife was somewhere in the middle. Nevertheless, even if my midwife had known how to deliver a breech, our current healthcare system would never approve an obstetrician or insurance company supporting her to use those skills. Because breech is considered a higher risk scenario, it is automatically deferred to the doctors. So that was that. Prep the O.R.; I was having a cesarean section.

At the time, we didn't stop to think about it. There was no question or discussion of alternatives, like waiting a little longer to see if the baby could flip on his own. We didn't discuss an *External Cephalic Version*, a procedure to manually change the baby's position, probably because the baby was already so low. No options were presented, so no choice was considered. At the time, I didn't have bad feelings about it. In fact, because I was still contracting quite strongly through all of this, I was eager to get the birth over with in whatever way we "needed" to. I understood that this was going to be "that other way babies come out." In 1993 the national c/section rate was almost 23%[14], which seemed alarmingly high to us back then. (Today it is even higher, at nearly 32%.[15]) In 1993, like my providers and peers, I too had accepted the idea that a lot of people end up with a surgical birth. I thought, if we have to go to surgery, let's do it pronto. In fact, couldn't you have done it five minutes ago? I was probably at about 7 or 8 centimeters dilated and was clearly in transition. I was scared, uncomfortable and on my back for the monitoring; it was a tough combination of feelings. So off to surgery we went.

I was separated from my partner, wheeled into the O.R., anesthetized, reunited with my partner, and cut open. Jasper was here. I cried in joy and relief, and so did my baby. Thankfully, there were no surgical complications. I had a very healthy looking, 9lbs 3oz baby boy, with a thick head of dark hair. 10 fingers. 10 toes. I eventually breastfed well and had no further medical complications as I recovered. But believe me please when I say, recovery is a *process*. It doesn't just happen in days or even weeks.

Looking back on my surgery years later, I realize that I learned a lot from the experience. It was my first birth. The amount of love I felt, and the increased meaning in my life that came from my child's arrival, was ecstatic and indescribable. And although it took some time to heal, I was eventually able to find a connection between the love I had for my baby and the circumstances of a surgical birth. I learned to give myself credit for doing the best that I could, in the circumstances I found myself. It may seem obvious to you, but I had to learn to see that my surgery was *my birth*, and my birth brought forth my baby. I am grateful for the care I received and the skill of my surgeon. But my joy lives beside my disappointment. I had wanted to feel the power of my vagina opening wide to release my baby. I thought going through the sensations of childbirth would yield to feelings of empowerment. I knew the work was going to be hard and I was scared. But I was also eager to face my fears and test myself. I thought unmedicated vaginal birth was, in addition to being an extremely beneficial process for my baby, also a gift to my future self. Years later, I now believe that I could have birthed him vaginally if I had had the right provider. But I have made peace with the experience. I look back at my son's arrival—my birth—with joy and acceptance. And I recognize that we each strive to make the best decisions that we can, in the moment that we have to make them.

It wasn't until I was recovering from my surgical birth that I realized how deeply I felt about my Bradley® class. My recovery and breastfeeding were incredibly well-supported by my education and the people I had connected to in class. The surgery was an ordeal, but what I learned helped me through. All around me I had friends who were taking hospital-based classes and not getting anything useful out of them. Even when their births were very straightforward, they found the information from their classes essentially useless for labor and beyond. There are of course truly amazing hospital-based educators scattered about the country, so my storytelling here is not meant to be dismissive. Rather, it is meant to shed light on my own personal experience in contrast to many of my friends. My friends' stories really brought home my belief in the benefits of the comprehensive Bradley Method®. Moreover, my birth transformation led me on a journey to keep learning about birth, and family-life, and to figure out who I was now that I had become a mother.

Fast forward... and the process of becoming a Bradley® birth instructor was as joyful as it was empowering. I worked hard: went to births, took birth classes, and strove to find the balance between motherhood and other work. My second pregnancy came after several years of teaching Bradley® birth classes. Already a birth educator, one cesarean section under my belt and pregnant again, I was amped up and eager to plan and flex with this birth. Julian and I did quite a lot of fear processing, academic research, and provider interviews, which eventually led us to a planned home birth that ended up being spectacularly simple and fast.

Yes, a vaginal birth after cesarean (VBAC) at home.

Arlo's birth

Arlo came two weeks before my due date. He pretty much just flew out of me. All told, the birth was 2 hours and 13 minutes long. Having him at home was the perfect plan for us. But let's not start at the end; let's go back to the beginning.

I had several nights in a row with a lot of contractile activity during my sleep. I could feel many developing changes. Day by day he was getting lower in my pelvis. Then one day, after a walk, some errands, and a nap, I went into labor. That day, when I got up from my nap, I sat down at my desk and felt a strong kick. So strong I said, "Ouch!" Of course, then I had to pee. When I stood up, there was a trickle of fluid down my leg. I instantly knew that my water had broken. The kick had been so strong that I essentially felt it brake through my amniotic sac. After I peed, as I was throwing my toilet paper into the bowl, I saw that there, in the toilet, was my mucous plug. In all its mucous-y glory, there it sat, splat on the porcelain, above the water line—a full round circle of snot, veined with a bit of blood. It really did look like snot from my nose. While I was still in the bathroom, pulling up my pants, I called Julian in to see it; it seemed like an exciting birth development that I should share. As I stood there, I had my first strong contraction. Oh yeah, that was real. I knew I was now absolutely, for certain, *in labor*.

Julian called our midwife saying, "We think this is it." He gave her the details and she responded, "Great, keep us posted. We're here getting our birth kits cleaned and stocked from our last birth. We're ready to come to you as soon as you need us." Everyone figured there would be hours before the next call.

But the labor was off to a furious start and within 15 minutes we were ready to call again. Julian realized that he had better time the contractions before actually calling, so that he could have more specific details to tell them. The contractions were coming every two minutes and were lasting a good solid minute each. While it's hard to talk about the progression of labor in terms of anything "normal" based just on the timing of contractions, this pattern of timing typically occurs once a person is already very advanced into their birth process.

With Julian timing the contractions, I stayed focused on coping. I wasn't paying very much attention to him. But when I heard him on the phone saying that my contractions were coming every two minutes and lasting for a full minute, I had to interrupt him. He must have timed them wrong. Intellectually, it just didn't seem possible that I could be in such an advanced pattern of labor, because the labor had only just begun.

Two hours and 13 minutes from the start of that first kick my second baby was born, vaginally and at home. It was so fast that the midwives almost didn't make it! They got to our home at 5:00pm and my baby arrived at

5:13pm, while I was on my hands and knees on our kitchen floor. I had hoped to birth in the rented birth pool we had set up in the kitchen, but there hadn't even been enough time to fill it.

We were all eating pizza by 6:30, which was equal parts crazy and awesome. The midwives joked and thanked us for keeping bankers' hours! We felt a bit dazed; it had just been so very fast. We also felt lucky, relieved, and incredibly happy.

For my work as a birthing educator, it was great to have had such different birth experiences. How our births unfold and how we feel about them are important parts of our development. They inform our identity and help mold us into the parents we become. And my births have undoubtedly affected my perspectives on teaching childbirth to others. Consequently, this is why I take the time at the start of all my classes to introduce myself through my births. Who I am, what I value, and the motivations I hold are all important disclosures. They make the curriculum more meaningful, more useful, more transparent, and more applicable.

Now that you've had a glimpse into what my physical birth experiences were like, you can understand in part why this book and its lessons will prioritize education, choice, and individual empowerment. Plus, you've discovered that I really like ice cream.

Conscientious breath awareness

Actively listening to your own breathing is not only an effective tool for good physical and mental health; it works well for birth, too. Breath awareness doesn't erase labor pain, but tuning into our breath helps us make the pain more manageable. Breath observation sessions are a wonderful way to work through the emotional challenges and physical discomforts that are so common throughout the childbearing year and beyond. Developing skill at breath-awareness helps to reduce stress and improve overall health. And when practiced together with your partner, this tool helps build trust between you, helping to deepen your non-verbal communication skills and training you to better listen to each other.

The kind of breathing that I want you to practice now is a *passive observation exercise*, one through which all your muscles (especially your abdominal muscles and the muscles of your pelvic floor) relax easily and deeply as you inhale. When we inhale, our bellies softly puff out, and when we exhale our bellies gently sink in towards the spine. As your lungs fill and empty, the lower belly rises and sinks. All this breathing action comes as a result of the diaphragm, that magnificent, dome-shaped muscle that bisects the torso. When the diaphragm contracts it pushes down and flattens out. This action creates a void above the diaphragm, the thoracic cavity that houses the lungs. That void then pulls air in, through the nose and/or mouth, to fill the lungs. As a general rule it is best to breathe in through your nose. The nose filters out more contaminants and better adjusts the temperature of the air going into your body.[16] Once the lungs are full, the diaphragm releases and rises up to push out the stale air. Meanwhile, the abdominal muscles engage in our breathing when we need to increase the force of our exhalations or increase the speed and quantity of our inhalations, like we do during hard physical labor. When we are relaxing, we do not need to use the abdominal muscles. In the relaxed abdominal breathing exercise that follows—the first birthing exercise to start you on your journey—the chest should appear to move very little even as it seems to fill with air after the belly. The idea in this work is to find the easiest and smoothest rhythm. Think about calm waves at low tide slowly rolling up onto the shore and then slowly rolling all the way back out to sea. Relaxed abdominal breathing allows for the best exchange of gases while using the least amount of energy. Relaxed belly breathing is how we breathe when we are asleep: calm, peaceful and restorative.

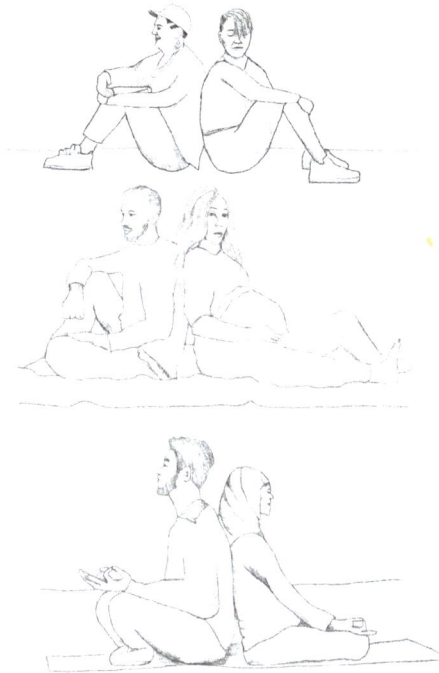

EXERCISE: CONSCIENTIOUS BREATH AWARENESS

Directions

After you read through the directions that follow, put the book down and sit back-to-back with your birthing partner or supporting object and practice from memory. Or, if sitting isn't best, lie down next to each other and practice. Or, read this script out loud as a guided exercise. And if you don't have a birthing partner, or you would both prefer to listen, record it on your phone and play it back to yourself. Feel free to use pillows for enhanced comfort. If you choose to read the script and then practice from memory, I recommend that you set a timer so that you don't have to bother wondering how long you should continue and you can more easily focus on the task of observing your breath. Start with short amounts of practice time, maybe one minute or two, working up to 20- to 30-minute sessions or longer. Be compassionate with yourselves and know that what is long for you is an individual preference; you get to decide. Please read the following script slowly, taking ample time for your breath.

Breath Exercise Script

"Close your eyes. Exhale fully. Allow your body weight to be supported by whatever or whomever you are leaning against. Settle. Spread out. Place your hands comfortably on your own low belly and with a gentle sigh, exhale again and encourage yourself to settle and soften more."

—Reader should pause—

"Notice and listen to your breath. Relax your chest and shoulders. Feel yourself open, calm and soft."

—Reader should pause—

"Allow your belly to rise and sink gently. Let go in your abdominal muscles, relax in your organs."

—Reader should pause—

"Notice any changes in shape you may feel. The idea is not to change your breathing, but rather to allow it to happen. Follow your easiest rhythm."

—Reader should pause—

"Experience what it feels like right now as you connect to your breathing. Invite your breath to slow down even more, follow your breath in and follow your breath out."

—Reader should pause—

"You may become aware that you and your partner are breathing in a different rhythm. That is normal, just notice the differences and try to stay true to your own comfortable rhythms. You and your partner are different, invite appreciation of those differences. Settle."

—Reader should pause—

"Feel support from what you are resting on. Feel the support of your breath from the inside. Observe your feelings as you notice them and then bring your attention back to your breath."

—Reader should pause—

"Your attention will wander and that is fine; there is no need for judgment. Bring your focus back to your breath."

—Reader should pause—

"Follow your breath in and follow your breath out. The mind wanders and we retrieve it. Follow the breath in, follow the breath out."

—Reader should pause—

"Now gently let some movement come into your toes and fingers, give them a little wiggle and a gentle stretch. Then gently let some light come into your eyes as you slowly open them and ease out of your focused awareness."

—End of exercise—

How was that? Investigate your experience by asking yourself such questions as:

O   Could you feel your belly moving?

O   What else did you feel?

○ Was your chest calm?

○ Did your mind wander?

○ Did the time go slow or fast?

○ Could you feel your partner's breath? Or the movement of air in the room?

○ How are you now?

○ Do you feel different than you did before?

○ Would you like a sip of water?

○ Do you need a little stretch or change of position?

This week please **practice this simple breath observation <u>twice a day</u>**, once in the morning before you get out of bed and once in the evening before you go to sleep. I encourage you to get curious about the ways meditation can change your brain and improve your health.

Peer introductions

Now that you have had a chance to get to know me a bit, in the context of these lessons, and you have begun to settle into your own breath, I want to introduce you to an amalgamation of some past Bradley® students. Throughout the remainder of the book your class peers will be a compilation of different real people representing a variety of perspectives and concerns. I know you will benefit from their perspectives. And I encourage you to write notes on your own perspectives as they emerge. Let's start with something you hope to learn from reading this book. Please write or draw your thoughts in the space below.

Todd: "My wife told me I had to be here (much laughter in the room). I would just like to go into labor with a better sense of what my role is going to be. I am a fairly stubborn guy I guess, and I usually kind of see how things should go. But I have absolutely no clue how this one should go, so I would like to take a step back and [leave it] to the experts."

Jonah: "I want as much information as I can get. Kealee has had a couple of bad experiences with doctors in the past, and I am in medical school and have had an opportunity to get an inside look at some of the shortcomings of the medical system. So I wanted to take a class. This one looked like the best of them."

Kealee: "I have a lot of severe allergies, so medication isn't really an option for us. We were looking for something to help us outside of medication. I am a little nervous about the whole process and not being able to take anything. So we are working around it and trying to find another way to cope in labor that we are comfortable with and can feel like we will be able to handle."

Imani: "I had a friend about 10 years ago that had a baby and she had an epidural. Then she developed a spinal headache. I spent a lot of time with her through that process. I was traumatized. She wasn't able to nurse. They thought [her headache] was meningitis, and she had to have a spinal tap and there were all of these problems. I thought, 'Who knew that could be part of an epidural?'

My friend's spinal headache lasted three or four days, and it took the doctors a long time to even figure out what was happening... I thought, 'I need to really understand what this process is all about.' Since then, I have been devouring as much information as I can about all the potential side effects of an epidural and everything else that comes along with interventions. I had actually read about the Bradley Method® before I was even pregnant and then my midwife recommended this class."

Jalen: "I want to learn how I can be supportive of Imani... And from talking to other people who have utilized the Bradley Method®, I have learned that I might have to run some interference... Also, I hope we can learn how to do that together with an informed perspective."

Jean: "I picked this class because everything in our marriage is such a partnership, it seemed really weird that I would be going into birth by myself without a lot of support, not from my husband's perspective, but from the medical perspective. For me it was like, well, of course we are going to go do this together."

Seth: "We have several friends that took this course. One man was telling me how helpful the class was for him even though he was well trained; he's a chiropractor. He had the knowledge about birth, but not necessarily the tools for how to support his wife and he found the class to be really helpful. So that sounded good to me. I am a supportive person, but I have no idea what to do, how to support in birth. So I would like to get a clue, in a constructive way."

I feel for the people these days who want to be a supportive part of the birth, who have the weight of so much expectation that they will be there to support their pregnant partners, yet don't know what they are actually supposed to do. Very few hospital-based birth classes really focus on giving partners helpful information. And clearly there is little information that is helpful in popular culture—and too much that is so incorrect it is harmful.

To birth partners, I ask: Have you ever seen a birth? How will you be able to help your pregnant partner if you are afraid or uncertain yourself? This is a heavy burden to carry: the expectation that you can be helpful when you do not have good information about *how* to help. We have all been indoctrinated by endless sitcoms and other popular media sources. We always see women in labor being mad at their partners: yelling at them, blaming them, or even hitting them during birth. I think it puts the partners in an uncomfortable place and does nothing positive to help them become parents. So good for you for doing the hard work of choosing education! The following information should help you provide useful support to your pregnant partner, while you become part of the birth experience. This in turn can help you build a solid foundation for parenthood.

Prior to the birth, we can't know for sure what any individual pregnant person will find most useful for birth support. We don't know whose baby is going to come first, or where they will arrive, or what kind of support they will require along the way. Even if you have already birthed a baby, all we know is that this time it will be different. Nevertheless, there *are* some time-tested birth positions and support techniques that can help. There are also some very useful things we can understand about how a person's feelings impact their body's functioning that can really help a caring person lend effective birth support.

Pregnancy is more than just growing and birthing a baby. Pregnancy is, amongst other things, your orientation period for parenthood. Your birth and your adjustment to parenthood will be affected by what you eat, how you move, who cares for you, even what you watch on TV or online. How you are communicating with your partner and how you feel about your baby and your plans for birth will also have significant impact on your health and the health of your growing family.

Nutrition and the work of baby building

You *and your baby* are what you eat. Trying to build a healthy baby without enough of the right kinds of nutrition is like trying to build a house without enough 2x4's: you might be able to do it, but it wouldn't be very safe in a storm. What you eat matters more than how much weight you gain or don't gain. What you eat directly impacts how well you can build a baby, how well you can sustain your own health, and how well you will handle the rigors of pregnancy, birth and breastfeeding. If you tell me that you have gained 35 pounds, I don't know if you have been eating a well-balanced diet with an ample supply of the whole foods you require or if you binged on doughnuts and sodas and other sugars and low-nutrient calorie sources.

We all come to pregnancy with a different health history. A lot of people in the United States are overweight while some people are underweight. Many people struggle with body image unhappiness, incomplete nutritional information, or inadequate access to good food. Many of us have deeply inherited and indoctrinated views that our body parts are too big, too small, or just plain wrong. These views can complicate our relationship to food. Body image and beliefs will probably affect you in pregnancy just as much as they did before conception. I encourage you to share your concerns through discussion, writing, and possibly professional counseling. Eat healthy food, but also feed yourself as much love as possible!

Obesity or being underweight will create serious risks for you and your baby. But what matters is what you are eating now and in what quantities. Again, it doesn't matter how much weight you gain or don't gain during pregnancy. **The right nutrition within the right mindset are what matters.** Weight is just one piece of the puzzle.

Evaluating your diet through diet charting can help you to identify previously unrecognized patterns. Then you can work toward making informed adjustments. Or, if you discover that you're already making good choices, you can relax into your routines. If the body is getting what it needs, then the body can gain or lose as it requires. Remember, you and your baby are vying for the same supply of nutrients.

During my first pregnancy, I had a nurse that would gasp in horror at each of my weigh-ins. It was humiliating and I resorted to wearing the lightest-weight clothes I could find on appointment days. It was late fall in New York City. It was cold, but still I would wear little summer dresses. I would also sometimes skip breakfast before the appointment. I was within 10 pounds of my "ideal" weight when I got pregnant and gained 50 lbs by my delivery date. What does that tell you about my health during that pregnancy? Not much.

Toward the end of that pregnancy I finally pressed my doctor to explain what was so awful about my weight. All he could come up with was that I might be left with some unwanted pounds after the birth. (I was, and then I lost them.) He never asked me about what I was eating or if I exercised.

Improving your lifestyle choices now not only improves your and your baby's health and birth, it also helps to establish a healthy family. Your children learn about food from you, before, during, and after pregnancy.

Breastfeeding will provide all of your child's nutritional needs for the first 6 – 12 months of her life. Breastfeeding is also a positive preventative for future obesity in children as they age. But once solid foods are introduced, being able to provide a well-balanced diet based on whole foods is clearly an important parental responsibility.

Learning to assess your nutritional intake over the course of a week sets you up well to be conscientious in meeting your child's nutritional needs. Additionally, small children seem to have a keen interest in learning about diet choices from someone other than their birth mother. (In my house, my boys were most interested in what their dad ate.) So it is helpful if both partners and other close support persons consider their food and additional lifestyle choices during pregnancy.

Do you know how to cook? My partner and I and many of my clients have found that pregnancy was the time that we started to really learn about food preparation and nutrition. Your child will need three meals a day plus snacks for the next 18 years or so. Children's nutritional needs are critical to their health and success. When you take the time to learn some good recipes and balanced eating habits, you lay an excellent foundation for a healthy family. Step one begins *now*.

Diet charting

During this Week 1, please write down *everything* that you eat and drink. Try to include your best assessment of your portions as well. A serving of meat or fish, for example, is generally considered to be a piece about the size of the palm of your hand, and average serving sizes of most all foods can be found quickly through online searches. The internet can also be a wonderful resource for figuring out protein values for foods and, of course, it offers endless recipe ideas too!

This week, after you write down what you have eaten, write down the approximate protein value next to it. At the end of each day please do the math and add up your protein grams. Please keep your chart with you all day and write down what you are eating as, or immediately after, you have eaten it. It is very hard to be accurate if you are sitting around trying to remember what you had for breakfast yesterday. Write as you go and tally up the protein totals each night.

Diet changes can be emotionally trying, so please go slow. No one is perfect every day. The point of the diet chart assignment is to see where you are at currently. (It will be beneficial to chart this week and then do it again later in the pregnancy, if/when you get to your Bradley® class. In my in-person Bradley® classes I usually ask couples to chart once at the beginning of the series and then once as they are completing the series.) This week I don't want you to try to make any big changes to your diet. This week's work should be about checking in and getting a week-long snapshot of your choices. Give yourself credit for the good choices you see. Listening to your cues for hunger and thirst are core components of a healthy diet. Please be conscientious as you do your homework.

Partners, please look for ways to get involved in your family's nutrition. You can help with support in planning, shopping and preparation. Your loving interest in this charting homework for your pregnant partner, as well as your practical help, can help them feel well supported.

When diet charting, please be sure to list all foods, snacks, water and other beverages consumed. If you prefer, you can also find various online resources and phone apps to help you chart your food intake. *(see sample chart on the following page)*

Babies are little, but they take up a whole universe of space, in and out of your body. Learning about and birthing babies also takes a lot of time and energy, which is still nothing compared to the adventure once they are born! You can start to make some of the needed emotional space now, with intention, and give yourself grace in your adjustments. This can help ease your transition later. We all adjust to this space invasion in our own ways and time; sometimes we hit bumps and struggles in prioritizing and time management.

With this in mind, I have another client introduction to share with you here. Meet birth class graduates Brian and Jill. Brian shares what happened when Jill signed them up for their Bradley® birth class:

SAMPLE DIET CHART

	Monday	Tuesday	Wed.	Thurs.	Friday	Saturday	Sunday
Food/ Protein							
Snack							
Breakfast							
Snack							
Lunch							
Snack							
Dinner							
Snack							
Total Protein							

I remember the whole process with our first son. It started out with this idea of taking a 12-week birth class with my wife on Sunday afternoons. That does not sound so bad except that the first class was the opening day of the NFL season and then, well, you see where it goes from there. So, the start of this whole process was a little rough for me. My first thoughts on birth were very simple. I mean we go to the hospital, she pushes for a little while and the doctors take care of the rest. I mean this birth thing happens all the time in hospitals with people who do not have a clue what they're doing. So why couldn't we be one of those couples? Then I can just watch football. Wow was I wrong...

My thoughts on childbirth started to change with the first class. The instructor said that this is a two-person event, and she wasn't talking about the baby. My role is to be there for my wife and to help this birth process, and this can only be done if I know what is going to happen and how to support my wife in the ways that she needs, without her having to tell me every little thing, since she will be busy. This is only accomplished through education. I have since told one friend of mine that if there was one thing he could do that was the most important it was to go to a birth class. One of the things that I learned in class is that this is our experience and we can make it be what we want. Now you might ask, how do I know what we want? Well you need to learn what the options are and what the risks and benefits are to these options.

Jill also wrote of their birth class experience:

Brian and I had GREAT conversations after class. He still loves telling everyone about the great sacrifice he made to attend a birth class on Sunday afternoons during football season, but the truth is he enjoyed the class as much or more than I did. I think the most important aspect of the class was the fact that we did it together. Brian went from a skeptic of natural birth to informing a couple we'd met only minutes before that squatting is a wonderful position to push in because of the way it opens up the pelvis.

These testimonials help to illustrate the importance of education and information gathering. They also reveal what will become a repeated appeal throughout this book: give yourself grace in your adjustments. If you can connect the time you prioritize to read this book with time to practice the provided meditation techniques and the focus of connecting deeply to the baby (and each other, if you're partnered), then you are utilizing and training valuable multitasking abilities that can, in turn, help you transition more easily into parenthood.

In the weeks to come I encourage you to fully participate in this book, including with your own notes and doodles. Both writing and drawing—at any level, from raw brainstorming and doodling to producing meditative masterpieces—can help you cope with any feelings (and can be especially useful for any feelings of dread or angst or impatience that may surface from time to time[17]). Above all, I encourage you (and, as promised above, will encourage you again and again throughout this book) to be compassionate with yourselves and to stay determined to prioritize selfcare, baby-care and healthcare. I also hope you find fun and humor while creating space in your life for your new baby. Certainly reading this (baby-sized!) book will be great practice.

Congratulations! You've already completed Week 1! I wish you a wonderful week.

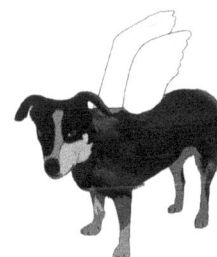

HOMEWORK

A) Birth History Investigation

Investigate your own birth history and the birth history of your closest family members or any other important adults in your life. Interview your parents or anyone that might have interesting information about your own birth. If you are lucky enough to have a parent to talk to about your own birth, notice the words they use to describe the event. These may provide clues as you search to understand the birth values that surrounded you during your upbringing.

B) Social Support Evaluation

Please begin to evaluate your life for social support. Are there friends and/or family you can turn to for emotional support and/or physical support, such as providing a meal, washing the dishes, holding the baby while you shower, or to help with laundry or pet care? Try to identify the kinds of support that will be most helpful for you. Identification of what your stressors are will be helpful as you determine what kind of support you will need/want. Who can you confide in? Who in your life helps to build your self-esteem and who doesn't? You will be learning so much as you begin your journey as a parent. Having people around who lift up your confidence will be hugely beneficial.

C) Build Daily Routines

Practice conscientious breath awareness at least twice a day, once on your own and once with your partner, if this is an option. Try to be physically active, get adequate rest, and eat good food. Look for opportunities to smile, but also don't be afraid or embarrassed to let your tears flow.

THIS SPACE IS FOR YOUR NOTES AND DRAWINGS

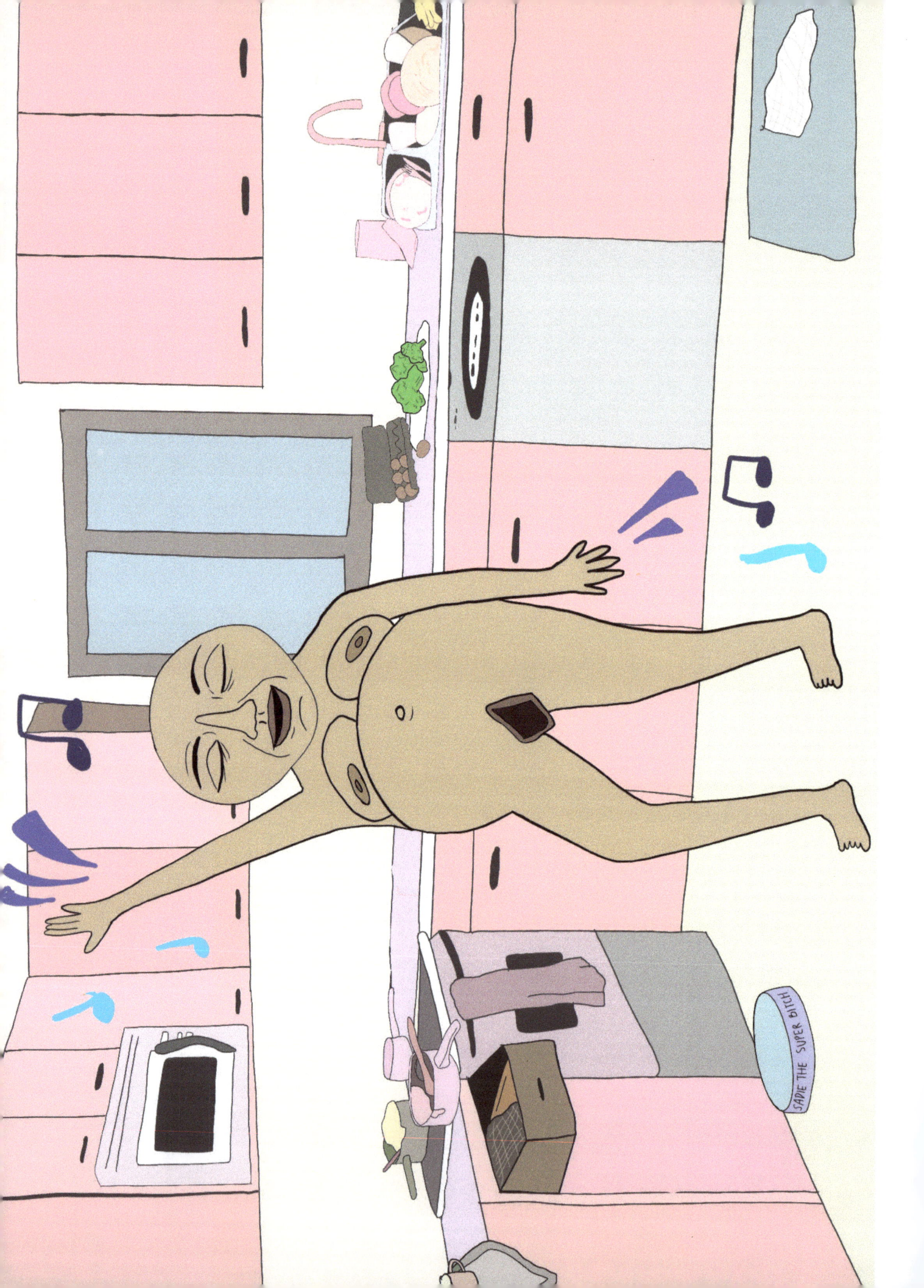

WEEK 2

Eat
and
Relax

Chapter contents:

O *Wholistic prenatal health assessment*

O *Diet development*

O *Relaxation/meditation/ breath awareness*

THIS SPACE IS FOR YOUR NOTES AND DRAWINGS

THIS SPACE IS FOR YOUR NOTES AND DRAWINGS

Welcome back! How was your first week? Feel free to write and draw in the margins and any open or shaded areas of this book. I love asking questions of my students, so the questions that follow are a great way for you to check in with yourself from week to week. Plus, your responses will be helpful touchpoints for you to reflect on as you move through the class:

Did you do any homework this past week? I am not asking to cause stress, take a breath. —pause— Congratulate yourself for picking up the book now!

Did you find time to practice breath awareness? If you did, how was it? When during your day did you try and what did you learn?

If you did not find the time this past week to tune into mindful breathing, maybe try it briefly now? You can also examine your long-range goals and review your motivations. Try to allow your priorities to shift into alignment with your goals. Development of a regular practice takes commitment and time, so be patient with yourself. Ideally, you are practicing breath observations once every morning before you get out of bed or perhaps after peeing (I remember needing to pee so much during my pregnancies!), then once every evening just before you go to sleep, and anytime throughout your day that you feel stressed or uncomfortable.

How was your appetite this week? How do you feel about your food choices? Were you able to chart your diet? If you did write down your diet history and did the math, how was that work? Were there charting challenges? What did you learn?

If you didn't start charting yet, don't worry, there's always this week and the weeks to follow. Of course, starting this sooner rather than later is strongly encouraged because tracking your diet history and being able to address any deficiencies is really important for your health and for the health of your baby. Regardless of your likes, dislikes, and access to food sources, knowing what you are eating is the best way to begin to figure out what you can try in order to optimize your best outcomes.

Were you able to investigate your family's birth history? What about your social support? Who did you identify to ask for help when you need it? Who supports good self-esteem for you?

Actively working to develop a list of people who can help to support you should be a continuous and adaptive process. And offering your help now to other new parents you know is a great way to pay it forward for when your baby arrives.

Prenatal health

When you're pregnant, your health matters in new and more critical ways. Before a pregnancy, you can endure quite a lot of inadequate nutrition and sleep and still manage, albeit sub-optimally, to get through your days. But getting through a pregnancy with stress from inadequate nutrition and sleep is a different, more serious beast. Your baby's potential cognitive abilities and neurological functioning, as well as any potential health challenges they will face as they age, are vitally connected to *you* and the circumstances and choices of your experiences while pregnant. But it's not just the baby's needs that matter during pregnancy, yours do too! When you work to optimize your prenatal health, you positively impact your safety and comfort before, during, and after birth. Taking a proactive approach to your prenatal health now will also make it easier to raise your child to develop their own healthy lifestyle.

Chances are very good that if you are pregnant and reading this book, you have a solid base level of good health. Pregnancy is a healthy human function; in other words, you need to be a reasonably healthy human to get pregnant and then maintain a pregnancy. Good health comes from being able to access good food, clean water, time for rest and sleep, enjoyable physical activity, positive social connections, and access to factual information. You deserve access to these securities, and I am sorry for the real-world challenges that get in the way. Access is everything, but many people with access still have challenges and/or misinformation that can impair their ability to maintain or develop healthy prenatal habits.

What motivates you, and what are your challenges?

Whatever you think about your current health, and whatever challenges you face, it is important to strive towards balance: balanced diet, balanced ratio of work to play (yes, playtime is healthy for adults too!), balance between rest and being physically active, and balance around social interactions and time to yourself. I encourage you to continue defining your motivation and refining your habits. Health is a dynamic state: the body is resilient, you are resilient and constantly changing in an effort to achieve good health.

Following are some questions to consider as you evaluate your motivations for making healthy decisions. Please try to answer each question, even if the answer is, "I don't know." Stop, think, and talk about these questions. Explore your thoughts even if you may not have answers. There is a good deal of information to gain from exploring life's open-ended questions and the "I don't knows." When we start to define what we don't know, it can help us to define what we do know and what we want to seek out. Being clear about what we know and don't know can help us grow.

First read through the following list of questions, then go back and attempt to answer them one by one by writing them down. (Note that I have provided a separate section for a partner-in-parenting to answer as well.)

To be answered by the pregnant person:

○ Share some feelings you have about becoming a parent.

○ From my perspective, parenting is at its core creative: you create a baby and then you have to use creative ingenuity to figure out how to raise that child within the context of your circumstances, dreams and education. I believe all humans contain creative abilities. What do you think about the connection between creativity and parenting?

○ Are there any selfcare habits you would like to develop or alter?

○ Will you teach selfcare routines to your child, and if so how?

○ When you take on parenting, I believe promises are made. Do you think so too? If so, what promises—or, social contracts—are you making with your baby, with yourself, and with your community?

○ What do you see as your main responsibilities as a parent?

○ What are some things you will teach your child, and what are some things your child might teach you?

○ Do you have positive parenting role models? If yes, name and describe.

○ Do you have negative parenting role models? If yes, name and describe.

To be answered by the non-pregnant partner who is becoming a parent:

○ Share some feelings you have about becoming a parent.

○ From my perspective, parenting is at its core creative: you create a baby and then you have to use creative ingenuity to figure out how to raise that child within the context of your circumstances, dreams and education. I believe all humans contain creative abilities. What do you think about the connection between creativity and parenting?

○ Are there any selfcare habits you would like to develop or alter?

○ Will you teach selfcare routines to your child, and if so how?

○ When you take on parenting, I believe promises are made. Do you think so too? If so, what promises—or, social contracts—are you making with your baby, yourself, and with your community?

○ What do you see as your main responsibilities as a parent?

○ What are some things you will teach your child, and what are some things your child might teach you?

○ Do you have positive parenting role models? If yes, name and describe.

○ Do you have negative parenting role models? If yes, name and describe.

Over the next days and weeks, please mull over and reflect upon your responses to the questions above. Ponder the different facets of your health: nutritional, physical fitness, emotional, creative, and social health. In addition to a balanced diet, safe housing, and space and time to move your body, good health flourishes with emotional well-being. While the details informing emotional well-being are defined individually, its general components often include a combination of social support (love, help, friendship, community), stress-reducing practices (relaxation and playtime for fun), confidence-building efforts (frequently a by-product of hard work and education), expressing your creativity, and connecting to your sense of purpose and hope.

Below (each of you, if relevant) list 5 things that you already do as part of your self-care:

1._____   1._____

2._____   2._____

3._____   3._____

4._____   4._____

5._____   5._____

Refining your self-care habits will help you to avoid unnecessary pregnancy/birth/childhood complications, while also leading you towards your most comfortable pregnancy possible. More physical comfort in pregnancy will put you in a better mood and with more reserves for the birth and your postpartum recovery. But your need for strength doesn't fade once you get the baby out or during your postpartum transition. Parenting takes strength, too. Gosh my kids were heavy and occasionally flailing! And then there is the work of keeping a partnership together. Partnerships require a reserve of energy and a lot of resolve to keep trying to work together. Don't forget courage. And, of course, there is the strength needed to cope with the rest of life, such as work, bills, cooking, cleaning, etc. Good nutrition, rest, and physical activity will support all that work, too. For solo parents, prioritizing your health is perhaps even more critical. Birth and parenting are some of the most physically and emotionally demanding challenges you will face in your life. But you can do this! Healthy habits help develop empowered parenthood.

And empowerment helps everything! I have found, and have experienced first-hand, that building physical strength helps me feel strong in my mind. Likewise, building strength in my mind, through meditation, creative expression, education, and social support, all help to bring strength to my body. All this strength helps to build confidence and courage, and who doesn't need more of that? The rigors of the journey before you are extreme: your baby is counting on you to do your best. Parenting is a tremendous responsibility; it scared me, and it likely scares you. But you can fortify yourself through self-care. Through a holistic and conscientious approach to self-care you can more clearly sort out and feel your individual feelings and fears. Where fears are felt, you can look for ways to express these feelings with the aim of releasing them. This again helps cultivate courage: the ability to be scared and to carry on anyway. Courage requires you to acknowledge your fear and to move through it and with it by your side. If you are expecting a baby, this is a great time to prioritize your health, face your fears and make your plans for coping and support, because your baby is already well on their journey here and into your arms.

As you let those thoughts on health and courage settle in, please consider this: your body and soul really were built to take this journey. It takes a special kind of strength to birth and parent, but don't worry because you have that strength deep inside you. And what you don't already feel you have, or have access to, you can grow along the way. The journey to parenthood can be viewed as a journey to meet your fears, find your courage, and develop your strengths for coping with your circumstances. However, as you evaluate your health and self-care practices, consider that sometimes what's needed for more strength is actually more softness: more rest, more self-compassion, more acceptance and/or more forgiveness, and more positive messages.

For the work ahead there will be high highs filled with more love than you ever imagined possible, and low lows filled with bleak, dark despair. Family life will take incredible energy, time, and work; but it's not super-human work, it's exactly human work. So, if you are not feeling strong at the moment, don't worry. Give yourself a hug, you may be tired. You have your whole lifetime to develop, redevelop, and repair, and develop again the strength and the skills that you will need. But if you can, why not start now? We can work on it together.

Consider this: a strong muscle is one that, when at rest, is relaxed, soft, and flexible; yet, when triggered, it is quick to contract, hard and powerful. A strong muscle can endure long periods of effort, and then fully relax again. As you assess your health status now, how can you use this fact about muscles as a metaphor for building your emotional strength alongside your physical strength?

Have you ever run a marathon? No? (Me either.) Well, what if you decided to run a marathon in just nine short months from today? What would you start doing now? You would strength-train your body and your mind. How would you train your mind? You would need to grow your confidence—psych yourself up. And if you have run marathons, and perhaps you spend much of your time striving for peak performance, maybe for this pregnancy it will be advantageous to ease up on your expectations, and to soften into a slowed tempo, as you look for ways to boost confidence and build emotional fortitude. Each of us must work to find our own balance in this new pregnant reality.

Below (each of you, if relevant) please list four things that can help *you* improve strength: list two items that will help you to develop emotional strength and two items that will help you to build physical strength.

For emotional strength

1._____   1._____

2._____   2._____

For physical strength

1._____   1._____

2._____   2._____

Working to build strength and improve health, with a comprehensive approach to bodily requirements and emotional wellbeing, is an affirmation of life. Prenatal health is all about affirming life.

My young self didn't quite get the long-term consequences

It wasn't until my first pregnancy that I started to understand that my nutrition, sleep and stress levels would impact my baby for the rest of their life and mine. Later, I read an article published in *Time Magazine* in 2010, by reporter Annie Murphy Paul. Her article, "How the First Nine Months Shape the Rest of Your Life," reported on research that linked heart disease with low birth weight.[18] Researchers found that people who were born under-weight (what we call "low birth weight") frequently develop heart disease later in life. The thinking is that if the fetus is denied adequate nutrition in the uterus, it will divert resources to the brain, the most important organ. This diversion to the brain then results in a deficit of supplies for the heart. This shortage of supplies for the heart then makes the individual more likely to develop heart disease later in life.

Murphy Paul's article also reports on the correlation between how a mother feels during her pregnancy and the mental health of her baby later in life. Scientists have found that times of *extreme* stress (their examples include the Six Day War in Israel and an extreme famine in China) correlate with higher levels of schizophrenia in the subsequent generation. In other words, the people that had been fetuses during those events were much more likely than the general public to develop schizophrenia in young adulthood. The article ties our individual health to public health and gives hope for how understanding can improve outcome.

> The Nobel Prize-winning economist Amartya Sen, for example, co-authored a paper about the importance of fetal origins to a population's health and productivity: "poor prenatal experience," he writes, "sows the seeds of ailments that afflict adults." And it makes the womb a promising target for prevention, raising hopes of conquering public-health scourges like obesity and heart disease through interventions before birth.[19]

In other words, what a pregnant person eats and how they feel are indeed important to them and their baby's long-term health, as well as their community at large.

It turns out that I am not that unique, and it is not until most of my clients get to their Bradley® class that they start to really digest the information that their diet and health choices are so important to how their own bodies function, and of the long-term implications for their baby's health. Like my story, for most of my clients their Bradley® class was the first time during their pregnancy that they were given both specific nutritional and exercise guidance plus emotional support to help them meet their health goals. Has your doctor or midwife asked you about what you are eating? Have they given you guidelines about how to make your best food choices? In my classes I always poll my clients with these questions, and most of them admit nutrition was only given a scant bit of attention, if at all, and they were never asked to do any diet charting. They were never told of the seriousness of the connections between prenatal nutrition and maternal and fetal health. The exception to this is for clients that are also working with homebirth midwives. Nearly 100% of my clients who work with homebirth midwives in my area report that their midwives ask about diet, supply at least some nutritional guidelines, and encourage diet charting.

When a provider (or healthcare system) fails to create the time to include nutrition in their prenatal check-ups, it sends the signal that what you eat doesn't really matter. "Here is a vitamin and don't gain too much weight" is not nutritional education. This gap in education is an unfortunate omission, but it is one that you, responsible parent, can make up for. (And then teach your kids as they grow!) Now let's get into some specifics. What food choices are right for you?

The Bradley Method® and The Brewer Diet

Dr. Bradley grew up on a farm and from a young age was intrigued by birthing animals. After arriving in medical school, he was so unnerved by how medicalized the contemporary (1940s) practices were that he went back to the farm to study the animals and their comparative ease with the birth process. He observed that animals preferred quiet and calm and they looked quite physically relaxed with their eyes closed. These observations were the foundation of what later became (and still is) the Bradley Method®. He also knew from his farmer upbringing that if one wanted to raise healthy animals, one had to feed them well, and it was this background that set him up well for a collaboration with Dr. Brewer.

Dr. Thomas H. Brewer, MD was born in 1925. He trained as an obstetrician at Tulane University, School of Medicine and went on to teach in the obstetrics and gynecology department at University of California Medical School, San Francisco. From 1963 through 1976, in Contra Costa County, California, he ran a county public health prenatal clinic where he oversaw the prenatal nutrition education of more than 7,000 predominately low-income pregnant clients. During this time, in a population previously considered to be at risk of preeclampsia due to low income, he had no cases of convulsive eclampsia and zero maternal deaths from eclampsia. Eclampsia is currently thought to be responsible for about 10% of maternal deaths (more specific information on the disease is coming later in this chapter).[20] Dr. Brewer and Dr. Bradley both believed that it was Dr. Brewer's nutritional counseling, including 80-100 grams of protein per day, that was protective and led to such excellent outcomes. Dr. Brewer's work from the 1960s and 70s is well supported by the 2018 book, *Real Food for Pregnancy: The Science and Wisdom of Optimal Prenatal Nutrition*, by registered dietician Lily Nichols.[21] Nichols also found that the average-weight pregnant person needs 100 grams of protein per day by their third trimester. This echoes primary research published in 2016 by the National Institute of Health (NIH):

> During pregnancy, an exceptional stage of life defined by rapid growth and development, adequate dietary protein is crucial to ensure a healthy outcome. Protein deposition in maternal and fetal tissues increases throughout pregnancy, with most occurring during the third trimester... The current Estimated Average Requirement and RDA recommendations of 0.88 and 1.1 $g \cdot kg^{-1} \cdot d^{-1}$, respectively, are for all stages of pregnancy. [This translates to about 60-74 grams of protein per day for a 150lb pregnant person.] The single recommendation does not take into account the changing needs during different stages of pregnancy. Recently, with the use of the minimally invasive indicator amino acid oxidation method, we defined the requirements to be, on average, 1.2 and 1.52 $g \cdot kg^{-1} \cdot d^{-1}$ during early (~16 wk) and late (~36 wk) stages of pregnancy, respectively.[22] [This translates to about 70 grams of protein in early pregnancy and 100 grams of protein per day in later pregnancy for a person approximately 150lbs.]

Backed by this more contemporary research, I am also heartened to have witnessed generally great results from the families that take a Bradley® course and follow Dr. Brewer's recommendations. Many pregnant people have reported that when they have increased their protein to meet Dr. Brewer's recommendations they found increased stamina. The Brewer Diet is an omnivorous diet that recommends eggs, dairy, meat, fish, fowl, whole grains, legumes, nuts, oils, and plenty of colorful fruits and vegetables. There is a focus on dark green leafy vegetables, animal proteins, whole grains, at least one daily serving of a fresh vitamin C-rich food, and at least one orange vegetable per week. Dr. Brewer's diet also includes drinking plenty of water and cow's milk and being encouraged to salt your food to taste. To repeat: **The Brewer diet emphasizes that pregnant people should aim for a goal of 80-100 grams of protein per day when pregnant with a singleton and 125 grams of protein per day when carrying twins.**[23] That is a lot of protein. It takes protein to care for our own bodies and even more to build new bodies, because protein is a building block for human life.

To reach the Brewer Diet target for protein, the following strategy has helped many people: Aim to eat protein-rich foods at breakfast, lunch, and dinner, and two additional protein-rich snacks throughout the day and evening. If each of your meals contains about 20 grams of protein each and your snacks about 10 grams of protein each, then you receive an average of 80 grams of protein total in a day. This exceeds the more common, daily pre-pregnant protein consumption levels. A typical American diet, in practice, is often simple-carbohydrate rich and protein low, especially at breakfast. Did you find any patterns when you charted your diet?

During pregnancy it may help you feel less nauseous and tired if you balance your protein distribution, making a special point to eat a protein-rich breakfast and a protein-oriented snack at bed time.

Dr. Brewer suggested that two eggs and one quart of cow's milk a day provide a healthy foundation for prenatal nutrition. I understand that a quart of milk per day could sound like a lot, but realistically it balances out to an 8oz glass with each meal and one more for a snack. It's also true that cow's milk isn't the only way to get that nutrition. The specific nutrition *you* are looking for in that glass of cow's milk, or it's alternative, will be helpful to consider. One cup of cow's milk (full fat, partial fat or skim) has 8 grams of protein and about 300mg of easily absorbable calcium, phosphorus, and many vitamins, including vitamin B12 and riboflavin (B2). One cup of raw spinach has about 29 milligrams of calcium and 1 gram of protein. Goats milk has 8.6 grams of protein per cup, and 327mg of calcium. One cup of Lentils has about 24 grams of protein and 38mg of calcium per cooked cup. Understanding what nutrients you want from a particular food can help you plan your diet. Yogurt, and especially Greek yogurt (which is higher in protein than other kinds of yogurt), are milk alternatives that may be more easily digestible than cow's milk. In addition to recommending dairy and eggs, the Brewer Diet includes two additional daily servings of protein from meat, fish, fowl, legumes, or from whole grains. The Brewer Diet also includes goals to reduce the amount of processed foods consumed and to avoid preservatives, other additives, artificial colorings, and any ingredients that you can't easily pronounce or wouldn't normally keep in your own kitchen.

As for eating two eggs a day, go for it if you can, or at least try to add in eggs if you are not currently eating many in your weekly diet. Eggs are a near perfect food. They contain all of the amnio acids (building blocks of proteins) that a person needs, and they are one of the best sources of choline, an essential nutrient many of us are deficient in. Eggs are also a good source of B vitamins, as well as the nutrients lutein and zeaxanthin, which are good for your eyes. "Eggs are among the most nutritious foods you can find, providing virtually all the vitamins and minerals you need."[24] Plus, eggs are a wise choice economically and they are also pretty easy to disguise in other foods if you are averse to their taste or texture. Some ways to disguise them are in French toast, stir fries, quiches, and baked goods where you can often add an extra egg or two without changing the texture too much. And if you enjoy or can tolerate eggs straight up, many of us enjoy a little salt on our hard-boiled eggs, which brings us to the topic of sodium.

Sodium is also an important nutritional element recommended by the Brewer Diet.[25] But if you eat a lot of processed and packaged foods, or rely on a lot of restaurant food, you are surely consuming too much sodium, which can be very trying for your system, so please work to reduce your consumption of restaurant and processed foods. If you are already eating a diet based on whole foods, then you should be encouraged to salt your food to taste. Did you ever hear the old wives' tale about pregnant women craving pickles? It comes from a pregnant person's need for salt. Many people have told me they crave olives, pickles, and other salty foods in their pregnancies. If you regularly steer clear of high sodium processed foods, then feel free to salt your food to taste. If you want to sprinkle some salt on your steamed broccoli, go for it. Good nutrition comes in a concert of various whole foods and flavors.

Prenatal vitamins

Prenatal vitamins can lend support to your diet. It's a bit like bringing your umbrella on a cloudy day: it probably won't rain because you are prepared for it, but you are prepared for it just in case it does. Rely on a well-balanced diet of whole foods, but think of the vitamin as your umbrella. Beware, not all vitamins are created equal! Research your options. If you have been given a prescription for a particular prenatal vitamin and it includes an iron supplement—most of them do—you may have trouble with constipation. If this is the case, please discuss with your provider the possibility of switching to a vitamin that does not include iron and then adding a product called Floradix®.[26] This is a plant-based iron supplement available in most health food stores that is more easily utilized by your body and is much less likely to cause constipation.

Vegetarian and vegan diets in pregnancy

The stakes of fetal development are as high as they come. All gestational parents will benefit from having blood work to check their iron and vitamin B12 levels. If you have been vegan prior to conception and/or you are maintaining a vegan diet now, it is especially helpful to check your status regarding these nutrients. Vegan diets are deficient in B12 unless the person is supplementing correctly, so if you have been vegan for some time prior to conception, you may have low B12 stores (and possibly low iron levels as well). Both too much or too little vitamin B12 can cause harm. It would be useful, therefore, to collaborate with a registered dietician or professional specifically trained in prenatal nutrition. As you will read later in this book, even many omnivores arrive at their pregnancy iron deficient. Supplementing correctly will be critical to your outcomes, not only for pregnancy but also throughout lactation. I do understand and respect that you've come to your diet choices from educated, heartfelt, and moral reasons. However, in my opinion, based on more than two decades of working with families as they chart their diets through pregnancy, I see much benefit to eating eggs and dairy during pregnancy and throughout lactation (and prior to conception when possible), Your goals for good health for childbearing are most simply met by including a variety of whole foods from a range of plant and animal sources.

Getting the supplementing correct, and having the information and motivation to really hit all your nutritional goals, takes a personalized plan that is grounded in solid prenatal and lactation information. While researching this book I have read many prenatal vegan resources and have found lots of nutrient-dense and yummy recipes. But rarely, if ever do they include exactly how much B12 should be supplemented or whether or not that should change as your nutritional needs vary over the course of pregnancy and while lactating. The Cleveland Clinic, for example, a well-respected medical center, has an article from 2020 that states that the recommended required amount of B12 needed per day in pregnancy is 2.6 micrograms (mcg).[27] In a paper updated in 2021, the National Institute of Health says that, for the first six months of lactation, the daily requirements for the lactating parent for vitamin B12 are 2.8 micrograms per day.[28] And in this doctor-reviewed Healthline article, the author states,

It's important to keep in mind that vitamin B12 is best absorbed in small doses. Thus, the less frequently you ingest vitamin B12, the more you need to take.

> This is why vegans who are unable to reach the recommended daily intake using fortified foods should opt for a daily supplement providing 25 – 100 mcg of cyanocobalamin [vitamin B12] or a weekly dosage of 2,000 mcg.[29]

With all this information in mind, I again come back to the need for an informed and personalized plan, based on your individual blood work. Caution in dosing is important, because again too much—not just too little—may also be harmful to the baby. A paper published by the National Institute of Health in 2017 stated that "another study in pregnant women showed that extremely high B12 levels due to vitamin supplements increased the risk of autism spectrum disorder in their offspring."[30]

I worry that most people don't have the resources (time, money, information, and energy) to sort out their own best supplementing choices and to really meet their individual nutritional needs. For vegans I also worry that too many won't get to a registered dietician with prenatal expertise or find ways to eat enough proteins, get the supplementing right, and get adequate calcium, which can be a challenge too. But, if you are willing or able to add eggs and dairy into your plant-based diet (preferably preconception), eating and supplementing gets a lot simpler. We can trust that the variety of whole foods will work in time-tested ways. I have seen many vegetarians, who eat dairy and eggs and are willing to track their diet, easily hit their nutritional goals and grow healthy babies. Through charting I have also seen some vegetarians realize that they weren't actually eating that many vegetables, particularly greens. I've seen some pregnant vegetarians also realize through diet charting that they weren't even getting to their pre-pregnant protein goals. Fruits and vegetables are a critical component of a healthy diet, but they are woefully low in protein. I have also collected a number of stories from vegetarians who, one day or night mid pregnancy, had undeniable cravings for meat. I applaud those who can listen in to what their bodies are communicating. I haven't always found that possible for myself, but I continue to listen in and try.

When cutting out animal proteins many people turn to soy (and often pretty large quantities of soy) as a replacement. While soy has some excellent nutrition, researchers have found that large quantities of soy can be problematic for various species of pregnant animal.[31] The research does not answer whether this could be true for human bodies as well, but it points to the fact that moderation is probably important. If you generally consume a lot of soy, please do your own research. To complicate the soy question even more, soy can be heavily laden with harmful pesticides, and so organic soy should be eaten when possible. Consequently, trying to sustain a higher protein pregnancy diet on a vegan diet, without too much soy, is a challenging process, and getting all of one's needed protein is not the only issue of concern. Vegan diets, as I mentioned, are deficient in vitamin B12. For example, at the beginning of *The Everything Vegan Pregnancy Book*, by Reed Mangels, PhD, RD, LD, FADA, the reader is told to take a B12 supplement every day.[32] Then soon after, on page five, the author suggests that if you are not getting enough from nutritionally fortified foods (processed foods that have additional nutrition added by the manufacturer), then you should take a B12 supplement. The author states that one should aim to take a supplement that covers 45% of your daily requirement. And again, I come away from my research thinking, *it's not a simple process to supplement adequately*. Eating an omnivorous diet based on a variety of whole foods is an easier way to get the needed nutrients.

B12 is critical to your baby's brain development. The following is from another National Institute of Health paper published on B12 supplementation during pregnancy and postpartum:

> Vitamin B_{12} is crucial for normal cell division and differentiation [during pregnancy] and necessary for the development and myelination of the central nervous system. Pregnant mothers in resource poor settings are at risk for poor vitamin B_{12} status. Poor vitamin B_{12} status in infancy is linked to poor growth and neurodevelopment. Brain development starts from conception, and pregnancy is a period of rapid growth and development for the brain.[33]

This NIH paper goes on to point out that a mother's B12 levels during pregnancy affect a baby's health and development during breastfeeding as well:

> During pregnancy, vitamin B_{12} is concentrated in the fetus and stored in the liver. Infants born to vitamin B_{12}-replete mothers have stores of vitamin B_{12} that are adequate to sustain them for the first several months postpartum. Consequently, vitamin B_{12} deficiency rarely occurs before the infant is about 4 months old if the mother has adequate vitamin B_{12} status during pregnancy. However, infants of vitamin B_{12}-deficient breastfeeding mothers are vulnerable to B_{12} deficiency from an early age.
>
> Maternal vitamin B_{12} deficiency has been associated with increased risk of common pregnancy complications, including spontaneous abortion, low birth weight, intrauterine growth re-

striction and neural tube defects. Children born to vitamin B_{12}-deficient women are at increased risk for adverse health outcomes, including developmental abnormalities and anemia.[34]

The US Center for Disease Control (CDC) points out that babies should get B12 from their mother's breastmilk:

> Vitamin B12 is transferred through the placenta to the fetus during pregnancy and through breast milk after birth. Infants who drink breast milk from a mother who consumes adequate amounts of vitamin B12 or infants who drink infant formula, will receive enough vitamin B12. However, if a breastfeeding mother is deficient in vitamin B12, her infant may also become deficient.
>
> Vitamin B12 is most commonly found in foods from animals; therefore, infants who only receive breast milk from mothers who consume no animal products are at greater risk for developing vitamin B12 deficiency shortly after birth.[35]

Given the import of such research, vegan parents should therefore investigate supplementation with B12 prior to conception, during pregnancy, and during lactation. Again, I make the plea, if you are vegan, work with a registered dietician who is familiar with vegan diets and has training in prenatal nutrition.

Appetite and nausea

In pregnancy, appetite can fluctuate wildly, affected by fetal growth, nausea, the position of the baby in relation to your stomach, the high levels of hormones circulating in your and the baby's bloodstream, and constipation. If the baby is applying a lot of physical pressure on your stomach or intestines, even though you may feel hungry, you may be quite uncomfortable after a few bites of food. If that is happening to you, then grazing (eating small amounts steadily throughout the day) will likely be more pleasurable than trying to eat three big meals. Some days you may just be insatiably hungry all day long, perhaps because your fetus is going through a growth spurt, or maybe she has shifted her position away from your stomach.

The causes of nausea during pregnancy are varied and not always easily understood. Nausea is sometimes worsened when a pregnant person is hungry and/or tired. In both my pregnancies I experienced a strange counter-intuitive experience with hunger and nausea. Sometimes when I was nauseous my gut would say, "don't eat or you'll puke"; meanwhile, my brain would respond with, "you haven't had any food for several hours." It was not a thrilling confusion to sort through, but when I allowed my brain to guide me, and I got some food into my belly, I usually felt much better. In fact, most bouts of nausea I experienced were calmed with a protein-rich snack, a nap, or combination of the two. Some pregnant people find solace from ginger, which they ingest by eating it in prepared foods, drinking it in the form of tea, or sucking on some ginger candies.[36] (Be sure to talk to your provider before taking any supplements or drinking herbal teas.) Perhaps surprisingly, people can also be made nauseous from their prenatal vitamins. And for some pregnant people, their unsettled pregnancy stomach can be directly related to their emotional uncertainty—i.e., fears of becoming a parent.

There may not be anything emotionally making you sick; it may be the hormones, or a digestive issue, or something unknown. Don't blame yourself. But do check in to explore what you are feeling. Be sure, too, to talk to your care providers about your nausea. If you are vomiting a lot, staying well hydrated and nourished will be a challenge. If you are unable to stay well hydrated and nourished, seek care. Engage your provider; optimum care will take teamwork.

How are you feeling about this pregnancy in your life right now? Is anything making you sick with fear or worry?

Sweets and treats

Over the years I have fielded many questions from pregnant people feeling burdened by their cravings for sweets and treats. If you make a commitment to eat great food, and you are meeting your nutritional requirements, and you still have some room in your belly, you can certainly consider having the occasional treat. But consider the nutritional value of your treat and try to avoid completely empty calories. Sugar and white flour can really be constipating, as well as cause huge fluctuations in blood sugar levels. Research suggests that it might be best to eat all starchy or sugary carbohydrates only after eating protein to achieve more even blood sugar levels.[37]

You can make great treat choices. Carrot cake, a slice of pumpkin pie, some cheesecake, or a fruit tart can pack a wallop of nutrition in addition to the added sugars and extra calories you will get. Any of those would be a better choice than say, a bag of Skittles, which has no real nutrient value and is laden with artificial colorings that have been shown to cause cancer in rats and negatively impact genetic material.[38] If you do indulge in nutritionally less-than-optimal treats, try to keep it to special occasions and try to eat them with or right after a good protein source. And always drink plenty of water.

Pregnancy is a time of great change. Your whole life, your body, all of your relationships, everything is changing and that has all kinds of repercussions when it comes to your mood. I don't believe that pregnancy is a good time to impose a harsh sense of self-deprivation. I personally would never suggest denying yourself an occasional serving of chocolate. Just try to remember to consider the nutrition of your treat. Dark chocolate is a better nutritional choice, for example, than other types of chocolate. One of my yoga teachers recently suggested an interesting approach for guidance in making food choices. She suggested that before you eat something, ask yourself if you are truly comfortable with this food choice becoming part of your (and your baby's) body. I encourage you to give it a try the next time you are selecting something to eat.

Building an adequate blood supply

A full-term, well-fed pregnant person can have as much as 50% more blood volume than they did at the start of the pregnancy.[39] Developing this extra blood supply is crucial for the good health of both gestational parent and baby. When a parent births their placenta, that amazing organ they have built to nourish their baby, there will be blood loss. This is by design. And when you have had a healthy diet based on whole foods with adequate protein, iron, and water, you will be able to build enough extra blood to recover smoothly from this loss. Likewise, the baby's safety is best supported when she has plenty of her own blood. The force of labor contractions on the baby will temporarily decrease the supply of red blood cells (which carry oxygen throughout the body) to the baby. This, in turn, will temporarily decrease the baby's oxygenation levels. A fetus that is nurtured by a gestational parent with adequate nutrition will have an excellent blood supply to carry plenty of oxygen. In the absence of adequate nutrition, therefore, both parent and baby are more susceptible to complication.

Malnutrition: Eclampsia, HELLP

Preeclampsia, as I mentioned earlier, is a serious pregnancy complication, with at least two medical names: Preeclampsia (and, once it has progressed, Eclampsia) and Pregnancy-Induced-Hypertension. These are both used to describe the same dangerous health complication for a pregnant person. Scientists and doctors don't fully understand or yet agree on what causes preeclampsia.[40] They can, however, now pinpoint the problem beginning, at least in part, with the placenta and its formation and growth into the uterine lining. The preeclamptic placenta doesn't alter the maternal blood vessels as it should. Instead of the placenta remodeling the maternal vessels into large vessels, as happens in a healthy pregnancy, the maternal blood vessels during preeclampsia remain small, thus causing the needs of the growing fetus to eventually effect an increase in maternal blood pressure. Preeclampsia usually presents symptomatically toward the end of a pregnancy and effects 3 – 5% of all pregnancies.[41]

The late Dr. Brewer believed that preeclampsia is a disease of malnutrition. By counseling pregnant people, at the county clinic he managed, to follow the Brewer Diet, Dr. Brewer achieved great success, reducing the incidence of preeclampsia to .05%. —and, as I mentioned above, with zero cases of severe eclampsia.[42] Dr. Brewer's work, however, was never seriously considered within the obstetrical community. Empirical research standards demand that a control group of pregnant persons without adequate nutrition be studied alongside those with adequate nutrition. Due to what he saw as the unethical realities of denying adequate nutrition to those who are pregnant, Dr. Brewer never endeavored to substantiate his research in this required way. Consequently, his work was never embraced by the medical community. Additionally, medical doctors are (still) not trained to appreciate the relationship between food and health and food and disease. From a review of literature published in the *Lancet* in 2019:

> 66 studies were identified by the search and 24 were eligible for full-text analysis. 16 quantitative studies, three qualitative studies, and five curriculum initiatives from the USA (n=11), Europe (n=4), the Middle East (n=1), Africa (n=1), and Australasia (n=7) met the inclusion criteria. Our analysis of these studies showed that nutrition is insufficiently incorporated into medical education, regardless of country, setting, or year of medical education. Deficits in nutrition education affect students' knowledge, skills, and confidence to implement nutrition care into patient care. A modest positive effect was reported from curriculum initiatives.[43]

In recent years, nutritional education does appear to be creeping into medical school training. This is good news. Let's hope the trend to improve medical education in this way continues. In the meantime, ask any farmer who raises animals how to breed the healthiest animals and they will tell you that it's nutrition, nutrition, nutrition. Some more good news is that by learning to eat a sound pregnancy diet and becoming aware of preeclampsia and its seriousness, you are being proactively protective.

The symptoms of preeclampsia include high blood pressure, protein in the urine, and remarkable swelling. Symptoms can also include dizziness, blurred vision, and searing upper abdominal pain. As the condition worsens, a serious disease state, medically termed HELLP Syndrome, can develop. "H" is for hemolysis, the destruction of the red blood cells. "E-L" is for elevated liver enzymes. And "L-P" is for low platelets. In HELLP Syndrome (also known to be called "Eclampsia") a pregnant person's body can either go into organ failure or seizure and coma. Clearly, neither scenario is good for the gestational parent or the baby. If preeclampsia is progressing, the only way to help is to get the baby and placenta out. A pregnant person must end the pregnancy through induction or cesarean section. Luckily this is generally a disease state that comes late in a pregnancy, so prematurity concerns are real but less pressing. If the pregnant person is not near their due date, doctors will try to slow their body processes down with bed rest and medications that lower blood pressure, such as the commonly prescribed magnesium sulfate.[44]

Tricking a person's body into early labor through induction interventions is difficult. It can work, but if the disease state is progressing too rapidly, the pregnancy must end in surgery. Platelets are the factor in your blood that helps your blood to clot. When preeclampsia is progressing, one's platelet count begins to fall. If a gestational parent's platelet count gets too low for them to clot their own blood, then the necessary emergency cesarean section becomes impossibly dangerous; yet it remains the only option. If left untreated, preeclampsia can lead to death.[45] Preeclampsia is the primary reason doctors and midwives check your blood pressure and ask you to pee in a cup at each of your prenatal appointments. (Note that checking urine is a protocol that continues to evolve. Your provider may no longer ask for that test, finding that blood pressure alone is sufficient. Yet many providers do still order urine tests. Maintaining open communication with your provider about their decisions is key.)

I have heard some obstetricians say that there may be a hereditary link to getting preeclampsia. But when considering a possible hereditary link, I think it is interesting to consider the fact that eating habits are passed on within families.[46] Following the logic in Dr. Brewer's approach, linking nutrition and pregnancy, maybe it's the shared eating habits that cause this pregnancy complication to get "passed on." While genetics will always play a part in the illnesses to which we are susceptible, eating the healthiest diet possible can also go a long way to alleviate emotional and physical stress on the pregnant body and mind.

Protein boosters

I have often been asked to offer my opinion on commercially available protein shakes (as opposed to protein shakes made at home with healthy, whole foods) as a quick fix. My answer is this: First work hard to get your nutrition from whole foods. If you feel you need an occasional supplement to your whole foods diet, consider your options carefully. Read product labels carefully; it is the only way to decide if a product is an acceptable one for you.

Greek yogurt; cottage cheese; whole grain bread with a glass of milk; brown rice with beans; high protein grains, such as quinoa, spelt and oats; whole grain pastas; and nuts and seeds, such as almonds and pumpkin seeds, are all whole food options for boosting your protein intake. If you do any baking, then you can usually adapt a recipe to include an extra egg or two, or some extra powdered milk, wheat germ, or flax meal to give your recipe a boost in protein without a noticeable change in taste. Nuts and seeds have a lot of healthy fats in them in addition to their protein. One of my new favorite foods is sunflower seed butter: it's delicious and has about equal protein to that found in peanut butter. (As with all value-added foods, be sure to read labels because some have added sugars, which you want to avoid or ingest only in small quantities.)

When it comes to eating your greens, romaine lettuce, spinach, broccoli, Swiss chard, kale, collard greens, mustard greens, and arugula are some of my favorites. When selecting fruits and other vegetables, I like to go for an array of colors. And to optimize my diet I like to consume a shifting variety of cooked and raw vegetables. I enjoy carrots and red cabbage (raw or cooked) grated up together with almost any kind of dressing—and almost entirely for their beautiful colors alone!

As I mentioned above, French toast, quiches, omelets, and stir-fries are all ways to make eggs more interesting—or palatable, if that's an issue. Try eating some of last night's dinner for breakfast or try breakfast for dinner. Have fun and think outside the box as you work to find your best nourishment. I encourage you to share recipes and food suggestions with other pregnant people when and where you can, like in a birth class.

Many pregnant people I have worked with report feeling better after they start to follow the Brewer Diet. They find they have more energy and more peace-of-mind when they take responsibility for their food choices. One of my clients responded with this when I asked for submissions for this book: "The pre-natal nutrition [information in my class] allowed me to have a healthy, low-risk pregnancy in support of a natural childbirth. Even though I tested positive for gestational diabetes, I was able, through diet, to control this and carry my baby to term without being induced."

Another graduate who offered up a testimonial for this book wrote that, "the prenatal nutrition portion of the Bradley® class was very helpful. It opened my eyes to the importance of eating well during and after the pregnancy. My husband jumped on board with me in this as well and provided constant support in ensuring I ate well."

Many pregnant people share that prior to doing the diet chart homework, they harbored deeply hidden concerns about whether or not they were eating well. Another Bradley® class graduate of mine, Robin, wrote that "tracking the amount of protein that we ate during a single week of the class was eye-opening: it showed me that I was getting plenty of protein, and that I actually had a very well-balanced diet. I could stop obsessing over whether or not my eating habits were up to par!"

How wonderful it is when we can allay fears with empirical evidence. It is equally excellent when the pregnant person can pinpoint specific areas for improvement. Tracking your diet is a win-win situation. Consider, too, that you and your baby are in competition for some nutrients, and some of these nutrients the baby takes in a bit easier and some you take in easier.[47] Working conscientiously, therefore, to eat enough of the right foods, helps to ensure that neither of you go without. Take responsibility for what you (and your baby) eat. It is one of the best ways to combat the concerns that so often creep up about the health of our growing babies. Being proactive can help to calm fears. If you feel a fear arise, take a deep breath, slow down your exhale and then plan for your next meal(s) with something that is chock full of great nutrition. And go for tasty too! The act of planning your meals may require you to develop new skills. Do the hard development work now and it will help you feel more assured about your body and baby. Planning your meals now will also help you to get a head-start on important parenting skills. It won't be long before you will have a toddler who will need to have healthy food at regular intervals. Remember that pregnancy is full of hidden parenting lessons; planning for your food is one of them.

Maybe you would enjoy spinach pie made with fresh spinach and feta or a burrito with brown rice, beans, and dark greens with a dollop of sour cream and salsa on top. Indulging in a special treat? How about a piece of homemade carrot cake and a glass of cold milk for dessert? Yum! Those are clearly some of my favorites. And remember: if you make the cake yourself, you can add an extra egg and some extra powdered milk to increase your protein intake. You can also reduce some of the refined sugar or replace it with dried coconut nectar, honey, applesauce, or real maple syrup (but always read labels and look to make sure there are no extra sugars or colorings added to your substitutions). And I usually use some or all whole wheat flour in desserts, instead of white (bleached) flour, and my family is none the wiser—shhh! I have also had success reducing my white flour intake by substituting all or some white flour with ground flax meal, wheat germ, ground walnuts, or a combination of these alternatives. I experiment with recipes all the time. Get creative! Nurturing your body and your efforts will be plenty good enough. You can then be comforted by knowing that you are doing what you can to give your baby the best chance possible for being healthy, strong, and full of love.

Please realize that once your baby is born, finding the time to take care of *you* will be a bigger challenge than it is right now. No matter what your pregnancy challenges are, it is generally easier to parent while the baby is still inside. So, use this time now to start to address and improve your nutritional habits. If there are any less-than-ideal food choices or patterns you're working with, they no longer really matter. Forgive yourself and move on. What matters now is what choice you make next. Each time you eat something is an opportunity to make a good or better choice. If you live somewhere where getting access to fresh produce is a challenge, consider that frozen vegetables are frequently more nutritious than canned (with less sodium), but eating canned vegetables (which you can rinse in cold water before consuming to remove some of the added sodium) is better than going without any vegetables at all.

Plan your menu with intention

Our bodies and our minds are one. Alongside the nutritional elements needed for a healthy pregnancy, birth, and postpartum, a diet rich in love, forgiveness, positive attitudes, good hard work, honesty, acceptance, and reciprocity strengthens our mind, which in turn helps to strengthen our body. Combining wellness practices for mind and body creates a nutritious feedback loop for you and the baby. Relaxation is a primary tool in this loop.

Relaxation/mindfulness/meditation/breath awareness

When we develop our skills for relaxation and then use them in birth, our bodies work more efficiently. Fear and excess physical tension deplete precious resources. In labor, when you relax your mind and all the muscles that don't have to work, such as around your jaw, shoulders, hands, butt, thighs, knees, and toes, you free up more resources, such as oxygen and nutrition, for your uterus to use.

From my own experience in labor, I learned that "letting go" and using relaxation really helped to make the labor sensations manageable. I believe this also helped my homebirth progress as smoothly and quickly as it did. When you use focused relaxation as a birth tool your body can do the hard work more efficiently. More efficiency means with less pain and in less time. A good goal, right? So I encourage you to believe it's possible for you.

Optimally strong and powerfully effective contractions might really hurt, but this is good pain because they are working so well. I found that a lot of the work in my two births was to try to not be afraid of the sensations. The act of letting my belly relax into what was happening took a lot of courage: it was challenging to release muscle tension while it hurt, but when I did, I was well rewarded.

What does it mean to you to use relaxation and mindfulness techniques for pain relief?

Do you believe relaxation/mindfulness can be an effective labor tool?

The concept of relaxation can mean different things to different people at different times. You come home from work, kick your shoes off, and sit back with a beverage and say, "Ahhhh...". That is certainly one definition of relaxation. Or maybe you love to whoop it up at a party and you go out hooting and hollering. This is another type of relaxation. But the type of relaxation I am referring to, and the type that the Bradley Method® puts forth, is different still. The type of relaxation that can best aid in labor is very mentally active and clear in focus. It helps to integrate a deep physical and mental connection: body awareness. This focus requires muscular awareness and relaxation in conjunction with a calm and focused mental state. In the Bradley Method® we use the word "Relaxation" to describe what some call Meditation or Mindfulness. These same relaxation/meditation/mindfulness principles also apply to the discipline of hypnosis.

Because we form our thoughts with our words, I want to take a moment and look at the dictionary definitions for "relaxation" and "meditation." Then you can examine how these words might connect to your birth preparation.

re'lax'a'tion (noun)
1. Enjoyable activity
    A form of activity that provides a change and relief from effort, work, or tension, and gives pleasure
2. Loosening process
    The process of becoming or making something less firm, rigid, or tight
3. Lessening of severity

Med'i'ta'tion (noun)
1. Emptying or concentration of mind
    The emptying of the mind of thoughts, or the concentration of the mind on one thing, in order to aid mental or spiritual development, contemplation, or *relaxation* [emphasis mine]
2. Pondering of something
    The act of thinking about something carefully, calmly, seriously, and for some time, or an instance of such thinking
3. Serious study of topic
    An extended and serious study of topic

Explore your thoughts about the possible connections between meditation and relaxation and birth. How can this inform your birth preparation?

List some of your ideas about using relaxation and meditation for pain relief. If you have any concerns that relaxation and meditation won't be able to help during birth, list those concerns, too. (Use extra paper or work in the margins if needed!)

I have found through my yoga practice that meditation and deep relaxation help me to create the emotional space I need to find my power to cope with the world around me. Meditation helps me to process my stress, which for me means to really *feel* it! This helps me to recognize and acknowledge that my stress often occurs because I am fearful of the future or second guessing or holding onto the past. But once I can become present, I can better observe my feelings and then more easily release what I don't need or can't control. This restores my emotional reserves. When I slow down, deepen, and feel my breath, I can figuratively and literally catch my breath. In a 2012 research paper by Robert Schneider et al., called "Stress Reduction in the Secondary Prevention of Cardiovascular Disease," the authors write:

> There are instantaneous benefits that come from even a few brief moments of conscientious breath awareness, such as a calming of nerves, conserving energy, and lowering blood pressure. When you practice over time you will maximize these benefits and develop useful skills for pain management.[48]

Practice builds reliable skills. When you are busy with the work of observing your breath, with a singular attention, you are also simultaneously busy *not* focusing on your stress or its causes. Your nervous system's attention is being "used up" or "anchored" by your focus on relaxation and your breath. Our focus fills up our attention and then we don't have room for stressful thoughts. In the nervous system, information gets transmitted by signals that jump across the gaps between nerve cells. We create pathways of signal transmission through practice. When we learn new things we create new nervous system pathways. By practicing meditation, you can create neurological pathways that will lead you to deep levels of relaxation. The nervous system is very plastic. We adjust and shift pathways of nervous system connections all the time. And nerve pathways develop over time. Therefore, the more you practice, the better you will get.[49]

In Hinduism and Buddhism, two religions that practice meditation, practitioners often use a mantra, which is a holy word or phrase to focus on during the practice. This acts as an anchor to help keep your thoughts from drifting. The Buddhist monk Thich Nhat Hanh offers many beautiful meditations in his book, *Happiness: Essential Mindfulness Practices.*[50] He says that if we are observing this basic function, our breath, we are not thinking. Turning off our thoughts, if you will, helps us avoid worries about the future or the past and helps us settle into the present mindful moment. In what follows, I will share one of his mindfulness phrases, or breath meditations, that you can try. But first, I want you to get really comfortable. (Do you need a pee break or to grab a blanket?)

The side relaxation position

Coping with the sensations of labor through the use of focused relaxation is a primary principle of the Bradley Method®, as well as most schools of thought on natural childbirth. The side relaxation position was designed for maximum comfort and relaxation potential. Many people find that it's not only great for relaxation practice, but it can also be a very comfortable position for sleep. If you are working with a partner, please make sure that each of you take ample time to explore the side relaxation position.

Lie on your side with a pillow under your head, then adjust the pillow height so that your head remains in good spinal alignment. Place another pillow between your knees, and another pillow supporting your foot, so that no part of you is dangling down. Try staggering the top leg either front or back so that it is not directly on top of your bottom leg. The major limbs should be in a mid-range of flexion. Your bottom arm can be in front of you, or behind you, which brings you a bit further over on your chest and belly. Some pregnant people also like a pillow under their belly and to support the top arm.

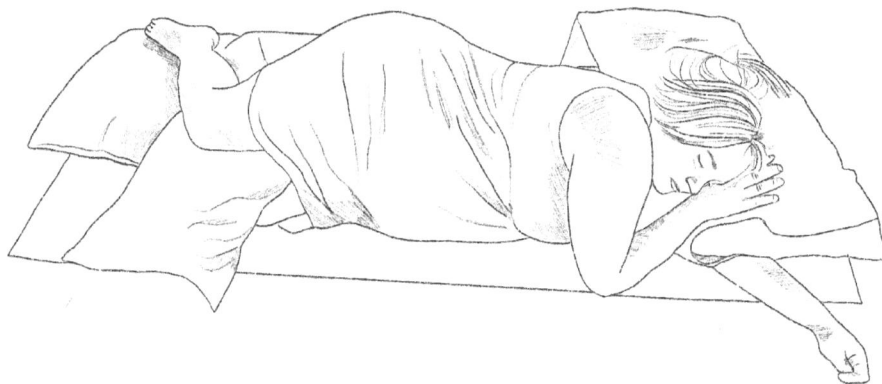

EXERCISE: BREATHING WITH A MINDFULNESS PHRASE IN THE SIDE RELAXATION POSITION

First, familiarize yourself with the following exercise and then get into the side relaxation position. Second, set a timer, starting small at maybe one or two minutes. (Over time you can build up your practice, and maybe 10 – 15 minutes will begin to feel short!)

Try to slow down and sync up your silent words with your breathing action.

As you breathe in think, "I am breathing in."

As you breathe out think, "I am breathing out."

With your timer set, or by giving yourself an approximate time allotment, begin to practice: "I am breathing in" fills your inhale and "I am breathing out" fills your exhale.

Close your eyes and repeat these mindfulness phrases until your timer goes off: "I am breathing in, I am breathing out."[51]

Breath awareness: A partner's tool for birth and a skill to develop for happy couple life

Breath meditation practiced together can emotionally connect the two people practicing. While listening to your partner's breath you can connect deeply to their mind and body. The benefits of breath awareness will develop in proportion to the amount of time you both dedicate to practice. If you are to become experts in observing and listening to each other's breathing patterns (which I recommend as a goal), it can help develop your intimacy and emotional connectivity. It will take a willingness to commit to the time together. This need not be a cumbersome commitment. It can be an easy, yet powerful way to spend a few moments together each day. Try once in the morning before you get out of bed and once in the evening just before sleep. The work will likely be soothing to both of you, and it will help you to deepen your connection through non-verbal communication. Relationships can be strengthened on deep visceral, instinctual, and intimate levels. What you are feeling and how you are coping are conveyed through your breath patterns and sounds. You are, at your core of humanness, your breathing patterns. In other words, what you feel emotionally, your thoughts, and how you feel in your body are expressed by—and responsive to—your breath patterns. In labor, when you the partner can tune into your laboring person's breath rhythms, it can help you assess how they are coping. This clue helps to create a pathway for lending useful support. When you tune into a person's breath pattern during birth, you remove (or at least reduce) the need for words. If the birthing person is starting to get tense, you will notice the change in their breathing. If they are breathing deeply and fully, you will know they are coping well.

As the intensity of the birth process builds, so does the rate of respirations. Fast, hard breathing is normal for very active labor. How hard do you breathe when you are running? Remember, we don't call this *labor* for nothing! Labor is usually butt-kicking hard work. If you have practiced listening to your birthing partner's breathing, you will know if they are breathing hard from hard work, or from panic, or if their breath is stilted from fear and gripping, or if they are focused and present and coping well; you will be able to improve the quality of support you can give them by how you respond to their breathing cues.

There is comfort to be gained through breath connection with a partner. Each person can settle themselves and that can improve communication. You, birthing partner, will be able to support them in their own release with the genuine support that comes from active listening. The birth partner also physically benefits from tuning into their own breath patterns as they work to notice their partner's. When each partner tunes into their own breath this helps to create a positive feedback system. When the partner calms down, it calms the person giving birth. When the person giving birth calms down, it further calms their birth partner, and so on. If a person in labor, for example, starts to get tense, their well-practiced and connected partner will generally be the first one in the room to notice. Likewise, if the partner gets tense, their breath will get tense and stilted and the laboring person will be receptive to that, too. Supporting a person in labor includes paying attention to your own (in addition to your partner's) stress levels. By focusing on breath—becoming mindful to the moment—you can observe your feelings, reactions, and instincts. These observations will generally help you to remain present with what is happening and aid you to make your best choices for your birth support tactics.

What you are thinking impacts how your body feels and functions. Emotional stress causes you to release powerful stress hormones that change your physiology. When you are tense in your mind, you tighten your muscles too. Love and happiness have different chemistry, and therefore a different body language with different muscle tone than fear and angst. This is true for the birthing person and partner alike.

Of course, this is all circular: your body's functioning impacts what you are feeling and thinking, and what you are feeling and thinking impacts your body's functioning. Which came first? To work towards optimal body function, for each of you, where should we focus our attention first, the mind or the body? The answer is: it doesn't matter. Start where you can. In a circle you will get where you need to be as long as you start somewhere. Our life is made up of many circular systems and the mind-body connection in labor is a beautiful example. The more we understand about what is causing the sensations of labor—what the work is—the less afraid we are. The less afraid we are, the more we can relax. The more we can relax and accept what is happening, the better the labor process works. And the better the labor process works, the more we can relax. Then the more we can relax, the more we can feel what our work is. Thus, the more we learn about birth and relaxation the better it all goes!

The mind-body connection

In our culture we know there is a mind-body connection for male bodies, and we apparently don't need science to prove it to us. Ina May Gaskin, renowned midwife and author, points out: "We accept the mind-body connection for men all the time. We know that the right thought can give a man an erection and the wrong thought can take it away."[52] Gaskin is correct. For male bodies we absolutely accept this. We understand it, experience it. We *know* it to be true. But when there is talk about a mind-body connection impacting a female body process, we tend not to accept that as real. We hear: "Hmm I don't know. Can this be proven? Is there science behind this? What does it matter what a woman thinks, the professional must manage this physical experience for her." How a female body *feels* is not necessarily seen or considered as a determining factor.

But there is a mind-body connection for all bodies. And how someone is feeling impacts how their birth process will work. Can you have an orgasm if your mind is not willing to let loose and follow along? Can you move your bowels if you expect someone to come bursting in through the bathroom door? The right thought can help to open you up to let your baby out, or to close you up to keep your baby in. Gaskin points out that our sphincters are shy and that the cervix could be understood like a sphincter muscle. **What you are thinking and what you are feeling will therefore impact your birth.** As I have mentioned (and Gaskin and others have written extensively on the subject), stress hormones have a powerful chemical effect on how your contractions work. If you were in a jungle in labor and suddenly a big hungry tiger appeared to eat you, you would need to suspend your birth process to get away to safety.[53] Stress hormones are behind this type of response.

What causes *you* to secrete stress hormones? Can you trust your body? Are you ok with yourself? Do you trust your doctor or midwife? What about your nurse, doula, friend, or relative who is planning to be in the room with you? Are you comfortable with your partner? Is there anyone planning to be at your birth that you don't feel comfortable being naked in front of? Are you comfortable with your location?

All of this is going to impact how your body works in labor. In labor, if you are embarrassed or overly tense or fighting, even fighting with yourself, you will likely have a more difficult and complicated labor. Of course, healthy birth is stress inducing (omg an actual baby is coming!) and not all stress is bad (omg an actual baby is coming!). Some stress can give us extra energy to complete huge tasks. Did you ever rage-clean the kitchen? I have and it's amazing to channel all that energy into something productive. But when the feelings take over, and we lose the ability to channel the surges of emotion, we complicate our process. Staying on top of or present with the feelings enough to work with them is the goal. A good birth strategy is to try and sort through your feelings and work out your arrangements and best plans *now, before labor*, so that when the time comes you can labor in peace, with meaningful support in an environment where you feel safe.

We humans really are one mind-body unit. We all have concerns, fears, inhibitions, and other emotional challenges. Allowing fears and concerns to surface—to feel them, sort through them and acknowledge their existence—is how you will start to work through them. Only then can you begin to make realistic plans for the future. A dark house is scarier before you turn on the lights. By expressing your concerns, you can shine a light into the dark corners of your heart and mind. In pregnancy, fears can grow like weeds. And where you don't grow your own fears, it seems that lurking down every supermarket isle is someone willing to scatter the seeds of their fears into your pregnant garden.

To truly know yourself, start by sorting through the chatter of your mind. This is the path to growth and emotional health and observation. Please do not feel obligated to have answers for each of your concerns—just keep exploring and expressing your feelings. Say them out loud and write them down. Think of it as diet charting for your psyche. Your issues will probably change and develop as the pregnancy progresses. Try to keep welcoming this work. Look for opportunities to reciprocate support amongst your friends and family. If someone listens to you, make the time and commitment to listen to them. Support your people and allow them to support you.

Preparing to birth and parent is an ongoing process. It takes time to grow. Using this book to write in and/or keeping another journal will help you to get to know what is in your heart. Knowing your heart can help you to learn to trust your instincts. Trusting your instincts is a critical component of birth safety, and an essential component of parenting. Furthermore, deciding to set goals and then having a place to write them down, such as below, can really help you to achieve success.

Thank you for your time this week. Please read your homework assignments below. I wish you another wonderful week to follow!

HOMEWORK

A) Nutrition

This week, try to make food choices that are responsive to what you learned from last week's diet charting. If last week you did not write down what you ate with a tally of the protein grams, please try to do it this week. If you did chart last week, you are welcome to chart again, but perhaps the lessons have been learned for the time being. If you are done with charting now, consider doing it again later in your pregnancy. The fetal brain goes through extreme development and growth right through to the end of the last trimester and beyond. Some pregnant people feel too huge and don't want to eat any more as they feel they have grown out of room, but clearly while all that baby brain development is going on, food choices still matter.

B) Conscientious breathing

Continue this week to build a daily practice routine for conscientious breathing. Please practice once in the morning, once in the evening, and at least once a day and with your partner, if possible. Be sure to practice relaxation in the side relaxation position to achieve maximum states of relaxation.

C) Sleep observations

Look for an opportunity to observe each other sleeping. When one of you falls asleep first or you get up before your partner, take a few moments and really observe them sleeping. What does their breath sound like? How does their belly move? What are their facial expressions when their muscles are completely relaxed in sleep? What do their bodies look like? What position are they in? When we sleep we are really relaxed. When we see what that looks like, we can better notice when someone is not relaxed. Being asleep is the gold standard of relaxed abdominal breathing.

THIS SPACE IS FOR YOUR NOTES AND DRAWINGS

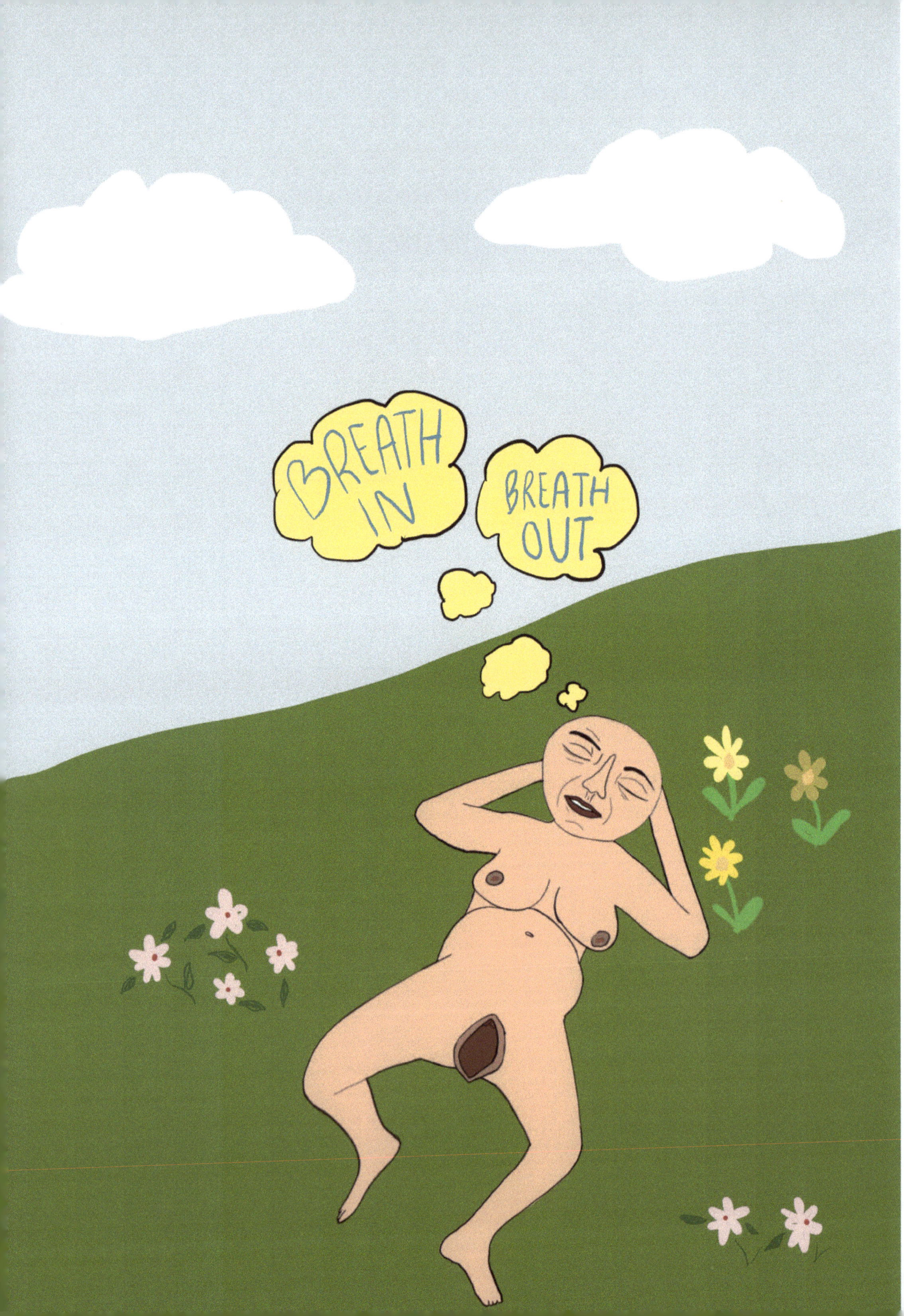
BREATH IN
BREATH OUT

WEEK 3

Chapter contents:

O *Prenatal general fitness*

O *Prenatal specific exercises*

THIS SPACE IS FOR YOUR NOTES AND DRAWINGS

Hello again, and welcome to Week 3! How did you do with eating this past week? If there were changes that you wanted to make from your first week of diet charting, were you able to implement them this week? Did you notice any difference in feeling or energy level this week? If you did not make the changes you wanted to... take a breath, notice and then release any feelings of guilt with your exhale... then ask yourself, why not? What were the challenges? What are your food goals for this coming week and how will you achieve them? Think, too, about how can you continue to release feelings of guilt. I know—and you know—that you are trying and that you care. This is what parenting is all about. My asking these questions here and throughout the book are meant to be a support, to offer myself as an accountability buddy. So please use the space below to write or draw your responses. Take some time to reflect on your thoughts and feelings.

Did you practice some form of focused relaxation/breath observation? What are you experiencing from this work? Are you taking turns at leading and following? If not, try to add that in this week.

Have you had a chance to observe your partner sleep? If you did, what did you notice? (If you didn't, there is always this week to try again!)

Cardiovascular fitness

Having good cardiovascular fitness means that your heart can pump more blood to the various parts of your body during sustained periods of physical exertion. Increasing your blood flow increases oxygenation throughout your body, which is necessary for building stamina (the ability to endure hard work over lengths of time). The more we challenge our hearts' ability to pump blood and deliver oxygen, by raising our heart rate, the stronger our hearts (and other muscles) can get, the better we can feel, and the longer we can work hard. A strong heart is a key component of good health. This is as true during pregnancy as it was before (and will be afterwards, too). Your birth is going to be grueling hard work, requiring both strength and stamina. And you can prepare yourself for birth (and parenthood) by approaching your preparation with an athlete's mindset.[54] Your work to this end is to cultivate cardiovascular fitness. If you have never before considered yourself an athlete, give it a try. If you must, fake it 'til you make it. Aside from the exceptional few, most athletes get to where they are through practice practice practice—and a healthy mindset. So practice good health habits and tell yourself over and over that you will be able to do this work; as tough as this work may be, you've got what it takes! Back up your words with actions: eat nutritious food, get enough sleep, and keep trying to increase or sustain an active lifestyle. Not only will you be helping yourself for birth and beyond, you will likely feel better overall, too.

Generally, any form of exercise you were doing prior to the pregnancy is safe to continue.[55] If you had not been exercising prior to the pregnancy, or you stopped because of the pregnancy, consider starting gently with activities you enjoy. Good health comes from having good fun. If you are able to, try walking. Our species evolved to do it, and it's free! I have even heard midwives say the longer one walks the shorter is one's birth! Maybe swimming is more fun for you, so check to see if there is a local pool you can access, like a public high school or YMCA. Specifically designed prenatal exercise classes and stationary bike riding are additional ways to improve your fitness. And one of my favorite ways to exercise: dancing around the house to some great music! I like to combine exercise and creativity through dance. I also like to dance while house cleaning. What's your sweet spot for being active? There are countless ways to have fun and build strength, stamina, and courage as you realize your healthy goals. Listen to your own instincts and decide what's best for you given your location and circumstances.

If you already consider yourself an athlete, beware: there may be some work to do to remind yourself that you are not actually training for an athletic competition. Instead, you are building a human being. You will want to be mindful of and probably need to replace calories being lost through strenuous exercise. You may need to make (sometimes tough) adjustments to reduce the amount and force of your workouts, and to allow yourself to gain weight and increase your rest times.

Physical activities that you enjoy can provide a great opportunity to practice listening to and then reacting to your feelings about exertion. For example, when I go outside for a run, I inevitably get to a point where I think I can't go any farther. At that point, I try to check in with myself to evaluate my resistance: Do my knees hurt? Is my breathing strained? Does *anything* seem wrong? Is it an energy issue? A mental challenge I can't overcome? Some days the answer is no to all of these questions, and then I think, "Okay, then maybe I don't really have to quit, maybe I can push through and actually continue." Other days I realize that I should have gotten more sleep, or not started out so fast, or that something does hurt in a bad way. If I allow myself the respect and compassion I deserve, I realize that the better health choice is to slow down and walk or just go home to rest or even call a friend for a ride.

When faced with your own resistance, whether it is resistance to doing more or to doing less, ask yourself why this is so hard, and then take time to listen to your gut (your heart, your vagina, your intuition); you just might hear something important. If you do listen (and you respond respectfully and with empathy), then there is a good chance you will be rewarded with guidance, improved energy, and increased confidence. Learning to assess the situation and then allowing your priorities to shift in response is another hidden parenting skill embedded in the work of pregnancy. Our energy ebbs and flows. What kind of day is today? What are my priorities?

There are some contraindications to exercise for those who are pregnant. Research published in the *Journal of Perinatal Education* shares the following contraindications:

The four most significant contraindications to beginning an exercise program or resuming one are (1) physical injury, (2) an acute bout of illness or a serious chronic disease, (3) onset of persistent or recurrent abdominal or pelvic pain, and finally (4) abnormal or heavy vaginal bleeding.[56]

Please consult with your healthcare provider to assess your personal risks before implementing any exercise program. Having this in-depth conversation with your provider will help you to better understand what, if any precautions should be taken.

Your sense of power, your stamina, and your courage will combine in varying amounts as you ebb and flow through the tides of birth and life. Surely there will be a time in labor when you will want to stop. In your parenting there will be times when you want to give up, to escape the burden of your responsibilities. In both cases you will need to dig deep into your life force to make honest evaluations and then problem-solve. By tuning into your challenges now, during pregnancy—pushing yourself where you need to be pushed and having compassion for yourself when you need to let up—you will develop new skills and build confidence. Please consider that, in birth, the physical work is about allowing the process to overtake you; yield to the fierceness of your sensations, as intense as they may be. It is not about needing super-human physical powers. Your body has developed to give birth. *Birth is a healthy human function.*

Monitor your exertion

The National Center for Health encourages prenatal exercisers to monitor their own level of "perceived exertion."[57] How hard does it feel like you are working? The Cleveland Clinic shares their Rate of Perceived Exertion (RPE):

The RPE scale is used to measure the intensity of your exercise. The RPE scale runs from 0 – 10. The numbers below relate to phrases used to rate how easy or difficult you find an activity. For example, 0 (nothing at all) would be how you feel when sitting in a chair; 10 (very, very heavy) is how you feel at the end of an exercise stress test or after a very difficult activity.

    0 – Nothing at all

    0.5 – Just noticeable

    1 – Very light

    2 – Light

    3 – Moderate

    4 – Somewhat heavy

    5 – Heavy

    6

    7 – Very heavy

    8

    9

    10 – Very, very heavy[58]

In most cases, you should exercise at a level that feels 3 (moderate) to 4 (somewhat heavy). When using this rating scale, remember to include feelings of shortness of breath as well as how tired you feel in your legs and overall.[59]

In short, listen to your feelings, in body and mind. Being active doesn't have to hurt or be awful to be useful. Being able to talk while engaged in your aerobic workout is a simple way to make sure you are not getting too short of breath. If you can't catch your breath enough to talk while exercising, you are pushing very hard. Reduce your intensity but keep moving gently until you can talk comfortably. Again, be sure to discuss your exercise goals and any limits with your care providers. Remember: I am not your care provider. I am more of a cheerleader and/or a grandma, with years of personal and professional experience to pass on.

Time for rest is a must for good health

In pregnancy it is critical that your exertion be followed by adequate rest. Muscle fibers need time to repair themselves. Build your strength and stamina steadily but slowly. The key is to carve out equal time for exertion and relaxation. The American Academy of Family Physicians points out that

> Sleep should never be seen as a luxury. It's a necessity—especially when you're pregnant. In fact, women who are pregnant need a few more hours of sleep each night or should supplement night-time sleep with naps during the day, according to the National Institutes of Health.[60]

Relish your rest and make it a part of your exercise, like an incredible feeling of accomplishment at the end. There is real joy in being done with your hard work/play. Cheeks flushed, blood flowing, work behind you. Completing your exercise goals can create happiness and pride, and this can in turn increase your energy levels. The goal within the goal here is that your life stresses can be kept in check, so that you can then take the necessary time to exercise and rest well. I know this will be a challenge for some, if not many, if not all of you. But keep trying day after day. Have confidence that every day you are working closer toward securing the balance you need.

The great feelings associated with post exercise come to us thanks to our wonderful endorphins, the hormones we release after hard physical exertion.[61] Our emotional feelings are inextricably bound to our endocrine system.[62] The endocrine system makes and regulates hormones, which are chemical messengers or catalysts—many of which are made from proteins.[63] (Another reminder to eat adequate protein!) Look for more on hormones as they relate to birth later in this book. For now, focus back to rest. Rest gives you time to daydream and to practice relaxation/concentration/breath awareness exercises. Rest creates opportunities to emotionally connect to yourself and to your growing fetus, and to physically cope with the rigors of life and baby building. From rest, sleep will come when you need it, but in and of itself rest has many benefits.

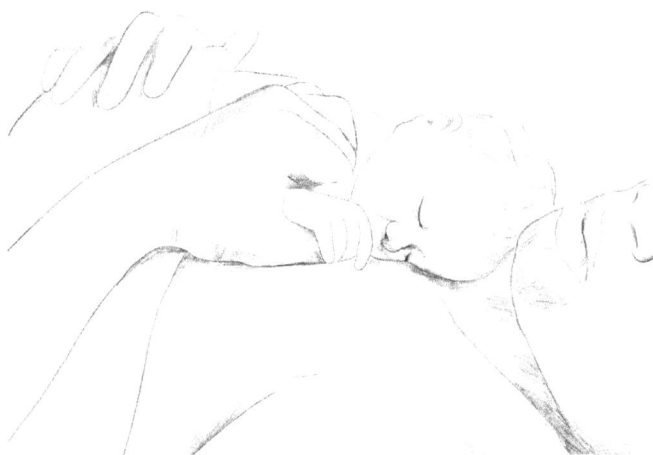

Flexibility

A flexible physical body will be more comfortable, less injury prone, and more easily able to open for birth. A muscle that is chronically locked in tightness cannot effectively contract further when called on for work. A muscle must be relaxed to be strong. A flexible body also supports a flexible mind, which as you're learning is very useful for birth.

Birth works best when a person utilizes their flexibility of body and mind to work with their sensations and circumstances as they develop. Increased physical and emotional flexibility help you to be ready for a full range of experiences and challenges. (I can also attest to the fact that being flexible has been critical to my success in marriage and parenting, too!)

As your pregnancy progresses you make a hormone aptly called Relaxin.[64] Relaxin helps to loosen up your pelvic joints by softening and elongating the ligaments around them. This enables the pelvic bones to shift to make room for your baby when you're ready to birth. During pregnancy, however, it is also common for the muscles around the loose joints to get extra tight, as they try to stabilize your structure. This tightness can result in soreness, especially around the hips. Undertaking regular stretching, gently and easily opening, closing, and rotating each of your joints with slow movements, can help to alleviate some of the discomfort from these tight muscles. Pregnancy is not a time to stretch hard or to try to jam the body into predetermined shapes. You can increase your flexibility best by moving within and exploring the boundaries of your comfortable range of motion at each joint. While stretching, you'll want to focus on breathing fully as you ease up to your edge—a place where you feel sensation but not discomfort.

Continue your focus on breathing while moving. Stretching takes time. Gently feel for your edge and then back off a bit and hold. By respecting your body's boundaries, and keeping your breath full, you will be safe. A safe body is more likely to soften and open with increased flexibility. For any static stretching please go close to your edge, and then SLOWLY, while breathing easily, creep further toward your limit. If you can't breathe fully, then you've gone too far. Once your limit is accessed, back off again gently and take a few deep breaths at around 97% of the full stretch, then release.

—Pause your reading here for about 90 seconds and take a stretch break,
focusing on any places that need some attention—

When you're done stretching, note here how you feel, what you were able to do and what felt good.

Prenatal yoga

Yoga means many things to many people. Overall, yoga is moving and breathing together with awareness of both. It provides the opportunity to practice being present with emotions and physical sensations. Yoga and childbirth both involve big sensations. Both activities are enhanced by having a conservationist's calm: don't use more energy than you have to and slow down your breathing as you can. The task of building muscle, increasing flexibility, and studying the coordination between your breath and movement are some of the components that make up a yogic practice. Prenatal yoga can be a terrific training tool for birth, helping to provide an excellent foundation to support the birth process. In yoga you can gently allow your body to open by learning to listen to your sensations.

While yoga can increase mindfulness, flexibility, and strength, as well as benefit your cardiovascular health, you can also push yourself into positions that stress your body and can cause injury. So take care when taking up a prenatal yoga practice. It's a good idea to research a potential instructor's prenatal-specific credentials and reputation before committing to a class, because if practiced incorrectly prenatal yoga can cause more harm than good. In addition to actual classes, there are many prenatal yoga and exercise videos available for use at home. The internet and your local public library can also be good resources.

Hydration for exercise

It is most beneficial to drink water one half hour prior to any exercise and then immediately following your exercise session. It is also important to have water available throughout the session. Never hesitate to stop for a sip of water. You can gauge your hydration level by your sense of thirst and also by the color of your pee. Your pee should generally be light in color. If it looks dark(ish) you should increase your fluid levels. In other words, your pee should look more like very light lemonade and less like apple cider. Also keep in mind that some prenatal vitamins can drastically impact the color of your urine. Have you ever had a vitamin give you neon pee?

Prenatal exercise is not for weight loss

Please do not try to lose weight through exercise during pregnancy. If you burn a lot of calories while exercising, you will need to replace them with nutrient-rich whole foods. For example, if you burn approximately 100 calories through exercise, you'll want to replace those and be sure to add the extra calories recommended in pregnancy. At Johns Hopkins Medicine they say, "To maintain a healthy pregnancy, approximately 300 extra calories are needed each day."[65]

To lose weight after your pregnancy you will do better by adjusting your food intake rather than rely on exercise alone. Exercise is helpful for maintaining a healthy weight, getting strong, and keeping a healthy heart, as well as having fun and feeling good. If you have concerns about weight gain, or loss, please fill out another diet chart this week for further evaluation. If you feel unhappy with your body getting large and it's making you upset or affecting your food choices, please *please* know that you are not alone and it's not your fault. Shame is a powerful emotion that can cause real obstacles to feeling better. But you must take care not to under nourish yourself or your baby. The website motherchildnutrition.org states:

> **Maternal malnutrition** increases the risk of poor pregnancy outcomes including obstructed labour [sic], premature or low-birth-weight babies and postpartum haemorrhage[sic]. Severe anaemia [sic] during pregnancy is linked to increased mortality at labour [sic].

Low-birth-weight is a significant contributor to infant mortality. Moreover, low birth-weight babies who survive are likely to suffer growth retardation and illness throughout their childhood, adolescence and into adulthood. Growth-retarded adult women are likely to carry on the vicious cycle of malnutrition by giving birth to low birth-weight babies.[66]

Pregnancy is a time to gain weight. If a person starts pregnancy at a healthy weight, it is recommended that they should gain in the area of 35 extra pounds, more if they were underweight and less if they were overweight at the start of the pregnancy.[67] But gaining weight and feeling fat can trigger some challenging body image issues. These can be common but can also negatively affect you and your baby's health. I encourage you to try and seek professional help if body image concerns are making you upset or affecting your food choices. I know it can feel impossibly hard to access professional counseling, but you are worth the work of trying. If such access truly isn't an option, and as a viable alternative, then it can help to talk to a friend about your feelings. Talking to a friend can help you to process your feelings and improve your mental health.[68] Again, please don't feel shame; we are a culture that has created very complicated relationships with our appearances. Healing is possible and you deserve to try. Many of us would do better to focus on the quality of our food rather than the numbers on a scale.

Looking ahead, after your baby is born, you can expect to be left with some extra pounds. This is normal and healthy. For some people the weight loss after birth seems to be effortless and for others the process is slower, and still others carry leftover "baby weight" at one year or longer. Rapid weight loss is not advisable during postpartum. There is evidence that some environmental toxins get stored in fat and that rapid weight loss transfers the toxins into the breastmilk fats.[69] If, after birth, weight loss feels arduous, remind yourself that your whole life is different now, especially your body. Finding the balance between baby care and self-care takes time. Try to find pride in your amazing ability to create and nourish life. Celebrate your best choices and keep setting positive food and exercise intentions. Strive for self-love and try to accept that this progress can be very slow, especially during breastfeeding when you still have a need for extra calories. From the Centers for Disease Control (CDC):

> An additional 450 to 500 kilocalories (kcal) of healthy food calories per day is recommended for well-nourished breastfeeding mothers, compared with the amount they were consuming before pregnancy (approximately 2,300 to 2,500 kcal per day for breastfeeding women verses 1,800 to 2,000 kcal per day for moderately active, non-pregnant women who are not breastfeeding).[70]

Likewise, the Mayo Clinic advises:

> Most women lose about 13 pounds (5.9 kilograms) during childbirth, including the weight of the baby, placenta and amniotic fluid. During the first week after delivery, you'll lose additional weight as you shed retained fluids—but the fat stored during pregnancy won't disappear on its own. Through diet and regular exercise, it might be reasonable to lose up to 1 pound (0.5 kilogram) a week."[71]

Note that the quote above states that it "might be reasonable" to lose a pound a week, which means it also might not be reasonable. I encourage you again to focus on how you are feeling and the food choices you are making out of what you can access, rather than dwell solely on the scale.

Pregnancy specific exercises: Let's start with the intimate bits

The pelvic floor is made up of an intricate assortment of muscles that form the foundational base of our bodies. In biological females, the pelvic floor has three openings: the urethra, the vagina, and the anus. The area in between the anus and the vagina is known as the "perineum." The muscles of the pelvic floor, like any other muscles, can have good tone or poor tone with weak spots and tight spots. The perineum will take quite a lot of stretch during birth. When one works toward good tone in the pelvic floor, and alignment in the pelvis and spine, one can better enjoy optimal function.

The pelvic floor is the bottom of our torso, on top of this bottom sits all the pelvic organs, and then on top of that the abdominal organs. Therefore, if the bottom of your body has poor tone and misalignment, then everything inside the body will start to sag. When this happens we can start to have problems with urine and bowel control, the ability to enjoy sex and/or have an orgasm, and/or prolapsed organs, which is when they start to slide down and out. The uterus can actually start to fall into the vagina and right out of the body.[72] For biological males with poor pelvic floor tone, incontinence can occur along with issues associated with an enlarged prostate.

For optimal function, muscles need to live at their full relaxed length during rest so that they can contract with force when needed. Sitting in chairs all day, poor posture, wearing high heels, and even emotional tension can all contribute to shortened muscles and imbalanced holding patterns. Pelvic misalignment, weakness, and/or chronic clenching of muscle can cause dysfunction. Lengthening and strengthening the gluteal muscles, learning to untuck the tail bone, developing abdominal tone, and gentle stretching that opens up the back of the legs can all help someone achieve improved pelvic alignment. A physical therapist that specializes in female anatomy can be an excellent resource.

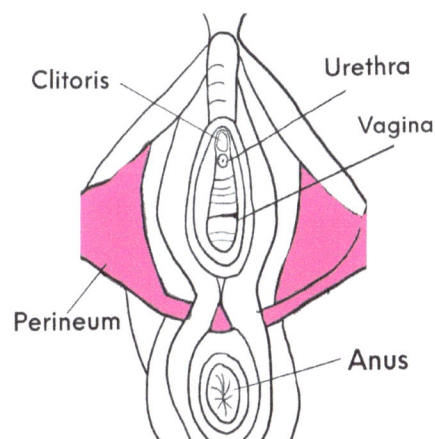

Vagina power

The vagina deserves special attention always, and especially during pregnancy. The vagina is a muscular organ that has seemingly magic powers. It is a sensory organ that self-lubricates, receives and gives pleasure, and beautifully accommodates the birth of babies.[73] The vagina has a mysterious allure. I was 51 years old before I started to fully get to know the intuitive, creative, and functional powers of my vagina. Since the age of 14 I've always had a pretty satisfying and diverse sex-life. By age 38 I birthed a child through my vagina and had already taught hundreds of other females about their own vaginas during birth classes, and still my vagina's full potential was unknown to me—even as I was beginning to suffer from some typical American female health issues.

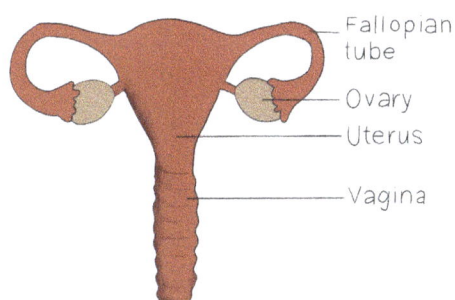

Over a billion dollars are spent annually on adult diapers and medical procedures related to incontinence and prolapsed pelvic organs in the U.S.[74] As a middle-aged woman I had low libido, and I was struggling with stress incontinence. My vagina was dry more often than not (except from pee), and I had the expectation that menopause would bring nothing but less good moisture and more bad moisture. I had been teaching people about pelvic floor health, and yet had somehow neglected the entire vagina. As I struggled with my own vaginal health issues, I knew better than many that there were answers connected to muscle tone and posture, and yet still I struggled. Something was still off. I gloomily embraced the party line: busy moms don't want sex and vaginas get old early. Then one day, as I was browsing through an online newsletter, something caught my eye. The newsletter was sponsored by Debra Pascali-Bonaro, the film maker who made the spectacular film *Orgasmic Birth*.[75] The film explores some of the many ways that birth can happen, including ecstatically. I recommend this film to all expectant families; it's important to see images of real people having empowered experiences. But what caught my eye that day was the offer for a free webinar about jade eggs and pelvic health. It was starting in 15 minutes and I had the afternoon available, so I logged in.

The webinar was taught by a woman named Kim Anami who, I learned, teaches a variety of online courses on sexual health and intimacy. I didn't know what to expect but I was intrigued. I had never heard of jade eggs as a tool before. These are polished, egg-shaped jade rocks with a hole drilled through them, through which you can tie a piece of silk or dental floss.[76] Right from the start Anami made solid good sense to me. She discussed that Kegels alone don't work. (Kegels are an exercise for strengthening the pelvic floor, named after a medical doctor, and taught in birth classes, including the Bradley Method®). Or, at least they don't work as effectively in isolation. The Kegel exercise is typically taught by telling women to repeatedly clench the vagina closed. Unfortunately, this is not enough information, which makes Kegels alone insufficient to best prepare for birth. Moreover, they don't often bring real change and relief for people already suffering with symptoms of dysfunction. Anami spoke about jade eggs for strength training. You insert the egg into your vagina. The string helps aid removal, and also adds strength training. You can pull on the string, or even attach a small weight to increase resistance, just like you would add weights at the gym. (There are, in fact, vaginal strength training contests. I haven't researched deeply, but supposedly the world champ can lift something like 35 lbs. with her hooha!)

Anami spoke to the fact that many people with vaginas suffer from the inability to fully relax their vaginal and pelvic floor muscles. Most enlightening for me, and yet perhaps most obvious, was when she highlighted the fact that people have a deeply complex emotional component to our sexual health. She explained that some variation of emotional disconnection and/or energy blockages from our vaginas can be a component of our overall pelvic health—or lack thereof. She went on to say that people with vaginas were at an increased risk of chronic tension and emotional disconnection from their vaginas if they have suffered any sexual violence and/or if they have had medical procedures on their cervix, uterus, vagina, or anus. Additionally, people can have emotional blockages from feelings such as shame or even disgust. (Aha! I thought. My cesarean section. Did this medical procedure leave a residual tension in and around my vagina? Do I have scar tissue or adhesions that may be impacting how I feel and function?) She said that many women were walking around with numb vaginas. (Aha again! I wouldn't say mine was numb, but I could sense some disconnection.) Anami went on to reveal that for birth preparation, and for optimum health thereafter, there is a need for a more multifaceted approach, something more than just clench-and-release Kegels. Her words resonated inside me, so I signed up for her course, Vaginal Kung Fu®.[77]

Just by processing the idea that my struggles with incontinence could be related to chronic tension, and that, at least to some degree, I had cut myself off emotionally from my vagina, I started to see improvement in my ability to relax deeply, develop awareness, and improve my functioning. Through this course, my urine control improved, my sexual desire increased, and I felt better overall than I had in some time.

My partner fondly nick-named Kim Anami the "Cooter Tutor." Pulling perspectives from ancient Chinese, Tibetan, and Indian cultures, Anami and her course helped to broaden my understanding of the many wisdoms of the vagina, including the creative and healing powers of sexual energy. The multifaceted approach was successful for me. I now live with a deeper sense of my physical body and I try to honor the intuitive connections from my body, including what my vagina can provide. Akin to making decisions from the gut or heart, I also listen to my vagina. One of the single best things I learned from Anami's course was to conscientiously stay focused on my breath during sex. In particular I learned to focus on a 4-count breath during sex: 4 counts for inhalation and 4 counts for exhalation. (But I often like longer exhales, so this, too, reminded me of the importance to connect to your own rhythm.) She encouraged us to allow ourselves to relax deeply with the inhales and contract strongly with the exhales. Give this a try! (I hadn't known I was a sexual breath holder before this course. Nor did I realize how awesome it could be for me and my partner when I could breathe and relax fully and so deeply.)

As my own knowledge and experience base was expanding, I realized that I had to reevaluate and expand what and how I teach traditional Kegels and posture work. The "pelvic floor" work wasn't wrong; it was just incomplete. In my quest to put all the pieces together, I also found the work of physical therapist Katie Bowman quite valuable. Bowman also has spoken out against the inadequacy of Kegels alone and teaches that to improve function one must address strength and alignment.[78] This wasn't wrong either; it, too, was just incomplete. For our health to be good, including pelvic floor function, we do need strong muscles (especially the gluteal and abdominal muscles). We also need the ability to relax completely. And we further succeed when we connect to our feelings.

Following are some questions to reflect upon as you ponder your anatomy:

O Do you have feelings about the way your vagina looks? (Maybe now, or as a homework assignment, use a mirror and take some time to really see your vagina.)

O Do you feel connected to all or just part(s) of your vagina?

O Do you feel like your vagina is mostly awake or mostly sleepy?

O Are you worried about your vagina opening for birth?

O Can you think of any positive affirmations to give yourself about your body's abilities?

Take some time to express your thoughts and reflections here. Pause to consider your vagina. Perhaps you want to color in or take notes on or around Sheela Na Gig on the following page.

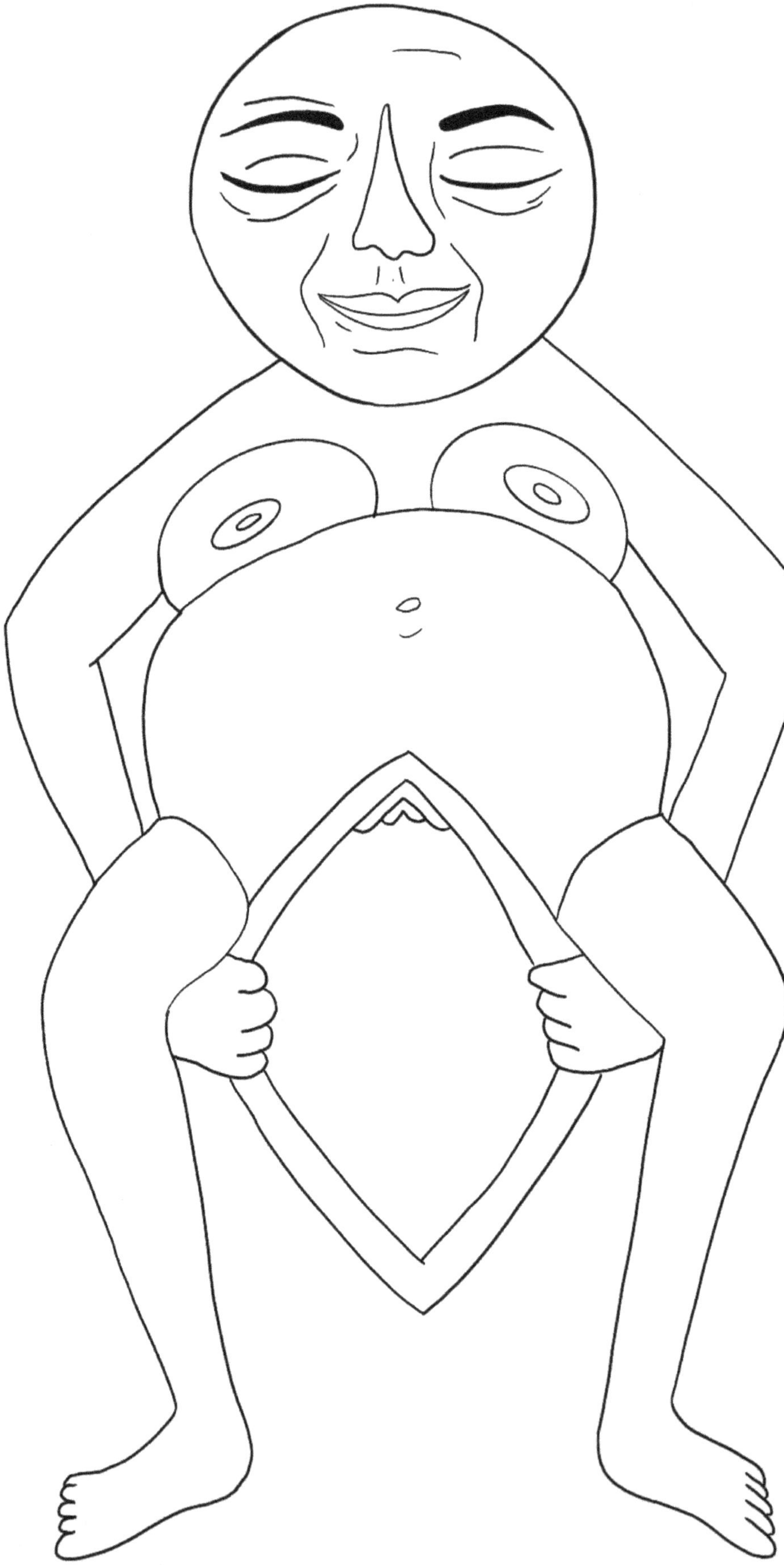

How a healthy (powerful) vagina and perineum aids the birth process

The muscle tissue of a toned vagina and pelvic floor helps keep the baby in good position as she starts her descent into the vagina. Ideally, you want the smallest circumference of the baby's head to come through the vagina first. This happens when the baby keeps her head flexed, chin to chest, as she enters the vagina.[79] If the vagina has good tone it is less likely to be sagging ahead of the baby's decent. Poor muscle tone would make it easier for the baby's head to extend earlier in the process. This early extension can create complications and cause the birth to be delayed. But with good muscle tone, the baby's head is more likely to be tucked in as she enters the vagina. This means *you* have the ability to improve your chances of an uncomplicated birth by learning to relax deeply, open and strengthen, and by learning to really connect to your vagina.

By exploring and exercising your vagina and perineum you will also increase circulation, which promotes good healthy tissue that can stretch and regain tone. Blood to the genitals makes them grow large. To birth your baby, you need to get large. When you learn to consciously relax and contract your vagina and pelvic floor, you can improve circulation and really help yourself open wide for the baby's passage. This will not only help the birth be easier, it will also reduce perineal tearing. Begin to build a daily practice now.

EXERCISE: THE VAGINA WORKOUT

There are several ways to test and develop your vaginal and pelvic floor strength. Start by waking up your awareness. Visualize your clitoris and try to move it side to side, without using your hands or any other manual assistance. If you can't feel it moving, that is okay, just imagine the movement; see it moving in your mind's eye. Using your imagination will begin to get the area engaged and grow your awareness. Think through the movement and you begin to lay the neural pathways that can one day actually make the movements happen. Next try to stretch your clitoris down and back towards your tailbone. Now try to visualize the opening of your vagina softening to open wide. And then, by pulling in and up, as if cinching up a pouch, visualize your vaginal opening contracting closed. You can coordinate opening and closing with your breath: relax your vagina open as you inhale for two counts and then contract up and in as you exhale for two counts. (Thank you to Anami for teaching this two-count pattern in her course.) Try it with your eyes closed.

Building awareness is useful because sometimes we think that we're contracting the vagina and perineum, but what we're primarily doing is contracting the abdominals or buttocks or even the thighs. You can test strength in your vagina and pelvic floor if you try to stop the flow of urine while you are peeing. (If you already have compromised muscle tone, this may be very difficult, especially if you're already very pregnant, which puts a lot of extra pressure on the entire bottom of your body.) Trying to stop the flow of urine is a simple way to engage and feel the lower segment of the vagina, so go ahead and test yourself if you are inclined. Note, however, that I do not recommend any actual strength training while on the toilet, because practicing (opening and closing) while peeing can increase your chances of developing a urinary tract infection. And a urinary tract infection is a bummer anytime, but especially while you are pregnant. Likewise, please do not try to test your strength when your bladder's really full, like first thing in the morning. Better to try in the middle of the day, when you're not super full. At that time, you can better observe your release and contraction. (It is also important to mention here that all human voiding processes seem to work better when uninterrupted.)

Sex and sex play (including self-pleasuring) are additional ways to test and learn about your vagina and pelvic floor. They provide a lot of wonderful benefits, such as muscle development, muscle release, emotional stress relief, cardiovascular exercise, improved nonverbal communication, excellent opportunities for breath awareness, and the chance to practice letting go of your inhibitions so that you may follow your body's sensations with carefree abandon. Incidentally, this all lines up directly with the best way to birth your baby: to repeat, let go of your inhibitions and follow your body's sensations with carefree abandon.

Like birthing a baby, consensual sexual activity is a healthy human function and very educational. Intercourse during pregnancy and birth is safe as long as the amniotic sac is still intact and you're in the mood. You need not worry that intercourse will harm the baby or bring on early labor. (Please do talk to your healthcare provider should you have any individual concerns.) However, in the absence of contraindications, if you are due and you want to encourage labor, sex is one of the most enjoyable ways you can try to get birth started. So test away... and read on as I discuss more on inductions in Week 12.

The nuts and bolts of exercising your vagina

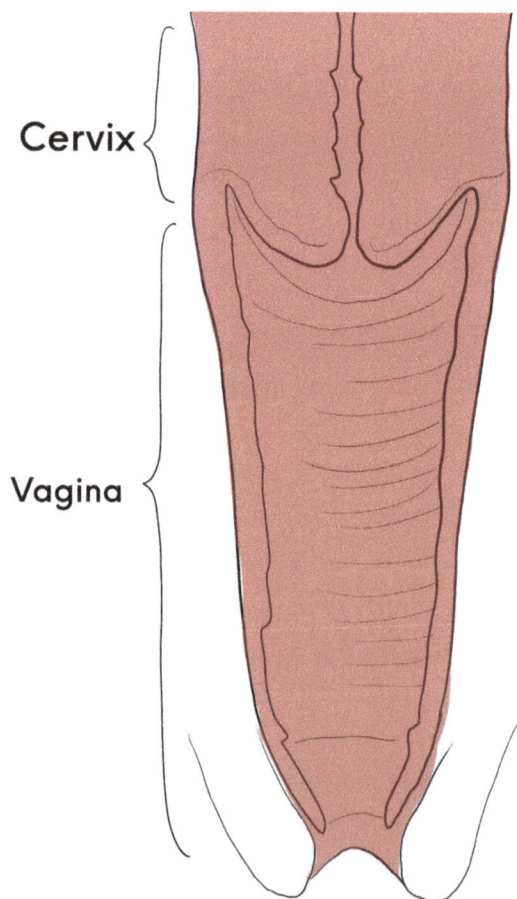

Cervix

Vagina

The vagina has an elongated, triangular tube-like shape. Consider the vagina in three segments: the opening, the middle, and the upper section that surrounds the cervix. It is useful to understand that the vagina is a muscular organ and that the segments of the vagina have articulation ability from top to bottom and side to side. There are circular muscle fibers that run horizontally around the opening and there are vertical muscle fibers around the outside. Your vagina also has both fast-action and slow-action muscle fibers.[80] These different types of muscle fibers enable you to clench quickly and with force, or to contract with endurance over time. **Make sure to breathe fully while holding any contractions and release your muscle action at the end of any conscious contraction,** then finish up any vaginal release with only about 10% of a full-strength contraction before letting your attention shift. Please experiment and incorporate both quick- and slow-muscle action into your daily routine. Always end by trying to deeply relax and open your vagina and perineum, then give yourself a gentle reminder of the 10% baseline of full-strength contraction to carry you throughout your day.

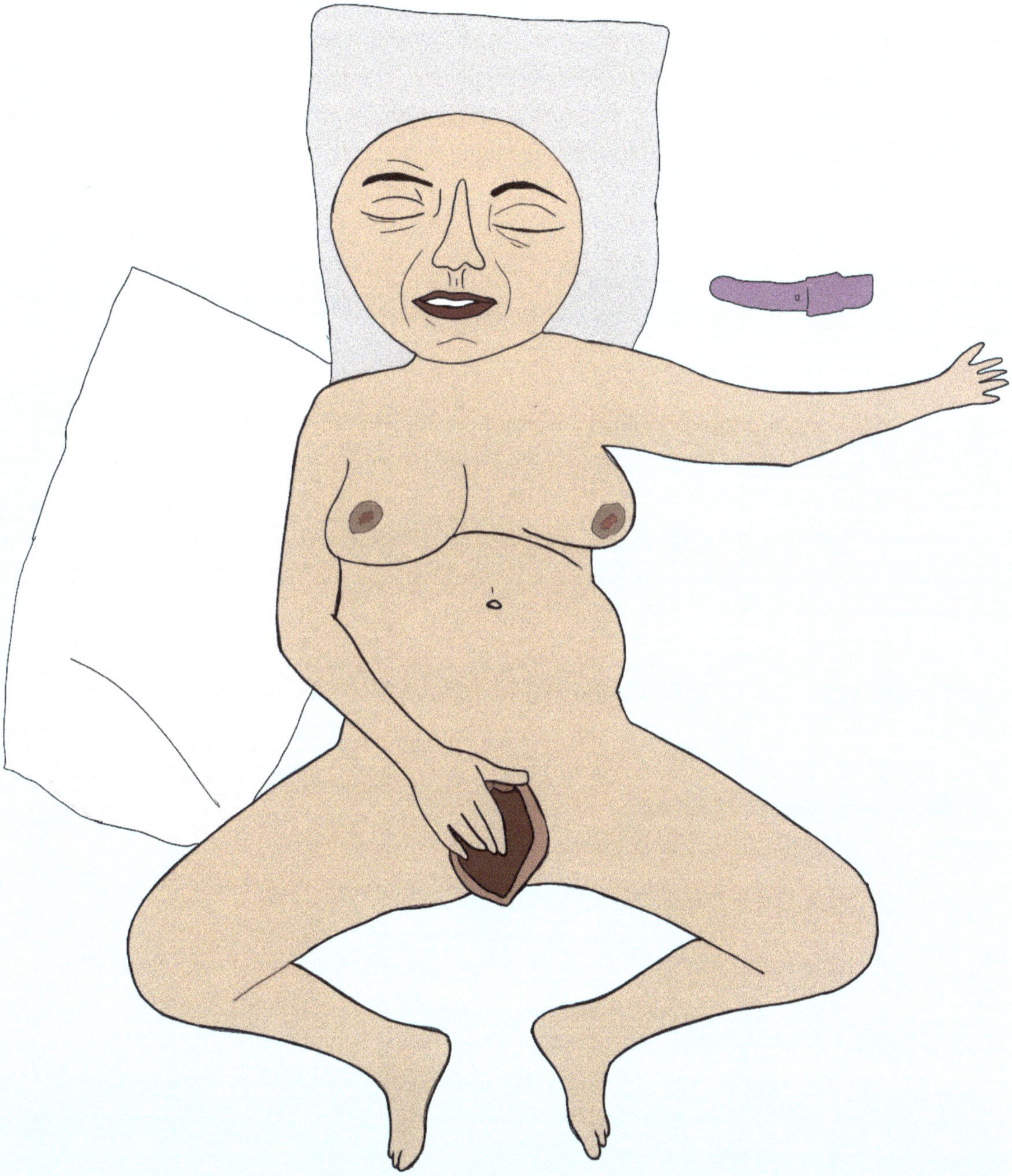

Vagina work

You can use (clean!) fingers (yours or your partner's), a penis, jade egg, or dildo to explore your vagina and perineum. Any of these objects can give you something to squeeze and tactile feedback for relaxation. A dildo, for example, can be a wonderful birth preparation tool. It can help a female really get familiar with the whole inside of their own vagina. However, I wouldn't recommend exploring in vibrate mode. Vibrating will add a lot of tactile chatter that can decrease your ability to focus on and feel the subtleties of the different areas of your vagina. A person with a vagina can use meditation to infuse any kind of energy they choose into a dildo; it need not be a male energy. A dildo can be saturated with an energy from the forces of nature, a female or male energy, or whatever strikes your fancy. With conscientious intention any object can be charged with any kind of spirit that suits you. It all depends on what you think and your energetic powers of imagination. If a dildo is being used, I encourage you to use one made from phthalate-free plastics only.[81] To infuse an object with your preferred energetic qualities, simply place the object in front of you and use your imagination to visualize the energy of your choice pouring over and saturating your object, such as a dildo. Ta daa! Object infused.

EXERCISE: EXPLORE YOUR VAGINA

To practice when the time is right: you'll first want to protect yourself from interruptions and then make yourself really comfortable. Maybe you'll want to lie in bed with pillows supporting your knees as your legs rest comfortably open. Take a few deep breaths and try to consciously relax your whole body. Take a few more moments to consider your intentions. Second, using some spit or other organic lubricant, if desired, place two fingers, a jade egg, dildo, or penis, into your vagina. Relax, open and inhale as you insert your object of choice, then try to squeeze it and pull it up and in with your vaginal opening as you exhale. Next, release your vagina as you breathe in and repeat your contraction; squeeze tight and pull up as you exhale.

Relax your vagina as you breathe in for two seconds, then exhale and contract forcefully for two seconds or longer. Use these two-second contractions to build strength and awareness. And if you are using something for tactile support, try and pull or suck the fingers, dildo or other object into the vagina with your exhales. Start by concentrating on the opening of your vagina. You can aim to do 5 or 10 or 15 repetitions in a row. Pace yourself. Start slowly and aim for an amount of repetitions that you can perform well, with good, focused contractions, then build up as ready. Next you can try to squeeze your vagina or your fingers or other object from the middle of your vagina. See if you can contract the mid-section of your vagina's front, back, and sides separately. Aim here for another set of two-second contractions, squeezing in the midsection of your vagina. Relax completely while you inhale, then exhale deeply while you contract with strength.

Now bring your attention to the uppermost area of your vagina, the area that goes around your cervix. Try to contract here again for another set of 5, 10 or 15 contractions. (Personally, I need something other than my own fingers to really reach into upper areas of my vagina, but everyone is different, and practicing without any external objects is beneficial too.) Relax completely as you inhale and contract with strength as you exhale. Now try to expel your fingers with vaginal articulation. If you are working with a partner, your partner can and should give you feedback about whether they can feel your contractions. If they can feel them, can they then differentiate your attempts at contracting different sections of the vagina? That feedback can be helpful as you are learning to increase awareness.

Sometimes you might think that you are still holding a contraction, but in fact the muscle action has greatly released and that contraction is really over. It's important to practice releasing contractions as well. How deeply can you soften and open, how far in can you let go? Your partner might really enjoy helping you to learn, plus they can provide information that you might not otherwise have. Don't get discouraged if you don't feel much in the muscle walls, or if you feel like you don't have any control. This work is about discovery. Strength, sensitivity, and articulation can all be developed over time. Your body and *every* body is amazing.

Meet your perineum

It's not just your vagina that you'll need to relax and open wide for your baby to pass through; your perineum will undergo a tremendous amount of stretch as well. Learning to release your perineum now will increase your tissue health from increased circulation. This will also reduce the possibility of developing any perineal tears during birth. What follows is a way to get to know your perineum a bit better.

While lying down or standing with a foot propped up on a stool or on the side of the tub, if you're in the shower (which, by the way, is a good place to do these explorations), insert your own thumb into your vagina and push down into your perineum (the area between your vagina and rectum). Explore. Feel your rectum from inside your vagina, feel the muscles and ligaments. While pushing your thumb down try to tense your muscles with strength and then deeply relax against your thumb's pressure. Also try to give yourself a bit of a stretch. How much can you relax? It may be scary to think about, but it's probably useful to try to imagine getting really big and open, like passing a grapefruit while big and open. Did I just scare you with the image of a grapefruit? Okay, feel that and take a breath. I am sorry, but a grapefruit is comparable in size to a baby's head. I hope you can find comfort in learning that birthing the head is a gradual process with time for stretching open. More on that later in the book. For now, take another breath, honor your concerns, and exhale slowly and fully. Feel your tension and invite yourself to release it as you can.

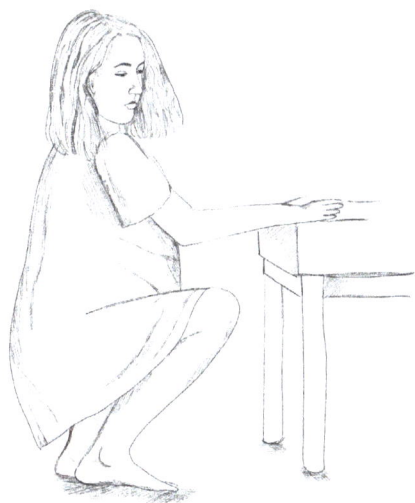

If you suspect that your perineum is very tight, and certainly if you have ever suffered from painful intercourse, you might benefit from going to a physical therapist that specializes in female anatomy, functional movement and pelvic health. There are ways to help you regain some stretch and mobility to the perineum prior to birth (and after). Sitting into a deep squat is one such method. Preparation, physically and emotionally, will aid your process of opening up in birth and it will help you to return to good tone after birth.

Develop your practice routines

Once you have figured out what vaginal and pelvic floor contractions feel like, you can strength train anywhere or anytime and nobody needs to know. I had a client who recently got our class laughing. She shared that her job was full of boring administrative meetings, which stopped being so boring once she started using her meeting time to get some vaginal and pelvic floor exercises done! During what part of your day will you explore and practice your exercises?

Finding a few times throughout your day will really improve your tone and can energize your emotional connection to your vagina. You might find success by trying to sync up the practice activity with some other daily activities to help you create new habits. If you take a Bradley® class, ask your teacher for some "Kegel" stickers. You can also leave little notes for yourself around the house, even make your own stickers, to help you to remember. I've had clients put "Kegel" stickers on the rearview mirror of their car, so that when they stop at red lights they are reminded to engage and release their vagina and pelvic floor.

EXERCISE: PICK UP A PEARL

Can you imagine that the lips of your vagina can pick up a pearl? Let's try now. Read the following exercise and then close your eyes and try.

Take a few deep abdominal breaths to settle down and prepare for the visualization. In your mind's eye visualize picking up a beautiful pearl aglow with creative energy. Use the opening ring of your vagina to lift the glowing pearl up. Feel your vaginal opening work hard to pick up and pull in your pearl of energy. Then pull the pearl up to the midsection of your vagina. Feel the glow of the pearl's energy as you squeeze the middle section of your vagina. Hold the pearl in place and gently raise your imaginary pearl up to your cervix. Can you imagine that your cervix softens as your pearl gently makes contact? Breathe fully, hold your imaginary pearl there for a while as you marvel at your pearl's glowing beauty, then slowly, slowly release it back down and out. As you completely release the pearl, allow its energy to dissolve its pearl shape and be reabsorbed through your vagina, floating up and into your low belly and up to your heart. You can store this energy and it will be ready for you when you need it. Now again, inhale and try to fully relax all of your vaginal muscles, and then release even further with your exhale.

Your exercise is over. Once you have completely relaxed, finish with a small contraction restoring about 10% of your full contraction strength, before letting your attention go on to other matters.

How do you feel now? Can you feel the warmth of blood flow that returns when your contraction releases?

It bears repeating: Learning to conscientiously relax and contract your vagina and pelvic floor will help you to let your baby out.

Abdominal bracing

Abdominal bracing is another exercise for pregnancy, post-partum recovery, and for the rest of your life. Abdominal bracing is a simple spine-stabilizing exercise for the innermost layer of abdominal muscles, the **Transversus abdominis.** This muscle forms a corset around your midsection. Good tone in this muscle is an essential component of core strength. Good core strength is critical to good posture, health and birth. Here I will guide you through learning the exercise, followed by an explanation of how this exercise will help with your birth.

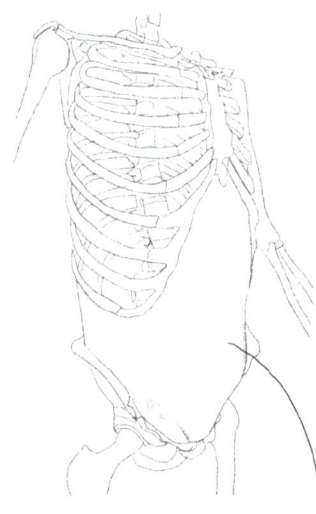

Transverse abdominis

EXERCISE: ABDOMINAL BRACING

Sit at the edge of your chair with your feet flat on the ground (if your feet don't reach the ground use two equal-sized books or stacks of books under them). Sit up tall with the crown of your head reaching up to the sky. Roll your shoulders gently back and down. Place your hands on your belly, between your belly button and your pubic bone, and take a few nice easy belly breaths. Breathe in and out, fully encouraging your belly to be relaxed. Invite your belly to expand as you inhale and to gently sink back toward your spine as you exhale. Take a couple of full relaxing breaths in this way. On your next exhale, as you feel the belly sinking back, engage your abdominal muscles to fully squeeze in tight and back toward your spine. Hold the contraction in. Feel the strong contraction pushing out any remaining air as you exhale completely. When all of your air is gone, hold the muscle contraction in, but do **continue to breathe**. Your inhale will probably feel a little different. You will likely feel the back of your lungs fill up. Continue to hold in your belly (Transversus abdominis) contraction as you slowly breathe in and out for a slow, count-out-loud of 30. When finished, relax your belly and breathe naturally. This is an endurance exercise. Practice daily, working toward extending the time you hold the contraction and the strength of your effort. See if you can work up to a slow count of 100.

Another strength-building variation on this exercise looks like this: As you exhale, squeeze your belly in tight, now release your contraction *just half way* and then squeeze in fully again. Count "one". Release your contraction *half way*, then squeeze back in completely and count "two." Continue to work this exercising action to a count of 30 or beyond.

It is critical for this exercise that you maintain fluid and continuous breathing and maintain good upright posture with your shoulders gently back and down. **At no point should you be holding your breath.** A specialist in women's health, physical therapist Debra Goodman, MSPT[82] taught me this exercise. She encourages all her clients to count out loud. When we are counting out loud, or talking in any form, we are breathing. Talking or counting out loud is a form of exhalation. If you remember to exhale, the inhales will naturally come. When practicing this exercise, also always keep your hands on your belly, between your belly button and your pubic bone. Your hands can provide important feedback that you are still contracting with strength.

How does the abdominal bracing exercise help the birth?

When we speak of "pushing" the baby out, we do not actually mean pushing. We mean squeezing or contracting the deep level Transversus abdominis. This squeeze action closes the space that the baby was in, which pushes the baby down. Think of squeezing a tube of toothpaste when you need to get out the last bit. You start at the top and squeeze all the way down toward the tube's opening. When you contract your deepest abdominal layer with strength and simultaneously soften and relax your pelvic floor, you can squeeze the baby out, just like the toothpaste. Once you are comfortable with this abdominal bracing exercise in a seated position, please experiment with it in various positions, such as standing, on hands and knees, and side lying.

Once the baby is born, you can use this same abdominal bracing exercise to rehabilitate your body in the postpartum period and beyond. During the pregnancy you have graciously lent out space in your body to your baby. After the birth it will be time to reclaim that space for yourself. Working to rehabilitate your body after birth will leave you in much better physical and emotional shape. Abdominal bracing exercises will be a key component of good health from here on.

One of the other ways to support your good postural health is to bring awareness to your **Rectus abdominus**, the outer most layer of abdominal muscle. The Rectus, a narrow band of muscle, which is sometimes called "the six pack," has a special feature: the center line of the muscle can separate to accommodate the growing abdomen. Nevertheless, it is best when this separation is as minimal as possible. **Protect your abs!** To minimize any rectus diastasis (the separation in your rectus muscle you may experience during or after pregnancy), take care to minimize any potential separation. To do this, you will want to pay special attention while lying down or getting back up from a reclining position.

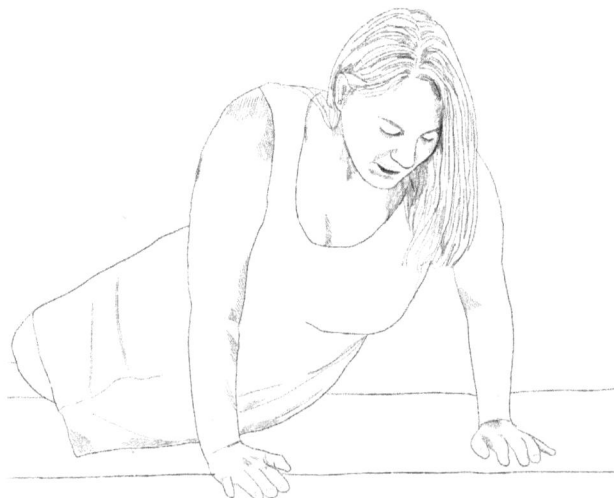

You can protect your abs and comfortably lie down or get back up, transferring down to bed, to a doctor's exam table, or the floor from your side, using your arms for support. The sequence goes like this: First, sit on the bed. Next, using your arms to "walk" your way down, lower yourself fully down onto your side. Once you are all the way down on your side, roll back onto your back (if that is your destination.) Reverse to get up. From your back, roll over onto your side and then use your arms to push yourself back up. Practice this now a few times, please.

The Pelvic Rock

The pelvic rock exercise is another excellent exercise to incorporate into your routine, for pregnancy and beyond, and even for non-pregnant bodies, too. Benefits of the pelvic rock exercise include relief of back pain, improved circulation, abdominal toning, and improved digestion. For pregnant people this exercise has the added benefit of improving fetal positioning by allowing the baby the room to adjust her position. Towards the end of the pregnancy, when the baby's position matters more and more, this exercise can help the baby to arrive at an optimum spot for decent.

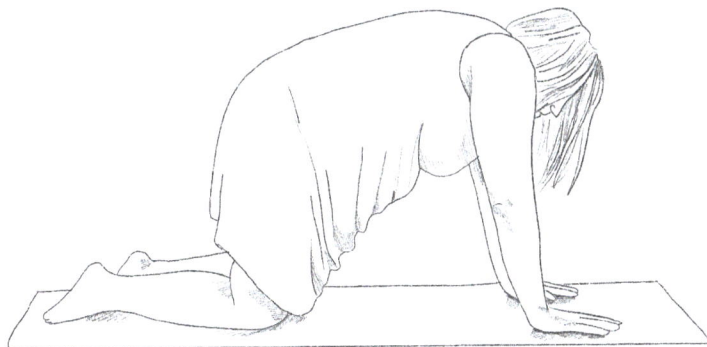

Once you are well-situated on your hands and knees, imagine that you are rounding your tailbone down under you, towards your belly button, and then trace the arc back so that you rock your tailbone up to the sky (or towards the back of your head). Breathe easily and fully. Find some flow as you explore your full range of motion. Experiment with speed and muscular effort. Explore this motion and see what your body tells you about it.

As a partner exercise, your partner can place one hand on your sacrum and one hand on the crown of your head. The partner should just hold their hands there, giving tactile feedback about the length of your spine. As the pelvis rocks, the hand resting on your sacrum just gets a ride as the tail moves up and down. As with almost any partner exercise, it is beneficial when you each try both parts.

Why pelvic rocks reduce back pain

When you are standing or sitting, gravity causes your baby to sink down. If your posture is at all slouched while standing or sitting, the extra weight of the baby applies pressure to the sacral nerves. When you get onto your hands and knees, in an all-fours position, the first thing that happens is that the extra weight of your belly falls away from the sacral area, instantly reducing pressure on the nerves. Pregnant people often feel immediate relief when they get into this position. As you then rock your pelvis forward and back, tipping your tailbone to the sky, you can start to visualize that you are dumping your baby, and all of her associated weight, out of your pelvic bowl and off of your sacrum.

I suggest that a gestational parent tell their baby as they rock to, "get off my sacrum, baby, get off my sacrum." They can imagine that they are spilling the baby out of the pelvic bowl as their tail bone goes up, and they can then think about the baby nestling back into a good position as they engage their core muscles and tuck their tailbone down and under toward their navel's center.

Incorporate pelvic rocking into your day

Ideally, you should do several repetitions of this exercise throughout your day and right before bed. The Bradley Method® recommends that you start with 10 pelvic rocks three times a day and 20 pelvic rocks right before bed, and that you work up to 40 three times a day and 80 right before bed. I think it is important to know what the expectations are; however, with any exercise during pregnancy, you should be listening to your own body and learning to develop your own ability to build physical self-awareness and strength. Please don't do more than what feels easy for the first week or two as you are learning about the impact this exercise has on you. Please remember that easy is always ok for your exercise, especially if you are pregnant.

Incorporating the pelvic rock into your bedtime ritual will improve your sleep as the pregnancy continues, when sleep can often become a challenge. The improved circulation and the relief of pressure on the sacral nerves can help you find comfort. Likewise, the physical massage of the gut will promote healthy bowel function. By the way, during your pelvic rock sessions, you can also work on your vaginal and pelvic floor exercises.

Cat/cow, the pelvic rock's cousin

For any of you that have studied yoga, or perhaps dance, you may know of the cat/cow exercise, which is similar and related to the pelvic rock exercise. In cat/cow you are initiating the exercise at both ends of the spine, head and tail, making your body into a giant U shape as your head and tail bone reach up. Cat/cow promotes spinal mobility and the full spinal stretch usually feels awesomely good. Cat/Cow is a good exercise during pregnancy or anytime. But to help you prepare for birth please focus on the pelvic rocks as your go-to exercise. In the pelvic rock you are only initiating movement from the base of the spine at your tailbone. This distinction gives you a chance to explore and understand pelvic isolation, as well as a clear sense of the bottom of your body—that place where the baby comes from. The pelvic rock exercise gives you clear and simple feedback, helps you gain comfort in pregnancy, and promotes optimum fetal positioning.

Squatting

When you squat during pregnancy you increase flexibility of the perineum, lower legs, hips and back. You also gain comfort and ease in the position, further creating the possibility that you might choose to squat during birth. It bears repeating, **squatting helps increase flexibility in your perineum.**

EXERCISE: SQUAT PROGRESSION

One way to get your body ready for squatting is to sit firmly on a chair near the outer edge of the seat. Use a kitchen-table type chair, if possible, or flat bench. Once seated, line your legs up so that your feet and knees are in alignment (pointing in the same direction). Sitting up nice and tall, with shoulders gently back and down, push down into your feet, allow your head to lead your spine slightly forward, and stand up strong on your legs, with the tail bone hanging down comfortably—not tipped back or rounded forward. From standing, you can repeat the action by tipping your tailbone behind you, then bend your knees and lower your bottom down toward the chair. Don't land on the chair, tap it lightly and push down through your feet to stand back up. Repeat this in a short series of repetitions that you practice throughout your day. This is a good exercise to help you get used to untucking the tailbone, and for strengthening the glutes (your butt muscles).

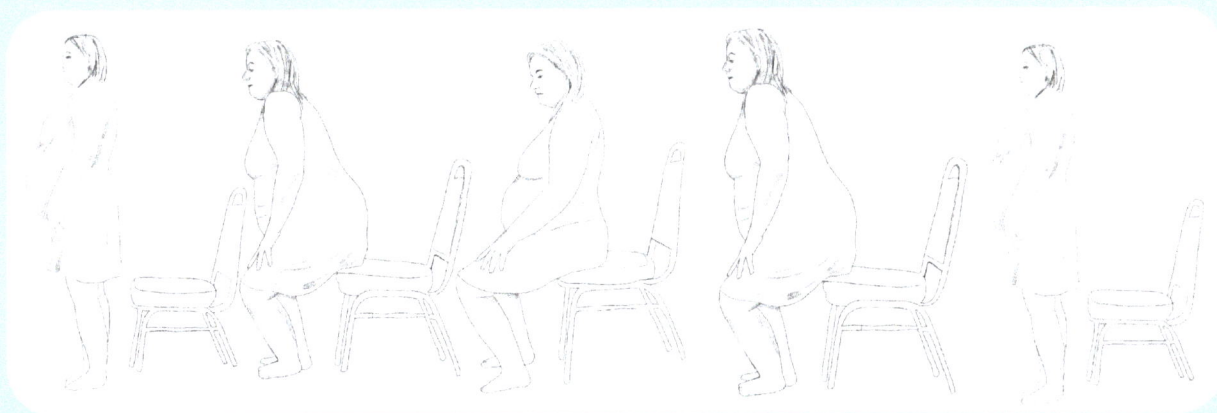

When you feel ready to squat lower than the chair, stand with your legs a bit wider than hip distance apart. Allow your toes to point out at about a 45-degree angle. Making sure that your knees are going straight over your toes and keeping your spine tall, engage your pelvic floor and core muscles as you allow your tail to sink down and back toward your heels. Your goal is to sit into the pose with your heels on the ground or sinking down toward the ground. You do not want to hold up your weight with your leg muscles. You want to settle your weight down through your bony structure, relaxing your thighs. If your heels don't easily settle to the ground, try wearing shoes with a low heel or placing a rolled-up yoga mat or two equal-sized books under your heels for support. Gradually, as you increase flexibility in your calves and hips, you can work towards being barefoot against the floor. If you feel gripping in your leg muscles, try using your partner or a solid doorframe for support. Work to relax your shoulders, arms, and chest, and keep your spine long with your sternum open and lifted toward the sky.

After your squatting explorations, how do you feel? These shapes may feel foreign, plus your body is changing day by day. Be kind and gentle with yourself and allow your feelings to shift as you learn and grow. This week, explore, strengthen and relax your vagina and pelvic floor. Tone your abdominals, explore pelvic rocks, cat/cow, and squatting. Experiment with different approaches to meditation and relaxation. Eat good food, drink water, be physically active, and get ample rest. Laugh and cry. Additionally, try to identify some of your stressors and see if you can find ways to solve problems that can reduce stress. Look into making plans to watch some birth videos. (See this book's Appendix for suggestions.) Reach out for support when you need it; don't be shy about asking for help. Likewise, look to help others, especially those with new babies. As I will say again and again, reciprocity is a lifeline. And perhaps most importantly, give yourself credit for what you have already accomplished today and yesterday. Forgive yourself any perceived shortcomings. With good intentions and a commitment to try, you will do great! You are already doing great now!

Congratulations on finishing Week 3. I wish you a fantastic week to come.

HOMEWORK

A) Physical exercises, including vaginal exercises, abdominal bracing, pelvic rocks, and squats

B) Breath awareness

Alternate positions for diaphragmatic breath awareness practice:

1. The partner sits and leans back against a wall, then the pregnant person sits in between their legs and leans back against their partner's chest. Both people face the same direction. The partner then lets their hands reach around and gently rest on the pregnant person's low belly.

2. Spoons in bed. The partner (the big spoon) should drape their arm over, so that their hand rests on the pregnant person's belly. Tactile feedback on the low belly can increase awareness and encourage deep relaxation.

3. Standing hug. Both of you stand facing each other and hug. Bring your torsos together with as much body contact as is comfortably possible. Try variations on this position that allow you to relax your shoulders and arms as much as possible. In standing positions, try not to lock the knees, try to keep them soft with a slight bend.

C) Meditation with visualization

Continue to build a daily practice of moving your body and breath awareness twice a day, once on your own and once with your partner. For this week plan to really build discipline into your practice routines.

Additional Visualizations for relaxation and meditation practice: Experiment with each of the following exercises in the side relaxation position. Also experiment in other positions.

1) **Progressive relaxation:**
   Start at the tips of your toes or the top of your head, then name and think through each body part as you consciously try to relax each area.

2) **Tense and release:**
   Systematically contract with maximum tension each area of the body, then soften and relax each area of the body. Again, start at the top of your head or the bottom of your feet and work your way through the whole body.

3) **A description of a beautiful location:**
   In your mind's eye, clearly see a beautiful location. Describe for yourself or for your partner this beautiful location. Perhaps it is one you have been to before, or perhaps it is made up. Include all the senses when you are describing this location. For example: Feel the warm sand or the cool breeze, taste the salt air or the chocolate cake, smell the spring rain or the roses growing, hear the ocean waves or the fire crackling, see the blue sky, etc.

4) **A favorite prayer or poem or song:**
   Insert your own here.

THIS SPACE IS FOR YOUR NOTES AND DRAWINGS

THIS SPACE IS FOR YOUR NOTES AND DRAWINGS

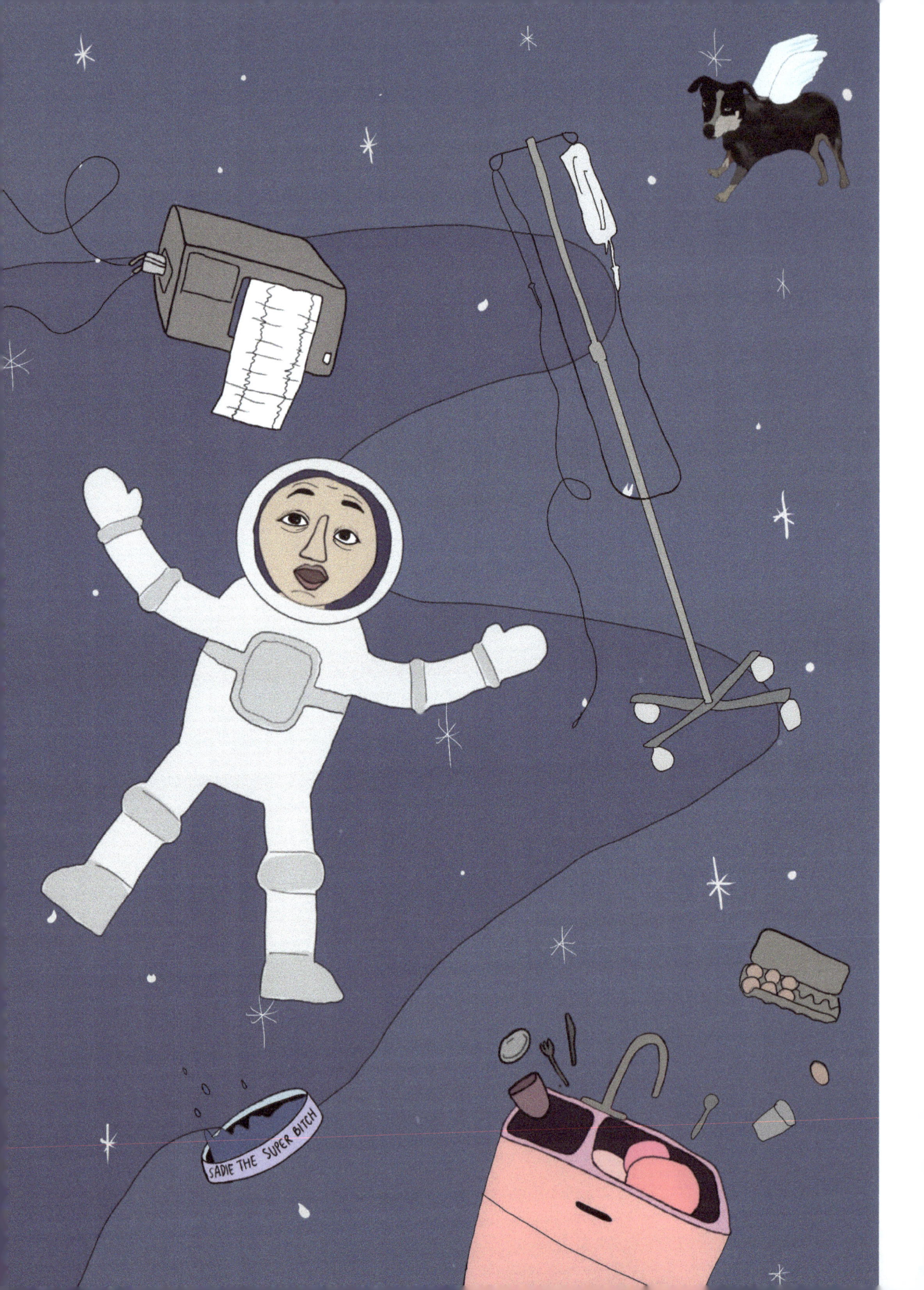
SADIE THE SUPER BITCH

WEEK 4

Take Responsibility

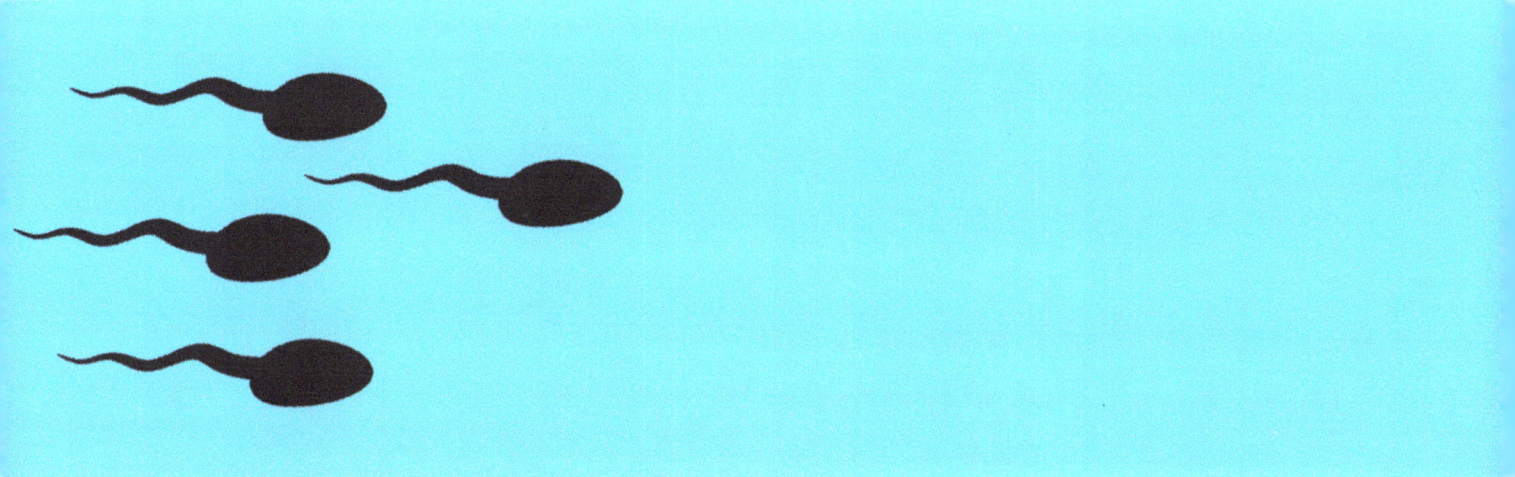

Chapter contents:

- Modalities of maternity care
- Interview skills and questions
- Prenatal ultrasound testing

THIS SPACE IS FOR YOUR NOTES AND DRAWINGS

Welcome to Week 4! I hope last week went well and that you enjoyed building your relaxation and exercise practice. Did you make time for that daily? If not, did you try anything out, even once or twice? If not, did you maybe think about trying some of these new exercises sometime? One of my favorite TV quotes comes from Bart Simpson. It's a quote about doing better in school: "I can't promise I'll try, but I'll try to try."[83] Creating space, whether it's thinking or doing or both, can be the first step toward implementing new routines using the practices presented throughout this book. And when you're ready, this book is here for you!

If you did some homework, how was it? Did you notice any changes? Whether or not you accomplished all that you set out to accomplish this past week or the weeks before, it is helpful to review your motivations. Ask yourself now: why do you want to do your homework? What specific gains are you hoping to achieve? What hurdles do you face? How best can you continue to try to make good choices?

Ruminate, too, on the chapter art presented this week: Sheela in Space. What do you want the physical space to be like for your birth? Who would you like to be present for it? What is the space between you and medical technology? What kind of space can you make in your life for this pregnancy and your baby?

Medical consumerism: Who you hire matters

When you hire a provider, you get the package deal: their training, ability/skill level, ethics (sense of right and wrong), values, biases, and fears. All of those factors will impact their practice and the decisions that are available to you in your pregnancy and birth. In fact, all of these same factors inform the content I'm presenting to you here, in this book! It appears to me that who you hire to care for you is perhaps the single biggest predictor of what happens to you and your baby during birth. The routines and expectations of your provider, as well as the way your provider views birth as a process, seems to impact your birth outcome even more than your anatomy and physiology. Look at it this way: if you hire a provider that has a 40% rate for performing cesarean sections, your odds of having a cesarean section seem to jump to 40% just by walking in the door. It is possible to birth, at least somewhat, independently of your provider's expectations; however, it's safer and arguably easier to hire someone that is already on the same page with you.

In my Bradley® class I teach the term "medical consumerism," and I focus in part on teaching students to be savvy consumers of medical services. When it comes to other types of consumerism, such as buying a vacuum cleaner or a TV set, many of us do our research. First, we collect information: What is out there? How many brands are available? What are the differences in functionality, size, cost, etc.? Second, we balance the pros and cons of our options before making our selection. Sometimes this is an annoyingly long process! If you need to hire a contractor for a building or repair job, as another example, hopefully you get references, you perform interviews, you compare answers, and you develop specific criteria for awarding the job. By contrast, people rarely follow this same process when it comes to hiring a healthcare provider. I often hear: "Dr. So-and-So has been my gynecologist for years, so I just stayed with her when I got pregnant." It is important to understand that a gynecologist is not necessarily the appropriate person for your maternity care. And, more importantly, just because a provider was meeting your needs prior to pregnancy, this doesn't mean they will still be the appropriate choice for pregnancy and birth.

Now that you're pregnant, you're a new kind of consumer of healthcare services. You'll want to decide who you can most trust to look out for your best interests and the best interests of your baby. Whose routines and expectations do you want to influence your birth outcome? Which providers are keeping up with evidence-based birth practices? Who is going to get your dollars and the insurance dollars that you represent? Who will you feel most comfortable with if they need to touch your vagina for a vaginal exam? Who do you want to be near you as you meet your baby? If you have hired someone you do not like, you can often fire them. You just need to verify the workings of your health insurance and what kind of flexibility it allows in terms of choosing your provider. Some of my clients have changed providers two or three times during a pregnancy before finding their best fit. If you can't change providers, you still want to retain some healthcare. You can continue to inform yourself and work to make *your* best decisions. Be fierce and birth your way, regardless.

When you can't change providers, there is good work to be done in discovering what the provider's routine birth practices are for the average, low-risk gestational parent. This information will help you to differentiate what in their recommendations pertain directly to your circumstances, and what doesn't. Learning about your provider's routines gives you a foundation from which to better see if those routines are evidence-based and appropriate to you. This foundation will also help you to advocate for your own needs, and help you to make your own informed decisions.

In an ideal client/provider scenario, you will have the longest time possible to develop a good relationship. But the ideal doesn't have to be met. I have one friend, for example, who changed her provider at 41 weeks pregnant. Her original provider told her that if she hadn't had her baby by the end of the week, then they would insist on inducing. This ultimatum not only ignored the fact that all of her medical tests were negative for any concerns; it disregarded her own wishes not to be induced. Consequently, she switched to another practice and ended up having an uncomplicated, spontaneous vaginal birth about 3 days past the arbitrary date of mandatory induction assigned by her old practice. She was quite lucky that her new practice was willing to take her on as a patient at such a late date. More than likely, it was helpful that she had also been working with a doula—a trained birth assistant—who had a good working relationship with the new doctor. The doula put in a phone call to the new practice to say that she had been working with this woman for months and that she seemed healthy in body and mind. That phone call helped to reassure the new team. In my opinion, if you find a provider that is willing to take you on, it's never too late to change practices. Nevertheless, you want to start researching your care options as soon as possible, careful also to include any network of resources you may have, to allow for the strongest connections to be made. Simply start now, if you haven't already or if you have any uncertainties about who you have already chosen.

Maternity care modalities: What are the choices?

There are different types of doctors and midwives, not to mention different personalities and practice styles within each. There are obstetricians, who are primarily surgeons (obstetrics is a surgical subspecialty). Gynecologists are also surgeons, but they don't necessarily practice obstetrics. Meanwhile, some obstetricians do practice basic gynecological care as well as maternity care and surgical procedures. There are also obstetric subspecialty categories, including high-risk obstetricians who specialize in pregnant people with significant medical complications. And there are family-practice doctors. Generally, these doctors are not surgeons, although some do obtain advanced training in cesarean section.

In midwifery care the choice is also nuanced, in part because of the variations in state laws and insurance mandates. Generally, midwives carry Certified Nurse Midwife (CNM), Certified Midwife (CM), or Direct-Entry Midwife (DEM) credentials.[84] While Certified Nurse Midwives are trained as nurses first, Certified Midwives are not nurses, and Direct-Entry Midwives are trained through apprenticeships. Whereas Certified Nurse Midwives can practice in hospitals or at home, Certified Midwives and Direct-Entry Midwives attend only homebirths. On the insurance side, Medicaid and most private forms of health insurance cover Certified Nurse Midwives.[85] Some private insurance companies also cover Certified Midwives. Midwifery certification and licensing is in a state of flux across the country and may well have changed by the time you are reading this book, so you will have to research what is available in your area and how it works (or doesn't) with your insurance.

My homebirth midwife, with the certification of Certified Midwife, was not recognized to practice midwifery in New York State in the year 2000 when I gave birth to my second son. (Ina May Gaskin, a world-renowned midwife, was also not recognized.) The law in New York has since changed, but back in 2000 my midwife would have been able to practice in other states, and in some states my insurance would have paid her. (In addition to wholeheartedly supporting a person's right to a safe and legal abortion, I also want "reproductive rights" to mean that all people can have options to birth how, where, and with whom they choose.) Regardless of her lack of NYS licensing, I trusted her credentials and I trusted her. I love her and I am forever grateful to her for having the strength and the dedication to endure the risks she took allowing me to have a safe and satisfying birth in my own home.

The category of nurse midwife, in my opinion, needs further subdivision, as I alluded to in the Week 1 lesson of this book. For instance, there are midwives who practice with a medical "management" perspective. These midwives are essentially performing the role of "doctor extender." Then there are nurse midwives who practice a more holistic midwifery model of care, as fully independent practitioners that care for the whole person and who will consult with their colleagues in the hospital as needed. Learning to distinguish the medical midwives, or "med-wives," from the *midwifery* midwives is frequently a challenge for my clients. I will address this challenge, but first I want to look at some of the broader differences between the medical and midwifery models of care.

The medical model of care, as it is currently being practiced, is based on the belief that birth is a risky and unbearable business, and that it should be managed by specialists. Obstetricians are trained to procedurally *manage* an unreliable, lengthy, and burdensome birth. The term "management" can be understood as medical speak for what the doctor does at a birth. In some cases, this can translate into a fearful and impatient approach to maternity care, one that relies on interventions to monitor, speed up, and then fix a supposedly problematic process. Such a medical mindset can lead to an exclusion of the gestational parent's emotional well-being as an element of the birth, instead placing primary emphasis on the provider's job to manage (read: control) the birth and protect the birthing person from the "horrors" of their (are we to assume, shameful?) experience.

Doctors are trained to view the process of labor by the measurements of the cervix, the strength of the uterine contractions, and the baby's heart tones.[86] Vitals from the pregnant person's heart, lungs, and blood pressure are also important, of course. But from what I have observed, nowhere in obstetrical medical protocol is there a place to pull all of a person's pieces back together—that is, to address the whole person, including their values and emotions. Nowhere is the practice informed by an understanding of a gestational person's holistic workings. The compartmentalization ignores, for example, the exquisite hormonal feedback system that creates a safe and manageable birth. Obstetricians, as a further example, disregard the endocrine system when they disregard a pregnant person's emotional well-being in labor. (In the obstetrician's defense, their training tells them that endocrinologists study and care for the endocrine system.)

One of my clients reported that she told her doctor she did not want to have an IV port put in at the hospital because it would "stress her out." (An IV port is an intravenous needle inserted into your arm that gets capped off and taped down in case it is needed later to administer fluids or medicines.) The doctor's response was that the patient's stress was "not her problem." The doctor's job was to keep her alive should an emergency arise. Although this doctor may be a very adept surgeon, after that comment they present as a dangerously undereducated birth attendant. The doctor went on to express her fears that my client (a healthy, low-risk patient) could all of a sudden have an emergency, such as a placental abruption (when the placenta prematurely separates from the uterine lining). She tried to convince my client that she "needed" an IV port. The doctor's coercive message was complete with a description of my client in a pool of blood on the floor. This doctor may well have been traumatized from a past experience, and is perhaps now caring for every person from this distorted view. Of course, there are rare medical disasters that could lead to this graphic nightmare, with placental abruption indeed being one. (Some of the risk factors for placental abruption include using cocaine, smoking cigarettes, multiple fetuses, previous abruption, and car accidents.[87]) In this scenario a person would need immediate surgery, but preemptive IV access—or the lack thereof—would not be the limiting factor. Please note, as a whole America does a really good job with emergency medical care in true emergencies. If a person needs an IV in an emergency, they get one (and there are multiple methods for gaining IV access, in proportion to the emergency).

What we don't much talk about are doctors being afraid. Doctors do seem to generally fear birth. They treat it as an intense medical procedure rather than a healthy human function. This fear is increased when they must take a disproportionate amount of responsibility for the safety of the birth process, while at the same time lacking some crucial education and skills needed to safely support it. Moreover, these doctors are often not allotted the time it would take to safely support the birth process. Yes, there are things that can go wrong in birth that no one can see coming, and outcomes can improve with useful redirections. (A diabetic with blood sugar trouble, someone with an infection, someone with very high blood pressure, or a baby in a very stubborn funky position that's just not descending, are some examples.) And sometimes there are other complications that don't have manageable solutions and seemingly no one can fix, such as a horrific congenital malfunction. Shit happens, we're human.

—Pause—
Close your eyes and take a few breaths, notice any feelings that may have arisen about things you can't control.
Life is full of things we can't control, such as pathological anomalies or our children's thinking.
Release any stress you don't need. Consider looking for gratitude in this moment of your full breath.

Our culture elevates the status of a doctor to superhuman, and we expect them to be able to ward off all ills. It's just not so. Yet many patients and some doctors continue to believe that if the doctor can just control things enough, no harm will come. However, not every problem can be fixed with "control." It is an intense stress when there are several people witnessing a birth and something seems very off. The doctor thinks, "Oh no! If something goes wrong here I will be blamed!" That *is* a huge fear, especially if you don't have an honest and open decision-sharing relationship with the client. After years of learning to look at birth as a set of risks that can lead to disaster, the medical surgeon becomes adept at viewing pregnancy and birth as a fearful complication needing to be "managed" and "fixed." Our profit-based, litigious healthcare system complicates this further.

The fearful doctor is also monetarily rewarded for each additional action of intervention, and this makes fear profitable. Cesarean sections, for example, become the gold standard because they are seen as the most "controllable" type of birth. Doctors make more money for performing a surgery over a vaginal birth. They also don't judge each other harshly for doing unnecessary procedures, only for not doing procedures. Every doctor fears the following questions: "What happened? How come you couldn't prevent this tragedy? What did you miss? What did you do wrong?" Even if the tragedy is a natural occurrence and there is no way the provider could have helped, they may still face a lawsuit.

Now the doctor is being sued and their job security and professional reputation are at stake. Hundreds of thousands of dollars in medical school debt loom over their future like a dark angry cloud. Moreover, the mother they couldn't save, for example, looks just like their sister, daughter, girlfriend, or aunt, and they have their own personal grief to contend with; yet, they have been trained to stuff those feelings down to the bottom of their soul. In her book, *Kitchen Table Wisdom,* Dr. Rachel Naomi Remen writes on the subject of medical training and the practices of stifling emotion and human connection.[88] She shares her story of becoming a doctor while also being a patient. Her book describes her being reprimanded for crying with a family that had just suffered a tragedy, and how she didn't cry for years after that on account of her being shamed by her attending physician. Happily, she did start to cry again and her work focuses on and illustrates the potential for healing that comes from being real with each other—provider to patient—and sharing and honoring each other's experiences and our stories.

> Everybody is a story. When I was a child, people sat around kitchen tables and told their stories. We don't do that so much anymore. Sitting around the table telling stories is not just a way of passing time. It is the way the wisdom gets passed along. The stuff that helps us to live a life worth remembering. Despite the awesome powers of technology many of us still do not live very well. We may need to listen to each other's stories once again.[89]

Remen's book encourages me to keep sharing my stories. I hope my story and the information I am bringing to these pages can help you to weed out the most controlling and emotionally disconnected providers, and instead seek out the most emotionally grounded providers who seek to engage in honest and respectful discourse and shared decision making.

Sadly, there are no, or certainly not enough, empathy and emotional support techniques that are taught to doctors in medical school, either for the care of their patients or for their own emotional needs.[90] And though the trend may change over time, for providers in practice today, it is not considered the surgeon's job to be a comfort. I should re-emphasize this point: Medical students who want to deliver babies and perform surgery go on to become obstetricians. That means that these such people who choose to specialize in surgery are currently defining and controlling the attitudes and accompanying protocols that dictate the medical modality of maternity care in U.S. hospitals.

By contrast, midwives, trained in the midwifery model of care, are educated to support and guide the whole person through the unfolding of their birth process. Midwifery students (at least in theory) want to work with pregnant people and their families. Midwives are trained to see birth as the healthy life process that it is. They are experts in normal and healthy function. Midwives are trained to stand by and witness the unfolding of a birth, almost like a lifeguard does at the beach. (It is worth noting here that economic pressures to care for too many patients weigh on all hospital workers, midwives included.) Midwives are trained to be independent providers. Likewise, because midwives are taught to identify the functioning of healthy people, they recognize when something looks off and will consult with other medical specialists (obstetricians, hematologists, infectious disease experts, etc.) when appropriate. They are also trained in emergency life stabilization and resuscitation techniques for pregnant and birthing people and babies, as well as a vast array of physical and emotional labor support techniques. A midwife will monitor the gestational person's and baby's vital signs to monitor health and progress. Simultaneously, this midwife keeps a careful eye on the connection between her client's state of mind and body functions. Midwives should also be trained to have patience for labor. A midwife should understand the importance of maternal stress reduction for optimal birth function. One generalized way to think about it: midwives seek to support life; obstetricians seek to fight death. The midwifery model of care is patient, while the medical model is impatient.

Of course, differences abound in medical doctors and midwives alike. We are all individuals, after all. There are some amazingly gentle, patient and wise doctors who both keep up with current research for their care perspectives and understand how to really care for birthing people. Yet, while they do understand the importance of compassionate and continuous care, even these doctors don't have the time in our current healthcare system to stand by a person's side from start to finish. And yet, we have scientific evidence showing that continuous care during birth improves the experience and reduces the need for medications and other interventions.[91]

Great providers value an educated and responsible patient who demands evidence-based care and genuine emotional support. One such wonderful doctor, a compassionate and skilled obstetrician I had the honor of working with in my professional capacity as a doula, once gently told me he didn't think anyone should give birth in a hospital without a doula. He said this shortly after we had just attended a birth together. It had been a long birth and we both knew that my doula skills had helped to keep the woman calm and feeling safe. This attention to her emotional well-being enabled her to yield to her sensations and work with her body to birth her baby. He hugged me with gratitude for my service to our shared client, and we rejoiced in the birth and in our respectful collaboration.

If you want or need to choose maternity care from a doctor, you will be better served if you understand that equally well-trained doctors can have vastly different routines, some manage to keep up with the research while others rely solely on how they were trained in school, such that Doctor "A" always uses every intervention and Doctor "B" never routinely uses any. They each "manage" a healthy low-risk pregnancy with completely different approaches. Which one of these two doctors will be a better fit for you? Or would you be better off with a midwife?

As mentioned above, midwives also come with different styles. Despite the specialty's reputation, there are some seemingly uncaring midwives out there, so you must screen them closely too. Some hospital-based midwives get burned out. They can't care so much anymore. They seem to want to speed up the process and get you out the door. There are also drug-happy midwives who are quick to medicate a patient; in hospitals it is viewed as compassionate to try to eradicate sensation with medication. Perhaps this also helps to reduce the amount of emotional care a provider will feel obligated to offer during their shift.

Interviewing midwives that are paid by hospitals and doctor's groups is a tricky process. All midwives understand and are taught the midwifery model of care, at least on paper.[92] So if a client of mine is asking conscientious and open-ended questions, it is quite possible for the midwife to answer with responses that really fit the bill of a wonderful model of midwifery care. The midwife knows what the pregnant person wants to hear so she sounds great in the interview, but in practice that midwife ends up really practicing like a doctor extender. She gains the person's trust through the interview and the prenatal appointments and then spends little to no quality time with them in labor. And when the midwife is in the room, she is actively trying to win permission to try and speed things along. (An educated partner and/or a doula can offer protection from this—keep reading!)

The economic pressures on hospital providers can and do blur the distinctions between care modalities. The influence of our insurance system takes its toll as well. In his important book, *Born in the USA*, Marsden Wagner points out that obstetricians in the U.S. have to pay $400 per day on average in malpractice insurance just to be able to go to work.[93] (This cost varies by state.) That creates a lot of pressure to make money. Can you imagine seeing 30 or more patients in a routine office day? Then there are procedure days, and patient rounds, and being on call for deliveries and late-night surgeries. Obstetricians work a lot of very long hours, and they are generally under a great deal of stress. It is a shame that our system is so off balance. Ideally, we'd like our surgeons to be rested and relaxed, right? The same should go for our midwives.

By now you're probably asking, "So how do I find the provider that is right for me?" Keep reading.

Defining your birth values is a critical step in making your best decisions

Take responsibility for your choices by exploring and developing your own birth values. What did your family teach you to value about your body, the pregnancy and the birth experience? (Do you remember that homework assignment to investigate your birth history from Week 1? If you didn't remember and haven't done your family investigation homework from Week 1, I encourage you to complete it this week.) What have you learned from television and movies, from society-at-large? Connecting to your birth history helps you prepare for your future birth.

What do you value about pregnancy and the birth process? What is important to you? What are you afraid of? Are you more afraid of the potential for pain or of the needles used for pain medication? Are you worried about your own safety or that something will be wrong with your baby? Ask yourself the tough questions; this is how you will face your fears. Say them out loud. Name them. "I am scared I won't be able to handle this birth. I think the pain will be too much. I think I will freak out and be hysterical. I think I might die from the pain." Or, maybe your fears are more about the baby dying or being malformed, or people being rude or coercing you into things you don't want, or that you might poop in front of your birth team, or that your partner will pass out or be afraid of your vagina afterwards. Perhaps your fears are more focused on the challenges of parenting: How can we afford to raise this child? Will the earth be too polluted? How will we cope with the dangers of our society? Will I be a good parent?

Consider your values, reflections, and fears. Speak, write, and/or draw them here.

Remember: it is ok to be afraid. It is ok to say it out loud. You can't make your fears come true by expressing them in words (or drawings, songs, dances, etc.). But you *can* work through them, once you acknowledge them. Defining your birth values helps you open for birth.

Before I got pregnant with my second child, I thought I wanted to have him at home. But once I was pregnant, my fears started to surface and I started thinking about a hospital plan. I interviewed many different providers and toured many different facilities, before I realized I should sift through my concerns to get to the bottom of what I felt. At first, I thought I didn't want a home birth because I was afraid for my husband. I thought, "What if something bad happens during the birth and he is somehow seen by the state as acting inappropriately because of his training and medical license?" (He is a Physician's Assistant). Then I thought it was because I was afraid if something went wrong at home people might blame me, call me selfish for wanting an idealized experience for myself over the safety of my baby. And then finally I arrived at the crux of it: I was scared for my baby's safety. I wasn't that scared of my birth sensations, and it wasn't that Julian's medical license or people's judgments were what really mattered to me. I was scared something would be wrong or go wrong with my birth. I was particularly scared of the "pushing" part of labor; for me it was the as-yet-unknown part of the birth experience. (Remember: I had dilated in my first birth but then went to surgery for a c/section before the expulsive phase began.)

Once I finally dug down to the seeds of my fear, I realized my chief concern was not simply for my baby's safety, but for my baby's safety *during the journey out*. That may seem logical or simple now as you read this, but for me it was the process of exploration that led me to identify the specific cause of my fear. Once I was there, and had said it out loud, I could untangle and confront it. I could ask myself the next question: Where will my baby be safest? For me the answer to that question would be the place where I'd have the most continuity of care with a trusted provider. I knew that if I had good continuity of care and good trust in my support, I'd have less stress, and less stress would be better for the baby and the outcome of the birth. Ultimately, I knew that by staying at home I would reduce interruptions—and then I could really get my work done.

For me, homebirth would create the circumstances necessary for the safest journey possible. I trusted that the homebirth midwife would really be able to get to know me. I knew that her services included planning to spend the entire birth by my side. I felt completely certain that if something were to start to deviate from normal in my process, she would be quick to notice. She explained in our interviews that she would work to get to know me, what I looked like, what my baby and I felt like, what my fears and challenges were, and what my thoughts were about my birth process. She would learn about what I ate, how I exercised, how I slept, and how I was handling the emotional aspects of pregnancy. She would get to know Julian, my husband, and what his health was like, too. She would get to know my older son. She would come to our home. She would meet our dog. She would see our kitchen and learn about the foods we ate. I knew in my heart that she would be the best one to monitor me, my baby, and my process.

Once I identified that my main concern was for the baby, I was able to understand that bad things do happen to babies in life, but that is as true in hospitals as it is in homes. I understood that sometimes babies need oxygen and that my midwife would have that. Sometimes babies need their lungs suctioned; my midwife could do that. I faced the reality that sometimes things go wrong even in hospitals with a very high level of care. Sometimes babies and gestational people die. Being in a hospital couldn't really protect me from being human. Given my own pregnancy and birth plan, I trusted that my midwife would have the tools and the skill necessary to stabilize us if we needed to transport to the hospital in an emergency. I also knew that if I could create my birth plan to proceed as smoothly as possible, with as little extra stress and interruption as possible, I could give my baby the best chance. Once I accepted my fear, I made the plan that intellectually and emotionally suited us. If my primary fear had been something different, I may well have made different decisions.

Realizing your goals for your safest and healthiest birth is about understanding your personal beliefs and concerns as well as your unique health history. It's also about understanding normal healthy birth and the negative effects of excess stress and interruption. Furthermore, your plans will be fine-tuned when you evaluate the beliefs and fears of those around you. With this understanding, you are closer to being able to evaluate your provider's practices in relation to existing research on best birth practices. Then, in turn, you will be ready to really participate in your care decisions.

Once you learn accurate information about birth physiology (which I provide later in this book!) and combine that with a connection to your values and emotional concerns, including an understanding of what your specific fears are, only then can you begin to accurately evaluate your needs in a birth provider, a location, and coping approaches. Once you decide what you think your birth should look like and how you should be treated by the people around you, you can begin to measure your options against your needs. Who helps you to feel safe and why? What will your insurance cover? Don't just make this up in your head: do your research. Just as you can contact your insurance provider to further explore your options, you can seek out real films of real images of as many different settings and types of birth as you can find. (See the Appendix for some film suggestions.)

Choosing between hospital and home birth

There is no one best place for everybody to have a baby. The best place for you to have your baby is the place that you will feel safest and most comfortable. If you have access to both homebirth and hospital birth providers, and there are no known outlying medical concerns that would rule out homebirth, I encourage you to fully research both options before making your selection. At the time of this writing, there are woefully few genuine birth centers around the country (meaning, out-of-hospital birth locations). Genuine birth centers rely on midwives, usually don't have the staff to administer pain medications, and therefore rely on non-medication pain relief techniques, such as emotional support, showers and tubs, massage, and mindfulness techniques. Should you have access to one or more of these birth centers, I encourage you to investigate this option as well. But beware: many hospitals call their maternity care floor their "birth center." The majority of these bear no resemblance to actual out-of-hospital birth centers. These hospital departments refer to themselves as a birth center, typically as a marketing term, to make it sound cozier, when in fact there is little to differentiate the care received there than from the Labor and Delivery department of a "regular hospital."

Even if you have already made your decision as to where you will birth and whom you want to hire, I encourage you to keep an open mind. **If you have any uncertainty about the choices you have already made, you've got nothing to lose by continuing to investigate other providers or locations.** If, in your family, one person feels drawn to a homebirth and another person feels fearful, as is a frequent scenario I have witnessed, I think it is fruitful to have both people meet with a homebirth midwife for research. I encourage the person with homebirth concerns to think deeply about their concerns and then write them in a list to share with a potential homebirth midwife and allow them to address these worries directly in the interview.

When planning for a homebirth one never knows in advance if they might need to transport to the hospital; that is always under consideration in a homebirth-midwife's mind. Going forward in this book, remember that even if you are planning a homebirth it's important to learn about the hospital routines and considerations, in the event that you end up needing or choosing to make a transfer. For those of you planning a hospital birth, please remember that it does not work in reverse; it is not safe or advisable to decide to just stay home. I do not support the plan of unattended birth. But as you likely still have time ahead to fine tune the plans you have already made, let's carry on with some pointers for your decision making.

When choosing a hospital birth: Provider or location?

If you are planning a hospital birth, your choice of care provider is generally more important than which particular hospital you are choosing. There are tremendous differences in hospitals and in hospital cultures. But it is the person (or group practice) who is going to manage your care that you want to review most carefully. I urge you to investigate both the providers and birth settings for tone and feeling and for the language they use when discussing birth. Also investigate concrete facts, such as the doctor's and the hospital's rates of cesarean section. (Note that laws vary by state as to what information institutions and providers are obligated to provide).

My clients have occasionally been caught in a muddle of finger pointing. While the doctor says, "Gee I would love to accommodate your desire to _____ but it's against hospital protocol," the hospital administrator says, "Gee, we would love to accommodate your desire to_____ but the doctor will not sign off on that." Ultimately hospital administrators want you to get in and out of the hospital quickly, happily and alive. They do not generally want to get involved in the micro management of care; they rely on the doctor to make those decisions. The doctor wants to get you in and out quickly, happily and alive, too, but ultimately it is their job to make all judgement calls in treatment, and then to discuss your options with you so that you can make the final decision. I have observed that doctors who have more confidence in the birth process, and more confidence in shared decision making, are less likely to answer patient requests for low intervention with, "but I have to because the hospital says so." Likewise, from what I have witnessed, doctors who are less open to shared medical decision making are more likely to frame their decisions as out of their control. This is why I emphasize that although hospital culture matters a great deal, the provider matters most.

By the same token, when possible, visiting a prospective hospital remains an essential part of making your informed decision. I have had clients that picked a particular hospital because of a doctor they wanted there, but after touring they decided to find another provider because the hospital wasn't right for them; something about the hospital culture felt off. These are important feelings to balance in your decision, whenever possible. Take time to weigh as many of the variables within your control as you can.

Your questions matter

In life, the questions you ask lead to the answers you get. It is *you* who must figure out what things you will need to learn to be able to make your best decisions. How you word your questions and the attitudes you convey (the emotions you express) will directly affect the responses you get. I intend for you to generate many questions as you work your way through this book. Allow one question to give birth to another question and then another... and another.

- Why is the sky blue? Because it is daytime.
- Why is it daytime? Because you were up all night.
- Why were you up all night? Because you went on a moon lit walk with your lover that turned into a dance at dawn.

Are there different possible answers to each of the above questions? Absolutely. Seek out answers to the same questions from a variety of care providers—you'll be surprised at the variation in response! Be sure to compare and contrast these answers. Listen to your gut (and your heart, and your vagina) as you react to the answers you get. This process will help you to find the right care provider for you, and it will help you to build trust with the care provider you choose.

Interview Skills

In order to conduct a useful interview, and ask the questions that need asking for *your* decision-making process, you must first consider the following two general questions:

1. What questions should I be asking?

2. How should I be phrasing my questions?

What questions you ask may often depend on what type of practitioner you are interviewing and what you want to find out. But how you word your questions and the attitudes you convey are universal to the interview process.

<u>Interview rule #1</u>: "Don't lead the answer"

"Don't lead the answer" means don't give away the response you are looking for with the question. For example, imagine you are interviewing a prospective provider and you ask: "I want to have a natural birth, can you support me in that?" It's very simple for a provider to respond, "Yes, of course. That works for many people, but if I see something that concerns me, I will need to intervene." On the surface, this sounds like a great answer, but ultimately it tells you nothing about that provider's routines and birth perspectives (beyond their willingness to intervene—but when, how, and to what extent would such intervention occur?). You have no better idea of the provider's actual practice now than you did before you asked your leading question. Instead, you were likely told what you wanted to hear because of the leading question.

Instead, try the question another way: "I have heard many different perspectives on how I should plan for and cope with pain in my labor. I am still uncertain about the benefits and the risks of pain medication in birth. Birth is your area of expertise not mine, so how do you suggest I think about this decision?" With this type of phrasing you haven't given away what you are looking for and the person is free to share their opinions. You are deferring to their expertise, but also making your voice and your investment in doing your research solid parts of your birth plan. If you already know what you want, you may feel like you are playing dumb. If you honestly haven't yet figured out where you stand on the use of pain medication, you can consider this an opportunity for further research. Either way, when you keep your preferences to yourself, you allow the provider to answer freely without fear of alienation. This is how you get real answers.

Whether they are doctors, midwives, doulas, or birth teachers, providers will likely attempt to tell you what you want to hear whenever they can, especially in an interview situation. They have egos, like all humans, and they will likely enjoy pleasing you. You are probably a very nice person! Why wouldn't they want to work with you? Plus, you represent *dollars*. When you like someone's answers you validate their worth, build their esteem and put dollars in their pockets. Avoiding any leading questions can therefore provide you with the best opportunity to understand a provider's routines and perspectives (ostensibly free from your own biases), which of course is key to determining if she will be a good match for your care.

<u>Interview rule #2</u>: "Be friendly and positive"

You want the person you are interviewing to feel comfortable and encouraged to answer your questions honestly. If you can be cheerful, honest, and warm, then the person you are speaking with will feel more at ease and will more likely echo these traits in her responses. You are trying to get a sense of who this person is as a professional, while also gauging her capacity for compassion, kindness, and patience. When you are more relaxed, your prospective provider will be more relaxed and then she will be more revealing of her practice routines and perspectives.

Interview topics for maternity care providers

The following list of questions and discussion points may include information you have not yet covered in this book. If you don't know anything about some of the topics outlined below, you can read ahead first or you can let your provider's answers be your first level of information. These example questions are in no particular order:

○ "Please tell me what to expect from your care during my birth. What is the typical experience like when a patient first arrives at the hospital?" (Or, "What typically happens when you first arrive at a patient's home?" for a homebirth.) "I want to understand what to expect for my care—physically and emotionally—during my birth."

○ "I understand that there may be a lot of decisions to make while I am under your care. I want to be responsible and fully participating, so I would like to understand how decisions get made and what my role really is."

○ "What, if any, prenatal tests do you routinely write orders for throughout a pregnancy, including but not limited to ultrasounds and vaginal exams?" (The final decision to consent to a test is *yours*. The provider may write orders, but you can say yes or no.) Follow up questions should include asking about risks and accuracy rates of suggested tests and when in the pregnancy or birth they typically take place.

○ "I have been hearing a lot about IV's and IV ports in labor. It seems like some providers use them all the time and some don't use them as much. Is that a tool that you will want to use? If so, why? If not, why not? Please explain IV use in labor."

○ "What are your thoughts about VBAC?" (vaginal birth after cesarean)

○ "Do you ever make the recommendation to use pain medications during birth? If so, when and why?"

○ "If I am hungry or thirsty in labor will it be okay for me to eat food and drink fluids, or are there restrictions?"

○ "Are there any risks associated with the use of pain medication? I have heard that they are very safe. Are they really?" (You may want to push them to list specific potential risks.)

○ "What percentage of your clients end up needing a cesarean section? Is there any one reason that stands out as the most common indication for surgery?"

○ "Are there any time limits for the individual stages of labor? If so, what are they and why?"

○ "Are there times that it is helpful to speed up a labor with medication (labor augmentation)? If so, when are those times and what is your preferred augmentation protocol?"

○ "Under what circumstances would you suggest [or 'want' or 'write orders for'] an induction of labor?" (Different words may give different reactions.)

○ "Do you have any restrictions or expectations about what position I should be in when the baby is coming out?" Good follow up questions are: "Have you ever had a person stand up to deliver their baby? Have you ever caught a baby when a gestational person was in an all-fours position, or while sitting on a toilet?" (If asking about these positions feels awkward, blame it on the "crazy" things you see on the internet these days!)

○ "What happens if my water breaks and I am at home?"

○ "I have heard pros and cons about working with doulas. Have any of your patients worked with doulas? Is this something you recommend or discourage, and why?" (I prefer the word "client" to "patient" for healthy pregnant people. But if you are interviewing a medical provider, it might feel more appropriate to use "patient.")

○ "How many hours in a week do you generally work?"

○ 'What is the most common procedure that you do?"

○ "On average, how many births in a week or month do you attend?"

That was a long list of questions. Which ones jump out at you? I suggest that you start with those when you create your own list of interview questions. If you're asking questions during a prenatal appointment with a doctor, which typically lasts about 15 minutes, then it is likely that you will have only a few minutes for these questions, at best. Realistically, you will need to pick only two or three questions per visit. Depending on how the appointment is going, you may be able to squeeze in a few more, so try to be prepared. If it is a formal interview/consultation you might have more time. It is always good to be aware of how much time the provider is allotting for your visit.

I do think it is a good idea to write down your questions and then review the list before you go into the appointment. A list of questions can help you to keep track of all the things you would like to learn about. It is true that some providers will misread a list. They may see it, not as an empowering educational tool, but as a sign that you are nervous and controlling. (Rooting out those negative responses might be a good argument for bringing in a list, but you need to feel that out for yourself.) In addition to having an actual list in hand, I think it a good idea to bring paper and pen into your appointment, in order to take notes during or directly after. I suggest writing down the answers you receive as well as your first impressions of the provider and of the visit overall. As you meet other providers you can re-read and compare your notes.

Explaining that you are eager to learn is a wonderful way to introduce yourself and describe your motivations. But if you feel awkward about taking notes in an appointment or interview meeting, it's always ok to blame your "pregnancy brain." Decide how *you* feel about taking notes and making lists. If it helps you to have your list with you, then by all means bring it. If you squirm at the idea of making lists and taking notes, forget about it. Getting your questions generated and asked is the only thing that matters; do it any way that works for you.

The goal for your interview/prenatal appointment is twofold: to figure out if someone's routines and perspectives are consistent with evidence-based practices and to determine if their values can align with yours. For example, do they have a strong belief that one type of birth is better than another, and if so what are their criteria? Once you figure that out, you can hire the provider who is the best match for you. If you and your provider are on the same page about the birth process and how to best support it, you can further work on building trust, which is essential to a safe birth collaboration.

Far too often I meet people (who do have choices) that hire a provider who has different values about birth than they do. These clients often try to get the provider to change routines. That doesn't work well, and is even insulting to the provider. We must assume that any licensed provider is highly trained and that they believe in their own practices, be they a surgeon, physician, nurse, midwife, or doula. Your job is to investigate your options and then hire the person whose birth values and routines most closely align with your own views. Of course, you may not know your own views until you start to really learn about the birth process. As you build your education your views will likely change and develop, which is why it's good to know that often you can change who you hire to care for you.

Three interview stories from Emily's real life

#1 When I was interviewing pediatricians during my first pregnancy, I asked a prospective pediatrician this: "I am not sure if I am going to breastfeed. I have to go back to work soon after my baby is born and I have heard that trying to breastfeed as a working mother is very difficult. What do you think is best in this situation?"

This well-meaning pediatrician didn't want to make me feel bad (I assume), so he answered: "If you line up a bunch of three-year-olds, you won't be able to tell which ones breastfed and which ones did not." What I understood him to be saying was, "It doesn't really matter if you breastfeed, so don't worry your pretty little head about it."

I smiled and said: "Oh, ok. Thank you."

I finished up the interview with some polite chitchat about their office and left. Once outside, I crossed his name off my list. His answer proved to me that he did not value breastfeeding over bottle-feeding, and I did. I knew going into the interview that I wanted to breastfeed. I also knew that if I led with the question, "I want to breastfeed, will you support me in that?", he would likely have responded with what he now knew I wanted to hear: "Absolutely, yes. Breastfeeding is great!"

Learning that he didn't really value breastfeeding over bottle-feeding, even if it meant that I had to be slightly less than honest in order to ask a less leading question, was important. I knew I wanted to breastfeed, and if I had hired him and then presented with breastfeeding challenges during the postpartum period, I was now certain he would have counseled me to supplement with bottles or abandon breastfeeding altogether.

I also saw the problem in his premise. He was right, on the one hand, that "if you line up a bunch of three-year-olds," you can't tell who breastfed and who did not just by looking at them. On the other hand, if these same three-year-olds were also holding up copies of their medical charts, you certainly can tell which ones breastfed by reading the data on these charts or seeing the larger stacks of paper in the three-year-olds' hands, should the charts be printed out. Formula-fed children tend to have much larger medical charts because they tend to have many more doctor's visits than breastfed children. Breastfeeding really does help to protect children from illness, but more about that later.

I went on to interview another doctor who responded to my same question by telling me that, although it would be a challenge to breastfeed and work outside the home, the benefits were too overwhelmingly important not to try. He was sure that when I understood how important breastfeeding was, I would find the motivation to persevere. He recommended La Leche League, an international organization that supports breastfeeding, for information.[94] He also said that his office would be available by phone and would do what they could to help me through the challenges. He got the job. I had found my pediatrician.

#2 I once had a highly respected and well-to-do, local doctor tell a client of mine (after she asked her open-ended questions about pain medications in labor): "You would be crazy to try and birth without an epidural."

That was all he offered. He never mentioned any of the risks associated with the use of pain medications, nor any alternatives to try first. I believe this was highly unethical and a reportable breach of her right to informed consent. He knowingly gave her incomplete information and he used fear to influence her opinion. I have countless stories like this one from my years of teaching the open-ended question technique, including a sad one about a hospital midwife who recommends against doula care. (See Week 15 for more on the benefits of doula care.)

#3 One final interview story, from Bradley Method® client, Paul:

> One of the most helpful things the Bradley® class taught us was what questions to ask our doctor, as well as how to ask them [to] receive [her] honest answer and not just the answer [we wanted] to

hear. We were able to ask about pain medications, the timing and expectations she had about labor, and statistics about C-sections. Through these questions we learned that our doctor did not share our philosophy on the labor and delivery process. ... My wife and I felt confident enough in our Bradley® education to not be intimidated by the medical profession. We knew what we wanted and were educated enough to use medical professionals' advice to make our decisions.[95]

Group medical practices

Due to the ever-increasing economic pressures on our healthcare system, and the nature of being on-call for maternity care, most providers form groups. The group practices present a difficult challenge for the person who wants to build a relationship with their provider. Most groups know that knowing your provider in advance of birth is helpful, so they encourage you to schedule prenatal appointments with all potential providers. If you really like each person in the group, then there is no problem. But it is also quite common to gravitate toward one provider more than the others, or to like everyone except for one particular doctor or midwife, who you don't want anywhere near you, ever. I always encourage my clients to put the onus on the group; let them figure out how to respect your preferences and keep you as a client. You can try to explain to someone in the group that you would like to stay with the practice, but the group would have to agree to cover for the one particular doctor or midwife you are unwilling to work with. You can also ask the provider that you like the best to be on-call for you. They may not be able to accommodate you, but if you don't ask, you'll never know. I have had individuals and groups make allowances to support a person's preferences in order to keep their business. Go ahead and ask for what you want, as this can be another determining factor in your decision-making about providers.

At 15 minutes a session you are not getting time to really build real relationships. Therefore, if you want a medical doctor from a group practice *and* you want to develop a relationship with someone who can provide continuous support, you may want to hire a birth doula. (Again, see Week 15 for doula care.) The more realistic your expectations are the better you will be able to work with your providers.

Under the U.S. Constitution you have (or in theory are supposed to have) the right to privacy and the right to bodily integrity.[96] Both the right to privacy and the right to bodily integrity should pertain to your birth, your basic human function. A person's basic human rights, however, are sometimes threatened or denied completely in our maternity healthcare system. Respect for your rights, now more than ever, depends on which state you live in and your financial solvency. Birthing people are also being confronted with emerging legal questions surrounding the concept of fetal rights. Regardless of the variables, such as which state you live in or your finances, education can help improve your safety. There are various state laws and regulations that govern who can practice midwifery or medicine. No laws exist that specifically dictate where your baby is born.

Don't give your process away

As you consider your healthcare options realize this: getting any prenatal healthcare is your choice. There is no law written out that says you *must* obtain prenatal care. Most state laws, where they do exist, focus on attempts to govern the care of pregnant people only in relation to illegal drug use (and if it is considered child abuse) and abortion.[97] In theory (and this is just for argument's sake, because I do strongly urge people to seek out prenatal care!) you could get pregnant, eat well, exercise, get plenty of rest and love, and water, grow your baby, go into labor, birth your baby gently onto your own bed, deliver your own placenta, cut your own cord, recover from your birth, and then show up at your local town hall to ask for a birth certificate. Again, I am not suggesting that you deny yourself and your baby prenatal care; I relied heavily on my own providers and encourage you to do the same. To repeat: unassisted birth is not something I endorse, even if the choice does appear to work for some. Postpartum hemorrhage, progression and positioning complications, preeclampsia, and infections can all lead to tragedy if not recognized and dealt with; however, these complications can generally be treated by a midwife or doctor at home or in a hospital. I want to emphasize that throughout all of the above-mentioned steps you really do get to make choices. And you will remember your birth in myriad ways throughout the rest of your life.

To help illustrate the endurance of birth memories (and some of the ways that maternity care has evolved), I am pleased to present Barbara's birth stories, written at age 87. Her first child was born in 1944, when she was 21.

The night I went into labor we hadn't been in bed more than an hour when I woke up my husband Pete, saying the bed seemed to be very wet and I felt some pains in my back. I had never even heard about water breaking...

I clearly remember walking across the lawn leading to the hospital; water seemed to be pouring out, but no bad pains yet. As it was the middle of the war there was a real shortage of nurses. I was hustled off to a small room. A young nurse came in. She felt my stomach and asked how I was. She meekly told me I was her first patient ever. They let Pete come in for a little while. The pains were coming and going. There was talk of the timing, which meant nothing to me. Then they sent Pete out. Pete and mother spent the rest of the night at the hospital sitting on some hard benches. He speaks of that as the most difficult night for him. I remember the pains getting closer, and they hurt a lot, this went on for the rest of the night. Finally, they encouraged me to push, but weren't specific about just how. It was a pretty unpleasant experience. Toward morning they clamped something over my nose, and told me to breath. I didn't fight it, and soon lost consciousness.

Karen was born in the morning, July 1, 1944, but the first thing I remember clearly was opening my eyes and seeing a strange woman in a green dress and scarf (my first view of scrubs). She was holding a bundle and I thought I was in a Nazi concentration camp. My memory stops there, though I am sure I was reassured and eventually really woke up. When Pete came in I made him kiss me, he didn't mind except ether smells horrid.

They brought my baby in quite soon after I was fully awake, they had used forceps, so her head was strange, sort of slanted. But this went away quite quickly, and she was beautiful. They brought her in to be nursed every three hours I think. They weren't too helpful, but I was able to nurse her, without help, most successfully.

I was not allowed out of bed for nine days. On the ninth day I was supposed to dangle my legs over the edge of the bed to get a little strength back but the doctor forgot to sign the order, so I couldn't dangle. When I did get up, on the tenth day, in preparation for going home, I felt very faint and had to be helped.

My other births were similar, except I was out of bed sooner (doctors had discovered during the War that getting up soon after any operation hastened healing), but I stayed in the hospital at least six days. I felt faint, or fainted, after each one. One doctor later told me it was caused by my reaction to the anesthetic.

Pete was back home from the Pacific and out of the Navy when Jamie was born (1947). Jamie was over a week late, and I was weepy, so they thought labor should be induced. But the doctor wouldn't make the decision. I was already at the hospital in White Plains with Mother. They called Pete at his office in New York and made him decide. This was very hard for him, being a Christian Scientist and not used to doctors. He hurried to the hospital and was persuaded to make the decision. I wasn't too aware of what was happening and thought they were giving me a pain killer shot to calm me down, but what a surprise! It was a shot to start labor and it worked. This time it was a shorter process, but still pains, and timing again, and I had ether at the end, but was more alert when they brought him in to be nursed.

Douglas was born five years after that. The doctor wasn't in yet, he was watching an important baseball game! An intern came to examine me. She never spoke to me at all. She gave me a hurtful exam, spoke to the nurse and left. I remember being so angry. I paid more attention to her callous treatment than to the pains coming every few minutes. I was given ether again just before the baby emerged.

Nine years later, Suzanne was born. I remember my roommate's mother was younger than I. I was 39. I felt fine during this pregnancy too, but I was conscious of being older, and took good care of myself: napping, and trying not to overdo anything. Suzanne's birth was similar to the others. Always I was "out" at the actual appearance of the child. I am surprised that, though I do not remember ever having heard that an older mother had a greater chance of having an abnormal baby, as soon as I woke up I kept asking and asking if she was ok. I still can feel that worry.

Some details come and go, but we do remember so much of our births. And should you think Barbara is an outlier, I have spoken to many women in their 70s, 80s and 90s about their births, and they always are surprised to experience how many details come flooding back, even when remembering what they had for their current day's breakfast felt elusive. Taking responsibility now, as much as is possible, for who you hire, the plans you make and the tests you take will help you to craft empowered memories from a conscientious birth. We don't control our births, and we can't control the powerful systems within which we must function, but by working to participate in your decisions you give yourself your best chance at your most satisfying memories. And as I mentioned earlier, if you haven't yet gotten around to investigating your own birth history (the homework assignment from Week 1), maybe Barbara's story will inspire you to tackle that investigation now. Is there anyone around who remembers your birth? Ask them and you may be able to learn something about what you have internalized about birth, and this in turn can help you sort through your feelings and take responsibility for your best birth plans.

Prenatal screening, diagnostic tests and ultrasound

There is a good chance that by the time you are reading this book you have already had one or more screening tests, including ultrasound. Perhaps you are currently waiting on test results as you read this book. If you are, how are you handling the waiting? If you have tested and already received results, how has that process been? If you have so far chosen not to take any screening tests, what has that been like?

It is considered conventional American maternity care to have all kinds of tests during pregnancy. We are curious, we want assurances, and we hope for solutions when problems are found. When making a testing decision there are two basic things to consider: how useful will the information collected be? And will there be any risks associated with the test (or the test interpretation)? Screening tests look for possible problems, whereas diagnostic tests are used to confirm or dispute the possibility of problems found from symptoms or screening tests. Ultrasound can be used for both screening and diagnostic testing depending on what tests one started with and what has been found.

All tests come with their unique set of risks for false positives, false negatives and incorrect interpretations. All tests come with a dollar price tag that you or your insurance will have to pay. In other words, tests are billable procedures. Some tests are associated with physical risks, including miscarriage. Two such tests are chorionic villus sampling and amniocentesis. More generally, testing has implications. It is a big, grown-up responsibility to really consider the problems one is looking for in prenatal screening tests. I didn't process any of this before my screening tests in my first pregnancy, and most people I have met with haven't done that either. In my first pregnancy, I had the assumption that screening was *normal* and would keep my fetus and I safe. I thought that we would be reassured and could then get back to dreaming about happily ever after. I did intellectually understand that we could get positive test results, meaning there was a concern, but I reasoned that (in the seemingly remote possibility) if my child was going to have some kind of health anomaly, it would be useful to know ahead of time. But I am no longer convinced earlier is always better. From what I have observed, earlier too often means more time worrying and a lot more time spent testing. Rarely does knowing something earlier make an actual difference in treatment through pregnancy or birth. For the majority, more time worrying and testing means less time sleeping well, eating well, and moving well. These worries can impact family bonding, happiness, and overall health. After my own experiences and years of watching other families swim through the ups, downs, and in-betweens of screening tests, I think that getting through the pregnancy as unencumbered as possible is perhaps ideal. But of course this is real life, and there are no true, one-size-fits-all ideals.

According to the CDC about 3% of all babies born have some level of birth defect.[98] The range of what that means as it relates to quality of life, for your future child (and you), is almost as vast as the universe itself. Do you, or any family members, or friends have any congenital anomaly? Do you know anyone raising a child with a congenital anomaly? If yes, what are your observations about their lives?

If your baby has a congenital heart defect it may be possible that a vaginal birth is deemed too stressful and a cesarean section would be preferable. For these families prenatal screening can literally be a lifeline. But for the vast majority of problems uncovered there will either be uncertainty about what was revealed, little solution beyond abortion, or nothing to do until after the birth. Whenever one learns the news that their baby has a congenital anomaly, it will be some degree of shocking. When the news is discovered early on in pregnancy, one must untangle many variables, including uncertainties, before deciding to act, if action is even an option. If you wait, and your baby survives through birth, and news of anomaly is discovered at or after birth, you will automatically have more information about your baby's health and fortitude than you would have had had you learned the information earlier on. Now that the baby is actually here, she can be directly examined and/or treated.

When it comes to sorting through testing choices and your possible outcomes, know that your energy is finite and you should be protective of how you spend it. What *I* want for you is for you to be clear with yourself (and your providers) about why you are choosing any particular tests, what limitations or risks might be associated with the test, and also to give yourself some emotional space to choose to *not* test. Here is a list of questions and considerations to ponder as you think about future medical screening tests:

1) Think through all the possible outcomes of the test before taking it. What will negative, positive, or inconclusive results mean to you and the healthcare decisions you need to make every day? (Decisions including what to eat, how to move, when to sleep.)

2) Will any of the potential test results you are considering be actionable? In other words, will there be something to do differently once you know these test results? This includes your consideration of and/or having access to abortion.

3) Does the test you are considering frequently lead to other tests? If so, what other tests? And will you be able to act conclusively from those test results?

4) Learn about any/all potential risks associated with any test in question, and with any tests most likely to follow the test that you are considering.

Up to now I have been discussing prenatal screening in a general way, meaning to include blood tests, chromosomal tests, and sampling tests like chorionic villus sampling, amniocentesis, and ultrasound. But the use of ultrasound technology, specifically as a routine screening test, in the absence of unique symptoms or a medical history that warrants closer investigation, requires some specific attention.

As with any general screening questions, deciding to use ultrasound should be based on weighing the usefulness of the information collected against any potential risks associated with the technology or the interpretation of data collected, as well as how you feel about taking the test. In addition, there are some unanswered scientific questions to consider. First, let me state the good news: ultrasound does appear **not** to cause harm. By 2009, the World Health Organization (WHO) said in their comprehensive systematic review of ultrasound research that **ultrasound appears safe**. Phew. Big happy exhale. However, they also said that more research is needed because the majority of trials that they included had not been designed specifically to look for potential harms from ultrasound. Plus, all trials they included were on equipment made in 1995 or before. They noted that in 2009 equipment in use was using acoustic outputs that are up to 8 times more powerful than they were in the earlier equipment. The WHO paper also said that additional research is not likely to happen because it has already become such a ubiquitous expectation in maternity care. (Is that really a good reason to stop investigating?) From the WHO paper:

There have been few studies specifically designed to evaluate the safety of ultrasound on human pregnancies, many suffer from methodological shortcomings and few have analyzed possible long-term effects on *in-utero* exposure. To the best of our knowledge, up to the present [2009] there have been no large randomized controlled trials done for the specific purpose of investigating potential bio-effects of prenatal ultrasound in humans, and it is highly improbable that such studies will ever be performed in developed countries owing to the almost universal use of ultrasound in modern obstetrics.[99]

In a more current review of literature on prenatal ultrasound from 2021, it was still found to appear safe, but also to not improve outcomes, and also based on trials that used much older equipment.[100] Our acceptance of this technology, even with these gaps in research, brings to mind a long list of stories of medical harm. One such story of over-confidence in technology was the use of x-rays in shoe stores:

> Marketed as a scientific method for optimizing shoe fit, the fluoroscope [x-ray] appeared in shoe stores nationwide from the 1920s to the 1960s. But the machines not only didn't do what they promised, they also exposed children, their parents and store clerks to unhealthy doses of radiation.[101]

There are countless more stories of doctors and scientists thinking they have a complete picture and then learning they didn't fully get it right. In the field of obstetrics, we are in so deep with technology. It is a lot to sort out emotionally. And what of the dollar expense? Each new test is a billable add-on to your diagnosis of pregnancy. I believe in science. I am not anti-technology, yet I also know that healthy human gestation has worked remarkably well throughout time without technological assists. And so, I am led to the conclusion that testing should be questioned. I recommend that you gather your own best information, beyond "my doctor told me it was routine."

I am relieved that to date all large reviews of studies find that prenatal ultrasound exposure is safe. But I can't help but wonder what there is still to learn. When your kids are expecting their own babies, what might shock them about our current beliefs and practices? Following are some of the observations of ultrasound exposure that are not yet understood.

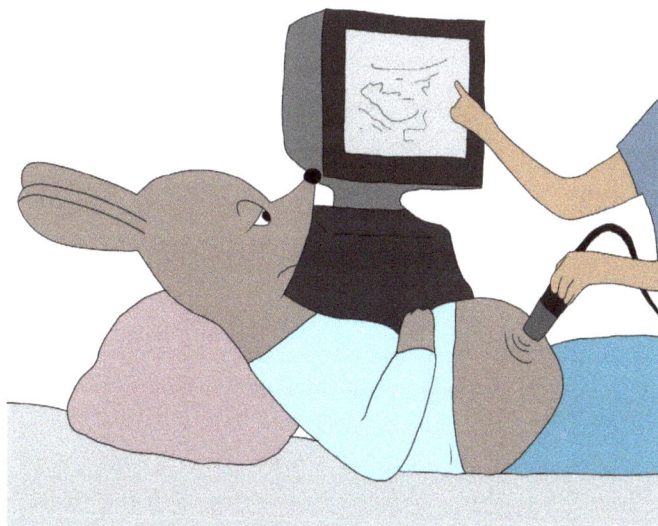

Ultrasound waves have been observed in experimental animals to heat up cells, cause gas bubbles in cells, cause something called "cavitation," which are indentations in cell walls, and potentially disrupt neural cell migration.[102] Scientists know ultrasound can cause these occurrences but do not understand what effects, if any, these observations may have on human development. Those observations are unsettling to digest, but I find solace that humans appear not to be suffering. I do wish there was research on the stronger contemporary equipment, and on any potential cumulative effects of exposure from multiple scans and/or long duration of exposure, but we don't have studies on any of that at this time.

Consequently, with organizations as powerful as the World Health Organization (WHO) stating that ultrasound is safe, what is an expectant family to do? Well, like making any other medical decisions, weigh what you know with how you feel and your personal health history, then make the choice that is best for you. Ultrasound testing, a billable test for your providers, is indeed a personal choice for you. Each of us must find our own answer, but to get an answer first we have to ask some questions. To help you consider whether ultrasound testing is appropriate for you, be it for the first time or additional times, here are some targeted questions (in no particular order) to ask your practitioners and yourself:

○ Do you have a medical indication to use ultrasound (beyond the diagnosis of "pregnancy")? Is there something concerning or abnormal going on? Does anyone involved in your care have reason to believe something is unhealthy or extra risky?

○ What prenatal actions can be taken in the event you get positive test results?

○ Will these test results impact what you are doing with the rest of your day? Or the rest of your pregnancy? If yes, how?

○ Can you sense if your baby is growing well inside you?

○ Are you feeling well? What does your gut, your heart, and your vagina tell you about your health and the health of your baby? (If you can't hear your intuition, try giving yourself some time to listen; a mindfulness exercise may help.)

Going forward in the pregnancy, especially when you are at or near term, ultrasound scans are ordered more commonly/frequently to assess amniotic fluid levels, fetal weight, and fetal positioning. However, when teasing out if a late pregnancy scan is useful to your care, please consider that ultrasound is not very accurate at gauging fetal weight at or near term. From a 2018 National Institute of Health (NIH) review of research it was found that current ways of using ultrasound to gauge fetal weight are not that reliable and that the most consistent errors were in over estimating the fetal size.[103] How might it impact you to be told you are having what appears to be a very big baby?

As for amniotic fluid assessment at term, many providers want to induce otherwise healthy gestational people for the diagnosis of low amniotic fluid. But in a review of research by Rebecca Dekker, PhD, of Evidence Based Birth, a research-based organization that helps families and providers follow the research, she found that the evidence to induce for low amniotic fluid in an otherwise healthy person at term is weak at best. She also found that being well hydrated at the end of pregnancy directly, and positively, impacts your amniotic fluid levels.[104] In other words, even moderate dehydration can make it appear as if you have low amniotic fluid levels. My advice? Drink up! Ponder these testing considerations and read on for some anecdotal stories that illustrate some of the challenges surrounding the decisions to use routine ultrasound testing. I share these stories, not to be scary, but to help you understand how complex the issues can be.

One family I know was told, after their anatomy scan, that their baby had several serious problems that had no solutions. They were told their baby would not survive until birth, through birth, or at best not much thereafter. This family, with their devastating news, having no options, carried on in grief, preparing to birth and then bury their baby. Remarkably, that frightening prognosis was incorrect. They birthed their baby alive, he received medical treatments, and they recently and joyfully celebrated their child's ninth birthday! Another family I have worked with was told their baby had a serious congenital heart defect. They were told that there was a surgery that could help repair the heart once the baby was born. However, the doctors feared that the baby would not be strong enough to survive a vaginal birth, so this family opted for a cesarean birth. The baby was born surprisingly robust and appeared to be well primed for the upcoming necessary surgery.

In another anecdote, a friend of mine had a routine early scan. They saw a cyst on her baby's brain. All her doctors and she could do was be uncertain, worry, and do more scans. The doctors had no idea what the cyst might mean for that fetus or the future. The mother went every two weeks throughout the pregnancy to see if the cyst changed size or made any other changes. There was no change until she got to term, at which point the cyst seemed to have just vanished. Another scan a week later, and still no trace of the cyst or any other abnormality. Days after that, my friend went into labor and gave birth to a healthy baby who grew into a healthy child that has achieved tremendous academic success. However, the stress on my friend and her family, throughout that entire pregnancy, was more than intense. The mother and her family were fearful for, and maybe also a little afraid of, her fetus, and this fear stayed with them for some time after birth. Long term impacts from that kind of stress are hard to measure but easy to feel.

In another one of my client's near-term ultrasounds, a "very big baby" was revealed. That mother panicked over the prospect of birthing a large baby, although she really wanted to strive for an unmedicated vaginal birth. During labor she had trouble dilating and ended up giving birth via cesarean section to an 8lb 10oz baby. (Not *such* a big baby after all, by average standards.) While she was recovering, this mother told me that she was sure she couldn't open during labor because she had been so concerned that the baby was too big. Another client of mine was told she was having a girl. She had asked the technician about the test's accuracy for sex and the technician assured her it was accurate. This client went on to emotionally bond with her supposed girl fetus. When the baby was born, they found out it was physiologically male. This mother went on to have a challenging time bonding with her baby boy. She realized, as she reported to me, that she had to grieve the loss of her little girl to be able to open up and bond to her new son. These such stories weigh on me, and certainly color my opinions toward testing.

In one final anecdote, from my own personal experience with near-term ultrasound, even when there is a medical indication for ultrasound use, doctors can't always obtain the information they seek from the test. In my second pregnancy I experienced some third trimester bleeding. I was frightened. I felt that I had a medical indication to use ultrasound. Possible side effects were balanced against figuring out why I was bleeding and where the blood was coming from. This time I heartily chose ultrasound. My test results were somewhat reassuring, although basically inconclusive. Everything appeared to be functioning as expected, but the bleeding remained a mystery. Of course, we were glad to rule out serious complications (a separating placenta, for example), but a visual check that blood was not pouring out of me (I was just spotting) gave us the same information. In the end, I felt stress from the inconclusive results and the understanding that the ultrasound wasn't predictive. No one could tell us what was going to happen. What we knew was what we knew before: there was some blood coming out of me; it appeared to be coming out of my cervix; it was intermittent and not large in quantity. The umbilical cord and placenta still looked well-formed and well-attached. My baby appeared calm and content. I had used the technology that was available and still our questions about what was happening remained.

Those are just a few of the stories you won't likely hear described as important to consider as you balance the risks and benefits of ultrasound scanning. But I think these stories should be included for you to explore your responses. Inevitably you will face further testing decisions down the road.

If you should develop a medical indication, or otherwise decide to use ultrasound in the future, consider asking the technician to limit your exposure time to just long enough to gather the necessary data. From my client's stories it seems that technicians frequently increase the time of exposure beyond what is necessary. The experience can be like watching television. A technician will go through the entire exam quietly, then once they have completed the initial exam, they turn the monitor towards the parent(s) and ask if they would like to see their baby. At that point the technician will do a duplicate scan pointing out the images on the screen, e.g., "There is your baby's heart, hand, lungs, etc." Some clients report that they had a third complete scan when the doctor showed up. I have heard stories of the ultrasound scan being left on for 30-plus minutes while everyone got their ample fill of seeing the baby. Maybe that will turn out to be absolutely fine. But with the unanswered technology questions that remain, I suggest that you consider asking the technician to be as efficient as possible with exposure time. If you do this, you will certainly have less exposure than had you not mentioned it. And because it's so important I will repeat myself: please be compassionate with yourself. You should never fault yourself for following your provider's suggestions and making decisions with whatever information or feeling you had at the time. What is done is done, and all that is left to do is look forward, knowing that if history has taught us anything, it is to be cautious. In this context, being cautious means considering closely your feelings about the test, weighing the potential impact of uncertain results, and, as a general rule, using the least amount of exposure time and amplitudes necessary to get the desired information you are after.

Before you finish up this week, let's pause for a relaxation exercise. Take some time now to get into the side relaxation position, or other comfortable relaxing shape.

EXERCISE: SENSORY AWARENESS

First pick one partner to lead/read the visualization, or record it on your phone, or read it through first and then take yourself through your sensory journey. Next settle into a comfortable relaxation pose.

"Begin by closing your eyes and tuning you're your breath. Follow it in, follow it out."

—Pause for several breaths—

"Now please bring your attention to your sense of hearing: what are the internal and external sounds you can hear?"

—Pause for several breaths—

"Now invite your attention back to your breath. Follow it in, follow it out."

—Pause for several breaths—

"Now please let your attention shift to your sense of smell. What can you smell? How does your nostril receive this information? What can you notice?"

—Pause for several breaths—

"Please now tune back into your breath. Follow it in, follow it out."

—Pause for several breaths—

"Now let your attention settle on your sense of taste. Can you discern any flavors from your last taste of food or beverage? What do your taste buds notice?"

—Pause for several breaths—

"Again observe your breathing process, tune into the ebbs and the flows."

—Pause for several breaths—

"Now to notice your sense of sight. Allow your eyes to open. What shapes, colors and textures fill your visual field? Experiment with soft and sharp focus."

—Pause for several breaths—

"Let your eyes close and return your attention to your breath. Follow it in, and follow it out."

—Pause for several breaths—

"And now, please bring your attention to your sense of touch. What can you feel? Are there parts of you that are bearing weight or feeling lightness? Can you feel textures of clothes or pillows or a partner? Can you feel the air? Notice what you can feel."

—Pause for several breaths—

"And now please bring your attention back to your breathing. Follow it in, follow it out".

—Pause for several breaths—

"And now, gently, as you are ready, bring some movement into your toes and ankles; give them a little wiggle and a stretch. Let some movement come into your fingers, hands and wrists; give them a little wiggle and some stretch. And gradually, as you feel ready, let some light back into your eyes, and using your upper body for support, work your way back to a seated position."

I hope you've found this sensory awareness exercise accessible. In labor it can be quite helpful to tune out your thinking by tuning into your senses. Inevitably your attention will return to your contractions, but the very fact that you have allowed your attention to leave them means that they are not swallowing you whole (which can sometimes be the experience). Training to tune into all of your senses in a focused, progressive exercise can help you to process in labor that the labor itself is only one part of your whole physical experience. This perspective change can bring comfort under the duress of hard contractions, just as it can bring focus to hard decisions.

Thank you for your time and attention this week. I understand that coming to terms with prenatal testing and the surrounding unanswered questions can be disconcerting. Be gentle with yourself. Remind yourself that you are doing the best you can, and that is all that you can really ask of yourself. Try to carve out some moments for selfcare and fun this week. Talk with your baby and think about the providers and birth space that will make you both feel most at ease. I wish you a wonderful week.

HOMEWORK

A) Research your care options

Consider your interview language carefully. Start to try and visualize what you think your birth should look like. Start to watch birth films.

B) Nourish yourself

Eat good food and take time for play. Exercise and practice relaxation skills. Dive into the scary places in your heart as you ask yourself the big questions about your fears, your dreams, and your values.

THIS SPACE IS FOR YOUR NOTES AND DRAWINGS

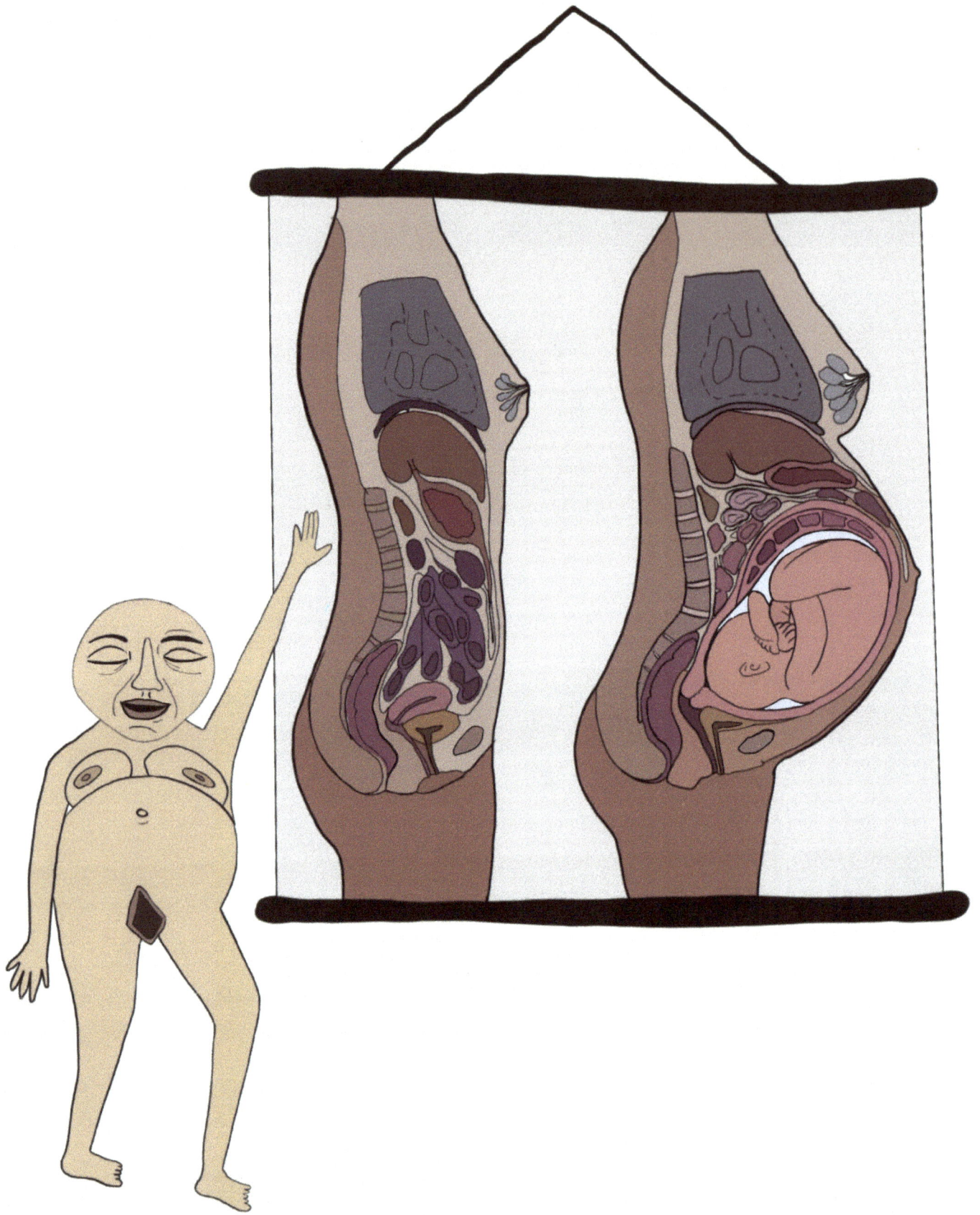

WEEK 5

Your Pregnant Body

Chapter contents:

O *Some basic anatomy*

O *Common pregnancy challenges*

O *Birth physiology*

THIS SPACE IS FOR YOUR NOTES AND DRAWINGS

Great to see you back for Week 5! How did your last week go? Are you happy with the food choices you have made this past week? Are you getting adequate rest? Basic self-care makes everything better. If you've been having challenges, please try to evaluate what the obstacles are so that you can get creative about making some changes. If you haven't been feeling any particular challenges, celebrate that. There is no need to expect any negative feelings to develop, and you'll deal with whatever comes your way if and when you have to. Please take a breath and, as you exhale, smile and try to enjoy something about whatever you are currently feeling—even if the positive is just that you are able to take another breath in and feel your challenges.

As I have mentioned, pregnancy and parenting require physical and emotional strength. I have been challenged in extraordinary ways. Every parent I know has been challenged the same. I have had to find endurance and resiliency I didn't even know I had before I found myself in the thick of family life. My experience can provide you with foresight! So please take a moment now to think about what kinds of emotional coping tools you already possess. What strengths do you rely on now that can help you in your pregnancy, during birth, and throughout parenting when obstacles arise? Reflect and then complete the prompt below. List as many positive attributes as you can! Go back and add details whenever you want. Be creative and compassionate with yourself. We all have strengths to rely on and to offer. Ask a friend, neighbor, loved one. Sometimes when we touch base with our low-confidence feelings the tears start to flow. That is okay: let them flow. Sometimes after a good cry we can see things a bit more clearly. From here on I encourage you to look for opportunities to identify your own positive abilities. Allowing yourself the room to accept your own strengths, and hold space for where you can improve, will help you to build confidence and trust in yourself. This empowerment will help you to trust your instincts, which is essential for good decision making.

Fill in the blanks with one or some of your own personality traits, skills and positive coping methods.

Statement for pregnant person: A coping mechanism, strength, or positive behavioral attribute I bring to this pregnancy (or this birth or for parenting) is:

Statement for partner in parenting: A coping mechanism, strength, or positive behavioral attribute I bring to this pregnancy (or this birth or for parenting) is:

A little bit of anatomy

It is not my intention to reinvent the wheel on this subject. I just want to highlight some important aspects of our amazing anatomy and the physiology of birth. There are plenty of sources on this subject; please take your interest as far as you like. Learning how your body functions can help you to build appreciation, which can in turn help you to reduce fear and inspire good health. In my Bradley® classes we look at charts and play with a model of a baby and pelvis. Being able to connect with people as you handle actual models is a useful educational benefit that comes from taking an actual birth class. My gentle reminder: if you have the opportunity to participate in a live class, I strongly encourage you to do so.

What follows are the elements of anatomy that I highlight in my own class:

Anatomy of the pelvis

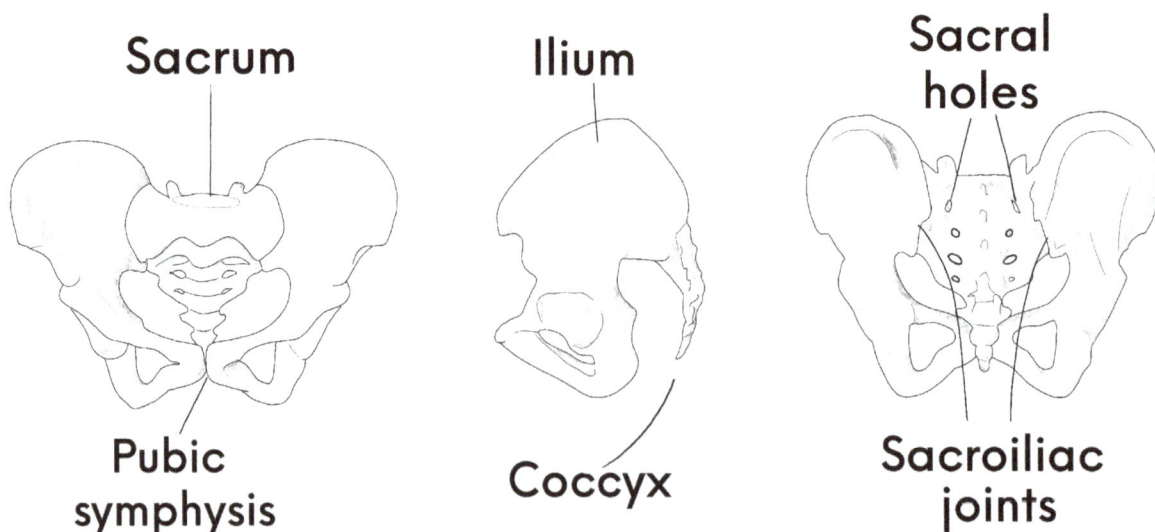

Sacrum

Pubic symphysis

Ilium

Coccyx

Sacral holes

Sacroiliac joints

The joints in the pelvis (the pubic symphysis, coccyx, and two sacroiliac joints) are classified anatomically as "semi-movable joints." In non-pregnant people these joints shouldn't move very much or at all. Remember, however, that during pregnancy the body produces Relaxin, the hormone that works just as it sounds: it relaxes the ligaments between joints. This allows for maximum movement within the pelvic joints during birth. Relaxin is produced by the corpus luteum.[105] (What, you ask, is your corpus luteum? It is a spectacular mass of yellow tissue that grows in the ovary and secretes hormones that help maintain a pregnancy, such as Relaxin and Progesterone. If there is no pregnancy, the corpus luteum degenerates, only to reform the following month. If there is a pregnancy the corpus luteum continues to secrete hormones.)[106] Thanks to Relaxin, your baby will fit through your pelvis.

You can build your confidence by understanding the positive effect from all the variables that make your birth process work. Your pelvic bones can shift, your baby's skull plates can shift. You can rock and roll your hips and open all your pelvic joints as you shift positions and allow gravity to help ease your baby down and out. There is so much movement potential. In the presence of good health and knowledgeable support, your baby will find their way through. Birth works, or the human race wouldn't still be here. In the journal *Midwifery Today* (2003), Gloria Lemay, a Canadian birth attendant, points out that African Pygmy women who average four feet tall successfully give birth to babies that are frequently 8 pounds.[107] Our remarkable anatomy makes this possible.

Your placenta: An extraordinary organ!

Please take a moment to honor your placenta. It's incredible that, in addition to growing a baby, we grow this other incredibly complex organ that feeds our babies, cleans up after our babies, and makes hormones that keep the whole process of procreation working. The placenta transfers nutrition and oxygen to the baby from the pregnant person's blood, while also transferring the baby's waste products to the pregnant person for them to carry away. I guess part of parenting is always to clean up, whether your child's waste is carbon dioxide or M&M® wrappers! As if all that feeding and cleaning weren't enough, placental physiology allows for the placenta to synthesize its own hormones to support the pregnancy. Parenthood is so creative!

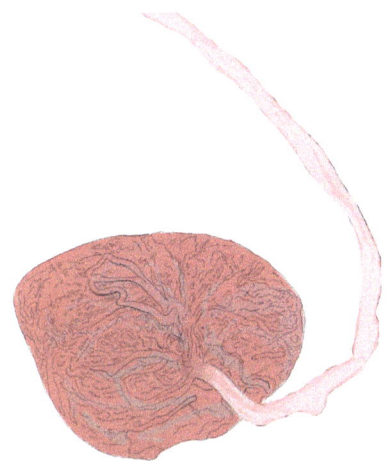

> In addition to its role in transporting molecules between mother and fetus, the placenta is a major endocrine organ. It turns out that the placenta synthesizes a huge and diverse number of hormones and cytokines [small proteins used by the immune system] that have major influences on ovarian, uterine, mammary and fetal physiology, not to mention other endocrine systems of the mother. [108]

Wow! Look at the work your own body is doing! (Cue the fanfare.)

The placenta is smooth and finished-looking on the side that is within the amniotic sac and next to the baby. After birth, when you can see your placenta, the side that had been attached against the uterine wall will look rough and unfinished because, essentially, it is sheared off from the uterine wall once the uterus gets smaller by continuing to contract once the baby is out.[109] The amniotic sac grows out of the placenta at the edges, and the umbilical cord grows out of the center. Placentas of singleton pregnancies (i.e., one fetus) generally weigh about one to two pounds. One client of mine, who spectacularly birthed two gigantic twin boys vaginally, was floored by the enormity of her close to *five pounds* of placenta! That's a lot of placenta doing a lot of important work. So eat well, because you need good nutrition to build a good placenta—one that stays well-attached and functions to its optimal, magnificent potential.

On a related side note: there are diverse ideas surrounding what parents do with their placental remains. I was told by a Norwegian that the direct translation from the Norwegian word for placenta is "Mother's Cake." Perhaps this references the belief by some people that a new mom should eat her placenta during the postpartum period. There is belief that ingestion of placenta creates an infusion of hormones; the iron-rich meat of the placenta helps to balance out a gestational person's hormones in the postpartum period. Over the years I have met doula's who will dry your placenta, grind it up, and place it in capsules for you to slowly ingest over time. And I have heard from a couple of people that it provided a powerful lift to their postpartum sadness. However, as of 2017, the Center for Disease Control warns against placental ingestion. The placenta, if not handled carefully, can transmit the bacteria Group B Strep, which can lead to a gestational person transferring the bacteria to the baby.[110] This can make a baby very sick, and even risk death. If ingesting the placenta is at all of interest to you, it is imperative that you thoroughly investigate your Group B Strep status, the processes used in preserving the placenta, as well as the skill and education of the practitioner offering such a service, well in advance of your postpartum period.

Of course, not all placental ritual is about eating it. There are so many interesting ideas around our placentas. Some Indigenous Peoples in North America have a ritual of burying the placenta. As described by Patricia Guthrie in an article from the *Chicago Tribune*:

> Among the Navajo Indians of the Southwest, it's customary to bury a child's placenta within the sacred Four Corners of the tribe's reservation as a binder to ancestral land and people. New Zealand's Maoris have the same tradition of burying the placenta within native soil. In their native language, the word for land and placenta are the same: *whenua*.
>
> The Indigenous Bolivian Aymara and Quechua people believe the placenta has its own spirit. It is to be washed and buried by the husband in a secret and shady place. If this ritual is not performed correctly, they believe, the mother or baby may become very sick or even die.
>
> The Ibo of Nigeria and Ghana treat the placenta as the dead twin of the live child and give it full burial rites.
>
> Filipina mothers are known to bury the placenta with books, in hopes of a smart child.
>
> Other cultures place a symbol of their people with the placenta when burying it, as a kind of heritage insurance.
>
> Among the Hmong culture of Southeast Asia, the word for placenta can be translated as "jacket," as it's considered an infant's first and finest clothing. The Hmong bury the placenta outside. They believe that after death, the soul must retrace the journeys undertaken in life until it reaches the burial place of its placenta jacket.[111]

My first placenta was disposed of by the hospital as medical waste and my second placenta is buried in my yard under a tree. What will you do with yours?

After any birth, it is important that, shortly following birth, a trained birth attendant examine the placenta to see if the edges look complete. In rare complications, a practitioner will notice that the placenta does not look whole and that means that some of the placenta is still inside. This is dangerous and must be tended to without delay.

A final note of caution: If you are planning a homebirth and you have a dog, you might want to consider keeping the dog away from the placenta, at least until it has been examined by a birth attendant. I once heard a crazy story about a family dog swooping in and gobbling up the placenta when it had been left briefly unattended in a bowl on the floor.

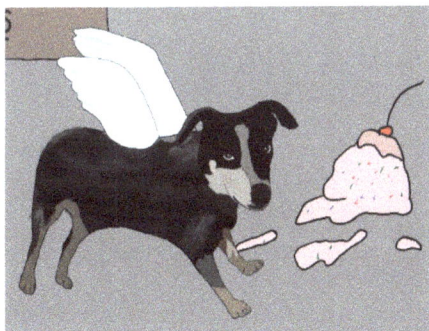

Your amniotic sac and fluid

(note: see Addendum meconium 1 page 498)

The amniotic sac is a protective, double-walled bag that holds not only your baby, but also your amniotic fluid and the umbilical cord. The amniotic fluid provides quite a lot of physical protection for the baby. It is hard to hurt something inside a water balloon, for example. Amniotic fluid helps to regulate the baby's temperature. Plus, the presence of the fluid is critical to the fetus's lung development. Your baby inhales and swallows amniotic fluid, then exhales and pees fluid out. Your baby is continuously circulating amniotic fluid and new fluid is continuously being made. Moreover, fluid composition changes and develops over the course of the pregnancy. Early on the fluid is mostly water, which comes from the pregnant person. (Another reminder to please keep yourself well hydrated!) As the pregnancy continues, the baby's kidneys develop and the fluid becomes more like fetal pee. The amniotic fluid also contains fetal skin cell debris and a variety of oils, stem cells, and electrolytes. (Stem cells have the potential to differentiate into different types of cells and electrolytes help balance fluid and pH levels to maintain an environment suitable for the electric impulses of nerve transmissions. How cool is that?!)

From the fetus's point of view, amniotic fluid helps to develop smells and flavors from the gestational person's diet. The breasts and the breast milk also secrete odors related to diet. When a newborn is immediately placed on their gestational parent's naked chest after birth, the baby frequently suckles their own hands, making a connection from the amniotic fluid smells and tastes to their gestational parent's nipple. This connection helps the baby find her way to the breast to establish breastfeeding.[112]

At the end of the pregnancy, it is common—in fact, *very* common—to be unsure as to whether you've just leaked amniotic fluids or peed your pants. The easiest way to figure this out, and perhaps the only way short of a litmus paper test, is to smell something wet by the fluid or to try and catch some of the fluid in a container. You may be able to see or smell the difference: urine is yellowish and has a distinct odor, while amniotic fluid should be clear or pink with no discernible odor, especially compared to the strong and recognizable smell of urine. When your amniotic sac ruptures at the end of your pregnancy or during labor, you may experience a big gush of fluid. At other times there may only be a small trickle of fluid, because the baby's head acts like a cork and stops or slows the release. When the amniotic sac ruptures it is often referred to as "the water breaking" or "ruptured membranes."

The umbilical cord: It lacks nerve, but it has a good beat!

The umbilical cord holds and protects two arteries and one vein. (Rarely, some cords only have one artery. Many of these babies do develop normally, although there is more risk of complication.) The casing of the cord has a spiral structure. It's built similarly to one of those old-fashioned, coiled telephone wires. Inside the casing, surrounding the arteries and vein, is a substance called Wharton's Jelly. (Wharton's Jelly was named after the man who identified it in the 17th century, Thomas Wharton.) This gel-like substance prevents kinks in the line, as the baby does her internal acrobatics. After the birth, Wharton's Jelly will dry up, naturally clamping off blood-flow between the baby and placenta, which is why there is no immediate need to cut the cord after birth.

The average umbilical cord length is 22 inches. Most of the time umbilical cords are plenty long enough for the baby to easily reach the birth parent's breast after birth, while the placenta is still attached. Occasionally, a short cord will mean the baby only reaches the parent's belly. That is okay, too: just leave the baby wherever they reach. You will all want to physically and metaphorically catch your breath after the birth. Placing the baby skin to skin on your belly is generally a comfort to you and your baby as you recover from the birth. And at the moment of birth some of your baby's blood is still circulating through their umbilical cord and placenta. If you touch the cord, you can feel it pulsing. This continued pulsing allows the blood to return to the baby. Once the cord has stopped pulsing the baby has gotten all of their blood back into their body and the cord can be cut. While the cord is still attached, it's important not to put any tension on the umbilical cord. One can gently test for slackness, but it is dangerous to apply tension. If the cord is pulled too hard, the uterus can invert (fold in on itself). This is an emergency situation for the gestational parent and requires immediate surgery to stem their bleeding.

Serious cord complications are rare, but potentially fatal. These complications are not well predicted with ultrasound, or any other means of screening. Cord tragedies can occur in any birth setting. (About 1% of all pregnancies end in stillbirth, and cord complications are suspected to account for about 10% of those deaths.[113]) In a healthy birth, it is fairly common for the cord to be around the baby's neck as the head starts to emerge. The medical term for this is "nuchal cord." Rarely is this a serious complication. Your care attendant will usually just slip the cord over the baby's head. In some instances, the cord may not slip freely over the baby's head, making it necessary to clamp and cut the cord where it is in order to allow the baby to be born. For the baby who has to have their cord cut early, they will not have gotten all of their blood returned, and so should be screened for anemia later in the first year of life.[114]

My son Arlo had the cord coiled twice around his neck, which prompted my midwife to ask if she could cut our cord. I consented, given the situation, but as my midwife reached for her clamps and scissors, I pushed Arlo right out before she had a chance. Apparently neither he nor I wanted to wait! It turned out that not only was his cord twice around his neck, it was also wrapped around his shoulder. Thankfully, Arlo's cord had enough slack, so there were no resulting problems. Given that the cord does not have any nerves within it, neither baby nor parent feels it when it's cut. (By the way, your baby's "innie" or "outie" belly button is genetically determined. It has nothing to do with the cord clamping and cutting process.[115])

Your uterus: A big, tough, stretchy bag!

The uterus is a formidable pouch made of muscle. The opening at the bottom of the uterus is called the cervix. The uterus has long muscle fibers that run from the fundus—the top of the uterus—vertically down to the cervix, where there are circular muscle fibers that go around the cervical opening (or "os," in medical-speak). The uterus has a special muscle skill called "retraction." Retraction is when the muscle contracts and then stays in its smaller contracted state as it relaxes. This is how the uterus expels the placenta after birth and then continues to contract back to its pre-pregnant size. (For more information on retraction see "third stage labor" in Week 10.)

Before and after pregnancy, the average uterus is about the size of a pear. Clearly the uterus grows markedly bigger as the pregnancy progresses, accommodating the baby as she grows markedly bigger. When providers are trying to measure the uterus, they are trying to measure fetal growth. During prenatal checkups, once you are least 20 weeks pregnant, your care provider will perhaps measure your uterine growth by placing a tape measure at your pubic bone and then finding the top of your uterus to measure your "fundal height." These measurements can let you and your providers understand if your baby is growing at a healthy rate.

From about 20 weeks on, the measurement of the fundal height in centimeters should be about the same as the number of weeks of gestation. For example, at 25 weeks pregnant, the fundus height should measure about 25 centimeters; plus or minus 2 centimeters is considered healthy growth. This hands-on measuring is a low cost, low risk, reasonably accurate way to measure fetal growth between 20 and 36 weeks of gestation. Before 20 weeks it's not accurate and after 36 weeks the fundal height may start to decrease as baby begins to settle into the pelvis.[116] As many of my clients have reported, however, their providers currently rely on extra ultrasounds to track fetal growth instead of a tape measure. If your provider wants to track fetal growth with ultrasound instead of a tape measure, you may want to inquire about just using a tape measure instead. This allows you to reduce ultrasound exposure in the absence of medical indication. If, while using a tape measure, there is a question about fetal growth (meaning, your weeks of pregnancy and fundal height are more than two centimeters off from each other between 20 and 36 weeks of gestation), then it may be appropriate to use ultrasound as a follow-up investigation.

It's time to consider your cervix

The cervix is like a mouth that stays closed, except when it has to open. It has some length, like when you pucker your lips—i.e., push them out. Generally, a cervix is about 4 – 5 centimeters long and its walls are thick. The cervical os (also known as the mouth or sphincter) is closed tight or opened just a bit for ovulation and conception or menstruation or opened wide for birth. In *Ina May's Guide to Childbirth*, Ina May Gaskin writes about our sphincters being "shy."[117] We open our sphincters more easily when we feel private and free from interruption.

When closed, the cervical opening is protected by a thick secretion of cervical mucus. In maternity care we have the unfortunate term of "mucus plug." Loss of the mucus plug is sometimes noticed as a sign that birth changes have begun. I always challenge my students to come up with a better label than "mucus plug." Imagine if we had a cool term like "Astroglide®" (currently the trademark of a personal lubricant product). Just imagine how different you would feel if you could declare that you just lost your "Astroglide": To me, "Honey, come see my mucus plug" feels icky compared to, "Honey, come see my [say it slow and flirty] Astroglide." Language matters because it can change the tone and feeling of your experiences. So why not make this change a positive one! And do note: a pregnant person will likely want to share the news of the passing of their "Astroglide," or mucus plug. Birth developments are exciting; it is normal to want to share them. So again, why not make it fun and inviting! What are some new terms that can replace "mucus plug" for your birth process?

Have you ever seen your own cervix?

With the help of a mirror, a flashlight, and a speculum, you can (which is not to suggest that you *should*—just that you *could*) see your own cervix. It would be useful also to have a friend help hold the speculum (an obstetric tool that helps hold open the vagina), mirror, or flashlight. Regardless of whether you choose to try and look at your own cervix, it is always helpful to look at pictures of real people's cervices. There is a lot of talk in maternity care about the cervical doorway, so it is helpful for a person to have a clear and accurate understanding of their own anatomy and the anatomy of their partner. If you or your partner want to use visualization to aid in labor, such visualization will work much more effectively if you and/or your partner can imagine the pregnant body's anatomy more accurately.

These cervix images are seen through vaginas held open by a speculum, which gives the vaginas a squared-off appearance.

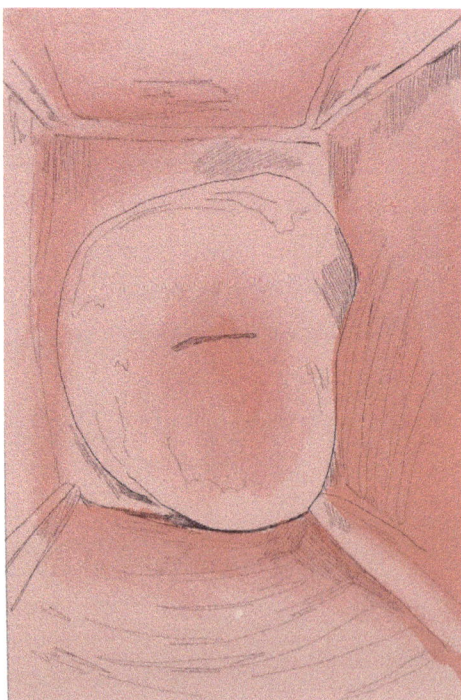

This cervix has opened for birth at least once before.

This cervix has not yet opened for birth.

Cervical openings look different in people who have opened up to have babies from people who have not had a vaginal birth. The people who have had babies have a horizontal slit of an opening as opposed to a person that has not had a baby: their opening is rounder. Everything in your life changes when the baby comes. Changes in your cervical os are no exception.

Structural protections for the baby

Your baby is well protected by your anatomical structure and amniotic fluid. The amniotic sac, your uterus, your abdominal muscles and fat, your rib cage, and your pelvic bones all provide a multilayered playpen in which your baby can safely romp and develop.

Ligament (noun)
1. Tough connective tissue connecting body parts
    A sheet or band of tough fibrous tissue that connects bones or cartilage at a joint or supports an organ, muscle, or other body part.

In addition to a female's bones, fluids, and muscles, there are two key ligaments that help support the uterus: round and broad. Have you had any sharp stabbing pains that seem to come almost out of nowhere, usually associated with moving, like taking a step, sitting down, or getting up from the floor? These discomforts are usually felt in the front of the hip-groin area under your belly. If you have experienced this, then it has likely been caused by a strain on the *round ligament*. This is a common discomfort mentioned by those who are pregnant. Some pregnant people report a nagging feeling of fatigue in the round ligament of their uterus, especially by the end of the day. It's a relatively small ligament charged with trying to support and help stabilize your giant growing belly. Adequate rest, regular exercise, staying well hydrated, and attention to proper posture all generally help. The *broad ligament* attaches to the uterus from the pelvis, behind the uterus, and is larger and less likely to announce itself. The pelvic rock exercise and posture attention can improve any discomfort you may feel from the broad ligament.[118]

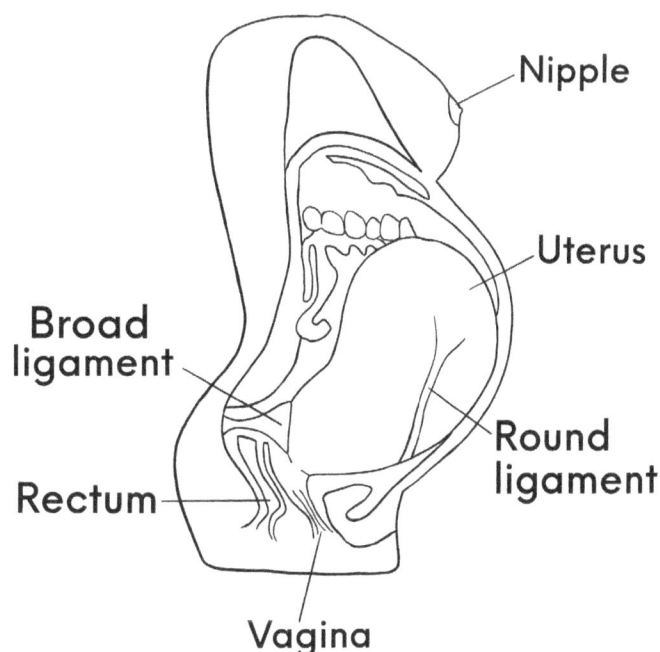

Common physical challenges in pregnancy

If you are pregnant, you are probably (and hopefully) at your healthiest, but pregnancy is a demanding state of being. Pregnancy is not an illness, but it does frequently present some hurdles. Consequently, I want to take some time now to discuss some of the challenges that can be a normal part of pregnancy. While any *one* symptom might be uncomfortable, many pregnant people experience several or all of these sensations. Of course, there are also many pregnant people who don't report any notable discomforts. If you feel good now, don't look for or wait for problems to develop. Enjoy your good feelings!

Backache

Remember the illustration of the pelvis earlier in the chapter? The holes in your sacrum, that large triangular bone at the base of your spine in your pelvis, allow the nerves that are traveling down your spine to go through the pelvic bone and down the legs, in order to innervate the contents of the pelvic organs. Increasing pressure from the growing uterine contents on the nerves that pass through the sacrum can cause a variety of discomforts, generally in the legs, hips, and back depending on which nerves are being impeded. Review the pelvic rocking exercise from Week 3 if your low back is bothering you. Remember that these rocking exercises can physically move the baby and help to reduce the pressure on your nerves. Chiropractic care, physical therapy, massage, and acupuncture are all additional modalities that can help improve comfort and support your process. (Be sure to use practitioners that are studied in prenatal care.) Ice and heat packs can also bring welcome relief.

Bladder pressure and frequent urination

Before you are pregnant the bladder is a nice-sized pouch with plenty of room to hold several hours' worth of urine. As your baby grows, however, the bladder gets more and more compressed by the weight of the baby. By the time you are near term the bladder is just a thin pancake-sized pouch, and the baby's head usually sits right on top of it. And what does the baby's head do? It moves! It moves up and down and side to side and even diagonally! For those of you *not* pregnant, please take a moment to imagine what it must feel like to have a small bowling ball rolling around on top of your full bladder.

For the pregnant folk, this fact of the baby's weight resting on the bladder is quite noticeable and often bemoaned. Nevertheless, try thinking of the increased frequency in urination as a benefit, rather than a bother, particularly at night. Could this be another parenting lesson embedded in pregnancy? Perhaps this helps you to begin to prepare for the sleep disruptions you will have once your baby is born? Frequent night waking during pregnancy can give you the chance to practice sleep-disruption acceptance and to improve the efficiency of your process for going back to sleep. Maybe this biological element also helps to facilitate some quiet baby bonding time.

Night waking and the journey back to sleep

If you don't struggle with getting back to sleep, hooray! Take a moment to be thankful for that. If you do struggle with getting to sleep or returning to sleep after nighttime peeing, I recommend trying to use that in-search-of-sleep time to practice relaxation techniques. I recommend "counting breaths" for sleep or anytime you are feeling stressed.

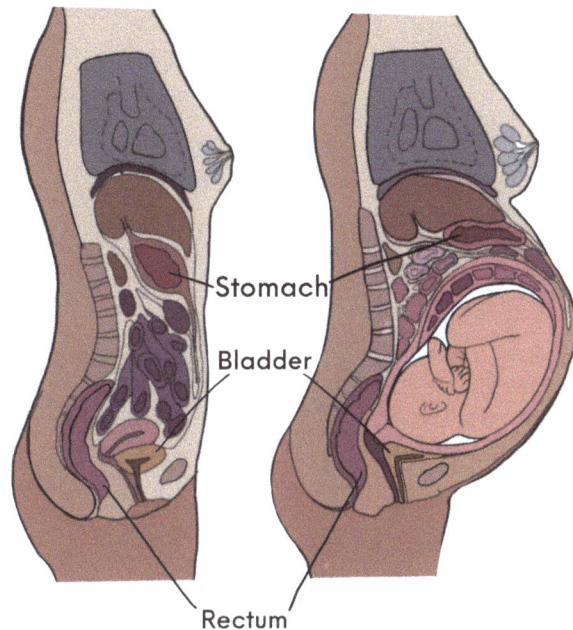

Stomach

Bladder

Rectum

EXERCISE: COUNTING BREATHS WITH FINGERS

Read this exercise and then try it.

In this exercise you will use your fingers to help you count your breaths. This added finger action will serve both as an anchor for your mind and as a useful release for some of your built-up tension.

Start by looking at the palm of your hand. Notice that each finger has horizontal lines that divide it into three segments. Now, with the tip of your thumb, lightly touch the tip of your pinky finger on the same hand. Breathe in and breathe out, and silently count "1." With your next inhalation move your thumb down to the middle segment of that same pinky finger and quietly count "2." With your third inhalation, move your thumb down to the lowest segment of that same pinky finger and count "3." With your next inhalation move the tip of your thumb to the top segment of your ring finger (the next finger over from your little finger) and again count "1." For the next breath move your thumb down to the middle section of your ring finger and count "2." Then again move your thumb tip down to the bottom segment and count "3." Repeat this sequence for your middle finger and then for your pointer finger. When you have completed the third breath on your pointer finger, use that same pointer finger to take over the role of your thumb, and now count out three breaths on your thumb of that same hand by placing the tip of your pointer finger first on the tip of your thumb, breathe and count "1," then to the middle of your thumb, breathe and count "2," and finally to the base of your thumb, breathe and count "3." Once you have completed three breaths for each of your fingers and thumb on your first hand, it's time to utilize the other hand. Begin with the tip of your other thumb touching the tip of your other pinky finger and repeat the sequence of three breaths per finger on the second hand.

You are now ready to try this exercise. Give yourself permission to breathe comfortably. You will want to observe your breath without forcing any changes to your rhythm and also set your intention to allow your breath pattern to slow and deepen.

—Pause to count breaths with fingers—

How do you feel now that you have tried counting breaths with your fingers? If you found the hand movement distracting or uncomfortable, you can try a variation of counting your breaths without your fingers. Count each breath quietly to yourself (but only as high as 3 per rotation), resting your hands and body completely: Breathe in and out, "1." Breathe in and out, "2." Breathe in and out, "3." And then start again, breathe in and out, "1," in and out "2", in and out "3".... repeat as long as desired or until sleep comes.

I am grateful to my friend Suryanarayana Chennapragada for teaching this technique at my children's elementary school and so generously encouraging all to share it.[119] I find this exercise (with fingers and without) very useful when I need to stop myself from perseverating on my stressors and get myself to sleep.

Your pregnant stomach

It is not just the bladder that gets compressed. The baby puts pressure on the stomach as well. During pregnancy, especially for those of you further along, have you ever felt intensely hungry and then just after a few bites of food you feel full and a little unsettled? Then, two hours (or maybe just 15 minutes) later you are hungry again? The pressure on your stomach will vary according to your baby's size and position. If you cannot comfortably eat your whole meal and your portion sizes tend to be reasonable, you may benefit from switching to that pattern of grazing I mentioned earlier. By eating a small amount of food frequently throughout the day, you may be better able to get the nutrition you and your baby depend on.

Digestion and the intestinal tract

One of the most amazing mysteries in pregnancy is: where have your intestines gone? Before you were pregnant, your torso was filled completely with your intestinal tract. And now, where is it? (It's pregnancy magic!)

Logically, we know that the intestines are pushed up against the back and sides of your torso. It would also seem logical to assume that this displacement would influence changes in your digestion and bowel function. Add to this that your increased levels of pregnancy hormones also directly contribute to a digestion slow-down and it becomes easy to understand why many pregnant people suffer with digestive woes during pregnancy.[120]

Some of your pregnancy hormones, primarily progesterone, slow down the action of *smooth muscle*. Peristalsis, the action of moving food through your gut, is a smooth muscle function. This slowness improves your absorption of nutrients.[121] Further complicating digestion is the fact that most gestational parents are prescribed prenatal vitamins that contain iron, and many sources of iron can be very constipating. If you are taking a prenatal vitamin that has iron and you are suffering from constipation, consider talking to your care provider about switching to Floradix®, the plant-based iron supplement that I mentioned in Week 2 that tends to be easily absorbable and non-constipating.

You can also reduce your risk of constipation by drinking plenty of water, eating plenty of vegetables, fruits, and whole grains, and by getting daily exercise, including doing the pelvic rocks explained in Week 3. Constipation can also be caused by overeating. Be aware that if you stuff your gut, it's going to take more time to digest.

Stress or holding in your bowel urges can also increase constipation. If you are under a great deal of stress and/or do not or cannot take the time to follow your body's signals in a regular manner, you can further complicate your bowel function. For optimal health, try to keep to a reasonably regular schedule.

Hemorrhoids

A bulge in veins typically at the anus or just inside the rectum, hemorrhoids tend to be the result of forceful voiding from constipation or from forcefully pushing your baby out. To reduce the incidence of hemorrhoids, try to avoid constipation and forceful pushing. When it comes to your baby's journey out of your body, try to do your work by following your own instincts. Current obstetric practices of encouraging birthing people to push as hard as they can, while holding their breath as long as they can, can increase the occurrence of hemorrhoids.[122] Additionally, such misguided birth techniques as this could work to create future issues with incontinence and other pelvic floor issues (but more about that later).

I live with a hemorrhoid left over from my first pregnancy. I find pads soaked in witch hazel tend to help relieve occasional inflammation. Please discuss what will be best for you with your care provider. I recently had a client who was suffering tremendously through her pregnancy and opted to have her hemorrhoid surgically removed. She was quite sore for several days after the procedure, but she found relief once she healed up. She got through the remainder of the pregnancy and the birth without developing any new hemorrhoid, which hadn't been a guarantee.

Heartburn

Heartburn likely results from the above-mentioned pressure on the stomach, plus the sluggish digestive activity. It might also be aggravated by specific foods. If you are suffering from heartburn, you might try switching from eating big meals to the pattern of grazing throughout the day. It might also be helpful to pay attention to the quality of your time while eating. Are you running around work or home with something in your hand that you are munching on hurriedly as you try to multitask? Try taking the time to put your food on a plate and sit calmly while you eat. Look—even create space—for gratitude for both your food and your time to nourish yourself and this baby. It is important to rest when you feel tired; nonetheless, try to refrain from fully reclining immediately after eating. Sit back with lots of pillows, keeping your body more upright until the food goes down.

Shortness of breath

Is it hard to take a big deep breath? Are you more winded by simple activities? Many of those who are pregnant answer "yes." It would certainly seem that your diaphragm and your lungs are a little cramped for space. Maybe it is time to slow down a bit. Listen to your breathing as frequently as you can. Take the time to close your eyes and observe how you feel. Use your mind to calm yourself by focusing on slowing and deepening your breath. No matter how big your baby grows in the uterus, there is still enough room for plenty of air to get in and meet your needs. Allow your breath to follow your natural, comfortable patterns, and try to remember that pregnancy thrives when a parent is able to slow their pace enough for genuine self-care.

Swelling (edema)

Mild swelling (or, edema) is often a part of a normal pregnancy. But any amount of swelling you encounter should be discussed with your care provider. In the presence of swelling, one's adherence to the Brewer diet should be reevaluated and improved if necessary. Treat swelling in the ankles and feet by elevating the legs. If there is swelling in the hands, please remove any rings. If you cannot get your rings off, then they may need to be cut off. Rings that are cut off can be repaired, but it is certainly better to remove them early on and avoid the discomfort and inconvenience. You can always wear the rings that you love around your neck on a necklace for the duration of the pregnancy!

Sudden onset edema, when you seemingly—out of nowhere—swell up all over and quickly, may be a sign that the gestational parent's body is struggling to tolerate the pregnancy. If you suffer from swelling that is pervasive around your body it is urgent to consult with a care provider to monitor your blood pressure and to reevaluate your diet and exercise choices. (See Week 2 for a review of preeclampsia.)

Enlarged breasts

This symptom is often one of the first signs of pregnancy for an individual. Although there are many cultural ideals and stereotypes surrounding large breasts, changes in our body image can be emotionally complicated and challenging. It is important to note that for many biological females the enlarged breasts associated with pregnancy are very tender and often quite uncomfortable. Learning to get used to a lot of sensations in your breasts is a part of pregnancy and good practice for breastfeeding. Ditching your bra, at least when you are at home, as well as self-massage, and focusing on breasts in sex-play are a few ways to acclimate to all the new sensations.

Nasal congestion

All mucus membranes are highly active during pregnancy, due to your elevated hormone levels. Many people have a lot of sinus trouble and increased vaginal discharge during pregnancy. It might feel like your mucus production has gone crazy! For thinning and clearing nasal congestion, I like to steam my face over a bowl of hot water with a towel over my head (which has the added bonus of an impromptu facial). If you try this, keep a box of tissues nearby with which to blow your nose, as this will help you to clear out quite a lot of mucus. Additionally, keep well hydrated by drinking plenty of plain cool water, as this will also help to thin and void nasal secretions.

Stretch marks and other skin changes

Whether or not you get stretch marks depends on your genetics, and not on whether you purchase the right skincare products. There are many products on the market that suggest you should rub them into your belly to decrease or even erase stretch marks. I say go for it, assuming you like the product's ingredient list. Many skin and beauty products have a lot of ingredients you won't necessarily want to soak in, such as mineral oil, propylene glycol, or parabens. By contrast, if you have confidence in the ingredients and you enjoy the smell, texture, etc., by all means indulge. There can be a very nice self-care pampering feeling that comes from rubbing a lovely lotion or oil into your belly. (I use plain coconut oil for a moisturizer. If you want to try it, know that a little goes a long way.). Do it because *you* like the overall feeling. In other words, do it for yourself regardless of whether it will prevent stretch marks (it won't). Stretch marks start from the inside of your body, long before they are visible on the surface of your skin. Again, whether you get them or not is a hereditary issue.

How you feel about your body and any markings left after your birth is an area that may take some processing. You are different after you have a baby. Your whole life has changed, your body along with it. Don't be shy to explore how you feel about your changes. Many of us have some complicated feelings surrounding parenthood, changing bodies, and aging.

Braxton Hicks

Braxton Hicks contractions are the practice work that a uterus does prior to the onset of labor. For those who feel them, they typically feel like a tightening of the abdomen. They tend to be uncomfortable but not quite painful, and irregular with no clear pattern. When I had them, I sometimes wasn't sure if I were contracting or if the baby was stretching out and causing everything to get taut. Generally, however, during a Braxton Hicks contraction the belly feels quite hard to the touch. The contractions help tone the uterus for the work to come and also help to encourage blood flow throughout the entire placenta. I like to think that the baby receives an important massage or hug from these pre-contractions, and that they help her to prepare for what is to come as well. Importantly, a Braxton Hicks contraction also provides a wonderful opportunity to practice your mindfulness skills. As you feel the contraction, take long slow exhalations and spend a few moments relaxing into the contraction with awareness of your breathing.

Some people are aware of Braxton Hicks contractions from early on in their pregnancy, while others don't feel them until they reach full term. Some pregnant people never feel or notice Braxton Hicks contractions. Braxton Hicks are a normal part of pregnancy. However, if you find that you are having a series of rhythmic contractions, especially if you are not near your due date, you should drink some water. Moderate dehydration will increase the concentration of hormones in your blood, possibly tricking your system into thinking it is time to labor. If hydration doesn't help calm your pattern of contractions, then please seek medical attention to rule out preterm labor.

Fatigue

Fatigue is when you are tired even after waking up. If you are tired in the morning or after a nap, then you should closely examine your nutritional intake, general health, workload, and stress levels. Pregnancy is hard work, but it shouldn't be so hard that after sleep you are still tired. Exhaustion is your body's way of giving you a clear message about your health needs. Your baby's health is dependent upon your ability to heed your body's signals. Your labor prognosis will be directly related to how well rested you come to this work. Your physical and emotional strength depend on your ability to be well rested. Fatigue may be the result of a dietary insufficiency, which can result in anemia (low iron) or low protein intake, or it may be the result of a medical illness, from overworking, and/or chronic or acute stress.[123]

If you are experiencing fatigue, then one of the first things to do is to spend the following week charting your nutritional intake. If your diet looks good and you are hitting your goals, it's time to look further. I encourage you to communicate with your provider about your exhaustion. There are blood tests that can diagnosis anemia. Plus, your provider may want to rule out other illnesses, such as cardiac problems or Lyme disease. If your nutrition is good and the healthcare provider has ruled out disease, yet you remain run down, then it may be time to do what for many is the most challenging: it may be time to evaluate your work and stress load.

You are pregnant. It is no longer business as usual. You and your new baby are depending on you. Do you have too much on your plate? (I know that you do, and I am sorry about that!) Take a moment to identify some, if not all of your stressors. Say them out loud. Then write/draw them on the following page.

Crossing off non-essential responsibilities from your list is the first place to start. Do you have many social obligations that weigh on you? Do you have family or friends who are used to depending on you to get things done for them? Are there any social boundaries that need reevaluation? It's time to brainstorm about what solutions you can find to nurture more energy for yourself. Meditation and exercise can absolutely help you to reduce the effects of negative stress. Can you get more sleep; maybe go to bed one hour earlier each night? Where are you pushing yourself? Where can you ease up? Are you prioritizing anything fun? Playtime is important for both adults and children. Doing something just for fun can give you quite a lasting energy boost. Get creative as you assess your fatigue level. Being rested is not just good for health and how you feel now. Showing up to your birth well rested is critical to a good healthy birth process.

Changes in balance, attention, and clumsiness

Your center of gravity is shifting. Your attention is shifting. Your body now contains a moving baby. So changes in balance, attention, and clumsiness happen. Many pregnant people speak of dropping things, walking into things, and being easily distracted and/or preoccupied in their thinking. During my first pregnancy I missed my stop on the NYC subway twice on the way to work in the same week. I had never even done that once before. I was lost in my own thoughts and didn't notice until I was pulling out of the station. This was a new behavior for me, and a symptom of my pregnancy.

I can hear the critics yelling at me now for saying people can be easily distracted in pregnancy, that this can be used as a rally cry for sexism. To those critics I say, yes this is tricky ground to navigate. I do not mean to imply that pregnant people aren't as reliable as non-pregnant people. Gestational parents can push through and do all the amazing things they need to—fly airplanes, perform surgeries, run the country, get the laundry done—all while pregnant. But why should you have to if you're feeling stressed or tired, or just ready to focus more on the pregnancy? Pregnancy is another amazing thing and hard work, too! When you're pregnant, your life is changing and your priorities likely need to shift.

The childbearing year is a unique time in your life. I think society should pamper you wildly for the greater good. Not because you are less than, but because you are *more than*. You shouldn't have to work so hard at other work while also creating and nurturing the future of humanity. If you drop a dish while washing it, be compassionate with yourself. You are very busy baby building and it can be a challenge to multitask while doing such important work.

Food cravings and repulsions

Strong cravings and strong repulsions are incredibly common in pregnancy. I believe in the body's wisdom and that you should listen to the messages you receive. Over the years, as I mentioned in Week 2, I have seen lifelong vegetarians wake up with undeniably strong cravings for meat. I have also seen meat eaters who are all of a sudden repulsed by meat or fowl. I believe these messages should be respected. Olives and pickles, for example, are a common craving when the body needs salt. I went through a section of my first pregnancy where I was absolutely repulsed by the smell of vinegar. Not only could I not eat anything with vinaigrette, I couldn't be near anyone eating it. Our guts and our sense of smell communicate important information to our brains, and give us more opportunity to follow our instincts. (Note: if you are craving any non-food items, such as ice, paper, dirt, etc., please consult a healthcare provider. In medicine, this condition is called "pica" and it is associated with nutrient deficiencies.[124])

Moodiness

All this change is challenging! Crying can relieve stress and is a healthy release, but also do try to schedule things that are just for fun. Seek out special activities that are pleasurable. Maybe try listening to music, visiting with friends, getting out into nature, or sharing massages. Prioritize something that feels special and fun. Writing in your journal is a way to connect to and express your emotional reactions to the challenges you are feeling. Seek out face-to-face connections with kind people. Hugs can sometimes help.

Never hesitate to seek out a mental health professional. Anxiety, depression, distorted or disorganized thinking, compulsive behaviors or thoughts, these are all serious health issues that can be triggered by negative stress.[125] Please do not suffer in silence. If something seems off, seek professional mental health support.

Sometimes when I am burdened by my workload and I start to feel inadequate, I make an "I've done" list for myself. It's the opposite of a "To do" list. Here's one that I kept from a few years back:

- I got out of bed, kissed my partner, hugged my youngest, woke up my oldest.
- I brushed my teeth.
- I made and ate breakfast.
- I got lunches made.
- I checked the weather forecast.
- I counseled family members on appropriate outer wear for weather.

- ○ I signed the school permission slip for next week's field trip.
- ○ I found the missing glove.
- ○ I wished each parting person a great day and said, "I love you," on their way out the door.
- ○ I paid several bills.
- ○ I checked my work email.
- ○ And it's only just now 8 a.m.! Wow, I am good. ☺

These lists are sometimes the perfect antidote for when I am feeling overwhelmed with the never-ending work at hand. My "I've done" list helps me to readjust my perspective. It helps me to realize how much I do, and that helps me to feel better about myself, which in turn gives me energy to carry on. Pregnancy is hard work! And so is parenthood. Nurturing uses resources and requires energy and time. Let's give ourselves a pat on the back as we work hard to do our best, which is and will continue to be good enough.

A strength that I bring to this process is…? Hmmm… what answers will I find today? Return to the exercise that opened this Week 5 and see what additional strengths or positive behavioral attributes you can add to your list! (No really, go back to the beginning of this chapter and add your new thoughts. What follows will wait.)

My most "glamorous" pregnancy memory

One night during my second pregnancy, while *very* extremely pregnant, I was sitting on a futon on the floor. I had just finished teaching a Bradley® class, so I had been sitting for some time. My clients had all left and I was finishing some notes. Julian came downstairs, just as I was ready to stand. As I was moving through a hands-and-knees position on my journey up, I suddenly felt a sharp, round-ligament jolt of pain. The cramp deep in my groin caused me to move my leg out to the side where I promptly knocked over my water glass. My dear sweet and loving husband found this hilarious. I did, too, actually. So I joined him in laughter, which made him laugh harder in turn. I was still trying to stand up, but I couldn't quite get myself up off the floor—between the pain and the laughter I was quite like a beached whale. This again made Julian laugh harder, which again made me laugh harder. But my round ligament still hurt, so my laugher turned into crying, and I still couldn't get up to standing.

The absurdity of it all encouraged more crying, but then I also laughed harder. Laughing harder made me pee my pants. I of course announce this to Julian, at which point we are now both in full-fledged hysterics. I'm still paused in my journey to stand. One knee up and one knee down, my pants were wet, my cheeks were tear stained, and my sides ached from laughing so hard. I tried to compose myself, there was work to be done. I had to get up off the floor, clean up the water, and change my pee pants. It took a few moments, but finally I steadied myself enough to get to my feet. Of course, this didn't happen without further incident: As I stood up I was caught by a sneeze. Oops, there goes a little more pee. And, uh oh, I now have a bloody nose! (Note that bloody noses are a fairly common pregnancy inconvenience, even if you don't typically suffer from them.[126]) There was blood and boogers all over my chest. By the time I got to the bathroom I was a total disaster and had to get completely undressed to clean up. Thankfully this was before smart phones with cameras. We laughed all night about it as we marveled at my enormous baby-belly and the process of pregnancy. As embarrassing as it sounds, this really is a cherished memory of how much and how hard I laugh with Julian, and how much love we have shared over the years. I have a pee-my-pants-from-giggling story from my first pregnancy, too. Eight months pregnant and in a canoe… but that is a story for another day.

Tears

Let your tears flow. Crying makes us healthier, just like laughter. I have heard that sometimes a pregnant person will cry to give voice to their baby's cries. It doesn't matter why you are crying. It's all a good release. Look for pride in your ability to release your tears. I respect the ability to cry as a powerful cleansing strength. Dr. Judith Orloff, MD writes:

> Our bodies produce three kinds of tears: reflex, continuous, and emotional. Each kind has different healing roles. For instance, reflex tears allow your eyes to clear out noxious particles when they're irritated by smoke or exhaust. The second kind, continuous tears, are produced regularly to keep our eyes lubricated—these contain a chemical called "lysozyme," which functions as an anti-bacterial and protects our eyes from infection. Tears also travel to the nose through the tear duct to keep the nose moist and bacteria free. Typically, after crying, our breathing and heart rate decrease, and we enter into a calmer biological and emotional state.
>
> Emotional tears have special health benefits. Biochemist and "tear expert" Dr. William Frey at the Ramsey Medical Center in Minneapolis discovered that reflex tears are 98% water, whereas emotional tears also contain stress hormones that get excreted from the body through crying. After studying the composition of tears, Dr. Frey found that emotional tears shed these hormones and other toxins that accumulate during stress. Additional studies also suggest that crying stimulates the production of endorphins, our body's natural pain killer and "feel-good" hormones.[127]

EXERCISE: SQUEEZE YOUR HANDS DURING INHALATION, RELAX THEM OPEN DURING EXHALATION

This is a simple coping technique for anytime you need to release some stress. Sit or stand comfortably and close your eyes. As you inhale, squeeze your hands into tight fists, continuing to squeeze with strength throughout the inhalation. As you exhale, fully release the tension of the hands. Melt your hands open, letting the palms be open and the fingers unfurl and have their full resting weight.

—Pause to practice—

The physiology of birth

Physiology (noun)
    1. Study of functioning of living things
        The branch of biology that deals with the internal workings of living things, including functions
            such as metabolism, respiration, and reproduction, rather than with their shape or structure.

The physiology of birth is a huge subject. There are many ways to think about the subject, from a host of different perspectives. For our purposes in this book, I will start with how labor starts, cover the basic medical language of the stages of labor, explore the muscular activity of contractions, consider the cervix and its status as a measurement tool, and then progress to the hormones and how they inform the process.

Scientists still aren't exactly sure how human labor begins.[128] I imagine a little pop-up baby thermometer, like ones found in those commercially raised turkeys that you might buy for Thanksgiving: Pop! "Hello, I'm ready!" But until we get more science, that is just my imagination. I find it intriguing that there are still such big, and yet basic, unanswered questions, like how does labor actually begin?

> In many animals (such as the sheep) the fetus sends a signal to the mother when maturity has been reached which precipitates the labour [sic] at the appropriate time. There is no such evidence of any such mechanism in human pregnancy though it is such an attractive mechanism in biological terms that it is unlikely to have been lost completely with evolution.[129]

Even in the absence of definitive evidence, it seems plausible that the onset of human birth might have something to do with the fetus's vital systems reaching maturation.

> Only a small percentage of women (4%) will deliver on the calculated date of delivery, with the majority being distributed within a period of 2 – 3 weeks around this date. The mechanisms governing the exact timing of birth are not known, though it is unlikely that they are designed to be specific to any 24-hour period, as the preliminary processes of labour [sic] occur over a matter of weeks.[130]

Birth takes time. The work is ongoing. And each little twinge and Braxton Hicks contraction helps, whether one is directly aware of the work happening or not. It's all part of the process.

> The term *parturition* refers to the process of giving birth. The process of labour [sic] is not well understood. It involves cervical ripening, uterine activity and membrane rupture. The processes that occur ... occur in parallel to allow the cervix to "give way" and convert the uterus from one which has incoordinate uterine contractions to coordinated regular contractions of greater amplitude and with greatly increased response to contractile stimuli.[131]

Hmmm... does that sound a bit like sex? Something lets go—gives way—and then little twinges grow to larger waves, getting more and more organized, louder and more sensitive... more and more and more...oh yeah! The birth process is a facet of our sexuality. Is that an idea you have considered before? I ask that you keep an open mind about this connection between birth and sex, and to keep your curiosity about these connections as you progress through this book and the rest of your birth education efforts. Seeing the link between our sexuality and our birth functioning can, I believe, help build trust in the birth process, and lead us towards our best support of each other through this incredible transformation to family life. With this in mind, I will continue with more birth physiology.

Labor is a process that happens over time, sometimes a very long time. Although there may be the equivalent of a flipped switch that begins the process, the work that follows is incremental:

> During the course of several days to several weeks before the onset of true labor [when noticeable contractions begin and don't stop until baby is born], the cervix begins to soften and dilate. In many cases when labor starts, the cervix is already dilated 1 – 3 cm in diameter.[132]

The "*Stages* of Labor": Ta Daaa!

In medical terms labor gets divided into three stages: first, second, and third.[133] **First stage labor starts with uterine contractions that work to thin and open the cervix. Second stage labor is the expulsive phase of labor. It begins when the cervix is completely open and completes when the baby is out of your body and into your arms. Third stage labor is the passing of your placenta, through the birth canal and out of the body.** That's it. 1, 2, 3 and you're done! All those things happen and in that order. Right? Be careful not to assume that the general medical description paints the fullest picture of your labor process.

Understanding the medical terminology can help you to better understand and communicate with medical providers. Understanding how medical language describes a limited view of what happens in the birth is also important. Medical language is a piece of the birth puzzle when you are with medical providers. Medical language is limited in scope because it often omits a holistic view of the gestational person and baby in their process. Instead, it suggests a segregated and disconnected understanding. Putting medical language and thought into a different perspective will make it easier to navigate interventions.

First stage labor, for example, does get further subdivided into early, or *latent labor* and *active labor*, which is classified as being once the labor has developed further. But those classifications are basically still all in relationship to cervical changes, or lack thereof. There is also another term used for later first stage: "transition." While it is not technically medical, it is commonly used among birth attendants to describe the end of first stage labor, just prior to the onset of the expulsive or second phase. (Transition has unique physical and emotional characteristics that I will discuss later in this book. It roughly correlates to the process of cervical dilation from 7 centimeters to 10 centimeters.) Second and third stage labor do not generally get characterized into smaller terms, such as early and late, because they are much shorter in duration than first stage.

Now that you have the basic language for the stages of labor, what does the *work* of labor involve?

Contractions: It's what our muscles do

A "contraction" is when muscle fibers shorten; they slide over each other toward the middle of the muscle, getting smaller and tighter.[134] When the uterus contracts, the action starts at the fundus and continues through the long vertical muscle fibers of the uterine wall. In labor, once the cervix has begun to soften, this contractile activity starts to stretch open the circular muscle fibers of the cervix, thus enlarging the os (cervical opening).[135] Just like other muscle groups in our bodies, when one group of muscles is contracting, another is extending, lengthening, stretching. Once the cervical door is open, the uterine contractions help to push the baby down and out through the vagina. And to help the cervix to open, just like other sphincters (such as the anus), the gestational parent should feel safe and preferably free from interruption to facilitate the opening up. Hey, that's true for sex too! I have always found sex to be better when I feel safe and free from interruption. How about you? Onward with the physiology.

Things that contract get smaller, harder, and tighter. This is the work of the uterus. By contrast, this is *not* what the mental work—in the bigger picture of birth—is really about. To birth, the emotional work is to yield, to surrender, stretch and open. To birth, therefore, seems paradoxical to the movement of contraction; to birth we need to get bigger, softer and looser (rather than smaller, harder and tighter). Yet birth necessarily involves contraction. The uterine muscle needs to work very hard to contract with full force and great endurance, with help from the abdominal muscles. Again, while birth contractions are the (mostly) involuntary work of the uterus, mental work during labor is the exact opposite: you will need to consciously soften, lengthen, and yield, to open wide with focus. (Yup, just like during sex.)

In medical textbooks, a mythical uterus has labor contractions that start out far apart and don't last long. As the textbook labor progresses, the contractions get closer together, longer and more challenging to endure. Eventually, during the end of first stage labor, textbook contractions are coming fast, lasting a long time and ferocious to contend with. (Contractions can last up to a full minute, and rarely, even a bit longer than that.) But please remember, this is a theoretical textbook definition. I have seen many people whose labors began with a bang and had fast and furious contractions throughout, and others who have sections of their birth that slow down and space out periodically during their process. I have heard stories from women who have had contractions begin at three minutes apart and lasting 50 seconds long, and they continued in that same pattern for the duration of the birth. We are not machines, and we are all individuals. Some of us are very fast; some are very regular; some of us take a long time to organize; and some of us never quite organize the way we are expected to. And yet we all get the work of labor done in our own way.

Nevertheless, during second stage labor the contractions often get farther apart than they had been at the end of first stage. This provides some much-needed rest time. You will need to rest when you can in labor (and in parenthood). The goal is to regroup and calm yourself emotionally as well as physically during the time in between your uterine contractions. The quality of how that time in between the contractions is spent may be one of the biggest predictors both of birth success and of how a gestational parent feels about their birth afterwards. But more on this last point later in the book.

Dilation and effacement

Your cervix will go through two processes during your first stage: "dilation" and "effacement." Dilation is when the uterine mouth opens. Once dilation is complete, the os will be at approximately 10 centimeters in diameter. As I noted earlier, the process of dilation may start many weeks in advance of recognizable labor.

Effacement, which starts prior to dilation, is the shortening, softening, and thinning of the cervical walls. Effacement is measured in percentages of softness and shortness. A laboring person will progress from 1% to 100% effaced.[136] But measuring the cervix is not directly predictive. In other words, if you measure at 100% effaced and 5 centimeters dilated you still don't know how much longer it will take until you complete your first stage of labor. (For additional discussion of these measurement issues, see Week 9 and the subject of vaginal exams.)

Before labor begins, the cervix feels like the tip of your nose (go on, touch your nose). The tip of a closed cervix is similar in size to the tip of your nose. As the cervix starts to efface, (soften, shorten, and thin) it changes to feel more like the softness of your lip (go on, touch your lip). At full effacement with partial dilation, a cervix might feel like a rubber band on its side. With full dilation your care attendant may not be able to feel your cervix. I have heard birth attendants proclaim that a person's cervix is "all gone." In fact, it is not gone, it just cannot be felt or measured at that moment in the birth process.

Is the cervix all that?

For obstetricians, first stage labor remains all about the measurable changes in the cervix. To start, changes in the cervix are "measured" with fingers not rulers. Next, the results of this measuring are interpreted. Math is put into play; it feels scientific. But what if we are wrong about what we are measuring, or how we are interpreting the data? What if labor is not just about cervical changes? What if we are collecting, measuring and interpreting the wrong data, leading us obviously to false conclusions? As you ponder these questions, I will add some additional perspective.

Trying to understand birth by focusing on the cervix is like trying to understand digestion by focusing on the anus. Think of all the physiology that happens from the first bite of food that goes into your mouth. You release saliva with enzymes, your taste buds are stimulated, your memories and associations start to connect, you chew, and you swallow, you start to produce insulin, you produce bile, you absorb, you discard, and on and on. From the first smell to the first bite, on through elimination, there is an incredible array of metabolic activity happening that is far more complex than the opening and closing of the anus (another body sphincter, like the cervix). Imagine how different going to the doctor with intestinal illness would be if we relied solely on the anal sphincter for our information about digestive health issues!

Why do some cervices open rapidly, in minutes, and others take days, even weeks? Do some people need more time to stretch open than others? Why, when you are making love, do you sometimes climax right away, while at other times you can take all night? Why is it that sometimes one lovely climax fills you up and at other times several lovely climaxes are barely enough? What mysteries our bodies hold!

The cervix can dilate very quickly, or it can take its own sweet time, which is why birth should be evaluated beyond just the muscular action of the opening and closing of the cervix. I want to encourage you to broaden your understanding of labor; to see more going on than just what is happening to your cervix. Some people are in labor for 15, maybe 20 hours and they have only gotten to 1 – 2 centimeters dilation. Then they can go from 2 centimeters to ten in 20 minutes. Once again: we are not automated machines; we are thinking, feeling, and reacting living bodies. What's more, during birth our bodies are dancing a duet with our babies, influenced by a musical score made from our thoughts and emotions!

"Labor"

Everyone refers to the process of birth with the term "labor." In keeping with the theme that our words really do matter, I think it's important to ruminate on the word labor a bit longer here. What does this word mean to you? Write/draw your responses below.

Now that you have thought about your own definitions, I encourage you to look up the word in any dictionaries you can access to consider as many definitions as possible. Taking the time to labor (!) over the process of defining this single word can help us more fully articulate our thoughts and deepen communication. We can also choose to accept, reframe, or reject someone else's words for our body process. The word "labor" can have many negative connotations. I know I don't want to think of my own birth process as something with so many negative associations. How do you feel about that word for your birth?

On the Farm in Tennessee, where Ina May Gaskin (renowned midwife and author) lives and works, they have chosen to use the word "rush" instead of "contraction." The concern with the word contraction is that it might make a person recoil or tense. The word "rush" lends itself to the perception that the experience is a rush of energy that passes through you. By this same thinking, what if we stopped using the word "labor," like we did with "mucous plug," and started using the word "transformation"? As in, "My child was born after a long and challenging transformation."

The words that a person uses as they define themself, or are preparing for birth, really do matter. For example, it is so important to discuss preferred pronoun use with our providers, friends, and relations. Our words and our definitions are critical to effective communication, which is critical to getting good healthcare and social support, and to knowing ourselves—our identities. Our words can lift us up, or they can be disempowering and misleading. Our words can scare us and undermine our confidence, or they can make us proud, hopeful and determined. What are we telling ourselves? What are the thoughts embedded in the thinking about this upcoming birth experience? What do we think we already know about the future from the associations we have with the words?

What happens to your experience when you use medical vocabulary that is narrow in focus to describe your own expansive birth process? Do you limit the experience by limiting your discussion to just a few elements of a birth? Can the medical terms be harmful? Can language be considered an "iatrogenic" (doctor-caused) intervention? The list of negative terms related to birth physiology in medical jargon is seemingly unending: cervical insufficiency, failure to progress, irritable uterus, geriatric pregnancy (for those over 35!), dysfunctional uterus, false labor, one can "fail" the glucose tolerance test, and on and on and on. Negative terminology causes us to internalize bad feelings.

Negative medical language shuts down confidence, implants fear, and leads to the release of excess stress hormones, which then complicates the birth. Imagine what positive language can do to reverse these feelings. If you were describing your body processes, what kind of words would you like to use?

"False labor" (My ass! There is nothing false about what you feel.)

In my opinion, one of the worst medical terms associated with labor is "false labor." This term is occasionally used to describe a common scenario in which many gestational people find themselves. Contractions begin and then fade, and this continues with several apparent starts and stops. This may happen over the course of days or even weeks. You seem to get a little work done, and then you stop. And then you get a little more done, and then you stop again. For many pregnant people and their babies this is a welcome way to get their work accomplished. I argue that if you are having a contraction, then there is nothing false about it! It is your body doing what it needs to do.

Birth is a process that requires patience (just like parenting will). Birth takes time; it ebbs and flows. If I had my choice, I would love to get some work done in smaller bits and pieces, with time to rest and recoup in between. Each muscle contraction is a part of your process. Any bit of work you are doing can be celebrated as good work, true work, real work done. Each contraction you have can be crossed off your to-do list, with a smile of accomplishment. Add it to your "I've done" list! Each bit of effort is work you won't have to do again. So please, feel free to throw the term "false labor" in the trash and embrace your *true* process and your *real* experiences.

And what about the baby in birth?

During birth, the baby goes through a significant physical transition to become an independent being. Contractions, for example, provide a tremendous deep tissue massage for the baby. This stimulation affects all of a baby's systems. Some babies may need more stimulation to be ready, hence they may need a longer labor.

During a contraction the baby is temporarily stressed by a decrease in oxygenation.[137] This causes the baby's vital processes to slow down. When the contraction ends, the baby's systems come back up to speed. This process helps the baby to make this enormous change-over from being a completely dependent system to being a completely *independent* system. I think of a train slowing down before it makes the switch to a different track. Think of all the metabolic changes that happen through birth, and then for breastfeeding, for both parent and baby. Humans have fluctuating metabolic speeds. With changes in effort and diet humans can decrease or increase metabolic rate. Birth embodies metabolic activity.

Fetal position is another logical variable in the length of labor. If the baby needs to adjust to a better position for decent, she may need to make many very small shifts to improve alignment. The baby wants to work in cooperation with their birth parent. (Who doesn't want their parent's approval?) The baby, in turn, relies on the parent to move their own body to help with this descent. There are many factors at play, some of which are known and some of which remain to be discovered. Perhaps, too, there are also psychological or spiritual developments for the baby (or parent!) that need to evolve for birth to complete. Likewise, birth also represents a tremendous emotional development for the birth parent and baby alike. Even a very long birth is still a rapid transition when you consider how big a deal being born or becoming a parent is. That baby is coming. Do you feel any angst over this upcoming transition? Do you feel elation? Both? What length of time will you and your baby need to process this transformation?

Hormones: The chemical feedback system of birth (or the "fizz" in "physiology")

Once the as-of-yet-unknown signals begin the process of birth, the pregnant person's body releases a dose of oxytocin. This hormone, often called the "love hormone," causes the uterus to contract. The contraction will be only as strong as the dose of oxytocin warrants. (In Week 12 you will discover that this "dose" may be more about numbers of oxytocin receptor sites turned on, rather than any actual quantity of oxytocin. But for now it's just as useful to think about it in terms of dosage size.) In response to the strong sensations the birthing person will feel, they will then release a dose of stress hormones. (The body says, "Oh ho! What is going on? What am I being called on to do?") In other words, the amount of stress hormone released will be directly related to the amount of physical stress experienced, which was determined in turn by the amount of oxytocin released in the previous dose. In response to the stress hormones, the birthing person will then release a dose of endorphins, i.e., natural pain killers. These endorphins reduce pain and help to energize the birthing person. With endorphins in our system, we calm down, so that stress hormones are reduced and another dose of oxytocin can be released. Thus the cycle continues—until the baby is out.[138] Oxytocin – stress hormones – endorphins, oxytocin – stress hormones – endorphins—until the birth is complete.

At least, that is the cycle that nature intended. But when a birthing person experiences stress from external circumstances, they cannot release enough endorphins to counter the increased amounts of stress hormones. This will reduce the overall amounts of oxytocin they release, which will slow labor and create dysfunction in the birth process. Excess external stressors negatively interfere with the internal chemical regulation of birth.

For a labor to progress well, one needs to feel safe and trust their surroundings so that the endocrine system can function optimally. But stress can also be caused by internal emotional forces. A birthing parent's own fears or negative attitudes can also create undue added stress, and therefore have a negative impact on their birth physiology. Different people will release different amounts of stress hormones in response to their particular circumstances, personal histories, perspectives, and expectations. Each person comes to their birth with their own memories, ideas, associations, fears, belief systems, and dreams. Each person is also uniquely influenced by the actions and emotions of the people around them.

Your pregnancy now—today, this week—is the time to think through these birth-facts, and birth-words, and your feelings in relation to them. With a deeper understanding of your process, you can better make plans that support your physiology. If it's overwhelming to consider any or all of this, try practicing the "Counting Breaths" exercise included in this chapter. It can help you make some emotional space to settle and get to know your feelings. Importantly, seek out ways to have a healthy and emotionally engaged week: eat, work, play, and rest well. And, of course, do your homework!

Thank you for your time this week. Take great care!

HOMEWORK

A) Identify potential issues that could cause excess birth stress for you

To help you to identify these such issues, discuss them, write them down, draw them, sing about them... explore them in any way you can. This will be helpful preparation. When you build awareness, in whatever medium(s), you can better strategize your ways to cope.

B) A Series of Four Massages

Each partner will give and receive two massages. If you don't have a partner, then it may be nice to try and exchange some massages with a friend or family member.

Step One: Each partner should visualize what they think would be a great massage for themself. Spend some time planning and thinking about it. For example:

○ Would you like to use any scented oils or lotions?

○ Would you like to be on blankets or on a mat on the floor or on a bed?

○ What kind of massage strokes would you like to feel: strong and deep kneading or a very light and gentle touch?

○ Is there one part of your body that needs more attention?

○ Would you like an hour on your head and three minutes on the rest of your body?

○ What do you think would be ideal for your own self-designed massage?

○ Would you like to play music or be outside?

○ Would you like your massage in the dark or with candlelight?

○ What would you really like to receive?

Step Two: Pick who will give the first massage and who will receive.

○ The giving partner will imagine—and work to create—the scenario of their own dream massage, and then give that to their partner. This will allow the receiving partner to learn firsthand what it is that the giving partner really likes. This is massage #1.

○ The receiving partner now becomes the giving partner, who must first visualize a version of their own ideal massage. This is massage #2

○ For massages #3 and #4 each partner will have an opportunity to recreate and give back their partner's ideal massage as it was learned by first having received it.

In sum:

Massage #1: Partner A gives their dream massage to Partner B.

Massage #2: Partner B gives their dream massage to Partner A.

Massage #3: Partner A recreates and gives back Partner B's dream massage.

Massage #4: Partner B recreates and gives back Partner A's dream massage.

Lather, rinse, repeat. This massage pattern is a great practice to integrate into your partnership. A couple can deepen and develop their nonverbal communication skills through massage. As with most things, if you practice you get better. If you are ever feeling cranky and disconnected from your partner, try agreeing to work on non-verbal communication and then quietly give each other massages. Your intention should be simple: to soothe tension and facilitate connection. Massage increases empathy. I find that when I give massages, my own breathing deepens; the focus of my task helps to center me. Listening to my partner's body gives me a singular task and, in this way, becomes a form of meditation.

Remember: non-verbal communication will be very helpful during birth. If a birthing person doesn't have to ask or explain things, they can conserve their energy and focus more readily on the birth process.

THIS SPACE IS FOR YOUR NOTES AND DRAWINGS

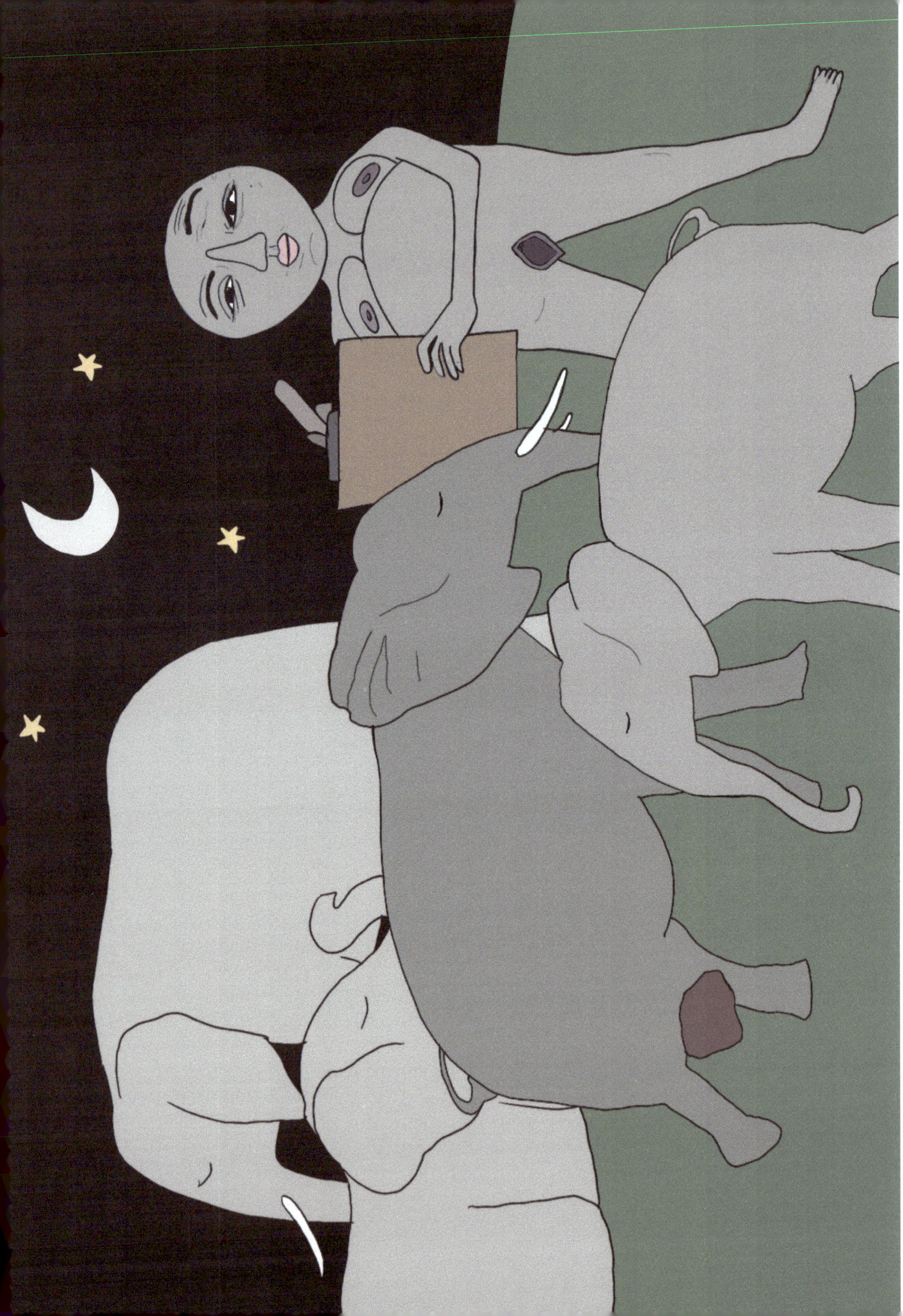

WEEK 6

Love
and
Service

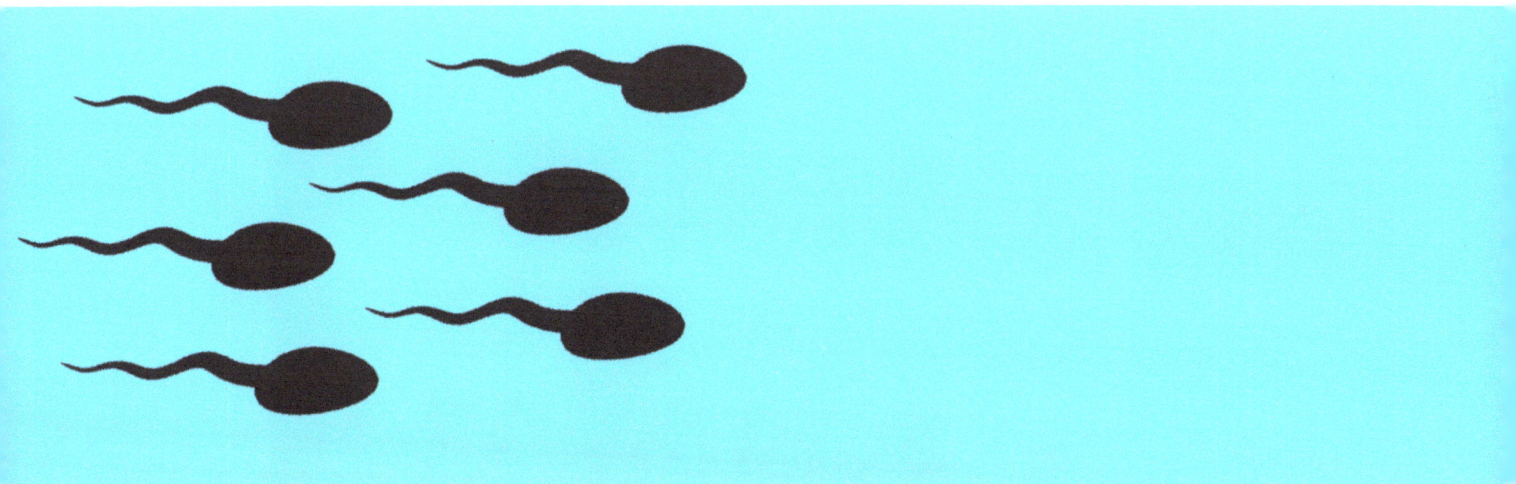

Chapter contents:

O *Building confidence*

O *Birth support skill development*

THIS SPACE IS FOR YOUR NOTES AND DRAWINGS

Hello hello! How was your week? Did you have a chance to exchange any massages? If yes, I hope it was enjoyable. Give each other some feedback on the massages now and make a brief plan for a future massage date! Did you identify anything that might become a source of excess stress during birth? Remember: identifying potential issues now will help you to plan and problem-solve later.

Skills for birth supporters

There are a lot of different ways to understand the role of a birth supporter. What constitutes meaningful support will be different for different people, with the exception that birth support always includes love and compassion—how you put these elements together and what form they take are up to you. Support needs will vary throughout an individual birth and from one birth to another. I like for birth supporters to think about having a metaphorical tool bag well stocked with an assortment of techniques and a variety of approaches, from which they can choose. But before we can fill this bag we must first examine some of the basics, i.e., the raw material of the task at hand.

Sup'port (transitive verb)
1. Keep something or somebody stable
    To keep something or somebody upright or in place or prevent something or somebody from falling

You know a healthy birth is well supported when the process can happen without you being fearful of or fighting with anyone, even yourself. Can you yield to your sensations and just "go with it"? In other words, can you relax all the muscles in your body during the strongest parts of your sensations? When you feel safe, for yourself and your baby, and you are surrounded by knowledgeable, happy, kind—read: supportive—people, your capacity to yield or surrender will increase exponentially.

Support can and should involve a multifaceted approach. It starts with you and your baby, then expands in circles out from there. By definition, a healthy pregnant person does not *need* anything or anyone to birth successfully. They do not need a medical expert, a birth expert, the right birth class, the right hospital; they do not even need to read the right book (says this author of a book on birthing!). You and your baby already have the information you need for birth deeply embedded in every cell of your bodies. The instruction manual has been there since human life first reproduced. Remember, if natural childbirth didn't work, we wouldn't be here!

I observe that in the U.S. there is too much emphasis on teaching pregnant people to be reliant on other people, things, and services for birth. There is almost always the expectation, including in Bradley Method® classes, that both a primary partner and a care provider play essential roles. Undoubtedly, the right helpers can aid in the creation of an excellent environment. Having the support of a well-trained and loving midwife can be an essential ingredient for birth's unexpected challenges. Having your lover, or loved one, friend or family, by your side can provide familiarity, comfort and powerful encouragement. External support, however, shouldn't be a pregnant person's first thought when they think of coping through birth; again, they should think of their own abilities and the work they alone must do.

Don't lose sight of the fact that you are preparing for your own body's natural function. Ultimately, *you* will birth your baby. That baby is coming out of you. Your muscles will be contracting and releasing, your nerves will be tingling, your blood will be flowing, your voice will be reverberating, and you will learn about your capacities for expansion, stamina, surrender, and growth. And don't forget the baby! She, too, is also an active, instinctive participant. I encourage you to acknowledge this continually throughout your process. Effective support involves confidence, not just in your partner or care provider or best-selling book (!); don't shy away from fostering confidence in yourself, in your abilities as a birthing parent. Be courageous!

How, you ask? How can you soften into your strong sensations and avoid the stress, fear, and routine overuse of medical interventions that dominate American birthing culture? Birth requires the release of your inhibitions. Ina May Gaskin refers to the process of "releasing your inner monkey": allowing your inner primate self to be free.[139] The process of releasing your inhibitions, of yielding to your sensations and finding your untapped power, will be easier once your courage and confidence are more developed. Birth education is a great place to start!

Remember: having courage doesn't mean you are not scared; it means you move forward anyway. Birth education can help you (*is* helping you) to examine your plans for the location of your birth and for who is on your support team. It helps you to better understand your legal rights as well as some of the many biases, traditions, and conditioning that you may consciously or unconsciously bring to your birth process. Ultimately, birth education (and, again, this book is just one of its many forms) helps you to identify and employ strategies that promote your best inner environment for working through the strong sensations of your transformation.

Courage (noun)

1. The ability to face danger, difficulty, uncertainty, or pain without being overcome by fear or being deflected from a chosen course of action

When you are pregnant you must face two immediate facts: 1) there is a baby growing inside you and 2) this baby is going to have to come out. Parenthood is *all* about courage. So how can you best tap into this important and wonderous resource? How do you find, build, unleash your courage? One way is to try to clarify your fears. What exactly are you afraid of? And why? By being reflective and introspective, you can try to understand where the fears you have come from. And then you can attempt to overcome them.

Write out a list of your fears and, if you can, explore where each of them comes from below.

Sometimes connecting to the source of a fear can help you to dissipate that fear. Other fears may not be as easy to let go. In these cases, it may be useful to build out plans that can help you to cope, should your fears be realized during your birth process. Creating routines to deploy when a fear is triggered, as well as working with a therapist or other wellness expert, if needed, can be important elements to help you through your fears. Nevertheless, fear remains a normal part of pregnancy, making your ability to identify your fears another one of your superpowers. When we explore our fears we learn more about ourselves. And knowing what you are afraid of can empower you to determine what you need to learn next.

Con'fi'dence (noun)
   Self-assurance or a belief in your ability to succeed

Admittedly, it can be difficult to maintain confidence when many of the messages you hear about birth are so scary. As a result, we may oftentimes feel disconnected from our magnificent abilities. As you prepare for birth, with your support team on board and your courage amped up, you may still need what social psychologist Amy Cuddy explores in her TedGlobal presentation: the stamina not just to "fake it 'til you make it," but "fake it 'til you become it."[140]

I highly recommend that you watch Cuddy's TedGlobal talk. She documents research that shows just how powerful our mind-body connection is. This research has discovered that by holding a powerful posture in our body, for just two minutes at a time, we can begin to change our hormonal chemistry and become more powerful within our individual selves. A powerful posture involves spreading yourself out open and wide, taking up as much space as you can. For example, stand up tall, with your legs in a comfortably wide stance, chest wide and open, and your hands on your hips with elbows out as wide as possible.

Cuddy's research reveals that such powerful posturing increases testosterone levels at the same time that it decreases cortisol (stress hormone) levels. Testosterone is known as a hormone that can produce strong, confident feelings, and these feelings often have a profound impact on both how you feel about yourself and how other people react to you. By the same token, if you make yourself smile, even when you feel down or angry, you will start to feel happier. Yes, Smile Therapy works! According to Cuddy, "Our bodies change our minds; our minds change our behavior and our behavior changes our outcomes."[141]

As you think about your upcoming birth, try telling yourself that you are confident and that you will be courageous now and when birth comes. Be honest with yourself about how you are feeling, of course; then push yourself, get into a powerful stance, hold it for two minutes, and "try on" your courageous voice. Announce: "I will get through this birth!" These simple actions will help you to embody confidence. Another way to think about it is to imagine that you are acting in a movie about a person courageous about their birth. What would your most powerfully spoken line be? How would you stand? What posture and body language would you project? Go ahead, play the part. See what it feels like. Get playful, laugh along the way, and *build your power*.

EXERCISE: POWERFUL POSES

Stand up and play with bold confident body language, stances and gestures. Explore different positions. Try making yourself as large as can be, stable and powerful. Stand with your feet apart (just wider than shoulder width), hands on your hips with elbows out wide, and chest lifted. Or, try hands in fists, raised up over your head. Find a stance you like and hold it for two minutes, or as long as you comfortably can. You can build up to two minutes through practice, in your own time.

What else can you do to build your confidence? You can build strength with physical exercise, more education, social support, good food, and adequate sleep. Try to surround yourself with people who have positive views of birth and who believe in you. Work hard to give yourself encouraging messages and repeated affirmations. I have seen affirmations work wonders for some while preparing for birth. I suggest you, too, give them a try. Try saying one or more of the following:

- MY BODY WORKS WELL.

- MY BODY IS MADE TO HAVE BABIES.

- I WILL BE SAFE IN MY STRONG SENSATIONS.

- I WILL GET THROUGH THIS NO MATTER HOW HARD.

- MY BABY KNOWS HOW TO FIND THE WAY OUT.

- MY BABY IS CAPABLE AND STRONG.

- I TRUST MY BODY AND MY PROCESS.

- I AM GRATEFUL FOR THE OPPORTNITY TO BIRTH.

- ACTUALLY, I CAN.

If you find it uncomfortable or false feeling to say such affirmations, then let it go. But if giving yourself a positive message helps to carry you forward with more confidence, then you've just identified another great member of your support team!

Accepting help is sometimes the hard part

While I am adamant in my own confidence that pregnant people have what they need inside themselves for birth, I also recognize the strength in being able to accept love and nurturing. For many modern, super-achieving wonder-people, asking for and/or accepting support can be difficult. Is it difficult for you?

Try to identify some examples of when you have welcomed support into your life. Try also to identify examples of when you wanted help but didn't (or couldn't) ask or didn't accept the help offered. Take a few moments now to write down your responses below.

When it comes to learning about birth support, elephants present an excellent model for us to consider. Elephants make a circle around the birthing mama.[142] In this way they are able to look out for danger while at the same time check in on the mother—assuming she can trust her herd. Humans attending a birth often create an analogously safe environment, full of helpful loving support. Just as often, however, the human environment created can sabotage birthing efforts. This may be done subtly or not. Either way, the result is an undermining of the birthing person's confidence through interruption, hurrying, disrespecting, threatening (even mildly), doubting, being fearful themselves, giving false information, etc. Your so-called support people can either be tremendously helpful or they can cause considerable obstacles.

Consequently, those in supportive roles should strive to fill the environment with love and enthusiasm for the birth process. They can provide physical, emotional, and mental support when, where, and how the birthing person wants it. They can be ready with water, a basin, or some tissues, for example, if you need to drink, vomit, or cry.

Perhaps it is helpful here to return to the role of language, and how it can impact who we appoint to be part of our support team. Think "coach," for example. What are your first thoughts when you hear this word? Maybe: horse-drawn carriage or person who trains athletes, performers, or students (think: soccer coach, voice coach, or debate team coach). Maybe you even thought about "Coach" as the name of a designer purse. Many of us think "sports" when we hear the word "coach." When I ask my classes what they think of when they hear the word "coach," I receive these common responses:

"A big guy with a whistle"

"Yeah, in a tight polo shirt!"

"Someone who motivates you"

"An authority figure"

"A role model or mentor"

Students have also shared their own experiences with a "coach," such as an authority figure who frequently yells at them and the other players on the team. I have gone on to ask if the coach *played* the game. Meaning, if the coach were ejected, would the game continue? Yes, of course! Everyone agrees: coaches are secondary to the playing of the game. Is it assumed that the coach knows more about the game than the players? Yes, the coach is responsible for strategizing and is perceived to know more about the game than anyone else. Coaches are charged with training "their" athletes, motivating them to do their best and to win their competitions—sometimes (and egregiously) with questionable ethics.

Hmmm... <deep sigh>. The sports coach may choose to motivate a player in a berating or threatening manner. If we transpose this over to the birth process (think: "birthing coach" or "labor coach"), is this appropriate for birth? No. A sports coach might punish a player, arguably for their own good, maybe with an extra set of laps to run or other additional activities that cause more physical and emotional strain. This would not be appropriate for birth (and is debatable for athletics as well). I think we collectively understand the power play: coaches tell us what we need to do—sometimes force us, as if they know something about our best interests that we do not.

One of my students once commented that she appreciated "the motivate part" of the coach idea. "I want my partner to motivate me."

My response was, "Ok, maybe motivation, but who is actually the most motivated to get the baby out?"

"I guess it will be me! I will be the most motivated to get my baby out," she replied.

Then another student added, "As the coach, isn't it my job to stick with the game plan of doing this [labor] naturally?"

Another course participant responded, "Yes, the coach will be there to remind me about what we agreed upon before the birth got started."

At this point in the conversation, I countered gently with, "The birth partner is the *partner*, not the gate keeper of birth plans or medications, etc. Sure, the partner can remind you how you felt earlier, but can anyone predict the future? Can we stick to a game plan in birth? As the birth progresses who will know more about what is happening and what might help? Not the partner. It is you, the birthing person. When you listen to your feelings, you will know the best way to proceed with your birth. You can directly dial into your baby and your process." As I said these statements, I made direct eye contact with each of the pregnant people in the room. I reminded them that "you will be the person who knows the most about your birth."

You may not feel like an expert now, nor in every moment during birth, but if given enough respect and encouragement, in a safe enough space, you will be plenty wise enough to get the job done. If you can find the courage to trust nature and listen to your instincts, then you really can be the expert in your birth.

Ultimately, the word "coach," with its deeply embedded sports associations, is not useful for birth. As I just illustrated, many of the word associations with "coach" are negative. Of course, there are many great sports coaches, amazingly supportive people (who can be great labor partners, too!), but birth partnering and athletic coaching are truly two different jobs. "Coaching," as we generally understand the word, is not only a misdirected way to support the birthing person; it's also not the best way to support the new co-parent. Think of it this way: a "coach" is disconnected, just outside the game. In birth this would be an unfortunate disconnection. I believe this exclusion, or even a subtle undertone of exclusion, does a terrible disservice to the start of family life. For both parents to be well engaged in parenting it is helpful for both parents to honor their individual evolutions into parenthood.

Nonetheless, one could argue that the partner *is* on the sidelines. In fact, I just did that above. And, of course, a birth partner may be asked by a laboring person to leave the room. (This does happen on occasion.) But this is not the same as being ejected from a game. The primary partner is still becoming the parent, regardless of whether they were in the room for the entire labor or birth. Sometimes the person in labor just needs privacy or the singular support of their trusted maternity care provider. If a partner is asked to step outside, they can shift their support to include protecting the outer ring of the birth environment—a larger circle, during which time they can continue to process their own transition to parenthood. In a way, the birth partner is birthing, too: not a baby, but their own baby-self as a parent, complete with their own fears and need for courage and loving, nurturing support.

The baby is coming. This is a big deal in both of your lives! Becoming a parent is a huge emotional transition, perhaps the largest one yet. On some level, your transitions start the moment that you learn you're becoming parents. But for some parents, that moment doesn't fully hit home until the actual birth. And for some it may take even longer than that. Regardless of when you open up, if you open your heart to parenting, each of you will be forever transformed. You both changed the moment you learned of the pregnancy. You both changed again with your decision to proceed with the pregnancy. And once the baby is here, you will both change yet again. Ahead of you is a life full of change-development and growth potential. This is your baby's birth and your birth as a parent. The doorway is open and you're walking through it! On the other side, there will be a new person—you—holding another new person—your baby.

This returns us to the importance of language and how it can impact your birth process, together as partners as well as singularly as parents. So what names for birth support do you like? My preferred titles are "Birth Companion" or "Support Partner," with my real favorite being "Birth Lover," because that is what the job is all about. The Birth Lover is there to love the gestational parent, the baby, and their process. The Birth Lover may or may not be the pregnant person's actual lover. Regardless, the job of the support partner is to **love**. When I work as a doula, I see my job as that of the Birth Lover as well. I am hired to come and love the birthing person, their process, their baby, and their primary birth partner, all of a piece and as individuals.

If you are in fact the pregnant person's lover, you are already well qualified for the work at hand. You are already practiced in reading their cues and understanding their body language. You will likely know them better than anyone else present. This intimacy sets you up well to provide excellent nurturing support. It gives you the confidence to support their courage!

None of us can really know anything about how a particular journey of birth will unfold, but there are basic known truths about birth. For example, there will be an exchange of chemical reactions between the baby and the gestational parent. As a result of this complex chemical feedback system, the birthing parent's muscles will contract and stretch, and they will eventually release a baby into the world. Beyond that, this journey is filled with unraveling mysteries, unknowns, and surprises. We need to be attentive to the gestational person's cues and treat them with respectful, confident love, and an enduring belief in their strength and ability to cope with the rigors of birth.

By approaching the task of labor support as a lover, we not only love and comfort the laboring person, we also effectively model appropriate nurturing behavior for them to bestow upon their baby. Labor partners, like birthing people, do best when they can embrace their role as servers. When your newborn calls you, you respond with love and compassion. This response is vital to the newborn's survival. When a birthing person expresses their needs, your response is likewise vital to their process and experience of birth.

Before we can assign actual responsibilities to the Birth Lover, we must first gain a deeper understanding of what the individual pregnant person considers to be useful in both general and specific terms. This is how we can better realize what exactly a Birth Lover does.

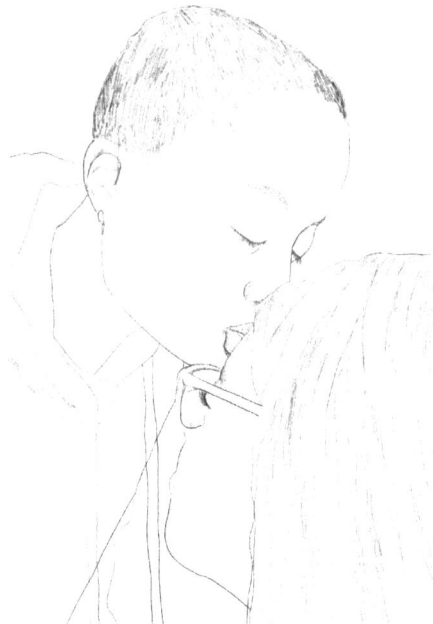

What will help me, the pregnant person, during birth?

Don't worry if your response is largely speculation. You can't possibly know for sure yet what you'll want. And your wants may change as your pregnancy and then your birth process evolves. No one will hold you to your thoughts now. You can certainly change your mind in the moment! Nevertheless, I think it's important to visualize some of your thoughts now.

What I think I will want for support during my birth is...

For additional insights into birth support, here are some of the thoughts shared by former students when I asked them the same question. As you'll see, the answer is not always easy or straightforward:

Client #1: "[My partner] is always very helpful, his calming words, his soothing tone. Rubbing my back, bringing in a sense of reality, it helps. He can remind me I'm not dying."

Client #2: "I don't know; I think about it a lot. I think I am going to be my biggest obstacle. I am not good at relaxing. He tries to do things for me, and I just say, it's ok. I don't want to be any trouble, I'm ok. He sometimes tries to really get out of me what I need. So this is something I am really going to have to work on. And he is very good about that, I know that if I say what I need he will be right there to provide it." [I interjected here and encouraged her to continue: "I want you to try and take a stab at it now," I prodded gently. "Tell us now about something that you think will be helpful in labor. There isn't a right or a wrong answer."] "My back being rubbed. I think touch will be important. I was amazed at how my body responded last week to the relaxation exercise we did. I never slow down like that. So I think touch and soothing words, simple things. I am just not sure, and I need to be able to receive it, his help."

Client #3 [preparing for her second child]: "I picture [my partner] making sure that I have my favorite blanket. There are certain things from home that they said I could bring and I want to bring. Once we get [to the hospital] I know Henry will set it all up. I hope we have time to do that. I don't want it to be so rushed that it's a whirlwind. I like meditation, it works so well. I do some yoga and I always like the meditation at the end. My response is just amazing. Sometimes I am almost half asleep when they wake me out of it. So that is really helpful. I hope we get so good at that. We discussed him coming so close to me and whispering and saying things that will help me get into that meditative state. But also getting into that state with me, which is what I hope for. That's what I hope will happen. I hope it isn't so fast that I get nervous, that I don't have enough time to do what I wanted to do."

Client #4: "I think my partner is good at helping me to relax. Sometimes if I am not really breathing into my abdomen, he notices and helps me to come back down."

I always thank everyone for sharing so openly, so thank *you* dear Reader, for taking the time to do this work in your pregnancy. Conscientious parenting is service to our planet, and I thank you for it sincerely. This is future work you are doing.

EXERCISE: LEARN ABOUT SUPPORT FROM THE PAST

This is a memory recall exercise. I want you to think about when you have received support in the past and what form it took.

Start by getting into a comfortable position and closing your eyes. Then check in with your breathing. After a couple of full, focused breaths, think about a time in your life when you had to make a big decision. Think about how you finally came to the decision you made. Did anyone help you? If so, how? What was helpful about the help you received? What form(s) did the support take? It may also be useful to ponder a time when you were sick and someone was around to care for you. What helped? Was there anything that was well intentioned, but not well received? Take a few minutes to complete this exercise, I suggest you set a timer. Then settle in, close your eyes, tune into your breath and dig into your memories. When you have finished write down any insights, feelings, or ideas that arose.

Very often my clients have shared that their support came in the form of someone being a good listener, i.e., being a sounding board, rather than *a solver* or *a decider*. They appreciated someone who helped them list the pros and cons of a situation, or someone who could be present and just witness their process. Often valuable was the presence of an encouraging person or someone who showed great confidence in their abilities to make good choices. For some it was helpful to have another person present with specific knowledge of the situation and able to provide information they hadn't considered. And sometimes support has meant help fitting the situation into a realistic context: guidance and reframing.

Categorize your support

With support being so multifaceted, it can be useful to break it down into three categories: Physical, Mental, and Emotional. (Note that the Bradley Method® uses these same three categories to classify types of relaxation.) Understandably, there is some arbitrariness to these categories, with each of the categories allowing for numerous crossovers and overlaps. For example, you might think of a hug as physical support as well as emotional support. When you hear your baby's strong heart tones during labor, this could feel mentally supportive as much as it does emotionally supportive. In the information that follows, I have made specific categorical determinations for individual actions and elements. It's ok if you don't agree with how I've assigned the categories; this exercise is a framework for you to adapt to your needs and understanding. You can use my suggested categorizations or create your own!

Physical support

Providing physical support can include helping the birthing parent bring attention to their breathing, helping them change position, and helping them work toward physical relaxation. Do they need to drink some water or need to pee? Are their pants feeling tight? Or are their feet cold? Offering them a snack, supporting them as they vomit (even cleaning up if a mess was made), giving a massage, hand holding, kissing, stroking, holding them up—these are all ways to care for their physical needs. Providing physical support also includes tending to the physical environment. For example, can you open/shut a window, get them a blanket, or chase out the stress-inducing person who just came disruptively into the room. Supporting them and caring for their internal and external environment is an ongoing process that requires you to monitor and assess the energy or feelings in the room to determine if they are supporting the work of birth.

The external environment, generally speaking, should be safe, private, and free from interruption, with low light or fresh sunshine. The birth space should be quiet, except for one's own birth sounds, the support person's encouraging words, or the music of your choosing. It may also be comforting to hear "everyday sounds," such as someone making food, older children playing, or loved ones chatting softly. Physical support includes being vigilant about who is in the room. What are they speaking about? Is it calming or tense? Are they loud or hushed? Do you need to clear the room of any distracting or tense people? You may also need to help the birthing parent to change environments; they may want to go outside or get into the bathtub/shower or they may need transport to a hospital or other birth location. All of these are just some of the ways to provide physical support.

Mental support

Mental support includes tending to the gestational parent's need for information. A person in labor might ask, "Is it dawn or dusk? What day is it? What time is it?" Or, "Did you call the midwife?" Or, "I feel all this pressure in my butt (hip or vagina, etc.), why won't that go away when the contraction ends?" Or, "How far apart are the contractions? How long are they lasting?" Or, "I don't understand what the doctor just said." Mental support is helping a person obtain and process the information they want or need.

Mental support might also include helping a person to focus their thoughts. You can use a distraction technique, for example, such as a guided visualization exercise, encouraging them to count their breaths or suggesting a helpful mantra. Mental support can help a person control, or focus, what they are thinking about. It can be particularly helpful if a person in labor is getting too far ahead in their thinking. Birth parents often report that the hardest part about contractions is not so much the work of the current contraction; rather, it is the fear of what is to come: "Where do I go from here and how long might that take? If this is so hard right now, what on earth is coming next?" This is an understandable fear, and mental support can help a person to stay clear and present in the birthing moment.

If a birthing person is expressing fear of what is to come, a Birth Lover might say: "How are you right now, are you okay right now?" If they answer yes, then say "Good." Smile and continue with honesty and gratitude in your heart: "You look amazing. I am so proud of you! I can't imagine how hard this is, but you're doing it and you're really doing great; right here, right now, you are really rocking this. That last contraction you just had got a lot of work done and you never have to have that one again. You can cross that one off the list. You are getting your work done. I am so impressed with your strength. Try not to worry about later. You are safe. We will handle later when we get to later. I am right here with you. Do you want a sip of water? I love you so much."

If the birthing person says they are not okay right now, encourage them to describe what is wrong. Your job is to listen and validate their experience; it is also to help facilitate communication with their care providers. Wherever possible, link up their sensations with progress and factual information. "You feel all that pressure between contractions because you have already moved the baby down so far." That perspective can help them to reframe their thinking. "This is good news; this is what needs to happen. You are safe, your baby is safe. Your body is amazing." If they feel tired, they may be thirsty or hungry. If they feel physical pain, they may find some relief by stepping up attempts to relax excess muscle tension in the body parts that do not directly support the birth action. As partners we can provide mental support by supplying the information the birthing parent needs and by helping them to keep their thinking on a positive track.

Emotional Support

How is the birthing person feeling about everything that is happening to them and around them? What impact does the mental information have on them? How are they feeling about the physical support they are receiving or not receiving? Do they feel safe? How is their self-esteem, how do they feel about how they are handling the contractions? How do they feel about their progress through labor? How do they feel about their transition to parenthood? Do they feel connected to the baby? Do they feel connected to you, the support person, or to one of the other care providers? Do they feel confident or insecure or vacillating between the two? (It's understandable for there to be no definitive responses... or responses that change from moment to moment!)

Does the birthing parent need to cry, scream, sing, or laugh to release any emotional tension? How are they feeling about the people in the room? Does the birthing person feel loved and/or respected by them? Do they feel secure in the quality of their care? Pain can be a very isolating experience. Being emotionally connected to their witnesses can help a birthing person to feel safe enough to release their baby. You, kind birth partner, can't make fears or pain go away. Your job is not to be a Solver. Your job is to tune into their emotional state and allow them the space and opportunity to express their feelings. When you, the partner, find your own confidence and trust in the process, you can be a more effective guide, and help the birthing person to find stamina and courage for the important release they are working through.

Each of the above classifications should give you a basic idea of how to categorize support areas, along with a host of supportive words and approaches to consider. With this understanding and common vocabulary, you can start to assess anticipated needs and actual abilities.

We each have natural strengths in some areas and challenges in others. Different people will anticipate needing different kinds of support for birth. By evaluating your own needs and strengths and then sharing the results with your partner, you can deepen your understanding of the dynamics at play. This increased understanding will help you continue to prepare for the work of birth and parenting.

Think about this hypothetical scenario as you think about your own strengths and support needs. Perhaps one person is comfortable giving physical support, but a hospital is outside their comfort zone. Now that they stop to reflect on it, they may realize that, during labor, giving physical support could be challenging. If you are planning a hospital birth, for example, maybe ask yourself, "Will I be comfortable holding my birthing partner if they have an IV in their arm?" If the answer is no, then perhaps you would feel more comfortable providing mental or emotional support. While the hypotheticals can be endless, the distinction between each of the three categories of support can become clear with a few honest thought experiments.

EXERCISE: SUPPORT ASSESSMENT

First read the instructions. Close your eyes and reflect on the three categories of support. Then open your eyes and take notes. Then share and discuss your findings. For the pregnant person: consider which support category (physical, mental, emotional) you can anticipate being the most important for you to receive in labor. Put this category first on your list and add a few examples of what goes into that category. Then make your best guestimate as to which category will be second most important, this goes next on your list also with some examples. Finally, with some examples, note which category seems least necessary and put that at the bottom of your list. For the partner: please reflect on which support category (physical, mental, emotional) you can anticipate being the easiest for you to give, which category goes in the middle as second most comfortable to provide, and finally which support category will go to the bottom of your list as the one that poses the most challenge. Then take your notes and add some examples for each category as well. After each of you has had a chance to reflect and take notes, it's time to discuss any misalignments of categories. (Note that this is a normal outcome from this exercise!) It is important to evaluate these needs and strengths without placing value and judgment on ability or category. *We are simply looking to balance your, the birth person's, anticipated support needs with your Birth Lover's anticipated ability to provide specific kinds of support.* If the pregnant person feels that they will benefit most from having strong physical support, and their partner assesses that their real strength will be in providing mental support, then you have uncovered an imbalance. Moreover, this is a great opportunity to address the imbalance *before* the baby arrives. This good work now allows you to plan accordingly for later.

—Put the book down to begin the exercise—

—Discuss your findings and conclude the exercise—

Because imbalances of need and skill are inevitable, there are myriad ways to confront and overcome any imbalance. No one person can easily and effectively meet all of another person's social needs. If life in general doesn't work like that, then why would it work like that for the birth process? We depend on a variety of people to meet our various social needs. This same variety can benefit you here. Think about, for example, hiring a doula or inviting a friend or family member to attend the birth in an additional support role. If, after completing the above assessment, you decide to bring in a trained doula or other support person, you can be clear about what skills you are looking for them to bring into the process.

By contrast, maybe bringing in another person is not the best option for you. Perhaps, then, this exercise will help you, the one who is pregnant, to clarify where you can address your own needs. Maybe you will adjust your thinking so that you're not planning to rely on your partner for those certain types of support. Maybe you will spend some time trying to figure out how best to navigate your own abilities to cope when those types of needs arise. Or maybe, for another couple, when they do this exercise, the outcome isn't that you will bring in another person, or that the gestational parent will try to build their own abilities; instead, it motivates you, the Birth Lover, to use the remaining time in the pregnancy to try to develop your ability to provide support in whichever category is less comfortable than another. You can use this time to strengthen perceived areas of weakness. In short, there is no one correct answer. The assessment process is meant to help you (and your birth partner, where applicable) more clearly understand your dynamics, and then to use this understanding to make practical plans.

Again, please remember, there is no way for a pregnant person to understand completely what they will need ahead of time. A gestational parent who thinks they are going to need a lot of physical support from massage and holding and hugs may not want to be touched when the time comes. A person who thought that they would not want to hear much talking in labor may find that they really want to hear continuous verbal support. Nevertheless, it does often seem that strong reactions during pregnancy provide important clues for birth. Experience has taught me to pay close attention to the labor support qualities that a person is drawn to, as much as the ones they strongly reject, while also remaining flexible as the process unfolds.

When the birth partner understands the uncertainty and unpredictability of what will be helpful, they can more easily avoid getting caught up in an ego funk from making "wrong" support attempts. In the end, it's impossible to know what will help until you try. Each of us is trying to do the best that we can and to make our own best decisions. If you are well intentioned and loving and present, you can easily let go of misjudged or "failed" support attempts.

Next up: it's time to address a specific and tangible support job.

Hydration and urination

I encourage the Birth Lover to be the person assigned to "fluids"—fluids in and out. In other words, it's useful to have some support and attention paid to encouraging the birthing person to drink and void regularly. But you might be thinking: if they have been doing just that on their own beautifully well throughout the pregnancy (which I assume is true!), then why would they need support around that in birth? Because the rigors of birth create extra challenges toward these goals. Sometimes the sensations of contractions are so enormous that they override the sensation of needing to urinate. And it doesn't take long, once that sensation has been ignored, for the bladder to become overextended. Once this point of overextension is reached, it is possible to lose the ability to urinate on one's own. In other words, a catheter may become necessary to insert to empty the bladder. In addition to being uncomfortable, this could slow down and thus complicate labor. Likewise, the strength of birth contractions can leave a person with an unsettled or nauseated feeling that can deter their interest in drinking fluids. Also, getting up and down, and moving to go urinate is often challenging from the end of pregnancy right through the birth. This, too, can discourage someone from staying hydrated. But it's important to work at hydration anyway. Birth is hard work, and even mild dehydration can complicate the process by causing headaches, dry mouth, chapped lips, unnecessary tiredness, and decreased amniotic fluid levels.[143] More severe dehydration can cause confusion, changes in blood volume, and changes in blood pressure (most commonly lowering it), and eventually even organ damage.[144] This is not good for the baby; lowered blood pressure and volume in the gestational parent can decrease the baby's blood pressure, and if this got bad enough it can cause distressing heart tones, neurological, and/or other organ damages for the baby.

Luckily this is all usually quite avoidable with a minimal bit of attention. Dedicating someone on the birth team to help is a great way to be proactive. If there is a Birth Lover, I like to assign them the job. In this role, the Birth Lover should do regular check-ins: about once every hour, suggesting that the birthing person consider a trip to the toilet to try to urinate. Even if no urination occurs, getting up, getting to, and sitting on the toilet can help to progress a birth. We have powerful muscle memories associated with sitting on a toilet. Think about it: it is where we were trained to open up and release, which is exactly the work of birth! When the birthing person has finished, offer them a sip of water, juice or broth. You can offer sips of water or other fluids after each contraction, before they get into the shower, before they lay down, before and after a walk, after they pee, etc. Of course, when it comes to offering a birthing person fluid, don't be a pest! Don't drown them, as it were, in your support. Just be vigilant and persistent and kind.

Note on vomiting: If vomiting is occurring, then hydration takes on even greater importance and water alone might not be enough. Vomiting can cause an electrolyte imbalance, and so it is crucial to include some salt and sugar with any fluid intake. A few grapes and a salty pretzel or cracker could do the trick, or a sports drink, such as Recharge® or Gatorade®, could help. Persistent vomiting should be discussed with your birth attendant.

Lastly, please do not forget to keep yourself, the Birth Lover, well hydrated (and well nourished) and take your needed time to void. You have a responsibility to care for yourself, so that you can continue to care for your birthing partner.

Timing contractions

What time is it? Time to realize that people birthed beautifully even before clocks were invented. Please discuss timing contractions with your birth care provider. Many providers encourage clients to time contractions so that when you speak with them on the phone you can fill them in on your process. I recommend that you make the task as simple as possible. Use a piece of paper and a pen to keep track or use one of the many phone apps available. Time a small series of contractions when you think labor may be beginning. Then stop for a while. Time again whenever you notice that something might be different about the contractions. Noteworthy differences might include: the contractions are coming closer together, lasting longer, seem to be farther apart, seem shorter, or the birthing person is acting differently. For example, maybe they seemed fine a little while ago and now they must concentrate or are crying or moaning. Because people are not machines, you should expect labor contractions to produce a regular or irregular pattern.

Whenever you time contractions, time several of them and then average out how long they are and how far apart they are. Take your timing cues from the birthing partner. When they say the contraction begins, note the time. When they say the contraction is over, note the time again. (However, I have attended births where I was also able to time contractions just by listening to the person's changing breath sounds.) The other key data to collect is the amount of time *between* contractions. You measure the time in between contractions by noting the time from the start of one contraction to the start of the next contraction. (The same way you chart menstrual cycles; day-one to day-one is how far apart your cycle is.)

| 8:05:30 | 8:09:15 | 8:11:25 | 8: 16:00 |
| 8:06:30 | 8:10:05 | 8:12:00 | 8:17:00 |

In the above scenario, the first contraction is one-minute long. The second contraction comes 3:45 seconds later and lasts for 50 seconds. The third contraction comes 2:10 seconds later and lasts for 35 seconds. The fourth contraction comes 4:35 seconds later and lasts for one minute. The average length of these four contractions is roughly 50 seconds long. These contractions on average are coming about every three and a half minutes.

After timing these contractions in an actual labor it would be time to put your pen down and get back to work supporting the person in labor. Partners need to be careful that they don't get too caught up in the task of timing. We don't want to lose connection with the birthing person. When I am timing contractions, I take a quick note at the start and then put the pen down to focus on the person through their contraction. Then I pick up the pen for a quick note of time at the end. I don't even bother to calculate the frequency or duration until I have timed a few contractions for a small sampling. It can be helpful to have some idea of what the pattern is, although not essential if this becomes too much of a distraction.

Honor your breaks

The time in between contractions is vital to a person's experience of their birth. This is the time that a person can regroup, regain their focus, rest, refuel with fluids and snacks, urinate, and prepare for the next contraction. Do they want (need) to change position, location, or activity? Do they need to conserve energy and rest?

In between the contractions the Birth Lover can also tend to their own needs. Do you need to use the bathroom, eat a snack, or call the midwife?

As the Birth Lover you can really help to bring this important time into focus. This is often the time for the most effective partner support. It could be an excellent time for massage, for example, which can help the birthing person to release the residual tension from the last contraction. Try to stay in the moment, rather than always be thinking ahead.

During each contraction the laboring person will be very busy with the work that is happening in their body. It may feel intensely private: the way you might feel if you were in the bathroom with diarrhea or vomiting. You might not want someone touching you or talking to you, or even in the room with you. But having them right outside the door and ready to help if needed could be a great comfort. Any interaction with a laboring person during a contraction can feel like a distraction; this may be a welcomed distraction or an annoying one. A laboring person may be especially sensitive if they sense you are trying to give them directions. A suggestion, such as "Breathe," might provide welcome support; however, depending on how it is received, it might just as easily make a person feel bossed. It could earn you the classic retort, "Hey! YOU go breathe! I am having a freaking contraction here!!"

Rather than feel offended, the takeaway here is that support techniques should be considered offerings not directives. Moreover, if given with this intention and presented *in between* contractions (not during), they can be far more effective—and help to avoid hurt feelings. When a contraction ends, a person may really want to hear loving and encouraging words or receive a fabulous shoulder or foot massage. When the next contraction begins, they may want you to back off silently. But stick close, as they'll want you nearby and attentive in case something changes, even if they don't say it out loud.

Value the contractions

Each contraction is a gift that brings you closer to the birth being over. At the start of each contraction, the Birth Lover can look for gratitude in the healthy process of their partner's strong muscle contractions. Each contraction should be honored for its contribution to the process. When you think of each contraction as a powerful gift, not to be wasted by stress and distraction, you can help the birthing person allow their work to happen. This will help the process be as effective, positive, and efficient as possible. Effective contractions get the baby out sooner.

Starting now, train yourself to equate "strong contraction" with "good contraction." Write down your thoughts here around what it means to "value the contraction"? How does this idea land for you? Does it sound doable? Not doable? What words can you attach to each contraction to help make it a positive experience?

No "no"s

Rule #1: Never say "no" to a birthing person. (Well, almost never.) When someone tells us "no," we retract as if on instinct. We shut down and stiffen up. If a birthing person says, "I want to eat a double bacon cheeseburger and swing from a trapeze before this next contraction," you need not say "no" out loud, even if you're screaming it quietly to yourself! A more appropriate response might be, "Okay, great. But are you sure you want a double bacon cheeseburger? It might be tough to digest right now. Also, it will take some time for one to be made or purchased. I do have some yogurt right here and that might hold you over while you are deciding. But if you really want a bacon double cheeseburger, I am sure we can make it work." As for the trapeze part of the request, don't dismiss it too quickly. You might ask how they think this would be helpful: "Do you need to swing, or rock, or float, or hang?"

By trying to understand what they want, you can help them to figure out what they need. Maybe the burger would cause them to vomit, and the expulsive forces of vomiting would actually help them to open up for birth. Vomiting, as much as it has the negative effect of causing dehydration, can often help the birth process move along.[145]

Vomiting and birth are both large, involuntary contractions that expel stuff out of our bodies. Who are you to say that a laboring person's strange craving or urge wouldn't help the process in some way not readily apparent? Remember: trust the birthing parent to know something about this birth, even if it may be cryptic at first.

In labor, as in life, it is often hard to know what it is that one really wants or needs, and it can be harder still to ask for it. How do you tell the difference between your needs and wants? Do you judge that distinction? As Birth Lover, your job is to remain positive, enthusiastic, and as calm and assured as you can be. Just assume the birthing person's wants *are* their needs. This will also be true as you care for your newborn. What a newborn wants is also what a newborn needs. (This is certainly not always true for teenagers, but that subject is for another book!) As you nurture a person in labor you want to help them assess and then respectfully attend to whatever they think they want/need. Asking for help is a sign of strength. And your support is life-sustaining.

EXERCISE: REVERSE SUPPORT ROLE PLAY

Now it is time to have some role-playing fun! In this exercise you and your partner will switch roles: the Birth Lover will assume a physically demanding position and hold that position for the duration of a mock "contraction." Meanwhile, the pregnant person will have an opportunity to support their partner through the "contraction." After you've read the following instructions, I will cue you to put the book down to try the exercise.

1. The non-pregnant partner will get into the Wall Sit position: Identify and gain access to a body-wide section of wall, with clear floor space in front of it. Depending on the flooring, choose sneakers or bare feet. (Sock feet could be slippery.) Lean your back against the wall, maintain back-wall connection, and slide down. Bend your legs at the knee to form a 90° angle. Your feet should point out away from the wall and either equal the width of your hips or be slightly wider. Your knees should be directly over your ankles, in alignment with your feet. Push down through your feet into the ground; push out through your back into the wall. These directional forces will help you to maintain the position. Ultimately, this position should be stable but challenging for the abdominals and quadriceps to hold. (Note that the quadriceps are long muscles along the front of each thigh. By activating—i.e., drawing in—your abdominals, you will distribute your workload.

2. Try the position first as a warmup, for just a few seconds. Stand up and recover.

3. Get into the Wall Sit position again. This time hold it for a full 60 seconds (longer if your level of physical fitness can handle it). 60 – 70 seconds is on average how long a natural labor contraction will last.

4. The pregnant-person-turned-support-partner acts as timekeeper. Announce "contraction begins," and start the clock.

5. During the 60-second mock contraction/Wall Sit, the timekeeper should tune into their "laboring" partner and get to the work of supporting. How are they doing? Do they seem challenged? Can you tune into their breathing? Do you have suggestions or actions to offer?

5. At the end of 60 seconds announce "contraction ends."

Disclaimer 1: Just to be clear, this exercise is a one and done. You do not switch back to your actual roles and try it again. Please do not ever task an actual pregnant person with unnecessary challenges.

Disclaimer 2: This exercise can be quite demanding on the legs. The actual birth partner will probably need to shake out and maybe massage some tension from their thighs. Some gentle quadricep stretching will probably feel good, too. Please don't stretch aggressively or be too zealous. Bend one knee so that the foot is going close to the butt. Keeping your knees together, hold onto the lifted foot, and allow the knee to hang straight down. This stretches out the front of the thigh. It may be that just holding the foot back behind the butt is enough stretch. If you feel some stretch that is enough. Hold your gentle stretch still for a slow count of 30. Repeat with the other leg.

Disclaimer 3: If the actual support partner has any injuries or other physical limitations that may prohibit getting into or holding these suggested positions, please modify the exercise. You know your body best. Two alternatives to try: hold a push-up position or place an ice cube on the inside of your wrist for the duration of the full "contraction."

—Please put the book down now and try this reverse-role exercise—

How did it go? Take a moment to discuss how you felt and what you were thinking during the exercise, or whatever else may occur to you now that it is over. In my classes I start the post-exercise discussion by addressing the pregnant people: "How was it for you? Did you know what to do to give support? Could you tell if anything you tried was actually helpful to your partner?" Feel free to use these prompts, too, and write your responses below.

Once the pregnant partners have had a chance to speak, I ask their support partners: "Were they helpful? If not, why not? And how did you handle that? Was there anything they didn't do that you think would have been helpful? Or, was there anything they did that you wish they hadn't?" Support partners, please take a moment now to ask yourselves these questions and write your responses on the following page.

Keep in mind that this is a learning exercise. Try to refrain from making value judgments about perceived successes and failures. Not surprisingly, pregnant people often feel surprised by the stress they feel when they realize the "contraction" is *right no*w! When reversing roles, many pregnant people have remarked that it was difficult to tell if their own support offerings were helpful to their "laboring" partner performing the exercise. By contrast, I am often told that it was easier to recognize if something was *not* helpful, leaving support partners feeling torn between providing the support they think their partner wants and providing the support they anticipate wanting for themselves during the birth.

One of the most important things this exercise can demonstrate is that often the most helpful thing the support person can do during a contraction is *be present*. When the partner is nearby and attentive and ready for work, the pregnant person can do their own work without distraction and still feel cared for and connected. Then, when the contraction is over, they can receive love, support, and/or guidance—whatever the situation requires.

"How can I help?"

Sometimes during birth, as the support partner (or the laboring person!) you can feel you're at a loss for what to do. It's okay to ask the birthing person questions, but be mindful not to overwhelm them with a barrage of questions. Furthermore, unless it is absolutely critical, *don't ask anything <u>during</u> the contraction*. (The exception to that rule is if you think they are responding well to distractions.) If, when you do ask and they aren't able to articulate their needs or desires, you may find it helpful to suggest a couple of options for them. Choosing between two options may be easier than coming up with ideas on their own. For example, you might give them a choice of trying the shower or going for a walk. They might be able to choose between the two. But if they still can't decide, pick something for them. "Why don't we go for a short walk?" It will be easier for them to say "no" than for them to get specific about what to try next. You can then cross walking off the list for now and go on to think about what to consider next.

Think of your support here as a kind of checklist:

1. **Ask them what they need/want**. They may be able to tell you. If so, great, go from there. If they can't, then go to step 2.

2. Give them a choice of two options. Perhaps the narrower scope of choices will enable them to pick something to try. For example, ask if the birthing person would like to take a shower or get into bed to rest for a while. If they can't seem to decide, then go to step 3.

3. Select something for them to try. "I will turn on the shower and warm up the bathroom for you to take a shower." If they want to take a shower, they will appreciate that. If not, they should be able to say "no."

As I go on to discuss the different stages and emotional components of birth, please think back to this discussion of support and start to imagine how different kinds of support might work during different parts of the labor process.

EXERCISE: GUIDED BEACH IMAGERY

Now it's time to give the support partner a chance to explore deep relaxation in the side relaxation position and for the pregnant person to read the following visualization script. It's useful to switch roles frequently while practicing relaxation exercises as this work is best learned through experience.

First, get the listening (non-pregnant) partner into a comfortable side relaxation position. Next, encourage the listening partner to close their eyes and take a few deep breaths to settle into this new position. The reader can begin once they sense the resting partner has settled. Note for the reader: please read out loud slowly. Take ample time for your own full slow and relaxed breathing. Please pause between sentences and try to see your own images clearly.

Reading script:

"I would like you to close your eyes and take a few settling breaths, and imagine that you are at the beach resting on an open expanse of fine, warm, white sand."

—Reader pause—

"You are being gently warmed by the sun. Feel the warmth on your skin."

—Reader pause—

"As you exhale, feel your weight sink into the yielding sand. The beach you are on is beautiful. The sky is a brilliant blue. There are small wisps of white clouds floating by."

—Reader pause—

"The air is fresh and flows freely through your nose. There is a hint of salty sea water in the air.

—Reader pause—

"The ocean is an amazing aqua blue. The color dazzles your senses. Relax onto this gorgeous beach. Feel the skin between your nostrils as the coolness of the air flows in. Invite your breath to flow without effort. In, and, out. Smooth, and slow, like the gentle ocean waves, rolling in and out."

—Reader pause—

"Watch a seagull soar overhead. Imagine the sound of the ocean waves, the sea gulls, and then some children laughing and splashing at the shores edge. As you relax a little deeper, settle further into the warm sand supporting your body."

—Reader pause—

"Let go and relax a little more with each exhale. Allow the sun's gentle warmth to smooth your brow and soften your muscles. Look out at the sea and notice a bright red and yellow fishing boat sailing by, just off shore."

—Reader pause—

"The salt air tickles as you feel the lightness of the sea breeze across your skin. It's so beautiful. The sky is such a brilliant, deep blue. The sunlight is dancing on the water. Your muscles are calm and pliable. Your mind is calm and graceful in the warmth. Allow yourself to drift into the deep beauty."

—Reader takes a longer pause—

"Please now gently invite some movement into your body by wiggling your fingers and your toes. Slowly begin to allow some light into your eyes. In your own time please bring your attention back to this room and work your way gently back up to a seated position."

—This relaxation exercise is now complete—

Please take a few moments to discuss the imagery and any other thoughts you have about this exercise. Note any parts of the imagery that were accessible and/or enjoyable, as well as any parts that might have been uncomfortable or difficult to relax into. Note how you feel now that the exercise has been completed. And for the reader, please note how it felt to read the words out loud. Plan to switch roles the next time you practice.

On the night that I was perhaps the most scared I have ever been, I led myself through this imagery with great success. This was when I was eight months pregnant with my second child, and I developed some third trimester bleeding. As I mentioned in Week 4, this was thankfully just spotting, rather than continuous or heavy bleeding, but it was still scary to me. After spending the day in the hospital for observation I was sent home. It had been determined that although I was still spotting, both the baby and the placenta appeared okay. My doctor could not tell me exactly where I was bleeding from or why, but he suggested that I go home and try to rest. With the exception of drugs to help me sleep, there was nothing that they could offer me in the hospital to assist my condition at that time. So I declined the medications and went home.

Before I left my doctor told me to pay close attention: if the bleeding increased or any other symptoms materialized, then I should return to the hospital without hesitation. Hmmm... rest, but pay attention. Antithetical recommendations. Not surprisingly, I was scared and unsettled. When I got home and into bed, I remember thinking that if I sleep I wouldn't be able to know if I were bleeding more. I even went so far as to ask myself the terrifying question of whether it were possible that I could bleed out in my sleep. I immediately tried to reassure myself that my doctor would not have let me go home if he thought that *that* was a realistic possibility. But that didn't really help me find sleep. Guiding myself through the above visualization exercise is what helped, bolstered by the courage to follow through with it during a time of extreme stress.

I remember clinging to the imagery as a lifeline. The beach imagery became my metaphorical life vest in the sea of my fear... and the next thing I knew it was morning! I hadn't even needed to pee. I had slept through the night. The exercise guided me to the peace I needed, and I had slept well. The sun was up, and it was a new day. I was alive and well, and so was my baby.

The next time I used this particular visualization exercise was several months after my second birth. It had nothing to do with childbirth, but worked well just the same! I was at the dentist's office having a cavity filled. I sat back, closed my eyes and decided to use the beach imagery to calm myself down. Initially it worked well; but when the drill sounded it jarred my attention and made the beach a hard focus to maintain. To cope with the distraction, I incorporated the sound of the drill into the image. I visualized my brother on the deck of an old beach house. He was turning on the blender to make a batch of frozen margaritas. Again, I was amazed by the powerful ability of visualization to support me through a difficult situation. All this is to say: don't hesitate to adapt the example imagery above to your own "happy place" creation.

A plausible labor scenario

The contraction begins. The partner begins to speak a guided sensory exploration of the imagined environment. If it's working, the laboring person is able to follow along and appreciates your help focusing their senses. As the contraction ends, they may breathe a deep sigh of relief. They smile. The beach was helpful. They get up and go to the bathroom. They return to the couch they had been resting on, have a sip of water, and begin another contraction.

You think to yourself, "Hey that just worked pretty well! I will try using another visualization exercise, or maybe I should try the same one again, or maybe I should ask them?" You decide to go for it and not bother them with a question. You decide to stick with the same imagined location, and you start to talk through the same visualization. This time they bluntly shush you. Their reaction may sound like a snap. Remind yourself that they are working hard and short on words. Their abruptness may sting your feelings; remember to tell yourself that they are probably grateful that you are by their side and willing to help. Nevertheless, they may want you to be quiet and they may not have a lot of energy to explain why.

So you take the visualization technique and put it back in your "bag of support." You pull out the next technique: a soothing shower. During their next break you suggest that they try getting into the shower. They say they're not in the mood to get wet right now and that they would rather go outside for some fresh air. You help them up, offer a sip of water, and head for the door.

Strong support, partner!

Packing the intangibles

What support tools will you bring to this birth? There are real items such as food, fluids, and a toothbrush. But I also want you to think about the conceptual items you will want to have handy. I encourage you to pack joy, encouragement, love, creativity, faith, and courage. I also recommend that you supply yourself with a list of loving phrases to say, for example:

- ○ *I love you.*
- ○ *You are amazing.*
- ○ *You are safe*
- ○ *The baby is safe.*
- ○ *Our baby is so lucky to have you for a parent.*
- ○ *I am so proud of you.*
- ○ *You ARE doing this work*
- ○ *You're making real progress.*
- ○ *You look beautiful.*
- ○ *It's time to let go and surrender to your process.*
- ○ *Allow the birth to take over.*
- ○ *You are healthy, your baby is healthy, your birth is healthy.*
- ○ *You are doing this amazing work now, that's why this is so hard.*
- ○ *You are laboring as well as any person ever has, and you will find power that you never knew you had.*
- ○ *Be brave.*
- ○ *Be soft, surrender to the feelings*
- ○ *I love you.* (Yes, repeat this often!)
- ○ *I know you've got this.*
- ○ *The number of contractions you'll have is finite. You never have to see that last one again. It's gone, let it go. There's less work ahead with each contraction done. Good riddance to that last one. Let's cross this next one off the list, too.*

You will also want to pack a variety of massage and relaxation techniques. Remember: *Practice now what you want to be good at later.* To effectively use relaxation techniques, work hard now to develop your concentration, guidance and meditation skills ahead of time. Practice on your own and practice with your birth partner. And surprise, it actually feels good!

When a tool doesn't work

If one tool isn't working in a particular moment, try another one. You can reintroduce the first tool later, when it may be appreciated. The support partner must be willing to roll up their sleeves and try, over and again. Note that sometimes trying to help means sitting there quietly, not touching, not doing, just actively witnessing with honest availability. The partner's roll is to be open and receptive and to witness. Trust your intuition. Your job is to serve the pregnant person's needs, and to believe in their strength and ability (your baby will need that too). The job of labor support, therefore, really comes down to this: open the flood gates of your compassion and *check your ego at the door*. Although you are critical to this family, and this is your transition, too, your focus shouldn't be on your own needs right now. And yet you do need to use the bathroom and eat and drink and rest to keep up your strength to stay present. This is not about you getting it right; it's about the laboring person and the rigors of this process. If they snap at you, let it go. Back off. Stay focused and attentive—just maybe from a bit farther of a distance (or get closer physically, needs vary and sometimes from moment to moment.) In my experience, those couples who prepare together tend not to miss each other's cues and can usually avoid getting snippy in labor. (Most of the couples I've worked with report that after they've taken their Bradley® class and built a skillset for birth together, they were then deeply rewarded with profound love and gratitude for the way they were able to depend on each other through their birth process.)

Different parts of a labor can require different tools, but not always. Don't shy away from utilizing the same technique or approach over and again with each passing contraction. When the same technique is used repetitively through each contraction, it can leave the support person amazed at the longevity of its usefulness—and the laboring person feeling grounded (supported).

I was once at a birth where, at the start of every contraction, I would talk the gestational parent through physical relaxation. Starting at the top of the contraction I would start at the top of her head. I would say, "Start relaxing your head, feel your scalp relax, let go behind your forehead, let your eyes be heavy and rest, feel your throat open and relax, let your shoulders go...." On and on I would continue down through her body throughout the contraction. I did this again and again. After a few hours I thought, surely she wants me to shut up. But no, she motioned me on. So I kept going, over and over, "relax the top of your head, feel your scalp relax...," and in that way we got through her entire first stage of birth. During second stage she did not want to hear as much talking. I would just occasionally remind her to stay with what she was feeling and to give in to her sensations.

Birth partners have fears, too

A few years ago, I had the honor of working with a loving young man who was quite concerned that he would pass out during his partner's birth. He was a grounded man and well connected to his feelings. Each week in our Bradley® class he would share that his number one concern was that he would pass out during the birth. He was afraid of not being strong enough to be there for his wife when she needed him. He expressed his fear of being a burden instead of a support.

I was grateful to him for sharing his concerns. We discussed the need for him to have courage, and we strategized. I told him that releasing his fears out loud to the group was part of freeing up vital energy that could be used to build up his strength for the actual birth. We discussed what it would be like if he did pass out. I suggested that if he started to feel light-headed, he must get his head down safely to the ground by getting on his hands and knees. I showed the class a film in which we actually got to see a man faint at the hospital. We saw how the person standing next to him (which happened to be the nurse) helped to catch him and lower him into a chair. The entire episode only lasted a few seconds and then the dad in the film was fine. (Interestingly, the film-dad passed out when his wife was getting an epidural, not during the moment of birth.)

My client continued to express his fears week after week, as he continued to attend class, learn about birth, and work through the process. And then, when the time came and his partner was in labor, he did just great. He was present, calm, and supportive. He didn't pass out. When his daughter emerged, he was helpful to his partner, just as he had wanted to be. He even helped to catch his daughter! This loving dad was eager to come back to visit his birth classmates and share his triumphant story. He proudly showed off his beautiful baby and even brought me a photograph he had taken of his wife's placenta.

Birth Partners: What are your current concerns?

Take a few moments now to reflect on this question and write your responses below.

EXERCISE: STANDING PELVIC BOWL
AND PELVIC FLOOR ISOLATION

Stand with your legs a little bit wider than your hips. Turn your feet out a little bit, about 45 degrees from parallel. When you gently bend your knees make sure that they line up to extend out over your toes. Put your hands on your hips and slowly begin to rotate your hips in a circular motion. Go in one direction for a while and then shift and go in the reverse direction—for example, right to left, then left to right.

Remember the pelvic rocking exercise? In that exercise we were isolating the pelvic bowl. Now we are doing that from a standing position. (You can also try this exercise sitting on a large exercise ball.) As you gyrate your hips, trying to make slow complete circles, notice if one direction feels smoother or easier than the other. Next try to make figure eights. Notice your sensations. Notice what your body is telling you about your movement. Making these circles and figure eights may feel helpful in labor.

As you are swaying your hips in circles and figure eights consider that, as the baby finds her way down, you will want to be able to help her shift with your movements. If you had a hollow container with a small opening and something small was inside that container, you would move the container around trying to line the object up with the opening to get it out. Imagine trying to get a guitar pick out from the inside of an acoustic guitar.

Now, let's have some more fun with this exercise! I have a male partner and two boys, all of whom love to pee outdoors. Occasionally, when they were little, they would turn peeing outdoors into a competitive sport. As a woman, I don't pee outdoors very often, and rarely if ever has it been for competitive sport or fun. But people with vaginas, here is your chance! Standing up, with your hands on your hips in a wide stance, with your legs out a bit farther than your hips, allow your knees to bed softly. Continue with what you were just doing in the above exercise, but this time, instead of making circles with your hips, *imagine that you are writing your name on the ground with your pee.*

This is your cue to engage your pelvic floor musculature. To write your name in pee (real or imagined!), you will need to both relax and contract the muscles of your pelvic floor and vagina. Assuming the first attempt at this exercise is imagined, think about how you would write your name in the snow, on a magically crisp and brilliant day. Or, maybe the ground is dry dirt and you can easily read the letters of your name while the sun warms your back. Try writing your name in block letters, then try cursive. Experiment. Don't forget to dot any i's or cross any t's! If your name is short, use your last name, too. Can you try calligraphy? Yes, this is funny and fun, but it's also effective! You must release and contract your muscles to make the shapes of the letters. You must *feel* what the muscles are doing. The more you can increase your body awareness, the better shape you'll be in for labor and for life. It all goes better when you understand how you work with deeper body awareness.

—Pause here to give this exercise a try. Let the hilarity flow! (pun intended)—

EXERCISE: SHOULDER ROLLS FOR POSTURAL ALIGNMENT AND GROUNDING

Remain standing and now do some shoulder rolls; allow your chest to open as your shoulders roll back and your back to open as your shoulders roll forward. We need to compensate for the closed and forward position that most of us are in so much of the time, like when we are driving, washing dishes, or sitting at a desk. These gentle circular motions in the shoulders will help your body to move within your range of motion. Performing repetitions of 10 – 12 shoulder roles can help you to realign your posture and find comfort.

Relax your arms down and bend your knees a little. Gently bend and straighten your knees to encourage your weight to drop down into your feet and to release into the ground. Feel the soles of your feet on the ground or in your shoes. Feel the soles open wide on the ground. Allow the weight of your body to drop down into those open soles and pass through you into the earth. This is *grounding*. This is releasing what you don't need to hold up. Allow the magnificence of your bony structure to support your weight. The crown of your head reaches up towards the sky as you look for balance and allow your muscles to soften. Your ankles, knees, hips, ribs, shoulders, and head all effortlessly balance over your big, open, wide, stable feet. Take a few more conscious, deep breaths. Allow your arms to float up in synchronicity with your breath. Then let the movement settle as you find a moment of stillness.

Please take this spacious and grounded feeling with you as you step out into the rest of your day or evening. Yay you, another week read! I am wishing you a wonderful week and hope you can have fun with your homework.

HOMEWORK:

A) Watch Ted Talk

Remember to watch (or, re-watch) the TEDGLOBAL presentation by Amy Cuddy, "Your body Language Shapes Who You Are," June 2012.

B) Birth affirmations

Try making up several of your own, personal birth affirmations, then pick one or two of your favorites to write frequently in your notebook, in the margins of this book, and to repeat out loud. One of my clients recently wrote out her affirmations and then taped them up all around her house. She put one on her refrigerator so that, as she made breakfast, she saw a positive reminder that she would be safe in her birth. As she brushed her hair in front of the mirror there was another reminder that she would be courageous in birth. A support partner might choose an affirmation like, "I can trust my partner's body to know how to birth" or "I will give compassionate support and my instincts will guide me." Again, revisit any of the notes and work you did earlier in this week's lesson.

C) Guided imagery and stretches

Finally, don't forget to practice the guided beach imagery. Roll your shoulders frequently throughout your week to create space in your body, alleviate tension and help you feel grounded. Continue or begin to practice relaxation alone and together *every day*.

Do your homework now, it feels good, and you'll be better prepared for later!

THIS SPACE IS FOR YOUR NOTES AND DRAWINGS

THIS SPACE IS FOR YOUR NOTES AND DRAWINGS

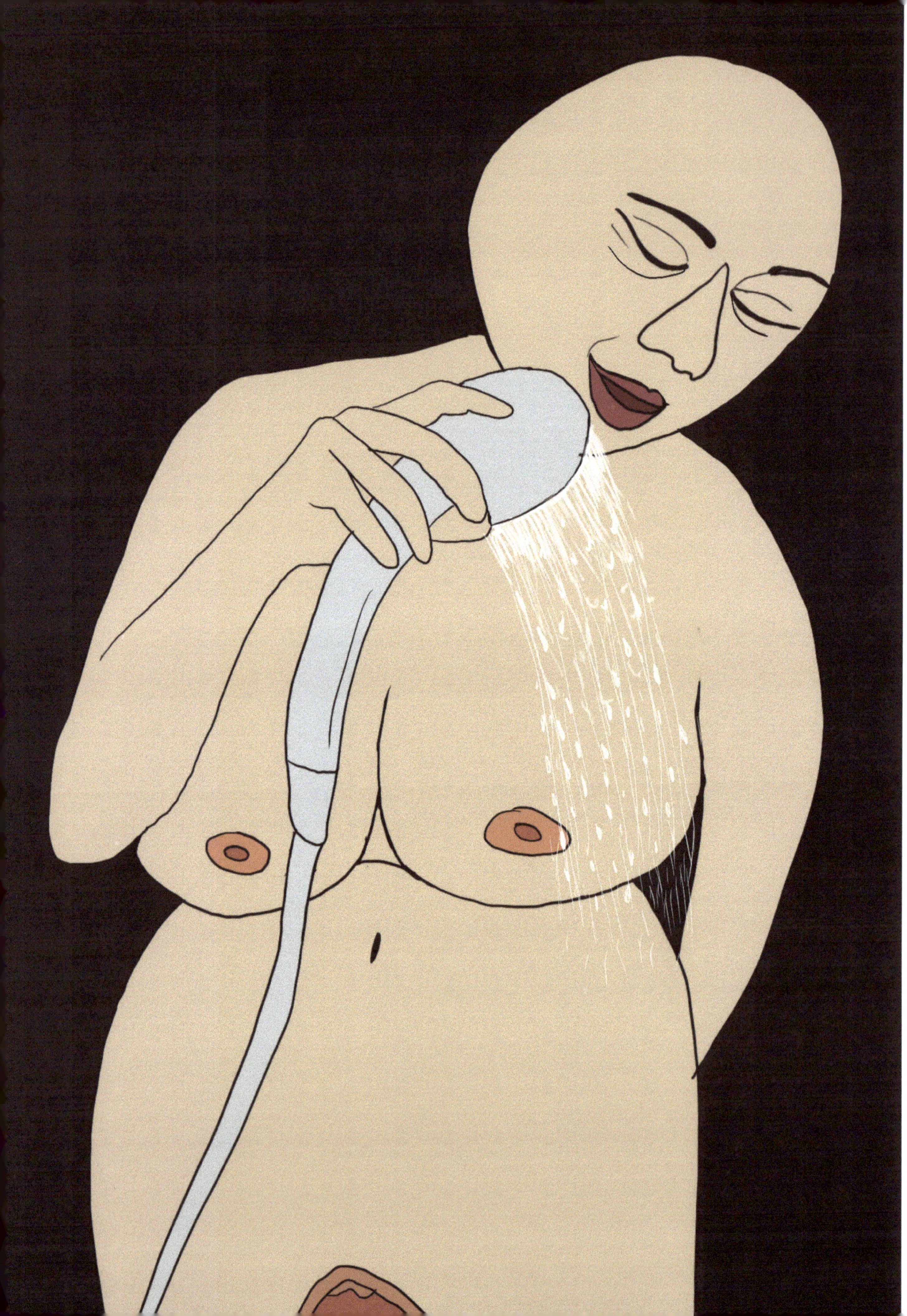

WEEK 7

Waiting
Wondering
Working

Chapter contents:

O *Waiting for labor*

O *Labor arrives*

O *First stage strategies*

O *Fetal positioning*

THIS SPACE IS FOR YOUR NOTES AND DRAWINGS

Welcome back! I hope you had a wonderful week working on support skills for yourself and with your partner, if applicable. Now, take a breath in... as you exhale take a moment to check in with your body. Take another breath in... and out. How was your week? What happened that put a smile on your face? What did you experience that made you stop and think? How were your stress levels? Did anything impact your selfcare? How have you been managing emotionally?

—Pause to reflect—

When was the last time you tried to use conscientious breathing to cope with an urgent moment, or for relaxation? I urge you to remind yourself that the next time you feel a tense moment, use breath consciously as a coping strategy.

What about exercise? Moving your body helps to release stress. Have you been able to try any of the exercises and birth positions I've covered so far? If so, which ones and how did they feel?

Obstacles to selfcare can feel mighty in the face of institutional oppression and financial stress. In other words, the demands of work, family, and friends can be fierce—life is packed. Know that compassion is out there (and in me) for those of you facing challenges unfair and well beyond your control. Learning to turn to our breath in times of stress is useful for childbirth and beyond. Take another easy breath in and easy breath out. And congratulate yourself for picking this book back up today.

When is this kid coming?!

The baby's arrival is always unknown. Remember, we don't control our kids... even from the very beginning! What follows are notes from a Bradley® pot-luck dinner centered around sharing birth stories. At the end of this particular evening, as a new mom was thanking me for all she had learned in class, she mentioned, "Emily, please spend more time in class on the possibilities of prematurity, and the massive surprise that it is."

This new mother's baby had been born at 35 weeks and a few days. There had been no warning signs of prematurity. Instead: Bam! A quick labor later and there's baby! Mom and dad had been sure they still had at least another 2 weeks, and likely another month. No bags had been packed. Their minds were blown when they found themselves in the hospital with a premature baby. Fortunately, for this family, their son was close to term, and at 6 lbs., a great weight for a preemie. Most babies don't leave the hospital until they reach 5 lbs. (Although weight in and of itself is not as important as gestational age for predicting viability, it is still considered an important factor.) This baby was breathing independently at birth and appeared to be doing quite well developmentally. Nevertheless, mother and father were shaken by the experience and had wished they were better prepared for the possibility.

Over the last several decades, while scientists have made many advances in keeping preterm babies alive, political and medical wills have not been strong on funding research into the prevention of prematurity.[146] Programs that helped ensure women, infants, and children could have access to food and healthcare, for example, have been slashed since the 1980s.[147] These changes appear to have directly increased the number of preterm births and the discrepancy between outcomes for babies of Color and White babies.

There are many ethical dilemmas attached to the technological advances in keeping the teeniest among us alive. Quality of life is uncertain for both baby and family. Babies born prematurely can struggle with high rates of long-term health problems. From the National Institute of Health (NIH):

> Although much progress in the treatment of infants born preterm has been made, many of the medications and treatment strategies used in the neonatal intensive care unit have not been adequately evaluated for their efficacies and safety. The high rates of neurological injury in preterm infants highlight the need for better neuroprotective strategies and postnatal interventions that support extrauterine neuromaturation and the neurodevelopment of infants born preterm.[148]

Neuroprotective = protect the brain. Scientists and doctors can keep babies alive better than they used to, but they don't necessarily understand the best way to grow them without injury. As the above quote illustrates, the emphasis is on finding ways to treat, not to prevent. Although the scope of this book is not meant to cover the subject of prematurity in any great detail, I do want to mention the fact that research evidence points to racism, not biology, for the difference in rates of prematurity and outcome discrepancies that families of Color experience in the United States. For a more in-depth exploration of prematurity and medical racism, I direct you to the book *Reproductive Injustice*, by Dana-Ain Davis.[149]

The emotional, ethical, and financial hurdles, combined with the uncertainty of developmental outcomes for the baby, can make coping with prematurity a difficult experience. As parents you will undoubtedly be consumed by the overwhelming rigors of parenthood. Therefore, while I am not suggesting that you plan for or dwell on prematurity, I do believe it can be helpful to think through some basic strategies for coping with the unexpected and with the chaos of life, prematurity included.

Take a deep breath and exhale slowly. Feel your connection to the earth. Take another deep breath, and let these thoughts go as you exhale. For those of you that are already dwelling in darkness: take additional deep breaths;

write down what is affecting you; say it out loud; allow yourself to cry; find ways to discharge some of your fear and anxiety. You are stronger than you know. Even in tremendous grief there can exist a great light of love. You'll deal with what you have to, when you have to. In the meantime, if you are having trouble living with your concerns and the emotions they engender, try meditation. Also, plan fun things to do, as these can help take your mind off the problems, especially the ones that don't currently exist. You are not alone, not now and not later.

I encourage you to put your energy, especially any worry-energy into self-care: eat your best nutrition, cope with stress through conscientious breathing exercises, and get enough sleep. Gathering information may be helpful too, so that should the unforeseen happen, like prematurity, you have some knowledge to guide you. For example, you can investigate Kangaroo care[150] for premature babies, a process of wearing the baby skin to skin. Kangaroo care has many proven benefits for premature and full-term babies alike. Also discuss any concerns about prematurity with your care provider. Above all, don't lose yourself in information and emotion. Again, reach out for lifelines, such as exercise, conversation, and conscious breathing.

Are you late?

Statistically, if you are expecting your first baby, you're more likely to go past your due date than before it. Watching your due date come and go requires patience and perseverance, like so much of parenting. Yet many a parent spends these last precious days with some frustration and angst.

Before reading on, take a moment and respond to this question: How do you think it will feel to see the other side of your due date?

When it comes to your feelings around waiting for birth, I suspect they'll change and develop over the course of your pregnancy. If you are very early in your pregnancy right now, then it may seem like a strange and future dream. But as you get near the end of your pregnancy, you may feel challenged by the uncertainty of when this major life-changing event will fully occur.

In general, human beings are creatures who like to schedule. However, birth without intervention isn't something that can be scheduled. Add to this that most of us are under the influence of the "television birth"—i.e., wham bam and it's over in half an hour, tops—that what we experience in real life leaves the potential for real frustration and stress because it is so different. The tension between what's real and what's popular misinformation or misrepresentation can make anyone a little edgy, especially in those last few weeks of pregnancy. Waiting for birth's imminent arrival is therefore best carried out with curious courage.

Feel the promise of being on the cusp of something new and primal. Acknowledge, even grieve for what is about to be lost—your old self and your pregnant self. All of your primary relationships are about to be altered, profoundly. Share your fears, share your dreams. What will this mean? Who will you be as a parent? Listen to your baby's rhythms. Can you sense what your baby likes and dislikes? Try to get plenty of rest for your body and mind. Focus on tending to the day-to-day necessities of life at the end of a pregnancy; eat, sleep, clean, rest, void, sex play, create, and rest again. Mindfully acknowledge your body's sensations and birth developments as they occur. If you can yield to the uncertainty of it all, you may find you can enjoy the mystery of not knowing. Look for joy. Look for silver linings. Try to listen to your body's sensations and think about what it means to communicate with your baby internally. Get in touch with your baby. This is precious time. You are a parent right now. Entertain the idea that waiting for birth to begin in earnest can be a playful time with your baby. This is your first game of peekaboo!

There are many common discomforts at the end of pregnancy; person-building is serious, tough, hard work. But learning to respond to physical and emotional challenges with courage is a requirement for life. Your toddler *will* accidently head-butt you; your acrobatic kindergartener might surprise you by jumping onto you from a staircase, while your back is turned, with no warning. (Trust me, it hurts. But it's also cool to marvel at your kid's agility!) Or, maybe you'll get a soccer ball to the head, step on a Lego®, receive an ear-piercing screech *directly* into your ear. It will all hurt, and sometimes heartbreak will follow. Parenthood is painful, but it also carries the ever-present potential for a truly ecstatic experience of love. Take care of yourself. Nurture yourself as you plan to nurture your baby.

If the waiting is challenging, then articulate what the specific challenges are. Remind yourself that you may have choices about how you respond. Seeing the positives may be a challenge. I am not talking about faking your way through misery. But can you find real relief by reframing your perspective? How can you build yourself some courage to see this through? When I felt the weight of my discomforts during pregnancy, I would sometimes remind myself that many people long for pregnancy and aren't able to conceive, and that they would switch places with me in a second—aches and all. Gratitude for the opportunity to have the experience often got me through the toughest times. (In fact, I find gratitude to be the antidote to a lot of life's challenges.)

At the long end of pregnancy there are more new sensations than you can imagine, and some might not be pleasant. (If this is a massive understatement for you, I'm sorry it's so hard.) Of course, it's entirely possible that you feel awesome all the way through, so please don't go looking for trouble where there is none. Many pregnant people report feeling fine even past their due date, yet report that they receive tremendous pressure and concern from co-workers, friends, family, and even their care providers. The concerns of other people can complicate the normal stresses of late pregnancy. If you can practice tuning out other people's stress you are well on your way to useful skill development; please practice.

If you're currently at the end of your pregnancy and this kind of external "noise" applies to you, remember that this is *your* pregnancy. You get to have your baby when your *baby* is ready. Try to tune out the concerns of family, friends, and co-workers; listen to your own proverbial gut, heart, and vagina. Hang on, slow down, eat some good food, take a nap, maybe masturbate, dance to some music, draw a picture, take a walk, cook and freeze meals for postpartum, and when the time is right your baby will arrive. Remember, no one has ever been pregnant forever!

Waiting for birth is another reminder that in parenting one doesn't control one's child. That child has a mind, body, and will of her own. Successful parenting is about raising a child who independently thinks for herself. Of course, there will be times when you will long to control your children's thoughts, feelings, or actions. I encourage you to tread lightly, starting in pregnancy. The issue of control will surely be a parenting struggle that arises time and again. My experience has taught me this: we all grow together in family life. It's a great idea to start now.

Ok, but *when* will labor arrive?

You can rest assured that active labor is not subtle. You will not miss your birth, even if you miss the early signs. Perhaps you've heard a story about a mother who didn't even know she was pregnant and then she went to the bathroom, and plop, out came a baby? I wouldn't worry about that happening to you. You are becoming more and more connected to your pregnancy as you work through the lessons in this book and your own feelings and actions toward birth. So just get on with your day(s) as best you can. Focus on the positives. Feel gratitude. And if your baby does deliver a truly surprise arrival, hooray! Just catch it and call for some help. (See Week 14 for catching a baby who chooses a surprise arrival.)

Ask yourself this: Can I trust my baby to be born when she is ready? If not, why not? Write or draw your response in the space below:

I urge you to consider the longevity of the human race as you continue to reflect on the question above. When it comes to waiting for the onset of labor, you are like an apple tree. When each apple is ripe, it will fall from the tree. One strong momma tree giving birth to differently aged apples. Each one will ripen and drop in its own time. Consider this, too: there is a 37-day range of when babies are "ready" in typical, healthy human gestation.[151] Your baby will come when she is ready, when she has finished her work inside or as some pathology brings her development to fruition.

As I stated earlier, you are more likely to go past your due date than to give birth on or before it. In France you wouldn't even be considered due until 41 weeks, so it will serve you well to plan for the long haul.[152] If this seems difficult to cope with, try the exercise of counting some breaths as a tonic for strength.

By the time you have reached late pregnancy, some of the most complicated work is already done. The sperm and the egg first found each other (no easy task), and then all those crazy early cell divisions happened (a massive amount of physiological specialization). The blastocyst, which is a blob of cells that represent both the future fetus and future placenta, found the right spot to implant and then you grew all the baby's other complex systems, including the placenta.[153] Now, as you approach birth, you are all systems go. Your baby is adding weight and undergoing massive amounts of brain development. Keep eating great food, move, stretch, rest, and relax. Your future work to birth is far less complex than what you have already accomplished. Please try not to fret away the end of your pregnancy. Embrace it and what's to come.

Signs of labor that you might (or might not) notice

What follows is a list of signs or symptoms that labor is starting.

○ *Repetitive aches*
A pregnant person might have repeating sensations that they do not experience as uterine contractions. Partners: please listen closely. If the pregnant person says anything about recurring sensations, especially sensations that repeat a couple of times within an hour or two, then this may be a signal that labor is arriving. I have heard women describe that their early signs were first noticed as repetitive gas pains or repetitive back aches from a "bad office chair." If a pregnant person says, "here is that back ache *again*," or, "here are those gas pains *again*" (or cramps, or pain in the cervical area, or pain down the front of the thighs, or belly hardening and squeezing), you should probably consider that this might be a signal of labor. Labor comes in waves. The ocean with all its tidal variations is a beautiful metaphor for the waves of birth: low tides, high tides, rough seas, and calm. Some waves are barely perceptible while others are powerful enough to move mountains.

○ *Contractions*
Contractions can come in a rhythmic pattern or have no clear pattern at all. Contractions might feel the same as the Braxton Hicks (practice) contractions you may have felt before, or they might feel totally different. Don't worry if you haven't yet felt any contractions. That's normal too! I commonly hear that early contractions feel like menstrual cramps. You might feel contractions in your low back, hips, vagina, anus, belly, or down the front of your thighs. Many people describe feeling a hardening in their belly, or like they are being squeezed. And sometimes a contraction feels like the baby is stretching out long, like you are being stretched from the inside out. You are!

○ *Rupturing of the amniotic sac*
When your amniotic sac, or "membranes," rupture at the onset of labor, contractions may follow immediately, or they may not follow for hours or even days. Statistically, your amniotic sac will break when you are well in the throes of labor and have dilated to about eight centimeters. Then again, you are not a statistic; you are a person, an individual. Membrane rupture could happen at the beginning of labor. Both of my births started that way.

○ *Mucus plug*

Another sign of labor that you may or may not see or feel is the loss of your mucus plug. You may remember from Week 5 that the cervical opening produces a mucus glop that seals the baby bag shut. As changes begin in the cervix, it starts to efface (soften and shorten), as well as to dilate (open). The mucus plug then falls out, or maybe just melts away never to be noticed. If you see it, you might see its slimy splendor in the toilet bowl, on toilet paper, or in your underwear. It's normal for the mucus plug to have a bit of blood in it as well; the area around the cervix is richly vascular. Losing your mucus plug means your process is working well. Nevertheless, you still won't know if it will be hours, days, or weeks before full-on labor arrives.

○ *Bloody show*

This is another weird term, isn't it? This is what birth professionals call spotting, or small bits of brief bleeding from the cervical area. Bloody show is a very common labor symptom; it, too, announces that the process is working but without any details toward whether it will be hours, days, or weeks before the full onset of labor. The gestational person can and should rely on their own instincts and training from their years of menstruation to decide if what they see/feel is *active bleeding* or just spotting. Bleeding is always a symptom to contact your provider about. If it seems like you are continuously bleeding, you should seek immediate medical attention. However, if the bleeding seems spotty, it is likely healthy and a conversation with your care provider can't hurt. Trust yourself to know the difference, and act on your instinct. If you ever have any questions, call your provider. (It is harder for them to care for you if they don't know what is going on. If you experience new symptoms, it's always a good idea to reach out.)

○ *Loose bowel movements*

Frequent watery bowel movements can be nature's way of helping the gestational person clean themself out so that baby has more room on the way out. This symptom generally signals that labor will arrive within a day. The baby will exert a great deal of pressure on the birthing person's rectum as she slides out into the world. This pressure causes feelings that let a birthing person recognize their urge to expel the baby. Regardless of pregnancy status or sex, we get the urge to poop when our rectum is full of fecal material. In other words, when we're literally full of shit we feel pressure on the rectum walls because the walls are being stretched to capacity. This pressure then signals the brain that it's time to void. In birth, when the baby's head travels down far enough, it too puts pressure on the rectum wall (but from the outside of the rectum wall), and so we recognize the same familiar urge to void. If anything is left in the bowel during the second stage of birth it will get pushed out just ahead of the baby. The birthing parent will likely not notice and is not likely to even care in the moment. As hard as this might be to imagine right now, at that moment in the birth the gestational parent generally has only one thought: *Get the baby out!* (If the thought of pooping in front of your provider, an assistant, and/or your partner causes you overwhelming stress, you may want to consider giving yourself an enema at the start of labor, if you haven't already cleaned yourself out naturally. Again, always check with your provider first.)

○ *Changes in mood or energy*

Some people report big changes in their mood or energy level at the onset of labor. These changes can go up or down from where you were. If you have been feeling cruddy and uncomfortable for days, you might suddenly feel great and energized. If you have been feeling great, you may suddenly find yourself tired and cranky and unable to get comfortable. These changes in behavior and energy are often indicators that labor is approaching.[154] Partners: if you notice that the pregnant person's behavior seems different, especially in combination with any other symptoms, you should consider that labor activity has begun or is near. This means that you could still have weeks to go or only a few hours before your work hits full frenzy. Some people also describe having had dreams that let them know of the baby's imminent arrival. Regardless of what symptoms you notice, you'll ease into birth if you can develop plans now and have a strategy for what to do when something changes enough that something needs to be done during birth.

Strat'e'gy (noun)
  1. Planning in any field
      A carefully devised plan of action to achieve a goal, or the art of developing or carrying out such a plan
      Biological definition: in evolutionary theory, a behavior, structure or other adaptation that improves viability.

Strategies for when you think you might be in labor

To repeat: you cannot plan a birth, per se. You won't be able to figure out exactly what you need until you need it. But strategizing and having a plan beforehand will help set you off in the right direction for when the time does come. Strategizing also improves your capacity to adapt to the situation as it unfolds.

If you think you are in labor, first drink some water and then change your activity. If you were resting, get up and move about. If you were up and about, try resting. If your birth work continues through hydration and an activity change, it is quite possible you are in labor.

When you think you are in labor, please go through the following checklist.

○ Am I well hydrated? If not, drink fluids.

○ Am I well nourished? If not, eat some food.

○ Am I well rested? If not, rest, even if no sleep comes. Rest like the world depends on it, which means make the room as dark and quiet as possible. Keep your mind busy with the work of finding stillness of body, slowness of breath, and limpness of muscle tone.

○ Is my partner thirsty, hungry, or tired? If so, please try to rectify those issues. Births, as well as the earliest days of parenting, go best when partners are in good shape, too.

○ Are there any necessary phone calls to providers, family or friends who need an early heads up that something might be starting (such as childcare, pet care, doula care, transportation, etc.)?

○ Do you have ice cream in the house? Oh wait, sorry, that last one was my own need, remembering my first birth! Replace "ice cream" with whatever special treat you want for yourself at the time of labor or soon after birth. ☺

Be prepared with your stuff

Hopefully you are well prepared ahead of time with your favorite music, important phone numbers, and enough water, juices, broths and nutritious snacks to get you and your partner through a few days of birth. Lotions, oils, a tennis ball for massage, hair ties, warm socks, etc. If you are traveling to a hospital or birth center, it's time to think about packing. Will you take pictures or video, or both? Are the cameras ready to go? Are phones charged? Chargers packed? If you are traveling to a birth location, do you have your transportation plans set, such as metro cards, gas in the tank, or cab fare? If you haven't pre-arranged your food supplies and other labor necessities, early labor is your last chance.

Pack an extra supply of determination

I suggest everyone start labor thinking that it could last at least 45 hours, and that you're strong enough to handle whatever comes your way. If you plan for 45 hours of birth (an improbable—albeit not impossible—length of time!), you will conserve physical and emotional resources with a much more focused intention. Note: if you should get to the 46th hour or beyond before completing your birth, it's okay to be mad at me for misleading you. I can take it! I know and you know that these lessons are a guide. Plus, the longest continuous active labor I've heard of was almost a full week! When I say this in class, everyone laughs, nervously. Everyone except me. I'm serious. You must plan for long, hard work—the work of feeling big things. Plan to be strong for the duration, however long it takes.

Say it now. Say it out loud: "YES, I CAN DO IT! I will survive, even through multiple days if I have to!" Now say it again.

Then ask, "How? How will I get through two or three (or more) days of very hard work?" Search for and lay out concrete answers; make a plan. For example: "I will sleep between contractions. I will look for opportunities to take longer rests where I can." Long births usually come with breaks, periods of time when the work slows down, that's why they're *long*. It is imperative to sleep whenever you can.

Likewise, ask yourself: "What will I eat? What will I drink?" Then make a plan and get the necessary supplies.

Plan to have a positive attitude

Do you have anyone that can help supply a positive attitude should your mood begin to falter? Remember the work you did last week, in Week 6? Think back to who you are turning to for support, knowledge, and/or spiritual energy. Who will you reach out to? Are they ready to be there for/with you? Plan to openly receive love, support, knowledge, and spiritual energy/good vibes from loved ones and birth companions. Maybe make yourself a poster with an affirmation on it or find an inspiring piece of art to bring with you, one that will fill you with courage and positivity. And, if/when your labor is shorter than 45 hours, you will be thrilled to have surplus energy reserves to care for yourself and your baby. Consider that even if your baby flies out in one hour, you will be working hard for the following 44 hours and beyond anyway. Newborns are challenging.

Throughout the birth I encourage you to welcome, maybe even *to will* for yourself strong, powerful contractions. Welcome the work that brings forth your baby. It is through these strong contractions that the baby will get out of you. The more work you can do with each contraction, the shorter the overall amount of time you will spend laboring. Wish or pray or dream for your contractions to be the strongest contractions possible. Visualize yourself melting open in response to that power. And remind yourself that the stronger the contractions are, the more you will need to surrender to your process. Then get ready to relax with the same sense of surrender.

In order to further develop your strategies for labor, think about the following questions. Allow your answers to develop and change over time. Start now and reassess weekly.

1. What body positions do I think might be good for my labor and birth?

2. Will I use showers or baths?

3. Where will I labor? What physical spaces will I be in?

4. What will I think about?

5. Who can give me good vibes/prayers/energy/smiles?

6. What kind of attitude will I bring to this birth?

7. Am I feeling up for this challenge?

8. Where can I find the courage to feel and yield to the birth sensations?

9. What can I do now if I feel overwhelmed by negative feelings about the birth?

10. Do I have goals or expectations for myself in labor? Are they realistic?

11. Is it reasonable to try to plan a birth? How can I build in flexibility?

—Pause here to consider what you can and cannot control during birth, and how you will cope—

Denial might be your friend

Some of my favorite midwives beg me to teach my clients to ignore labor as much as possible. I, too, have often thought that a healthy dose of denial can be a helpful labor tool. But only once you have gotten all your ducks in a row (hydrated, made calls, finished packing, etc.), do I recommend that you get back to living your life and ignore the birth as much as you possibly can. The difference between two people's labors, with regard to length of time, is sometimes the difference between when each person started to focus on being in labor. A person who has a six-hour labor may well have been able to just ignore the first six hours of work. A person who speaks of a 12-hour labor may have progressed in a very similar pattern, yet for the first six hours they focused intently on the process. Perhaps the adage of "a watched pot never boils" is a helpful reminder here, too. Once you have taken care of the basics, do your best to ignore your labor until you absolutely can't anymore. Try to get on with your day or evening as you had planned. Good plans include a commitment to trying to stay calm and restful. Try to stay out of the way of your body's functioning. Read a book, watch a movie, bake something yummy, make love, take a nap, go for a walk, and take another nap.

Strategies for when you just can't ignore your labor any longer

Focus on your exhalation at the start of each contraction. Try to stay focused on deep, slow, full breathing. Relax the muscles that don't have to work. The jaw, tongue, all the muscles of the face, hands, shoulders, abdominals, buttocks, pelvic floor, thighs, knees, and lower legs—these are all common places for us to tense up during a contraction as we try to brace against the sensations. Yet none of these areas directly help you open up for birth. (The abdominals will assist later in the process, for the expulsive phase. But in the first stage of labor it's best to let the abs relax.) When you tense indirectly related body parts during a contraction they use up vital resources, such as oxygen and nutrition stores. Any extra muscle effort will be competing with the work of the uterus, and other body systems, like the endocrine system, that must function optimally for labor to progress well. If you practice relaxing your muscles every time something physical or emotional becomes uncomfortable, you can train your body's response to follow your mind's direction.

Above all, rest when can. I can't say this enough. You can gain energy even if you only get to rest for seconds or minutes at a time. Use your power of visualization to help you rest. Pay attention to the time in between contractions, rest your mind as well as your body. Focus on something positive; this will help you with the work of feeling peaceful. Change your position before the contraction starts or at the earliest signs of it arriving. Try to rest in your chosen position. Focus on surrendering: soften all your muscles in response to the strength of the contraction as it is building.

Tools for the birthing person's tool bag

Read through the following list once and then consider which tools jump out to you, the birthing person, as most important. Then go ahead and number them in the spaces provided, making #1 your most important.

_____ Exhale at the start of every contraction. Slow down and elongate your breathing process. (Repeat this often to yourself.)

_____ Only work as hard as you have to. Think about softening and letting go of all your muscle action.

_____ Remind yourself that labor is good for your baby.

_____ Turn the lights off or turn the lights on, whichever makes you comfortable.

_____ Go outside and connect with nature where and how you can.

_____ Moan, sing, scream, and cry.

_____ Consider that pain is sometimes the result of fear, and that pain is always intensified by fear. Pain is caused by nerve stimulation; it is a product of the nervous system.

_____ Remember that birth happens through a series of muscle contractions and releases.

_____ Repeatedly tell yourself that contractions are good and safe.

_____ Utilize and release your creativity.

_____ Birth is sensual and can be very sexy. Oxytocin is a powerful hormone associated with uterine contractions. It is also associated with love! Consider masturbation. If you have a romantic partner with you, try kissing through a contraction.

_____ Rest, conserve your energy, and try to sleep.

_____ Use intentional relaxation exercises to stay calm, such as breath awareness, mental imagery, and progressive relaxation techniques. (What relaxation exercises have you practiced so far? Which ones are you enjoying? Which ones would you like to practice more? The more techniques you have available to you, the more able you will be to improvise and navigate through the developments of your birth.)

_____ Listen to your baby.

_____ Let your mind wander to a far-off place. Cultivate and visualize a happy place.

_____ Pray if your belief system includes prayer.

_____ Change positions. Try dancing, swaying, rocking, and moving with your sensations.

_____ Try stillness: real, complete, concentrated stillness.

_____ Use water: a shower or a tub, ice or heat packs.

_____ Meditate.

_____ Music is a powerful way to transform your environment. Music can relax the people around you, which will in turn help you to relax. Music can help you move in relation to your sensations. Rhythmic rocking and rolling can help to alleviate discomfort and aid the baby's journey. Music can soothe your soul and give you energy. Music can provide a focal point for your attention. (Note: most birthing people do get to a place in labor where they need to quiet the music, or they just tune it out if/when their attention can no longer tolerate distraction.)

_____ Use the time between the contractions with intention. Honor this time as an important element of your labor. Use this time to recover from the last contraction and prepare for the next. Use this time to assess your needs and concerns, to receive comfort and support from those around you, and to stay hydrated and well nourished.

Tools for the support partner's tool bag

Read through the following list once and then consider which tools jump out to you, the Birth Lover, as most important. Then go ahead and number them in the spaces provided, making #1 your most important.

_____ Believe in the birthing person's and baby's ability to safely navigate the birth process.

_____ Prepare with relaxation/visualization scripts/stories. What will you say if your voice is a soothing distraction?

_____ Have an intent to protect the environment: sound, temperature, light, and the energy of the people in the room.

_____ Be able to offer new labor positions (keep reading, as I will explain several options).

_____ Suggest the use of a shower, bath, ice packs, heat pads, and/or aroma therapy.

_____ Offer massages and sweet loving kisses. Help to generate some of that oxytocin.

_____ Tune into your own breath, slower will be calmer. Your birthing partner will respond to your body language.

Your support as Birth Lover comes because you are attentive, ready and willing to serve, to witness, to listen, and to love. Remember: you are not necessarily the solver of problems. Birth, although sometimes problematic, is not technically a problem that needs solving. Birth is a transformation. Sometimes your work will be *not* doing, i.e., not talking or touching or acting on anything. You can actively but quietly beam love in their direction, as you stand by as witness, attentively waiting to serve whatever needs arise. More support and coping techniques, including specific positions, are explored in later chapters, so please keep reading.

Baby's position impacts labor

There are various ways for a baby to present in the pelvic bowl. "Transverse" is when the baby is positioned completely sideways across the gestational person's body. This is a rare final presentation, and requires a cesarean section unless the baby can be jostled out of position.

And, as I mentioned in Week 1, "breech" is when the baby's head is upward, towards the gestational parent's head, and the butt or feet are down and "presenting." This position brings added risk and is commonly a reason for cesarean, yet as I also mentioned, not always. Some practitioners do consider a vaginal birth option for the breech position. And for review, "vertex" is when the baby's head is down. A vertex presentation is generally easier, simpler, and therefore safer. It is also more common.

There are also variations within a vertex position that can affect the ease of the baby's passage. Such variations have to do with the orientation of the baby's head inside the pelvis. When the large bone in the back of the baby's head, the occiput, is at the front of the parent's body, the baby is in an *anterior presentation*.[155] In this anterior presentation the baby is born looking down, behind the parent and towards their butt. A *posterior presentation* is when the occiput is at the back of the parent's body and the baby is born looking up towards the birth parent's face. The posterior presentation is often called a "sunny-side up, baby."

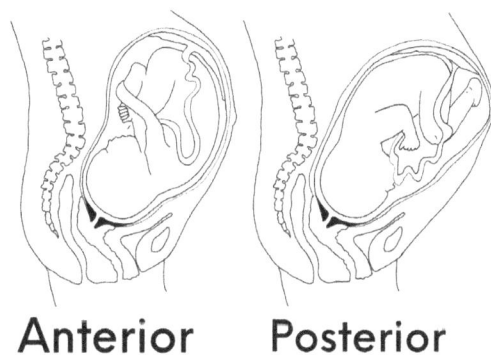

Anterior   **Posterior**

Generally, birth occurs the most smoothly when the baby is in a *vertex* and *anterior* position. When the baby is in a posterior position, labors tend to progress more slowly and cause strong sensations of back pain, during the contractions as well as in between them. We refer to this challenging scenario as "back labor." Some people describe their back labor as a terrible pain in one hip or the other, or even shooting down the front of their thighs, and not necessarily in their low back. Remember, again, that the pelvis has holes in its sacrum, the large heavy, triangular shaped bone in the back of the pelvis, which allows nerves to pass through. Back pain in pregnancy, and during birth, is usually related to posture (gestational parent's and/or baby's position) as well as to the extra weight of pregnancy putting pressure on these nerves. In a posterior presentation, a big bony baby head exerts a great deal of sustained pressure on the gestational person's sacral nerves. Try leaning back against something with the back of your head. You can put quite a bit of pressure there, especially in comparison to how hard you could push against your face.

Techniques to ease back labor pain should be tried regardless of whether the pain is felt in the hips, thighs, or back, because the pain is being caused by pressure from the baby's head on the sacral nerves. The better a gestational parent's posture and muscle tone prior to birth, the more likely the baby will maintain and/or arrive at an optimal position for birth. Of course, plenty of people with good posture have their babies arrive in funny positions. Don't blame yourself if your baby ends up in one such funny position. Our children have minds of their own!

EXERCISE: WHY BACK LABOR IS A PAIN IN THE BACK

1. Place your hand on the back of your head and then push your head and hand against each other as hard as you can.

2. Now place your hand up against your face and try pushing your face and your hand against each other as hard as you can.

You should notice that you can't tolerate as much pressure against your face as you can against the back of your head. Your baby would notice the same thing. If your baby, therefore, is in a posterior position, she is well motivated to lean back to keep her face away from your pubic bones, which she can do easily by pressing back into your sacral nerves. If your back or hip is hurting during birth, your baby is almost definitely in a posterior position. If you are not feeling low-back or hip discomfort, your baby is most likely in an anterior position.

In addition to pain in the low back or hips, one of the other drawbacks of back labor is that it tends to progress more slowly. In a posterior position the back of the baby's head can fit snuggly into the curve of the sacrum. In this scenario, the baby's head is angled farther back and the parent loses the direct downward pressure on their cervix that comes when the baby is in an anterior position. This lack of direct downward pressure can slow progress. Add in the sensation of back pain, and this creates a tough set of circumstances.

But fret not: should this occur in your labor, you can and will be able to handle it. Babies can and do come out vaginally from a posterior position, and there are some helpful pain-reducing techniques to use if you need them. Plus, there are techniques to help the baby turn out of a posterior position (which I will discuss later in the book). Lastly, it is helpful to remember that your baby may shift out of posterior position on her own. Back labor during part of your labor does not mean that you will have back labor for the duration of your labor.

Potential mismanagement of a posterior position

Mainstream American medical professionals do not always handle back labor appropriately. For example: I once had a woman cry in class when we started discussing back labor because, during her first birth, she had excruciating back labor and her nurse and doctor told her that she should stay in bed, on her back. Although this birth took place at a modern, upstate NY teaching hospital, the medical care in this scenario attempted to cope with the *symptom* of back pain, rather than the *cause* of the pain itself. The birthing mother recounted how the pain and immobility were traumatic. She said she tried all the medications they offered her and none of them helped, not even the epidural. She spoke of the fear that she had felt. She said that she was sure something was very wrong because of all the pain, even in between the contractions. After I described the causes of back labor in class, she said she wished she had known that the pain was a result of the baby's position; it would have been a lot less frightening. She also said she would have demanded to get up off her back. As you can imagine, it was a moving moment for all of us in class to witness. This woman of course did birth that posterior baby vaginally. And then, for her second baby, and after her Bradley® class, she went on to have a wonderful and more informed vaginal birth, thankfully free of back labor.

I also had someone relay the story of a woman that was induced and then given a cesarean section simply for the diagnosis of posterior presentation. Inducing a posterior baby, just for the diagnosis of posterior presentation, is unwarranted. Why would you want to rush this baby out, and take on the added, yet unnecessary risks of blood loss and recovery time associated with surgical birth? Why not work on trying to shift the baby's position? Even babies that stay in posterior position can surely be born vaginally as well.

Posterior presentation is another reason that your choice of birth attendant is so key to the safety of birth. Posterior position is not in and of itself a reason for medical intervention. Midwifery techniques that encourage baby to move may help.

Back labor relief

Follow your instincts. What is your body telling you to do? In general, most people in back labor report needing to get up and off their backs. Pelvic rocks (see Week 3) may help to encourage your baby to move. They may also be helpful for coping with back-labor pain. I also recommend that you try the following techniques:

The Lunge

From a standing position or from your knees, step one foot out, not directly in front of you, but at about a 45-degree angle to the side, opening your pelvic area. Bend that front knee and plant the raised foot firmly on a chair or on the floor. Notice the gentle opening you can create in your hips as you straighten and bend that front leg. If you are standing, allow your back leg to soften and straighten as feels good. Allow your weight to shift forward and backward, easing open your hips. Try it with each foot forward and look for the side that feels best. That is likely the side to which you should encourage your baby to shift. Try this position now, from both standing with a chair and without a chair and kneeling positions (to help you to determine what is most comforting).

—Pause to try the lunge technique—

The Belly Lift

As explained and named by Janie McCoy King in her book, *Back Labor No More! What Every Woman Should Know Before Labor*[156], the Belly Lift technique attempts to directly shift the baby's position up and off the sacral nerves. Not only do you actually lift and shift the baby's position to reduce pain; you will create more of a direct downward pressure on the cervix, thereby helping it to open. This improves the alignment of the baby and may help her to travel through the birth canal. The laboring person can do this technique for themselves, giving them a great sense of empowerment. It can also be modified for the partner. (McCoy King uses her training as a mathematician and her experiences as a laboring mom to explain back labor and her Belly Lift technique. She teaches about vectors, lines of direction and force, using math and physics to explain why the technique works.)

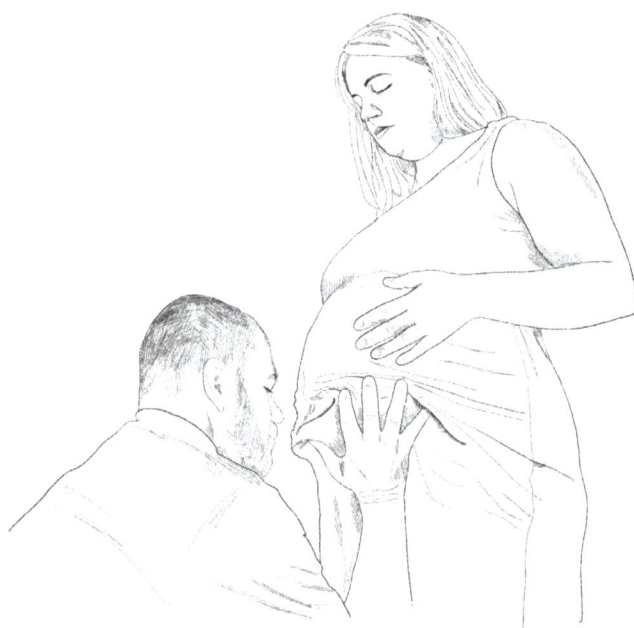

To self-apply this belly-lift technique: The gestational parent should stand up and let their arms hang straight down. Leaving their upper arms and elbows at their side, they should reach their hands together under their belly and interlace their fingers. Gradually they can begin to lift the belly straight up, shifting their baby's position. There is a good chance that they will feel quick relief if they get the baby's head redirected off their sacrum. They will likely want to hold the baby up for the duration of the contraction. This will help optimize the work of the contraction while it reduces back pain. Hooray all around! If it is not helping at all, they can move on to the counter pressure techniques that follow below. Then, later in labor, if back pain persists, this technique can be tried again.

For the partner to execute the belly-lift: The partner can help facilitate this technique. They can get on their knees in front of the birthing parent and ask for permission to place both of their hands gently on the underside of the pregnant belly, with their fingers pointing up towards the pregnant person's head. The partner should greet the belly/baby with intention and love and a very gentle first-contact. No fast or sudden movements. The motions should not ever be jerky or abrupt. You must have a slow and sensitive intention here. What you are thinking really translates. The gestational parent and the partner can and should try to visualize how the baby is laying and how she can shift. Firmly, slowly, and with the intent to listen to the birthing parent and the baby, the partner can exert pressure in an upward direction. If you can shift the baby's body up just a bit, it will alleviate the pressure on the birthing person's nerves and place a bit more pressure directly down on the cervix. If this technique is helping, the partner should pay close attention to their own body mechanics and comfort level. Do you, the partner, need something under your knees? Are you breathing fully?

This is a perfect moment for me to remind the partners that they, too, should be getting extra rest and making the time to exercise. They should be eating good food and tending to their own emotional needs. Remember: we need our partners to be in their best possible physical and emotional shape, too! Labor is hard work for everyone.

Question from one of my former students, and a support partner for a birthing person: "How will we know how hard to press or if it's really not working?"

Answer from me: "The pregnant person will have to be the one who answers that question, saying something like, 'no, not working,' or, 'please, try a little more pressure.'"

Remember that the baby is safe inside. I do understand that just touching the pregnant belly can be a little disconcerting for some partners. Always start by asking permission, greeting your baby, and remembering that your intention is to just move the baby a little bit. The amount of pressure that works or feels right may vary from contraction to contraction. Listen and adjust your pressure. Remember that your partner may not have a lot of words available for communication. You may have to rely on non-verbal cues.

I suggest that you go through the motions of this exercise now by preparing with your hands in the appropriate position and discussing each of your responses. (No need to exert enough force now to move the baby!)

—Pause to try the belly lift technique—

Counter Pressure

This is a technique that I have used on several birthing mothers with back labor, always with positive feedback. I've even heard it described as a "life saver." The pregnant person gets into an all-fours position, i.e., on hands and knees. The partner then applies pressure to the back of the gestational person's sacrum. The partner is looking for

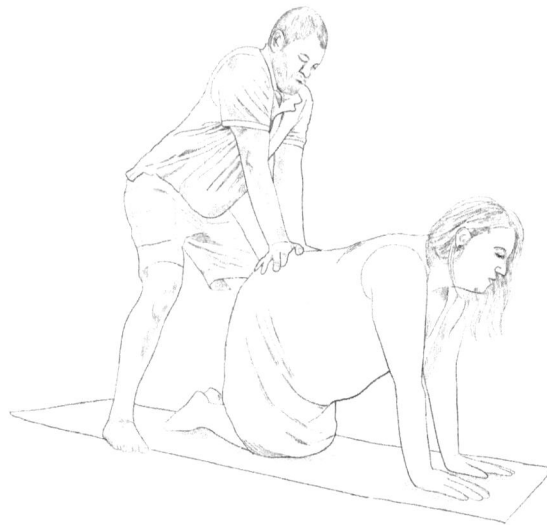

the exact area where the baby's head is. It seems that when the counter pressure meets the location and force of the baby's pressure the pregnant person feels relief.

In this technique, as in the Belly Lift, it is important to visualize the baby's position. Clearly imagine the baby's head pushing against the sacrum. You'll be looking to apply your force on the *outside* of the gestational person's body at the same location that the baby is applying force to the *inside* of the body. It may take some trial and error, but when the two forces meet the person in back labor will likely sigh in relief. You must always direct your pressure into the sacrum and then down and back toward their heels—*not* toward the center of the back. Giving them a sway back will cause discomfort and accentuate the back-labor pain. In sum, think consciously, clearly and purposefully about directing your force down and away from their mid back, toward their heels.

Support partners: here again, pay attention to your own body mechanics, too. These will affect the laboring person's perception of the technique. Proper body mechanics and calm, full breathing will help to generate a more soothing and powerful experience for the birthing person. And it will help you, the partner, persevere through the labor. If this counter-pressure technique is helping, you may find yourself at it for some time. Take care of your body so that you can provide the comfort and care you want to give for as long as it is wanted.

I have had to do this technique for hours. I worked with one woman who found this technique so helpful that she described it as the difference between bearable and unbearable. She needed counter pressure for every contraction over many hours. And yes, it was hard work for me. But when I got the amount of pressure and the location right, she would sigh in relief, and that was extremely motivating for all of us.

Partner, as you stand to apply pressure, bend your knees softly. This will keep your back loose and long. It's so important to keep your spine long to prevent your own backache. A fully extended spine will help you use your body weight instead of your arm strength. This will feel better for the pregnant person, too. Put your hands together with the inside of your wrists attempting to touch. The point of pressure should be comparable in size to the size of the baby's head. This is best done with the meaty parts—i.e., the "heels"—of your hands. If your hands are farther apart, the pressure gets diffused over a larger area.

If this is problematic for your wrists, you may want to try to use a tennis ball to apply the pressure. A tennis ball can provide a very intense pressure, which can bring welcome relief to both partner and pregnant person. By the same token, some people do prefer the touch of someone's hands and find the pressure from the ball to be too intense. Some birthing people hate the tennis ball during pregnancy and then find that they love it in labor. It is always good to have options. Add "tennis ball" to your supply list.

Once you have placed your hands on the gestational parent's sacrum, with full slow and easy breathing, allow your body weight to settle down through your arms. Start gently with just the weight of your arms applying pressure, stay with that until the pregnant person requests more pressure. Then use more of your body weight, as if you could pour or release the weight of your torso through your arms into the spot your palms are touching. If the pregnant person wants less pressure, back off by taking more of your weight back over your feet. You are not holding anything up. You want to allow your weight to drop down through your feet into the ground and down through your arms into the pregnant person's back.

When you explore this technique, it is important to realize that a pregnant person is not going to be able to tolerate nearly as much pressure now, during pregnancy, as they might during back labor. When a person is experiencing back labor, it's amazing to see how much force they not only tolerate but crave. I once had essentially *all* of my body weight going into a woman's sacrum when she said, "That's good, but could you press a bit harder?" I had to get someone to climb up on my back to increase the force!

Another note to remember: during the contraction, the pregnant person probably won't want a lot of movement in your hands. This is not really a massage technique; it's a counter-pressure exercise. Movements or changing pressure levels could be quite distracting during contractions.

Here's how it can work: the contraction begins and the pregnant person gets down, or up, into hands and knees position. The partner then straddles their feet over the pregnant partner's feet and lower legs on the floor. Once the birthing person is set, the partner can start by asking permission to place their hands on the sacrum. Obtaining consent is always a good idea. The birth partner should start gently, first with just the weight of the arms for pressure. Slowly, with the pregnant person's permission, experiment with increasing amounts of pressure. Both of you should be breathing fully and deeply, encouraging yourselves to be mindful of your breathing. Start with your hands placed at or near the top of the sacrum and then give the pregnant person options, moving in small increments down toward the tail bone. (Do not apply pressure directly to the tailbone.) The pregnant person can try to figure out where the pressure feels best.

Even birthing people who are not experiencing back labor may find counter-pressure techniques comforting and helpful during birth. The partner's tactile connection can be a good focal point for breathing into the low back area, which can help to reduce muscle tension, encouraging the gestational person to stay focused on yielding to their sensations.

—Pause to try the counter-pressure technique—

Counter-Pressure Massage

The same counter-pressure principles from above can be used in a potentially helpful massage technique that is often appreciated during pregnancy, although not necessarily during back labor. Regardless of fetal positioning, however, this technique may be especially appreciated between contractions.

In the same positions as the counter-pressure technique above (with the birthing parent on all-fours and you, the partner, with the heels of your hands together, touching their low back), allow your weight to flow through your arms. This time, instead of focusing your energy and attention into one part of the sacrum, slowly walk your hands around the entire back of the pelvis. The support partner should allow their weight to drop through one hand and then the other, each time shifting the location of the hands to slowly and mindfully "walk" around on the sacrum and iliac wings of the pelvic bowl. In general, especially in pregnancy, people tend to carry quite a lot of tension in their hips and low back.

This massage technique can help to reduce some of that tension. Explore the area around their sacroiliac joints and also around the iliac crests. This "walking massage" can bring a lot of welcome relief to an achy low back.

Note to the gestational parent: if your knees are prone to getting sore while kneeling, it is much better to try and prevent soreness than it is to try and reduce soreness once it has already arrived. Start off with a pillow or two under your knees. You can also purchase a kneeling pad: a very dense piece of foam, designed for gardeners, which works very well. If your wrists are prone to soreness from being in a hands-and-knees position, try making fists instead of leaning on your palms. You can also try draping over a birth ball, an ottoman, the side of your bed, a large stack of pillows, or the seat of a chair to support the weight of your upper body.

—Pause to practice the counter-pressure massage technique—

The Hip Squeeze

In this technique the support partner places each hand on opposite sides of the pelvis, on the upper ridges of the iliac crests (ilium), and then pushes in towards the gestational person's center. The hip squeeze can be performed by one partner or by two attentive birth companions who "tune in" to each other as they push from opposite directions. As above, the partner(s) should first ask permission to place their hands on the crest of the pregnant person's iliac crests. When permission is granted, slowly and steadily push in on their hip bones and listen for their feedback. This technique can be used while the pregnant person is standing or on hands and knees.

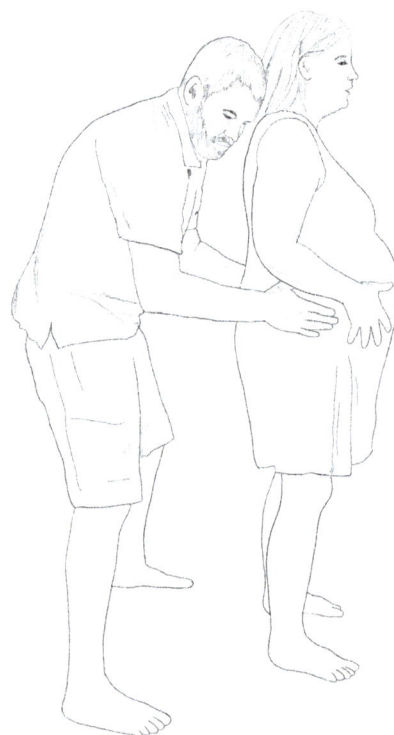

—Pause to practice the hip squeeze—

Back Labor Prevention

Now that you have had an opportunity to understand the positioning issues behind back labor and have learned some strategies to cope with it and labor in general, I encourage you to examine what you can actively do *now* to help avoid posterior positioning in the first place. Pay attention to your posture! When you schlump back in your chair, the back of the baby's head, the heavy part, can swing down towards the sacral area. When you sit upright, with good core tone, the back of the baby's head is more likely to stay in the preferred anterior position. Practice your abdominal bracing exercises from Week 3. They will help you to improve and maintain good posture. Additionally, the pelvic rock exercise done daily will help baby arrive at and maintain ideal positioning. Chiropractic care, prenatal massage, acupuncture, and/or physical therapy during pregnancy can all help you to maintain good posture and proper pelvic alignment.

Now it's time to let this information settle with some massage.

Stroking Massage technique

Sometimes massaging fingers can become a bit pokey, creating a ticklish response. This ticklish response is especially likely to occur when there is a lot of tension in the muscles. I have been known to jump excitedly if someone massaging me digs their fingers into the back of my thighs. Obviously, this would be less than desirable during labor. The stroking massage focuses on the palms of the hands instead of the fingers. This technique can be applied in any position.

For the person receiving the massage, please begin in a standing position. Keep your eyes closed with the crown of your head reaching comfortably up high towards the sky, your shoulders back and down, and your body in a relaxed and good alignment.

For the person performing the massage: rub your hands together, focusing entirely on the palms of the hands meeting. The goal is to generate some warmth in your palms. Ask for permission to begin and then start at the top of your partner's head and work your way down the length of their body with long stroking motions, sort of like petting an animal only with long, exaggerated strokes. One hand may follow the other or they may go side by side. Again, make your strokes long, slow and deliberate. Make sure that you have the intention of massaging the body, and that you aren't just rubbing clothes. Consider, too, that what you are thinking about really translates through your touch.

Work down the arms and down through the fingertips. Work down the legs, all the way to the feet. Give the tops of the feet a little extra push into the ground, helping your partner to connect with the earth. Come back up and start again: at the face, gently over the face and down the chest, abdomen, and front of the thighs, shins, and tops of the feet. Start again, this time down the back of the head, neck, back, buttocks, back of the thighs, calves and ankles, with a little gentle push down toward the earth when you get to the backs of the heels. Continue for as long as is desirable for you both. Let your breath be calm, full and soothing. Let your touch be calm, full and soothing. Take your time. Experiment with the pressure of your touch and the speed of your strokes. Try using strength and then lightness. Try slowing way down, and also try using really fast strokes. Visualize that as you are stroking you are releasing tension.

Once you have finished it is time to switch roles. It is so important to learn about relaxation and massage by both giving and receiving these techniques. Have fun and make this massage your own.

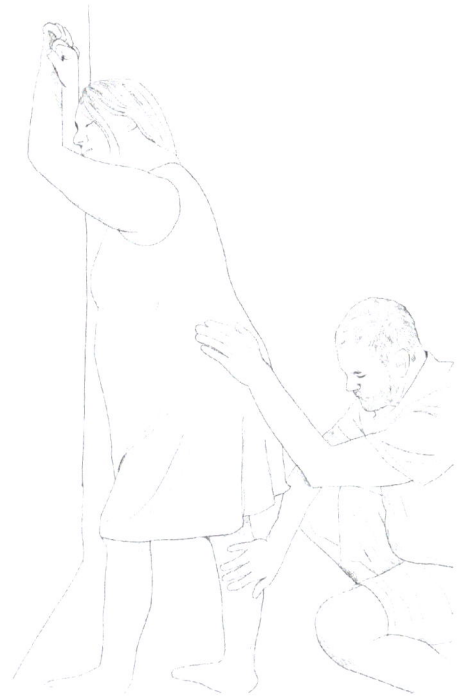

—Please put the book down now and try the stroking-massage technique—

Thank you for your time this week. I bet your belly is getting big. I hope you've been feeling well and find some happiness in the changes you are experiencing. Are you eating well? How are you doing with protein intake? As you now take a moment to review your homework, please look ahead at your coming week, what are the obstacles? Can you make plans to carve out some practice time? What you practice is what you will have available for birth support. Take great care and remember that I appreciate how hard you are working—and so does your baby!

HOMEWORK:

A) Continue to do your research

Consider looking up kangaroo care for preemies. And for fetal positioning consider looking up Spinningbabies.com, The Webster chiropractic technique, and Rebozo techniques.

B) Think about what you will do if you go past your due date

Consider what messaging you will want to give yourself, and how you might handle pushy friends, relatives or co-workers who may feel empowered to weigh in.

C) Begin to devise your own first stage labor strategies.

What are you going to think about during labor? How will you move your body?

D) Review back labor techniques.

Practice, practice, practice.

E) Enjoy the stroking massage

Practice, practice, practice.

THIS SPACE IS FOR YOUR NOTES AND DRAWINGS

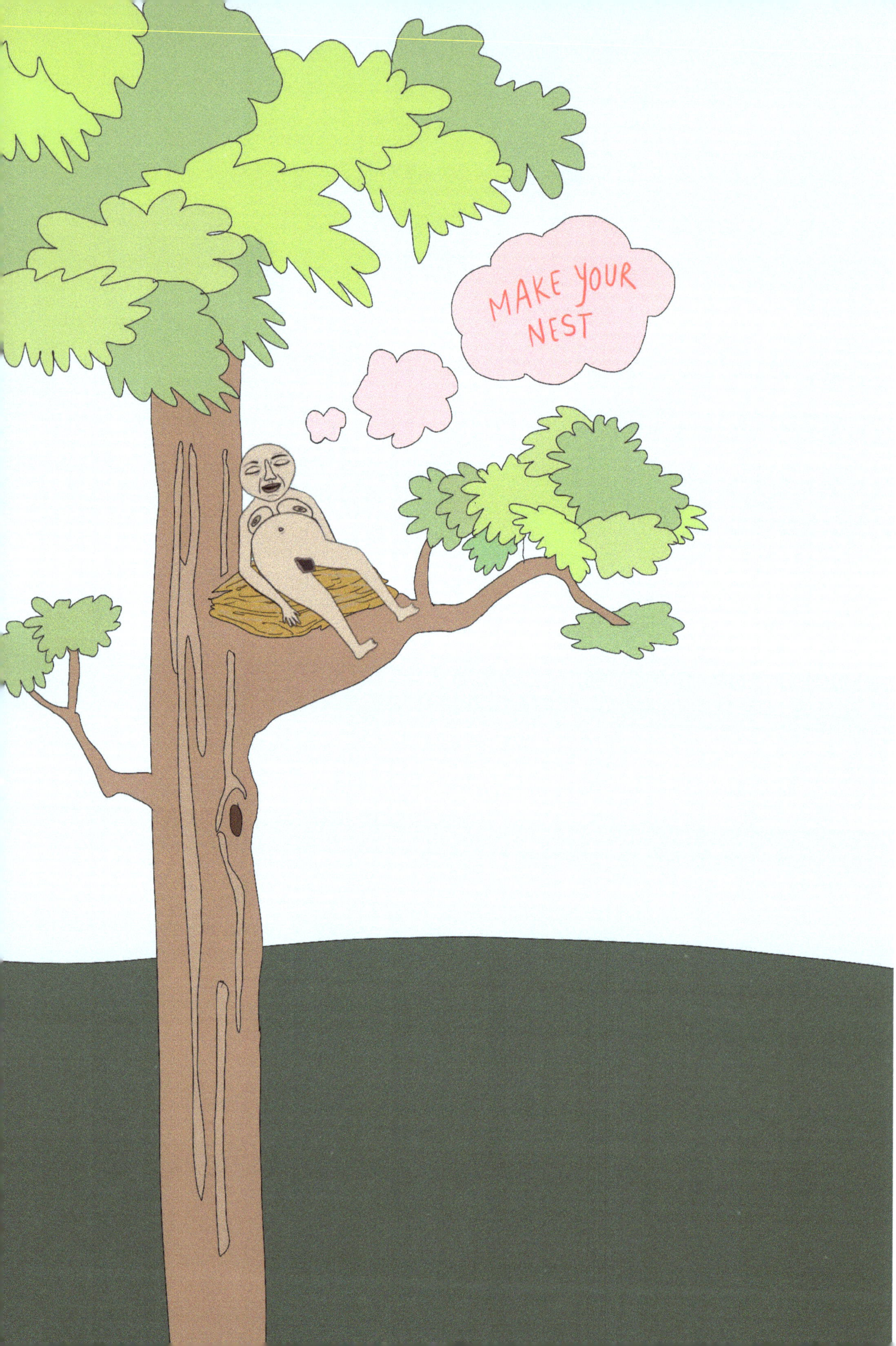
MAKE YOUR NEST

WEEK 8

First
Stage
of Birth

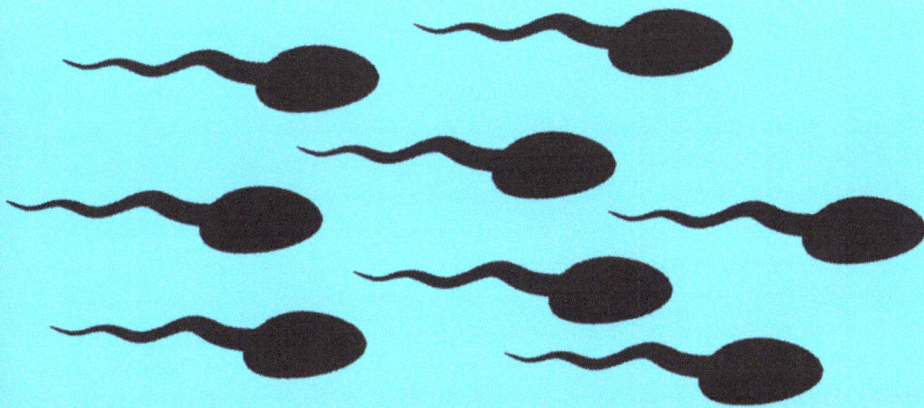

Chapter contents:

O *Develop your labor groove*

O *First stage labor positions*

THIS SPACE IS FOR YOUR NOTES AND DRAWINGS

Hello again! I'm so glad you are back! How did last week go? Were you able to carve out any time to ponder what your labor strategies will be? Did you get a chance to practice the back labor or stroking-massage techniques? If not, take some time now to review last week's exercises. Remember to continue to train yourself to exhale at the start of any practice contractions (Braxton Hicks) or during any other uncomfortable sensations or otherwise stressful moments you may encounter. Doing your homework will pay off. What you practice now will be easier later—feel more intuitive—when you experience greater sensations.

Develop your labor dance

When it comes to birth, particularly in first stage labor, there aren't any wrong positions or shapes to try. It's helpful to be active. Any way you want to move and any shape you want to pause in is a good choice for you. Move your body in exploratory ways, anything that occurs to you should be tried, and if it feels like it's working for you then, yay! In this forthcoming section, I focus on labor positions that are well suited for the first stage of labor. In the weeks ahead, you can read my offerings for second and third stage labor.

In first stage, in addition to your own experimenting and explorations, I am going to teach you some positions that may aid your ability to cope during your contractions. What I will explain can help to increase your labor-position vocabulary and practice. Note that these teachings are not meant to promote a "right" or "wrong" position to be in; I teach these only to support your creativity and to foster a conscientious approach to your independent exploration. I also teach some specific labor positions so that partners, who aren't directly experiencing the contractions, can have useful suggestions to contribute during labor. Many of the positions I discuss below are those that birthing people throughout history have found helpful. I'll explain why they are worth a try and what makes sense about them. Then you can explore and adjust them until they become your own; your birth dance. Be sure to continue investigating (finding your groove in) these positions—and adapt them to your comfort—as your belly grows! But first let's consider a few fun facts that can help you contextualize your labor position explorations.

The uterine shift, energy conservation, and gravity

As we discussed earlier, contractions cause the cervix to dilate and efface. They also cause the uterus to shift position. This shift helps to better align both the cervical opening and baby with the pelvic outlet. Understanding this alignment shift can help you to focus on releasing your abdominal muscles during contractions. When the abdominal muscles are tight and tense, this added effort forces the uterus and abdominals to work against each other, wasting your precious energy.

But, Emily, tensing is a common response to pain! Yes, it is. We pull in and brace around what we are feeling: "Ow, it hurts!" It's a protective response to the sensation, seemingly instinctive. But you can learn to relax through the pain. Try this now: Tense your muscles, squeeze your belly, pull your elbows in tight, and exclaim, "Ow, it hurts!" Then release, melt your muscles into softness, and breathe fully. Again, when we do this tensing, we are trying to be protective. In labor, however, this effort wastes valuable resources. When you brace against the work of the uterus, which you don't really need protection from, you engage muscles that do not directly contribute to the process of opening up the cervix. By contrast, when you soften your abdominal muscles, interior structures can soften too; they become more pliable. In this way, the uterus can shift freely as it contracts. No fighting necessary. This saves vital energy for better things, like kissing and laughter and having more contractions.

It is also helpful to consider the power of gravity while you explore your birth positions. If you are leaning backwards, bracing against the pain, then gravity pushes down on the baby, who in turn pushes down on your spine. This ultimately works against the shifting uterus. It prohibits you from taking advantage of the potential pressure of the baby down on the cervix to aid in the birth process. This doesn't mean you should never lean back during a contraction. The only time to think something is off with your positioning is if the baby gives you signals through her spastic, painful or disconcerting movements, her heart tones, or your own intuition.

Consider with me the following scenario: You are in your bed, and you are comfortable. You're leaning into a big stack of pillows or your partner's chest. You are resting well. If you have a contraction now it might be most useful to stay where you are and just relax into what is happening. Maybe the comfort that comes from resting where you are at that moment is more important than working with gravity or being concerned with maximizing anything. (Faster birth doesn't necessarily mean better birth.) By the same token, if you really need to conserve your energy, then you will want to try positions that acknowledge and respect gravity.

Regardless of position, your work will be supported by trying to soften your abdominal muscles and your pelvic floor, exactly during the huge sensations. Fiercely strong uterine contractions are what you want. That bears repeating. *Fiercely strong uterine contractions are what you want.* Strong contractions are not a problem. (Are you thinking a rather sarcastic, "yeah right!"? If so, hear that voice and acknowledge it as fearful. Remember: saying hello to your fears can help you to find added courage.) During birth the work is to match the depth of your relaxation (the amount of brain power you put into it) to the intensity of each contraction (what your physical body exerts).

As we go through possible labor positions, take note of gravity and how it will impact the gestational parent and baby. The partner's job is to look for ways to utilize massage and/or counter-pressure in all of these different positions. In addition to applying counter pressure to the sacrum or hips, applying gentle touch without pressure may at times be very welcome. The act of resting a single open hand somewhere on the pregnant person's body, with a calm and focused touch, can soothe. It can provide comfort without distraction. When a loving hand is placed on the sacrum or other bodily location, and left there with intentional stillness, it serves as a place or target to "breathe into." While it may not suffice during a tough, back-labor contraction, it can be quite effective during a "regular"—good and strong—contraction. Placing a hand with kind intention on the pregnant person's low back or foot or arm or head—again anywhere, and then just resting your hand there with purposeful stillness, can provide a great focal point. The tactile connection encourages deeper breath for both people involved. Through your focused intention you can reduce their pelvic tension and provide social support. This is all about providing comfort without distraction.

But yes, of course it could be that, during their next contraction, they will find comfort through lots of distraction. So stay tuned in!

Logic? Maybe not: What are you feeling?

Theoretically, starting labor with standing positions and then progressively getting lower down in space (from leaning to sitting to squatting to kneeling to lying down) is physically logical. But understand that real birth shouldn't—and can't—be weighed down by the rules. To pick your birthing positions you will need to balance logic, physics, body signals, and sensations *in the moments* of you doing the hard work. You will want/need to freely shift between up and down during the night(s) and day(s) of your birth.

For vaginal birth to happen, you need the baby to get down into the pelvic bowl. First, the baby enters the *pelvic inlet*, the opening at the top of the pelvis. Later, the baby moves through the *pelvic outlet*, the bottom opening of the pelvic bowl. When birth begins and a person is upright, walking, swaying, dancing, etc., it helps the baby move down into the pelvic inlet. As the birth progresses, however, and the baby moves lower into the pelvis, it gets harder for the gestational person to move around. Then typically they feel the need to get closer to the ground (though some people do prefer to stand through all phases of birth, including delivery). Often, when a birthing person feels the need to get lower in space, they either need to rest or to create more openness in the pelvic outlet. To really open up, they might need to squat down, pushing the bones of the pelvis apart. (More on squatting when we get to second stage, so keep reading!)

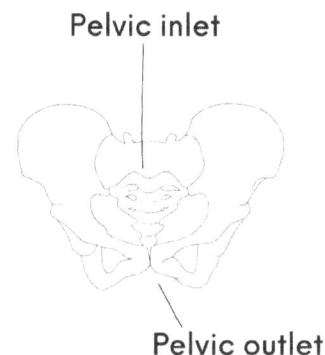

Pelvic inlet

Pelvic outlet

Choosing positions at the start of labor

Imagine it is 11:30pm and you are at full-term in your pregnancy. It's late, clearly, and it's been a long day. As you get into bed, you think to yourself, "Wow I am *really* tired. What if I went into labor now? I can't stay up this late again until after I have my baby. I better get a good night's sleep. I will be so good tomorrow night. Tomorrow I will go to sleep at 7:00pm, just to make up for this!" You pull the blankets up, settle into your pillow and think, "Ahhhh yes, bed." You close your eyes and start to drift off. Then…

"Ugh! Oh my gosh. What was that?!"

You have just had a massive contraction that feels way more intense than anything you have ever felt before. Labor has begun and you know it, or at least you strongly suspect it. A few minutes later you have another contraction, and any uncertainty fades. You are in labor.

Should you jump out of bed and speed through all your different labor positions, charging around your bedroom to get this thing going? No! Should you jump up and nervously start to clean the house? No! (But it does happen. One of my clients recently admitted that she did just that. She realized she was in labor, so she jumped up and started to clean the house, even though it was bedtime. She said she was too excited, she couldn't rest. But then she did become exhausted and dehydrated, and she had some regrets as she retold her story.) Again, don't do it. Try not to jump up if you need to rest, even if you are so very excited. Sip some water and try to stay in bed. Try to rest. If your mind must race, encourage your body to be still. Put your mind to work with a mindfulness assignment as you commit to stillness in your body. Try to ignore and let go of what is happening. Actively work to relax. Maybe listen to a bedtime story or try to visualize a small circle opening up to fill the screen of your minds-eye. Or, visualize your cervix opening up wide like a time-lapse video of a flower as it blooms. Even good old day dreaming with your eyes closed and your body still can be restorative.

Focus on relaxation like your life depends on it, find a way. Channel your surge of energy. Work your relaxation practice. Although not as restful as resting, if you really can't slow yourself down, maybe try cuddling, sex, or masturbation. While these activities can lead to dehydration and a depletion of energy, they can also help to reduce stress and promote rest. In short, have a plan. How will you cope with your excess energy and remain in bed? (Safety note: Please refrain from intercourse or putting anything into your vagina if your amniotic membranes have ruptured. Reduce the risk of infection where you can.)

The excitement/arousal/trepidation of early labor can be extreme, but rest is going to be of vital importance; there is a lot of work ahead. It doesn't matter that there is a theoretical logic to being upright at the beginning of labor. In this instance, if you're getting to bed too late or are otherwise already tired, follow the more immediate logic: if you don't get some rest now, then you'll be exhausted way sooner than need be. You have a long haul in front of you. Deeply relax your muscles and let be what will be. If you are unable to rest or sleep through the contraction, work to rest or sleep in between your contractions. Use whatever moments you have wisely, for positivity and for restoration.

In the example above, labor started in the lowest plane (lying down), and it made sense to stay there. Sleep, rest, sleep, rest, sleep, rest. When you simply cannot rest any longer, it might be time to move. Engage in the dance of your birth, yet actively continue to rest whenever you can, just in case!

Here's another scenario: Suppose you have just had a great night's sleep followed by a lovely breakfast, and as you are cleaning up the last of your dishes you get a strong contraction. You and your partner are well-rested and well-nourished. In this example it might be more appropriate to go for a gentle walk and/or do some light stretching before getting back into bed for rest. Perhaps here, being upright and moving, maybe engaging in a little dancing, is just the ticket to help ease your baby down into your pelvic doorway. Later you can progress to all fours or horizontal shapes. After some additional exertion it will be time to rest again. Then later you might get up again, eat a light snack, drink some water, go for a walk, and rest some more. Then up again, walk a little, use the bathroom, take a shower, rest again. And so on until the baby is out. The act of changing activities can help many (rested) people cope in labor.

Throughout birth there will hopefully be a lot of listening to your own instincts as you make educated guesses about your needs. Continuously assess if you need to conserve energy or if you need to help move things along by being more active. *You will learn your labor logic as your birth unfolds.*

As you explore the following positions in your own home, give yourself credit for actively preparing for birth. Congratulate yourself. You do this preparation so that when you are really in labor you can try to let go of thinking and release into the moment, well-armed with possibilities and practice. Be conscientious and make whatever adjustments you need to make.

Remember: having a strategy for labor promotes courage, which will in turn help you to surrender to the forces of birth. Experiment with the labor positions, be bold and adjust as needed. There is great learning to be done from this practice. You will gain confidence through familiarity. A person who practices more positions during pregnancy will have more options for finding comfort during birth. A support partner that practices their own role in different positions will have more support to offer. A partner cannot physically feel what might be helpful to try in labor. But by practicing birth positions with the pregnant person their tool bag grows, and the practice provides time to emotionally connect into what is happening. In other words, a baby is coming!

Please take a moment now to "get into your body" before you move into practicing the labor positions. I've included a warm-up exercise below to help.

EXERCISE: WARM-UP

Within this warm up, move each of the joints in your body in small rotations. Imagine that you can make some space in each of your body's joints, breathe fully and conscientiously. Think of "lubricating" each joint with your gentle movements. Together, this will enhance your physical experience. Read what follows out loud to your partner and then warm yourself up as well.

"Stand with your feet about shoulder's width apart. Take a few deep breaths. Relax your weight down into your feet and into the earth".

—Reader pause—

"Gently reach your fingertips, hanging by your sides, down and then out to the sides and then up and overhead as you inhale. Breathe in as your arms go up, exhale as your arms come down. Repeat this movement and breath a few times. You'll be tracing your largest half circles from the thigh (where the hands are at rest), out from the sides of your body, then up over your head. Feel and allow the shoulder rotation as you go from the arms extended at shoulder height to over your head. Relax your shoulder blades and try to leave them heavy. As you exhale and lower your arms down by your sides let them rest fully in between breaths. Try to sync your movement with your breathing. In yoga these are called sun breaths, because you are tracing a large round sphere like the sun."

—Reader pause—

"Now gently, slowly, circle your arms front to back a few times in each direction. Be compassionate with your body. Try not to force anything. Try not to rush. As you slowly circle your arms, bring your body-awareness down to your knees. If they are locked, gently soften them."

—Reader pause—

"Now sink your awareness further down to the soles of your feet. Feel them firm and relaxed on the ground as they root you down into the earth. Feel the weight of your sacrum and allow that to drop down your legs as well. Continue to trace a few more circles, arms extended long through the fingertips."

—Reader pause—

"Next, let your hands come to settle on your hips. Bend your knees gently and begin to isolate and rock your pelvic bowl front to back, side to side, and in a circular motion in both directions. This will help to increase awareness, warm up and lubricate your hip joints, and gently stretch your muscles.

These circles are an important range-of-motion exercise. Feel the weight of the sacrum and tailbone releasing down. Feel how the soles of the feet, ankles and knees all move as you rotate your hips. Let the heaviness drop down through your feet into the ground. Feel the gentle activation of your abdominal muscles helping to hold you upright. Explore your comfortable range of motion and try to notice your pelvic inlet and outlet. Gently engage the pelvic floor muscles and gently release them. Wag your tailbone in circles and figure eights."

—Reader pause—

"Relax your body weight down through your legs into your feet, into the ground, and find stillness, except for breathing. Feel your breath change your shape."

—Reader pause—

"Feel the energy that comes up from the ground into your body."

—Reader pause—

"Take this moment of stillness with eyes closed to feel the reverberations of your warm-up throughout your body".

—Pause to feel your stillness—

"Now, if there are any more stretches or movements that you would like to do, ones that might help you to feel more ready or more comfortable, please do them. This is also a good moment to practice the abdominal bracing exercise explained and practiced in Week 3. Warming up the abs will support all of your other movements. Follow your instincts to take care of yourself. When you come back to stillness you are ready to try some first stage labor positions."

First stage labor positions

Be sure to read through each of the positions detailed below before putting them into practice. Each position moves the laboring person lower down in space, starting from a standing position to a bent or draped over position, and on down into being seated, then on all fours, and finally lying down. When you do practice these positions, one at a time, try to do so without the book in hand.

As you work your way through, practice an audible exhale each time you arrive in a new shape. Spend a minute or two in each position before moving on. Experiment with any and all visualization techniques while in each position.

Slow Dance

If you are doing this exercise without a partner, then lean into a wall for support. Leaning into a wall is grounding, permanent, not as soft as into the arms of a trusted human, but the wall is reliable (in a way that humans sometimes aren't). It's empowering to be able to get support wherever it exists. Consider the words that you will want to tell yourself or have someone else tell you during labor. Consider how you can help yourself feel safe and protected and encouraged.

If you are working with a partner, stand and face each other. The pregnant person should place their arms around the partner's neck. The partner should place their arms around the pregnant person's waist. As you both settle into position, focus on long, slow, full exhalations. The birth partner can encourage the pregnant person, and therefore remind themself as well, to focus on relaxing both body and mind.

Both people should have their feet in a comfortably wide stance. The legs should have a soft bend in the knees. Like in the warm-up you just did, try swaying your hips gently side to side; imagine that you are swaying to a slow, romantic song. (You can even take some time later this week to practice while listening to music.)

The pregnant person should comfortably lean in towards their partner and maybe even burrow their face into the partner's chest. This burrowing provides a good place to tune into your pregnant body and tune out the external world. The pregnant person should try to relax the abdomen and pelvis. Both partners should continue to try and breathe slowly, and easily. The partner can whisper encouragements, sweet nothings or specific visualizations into the pregnant person's ear. In this slow dance position, the partner helps to support the weight of the pregnant person's upper body and can encourage good and empowered feelings. In this position the partner can usually also manage a bit of stroking massage if that is appreciated.

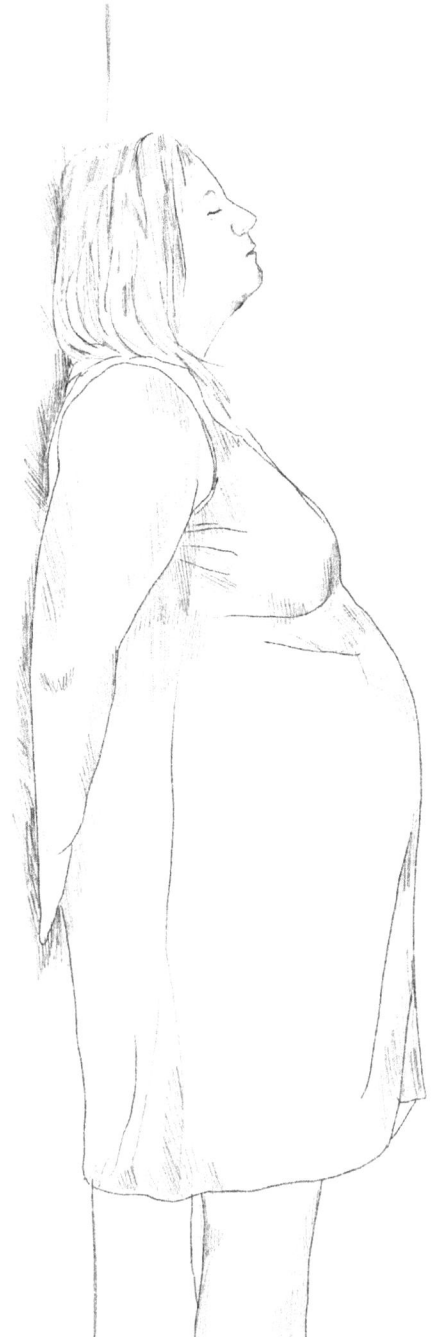

If you are practicing by yourself, again I ask you: what encouraging words do you want to give yourself? How will you be able to promote calm feelings of being safe and protected?

For all pregnant people with partners or without, it is your work to be in your own head with positive messages. What words would you like to hear?

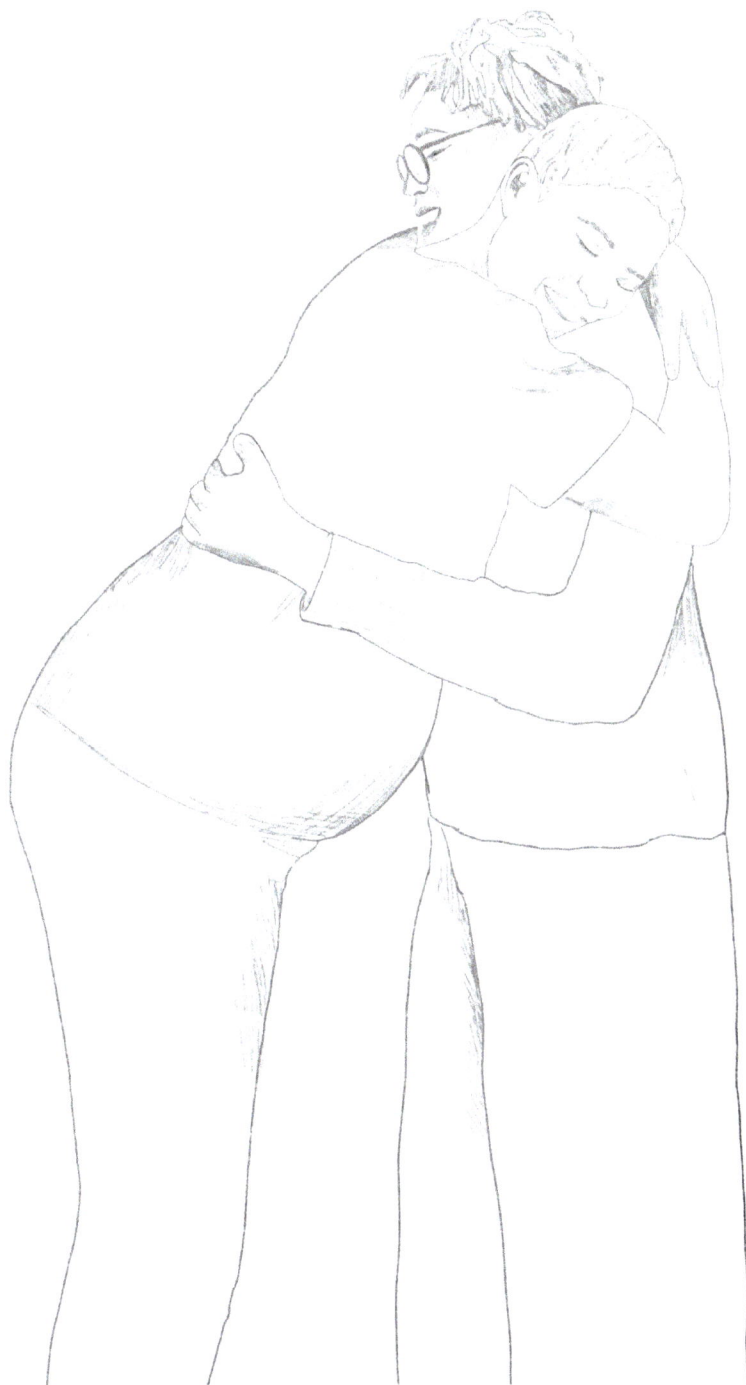

—Pause to practice the *Slow Dance* position—

If you are planning a hospital birth, or live in an apartment building with an elevator, imagine that you might be in a public space waiting for this elevator when you get a strong contraction. (Speaking of which, do you know if you will need to take an elevator where you are planning to give birth? Do you know what floor you'll need to go to, or which way to walk when you get there? These additional preparations can also help reduce any added stress from the uncertainty about which way to go while laboring.) There may be other people waiting for the elevator, each of them with their own story and energy. The slow dance position can allow you—the laboring person—to tune them out. You can sway and breathe and settle. You can hide in your partner's chest, as your own personal labor land. Think of this as a safe place with minimal awareness of or concern for your surroundings.

The partner can keep an eye on the environment, but they can also tune into the pregnant person and whisper into their ear, telling them how safe and amazing this birth is, how proud they are of them, what a great parent they are, and how much they love them. They can encourage them to let go, and to trust and allow the process of the birth to unfold as it needs to. And they can be quiet but dialed in emotionally.

What follows is a sampling of phrases that the support partner can use for verbal guidance and encouragement. Laboring people can also tell these to themselves!

- "Your job is to let your arms go... that's it, you're doing great. Let your arms be heavy, let your head relax."
- "I know this must be so intense, but you are amazing and you're handling it so well."
- "Breathe fully, deeply and with intention. Let your body weight drop down through your stable structure, down through your torso, down and out your body."
- "Let your breath wash away what you no longer need. As you inhale receive the new air as a gift of energy and strength."
- "Trust the ground to receive your weight. (Deep audible exhale.) Let go."
- "Trust your body to know what to do. Let go."
- "I love you. You're making progress. You're safe. You are so very beautiful, and I know this must be crazy, but you're doing it! And no one ever did it better. You're rocking this!"

Anytime and anywhere that you are upright, it's worth trying the slow dance position. In a hallway en route from the bedroom to the kitchen, in a parking lot, at a restaurant, on a nature trail, or in a hospital room—wherever. With an attentive birth partner at your side, you can slow dance through it anywhere. Without a partner by your side, you can close your eyes and tune into your own safe and supported place, hear your own music, find your own ways to tune out the world around you.

Reverse Slow Dance

In this standing position, the pregnant person will connect their back against the partner's chest. If the partner is leaning back against a wall, they can lean way back into them and give them a lot of their body weight. If the partner is standing in the middle of the room, they won't be able to support as much weight. (Practice both: against a wall and in the middle of the room).

In this position, the partner can put their arms around the laboring person. They might try to gently stroke their pregnant belly or hug/hold them from behind. Another option here is for the partner to place their bent arms under the pregnant person's armpits and around their shoulders, fingers pointing up. This provides a bit of a shelf, or two hooks, for them to rest their arms over. The pregnant person can gently lean or hang their upper body forward as they tip and release weight from the shoulders, arms, neck, and head. (The partner won't want to grasp their own hands across the chest, as it might feel restrictive, almost choking).

Please remember, the partner cannot support much weight here. Nevertheless, supporting just a little weight can foster a deepened sense of communion and yield tremendous comfort.

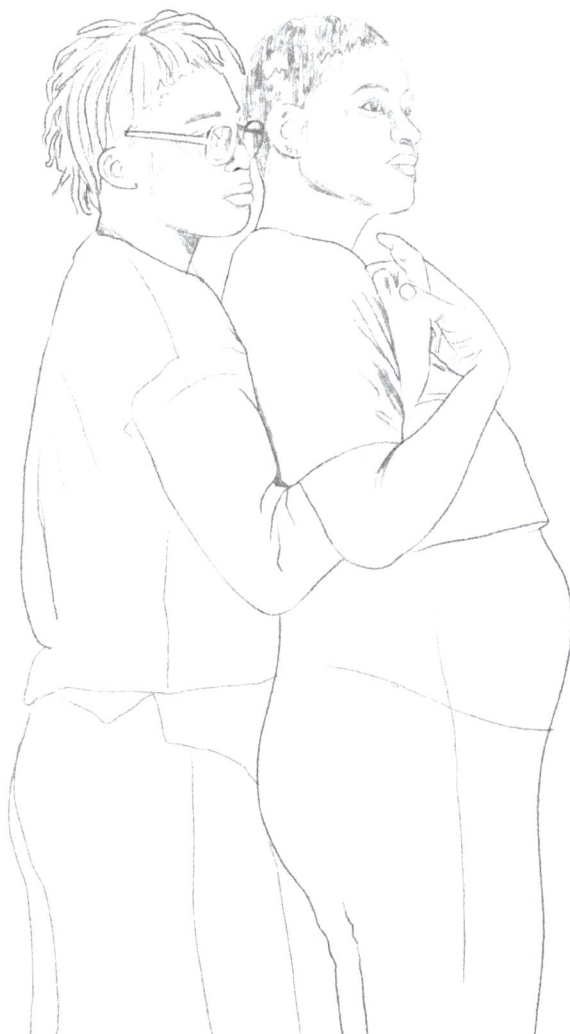

—Pause to practice the *Reverse Slow Dance* position—

The Drape: Standing Variations

Drape your upper body over anything solid, such as over a kitchen counter, bookshelf, or other solid piece of furniture. Or lean into a wall or stand in the shower while leaning into the wall for support. If you do not have a partner these standing drapes may be appreciated. If you do have a partner these standing drapes can free up the partner for other tasks, such as massage or phone calls to the midwife.

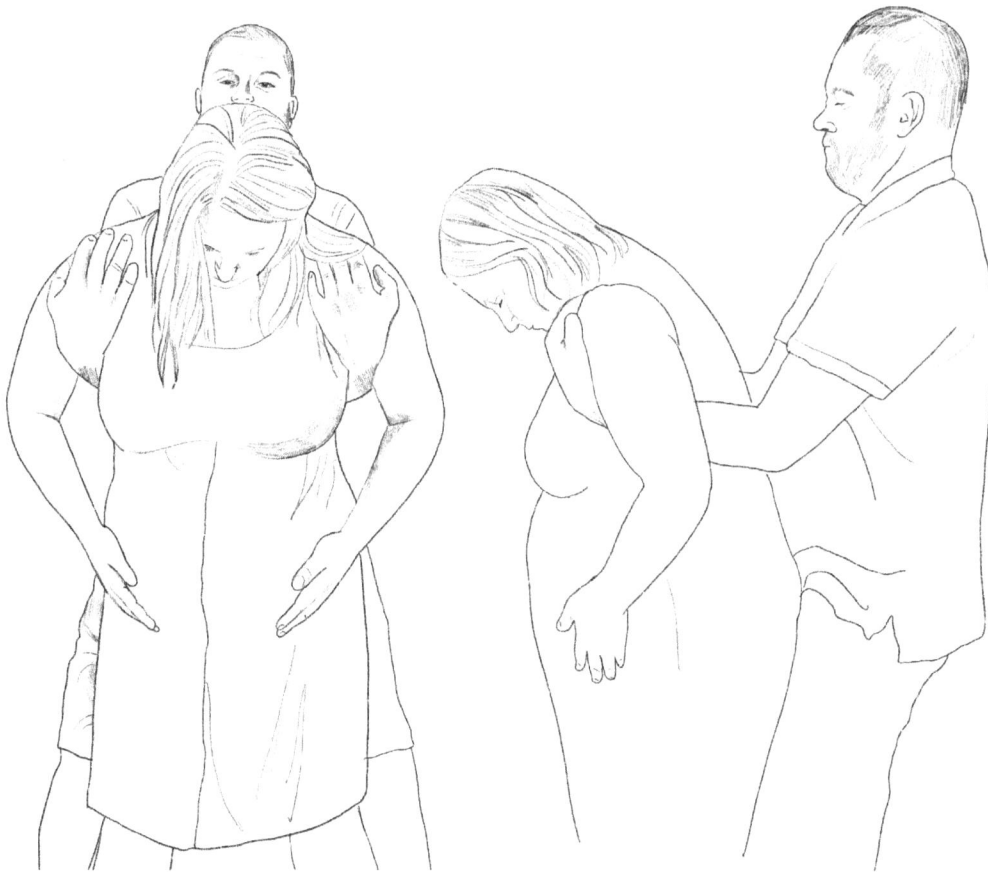

Once in position, let go, settle into the wall or furniture, and allow the work in your uterus to happen. Drop your belly down, focus on slowing your breath, bring your awareness to the soles of your feet—letting them be open and relaxed as your body weight drops through them into the ground.

Partner Drape

This shape will take you farther down in space, yet it is still a standing position. This one requires the partner to form a strong base of support so the pregnant person can drape their torso over the base partner's back, releasing their weight and allowing them to relax their upper body more fully. Hips can sway, and a close physical contact between the couple is maintained.

The partner should stand with their feet parallel and just a bit wider than hip's width apart. As they bend their knees, keeping a long straight back, they should hinge at the hip and really stick their butt way out behind themself, lowering enough to rest their forearms or hands on their thighs. Use trial and error to find the most comfortable variation—e.g., resting forearms or hands across thighs. A large height differential for a couple may also lend itself toward one variation or the other.

The partner's comfort and safety will be enhanced the more they can keep their spine long and let their own weight drop down through their legs, as opposed to trying to brace themself up with their thigh muscles. This is best achieved when they can reach their butt out behind them while extending energy through their upper back and out the crown of their head, while also gently engaging the abdominal muscles. The spine should be in a fully elongated neutral position. Again, in this position it is important for the partner to understand that their job is not to hold up their weight, or the pregnant person's; rather, it is to allow the weight to drop down through the legs to be released to the ground.

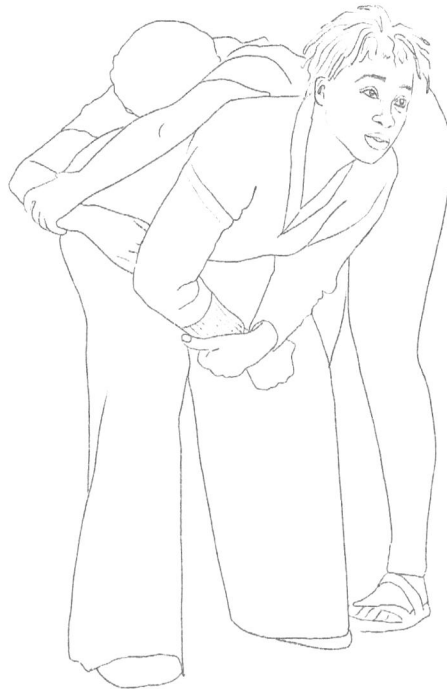

The pregnant person is now going to stand perpendicular to their partner, sideways to their body, so that when draped over, one breast will be closer to the base partner's shoulders and one breast will be closer to their butt. Once standing in position, the pregnant person can slowly drape their body across the base partner's long, straight back. The pregnant person will want to allow their chest, neck, head, and arms to rest completely on top of the support person.

Pregnant people: please be careful not to dig your chin into your partner's back! Keep your head to one side but change sides frequently so you don't get stuck in one position, which would cramp your neck. Relax into your partner's support. Allow your hips to sway and your belly to be free. In this position, the pregnant person can really think about slow dancing the baby out. Let your belly hang heavy. Let your vagina and butt be heavy, relaxed and open. Allow yourself to feel the sensations of your body.

The pregnant person may want to release through their contraction in stillness, or they might enjoy the base partner giving them a ride by gently swaying and rocking their base. Once the partner finds some ease in this drape position, they can try a variation where they release the arm closest to their pregnant partner, then reach around and place their hand on their pregnant partner's low back, and/or give some stroking down their leg.

Position notes for the pregnant person: If the pressure of leaning on your chest is uncomfortable to your breasts, step your feet out and away from your partner and then just rest your upper chest, shoulders, arms, and head on their back, leaving your breasts free to hang down between you. Again, please be careful not to dig your chin into your partner's back.

Once the contraction (or practice contraction) has ended and you, the pregnant person, are ready to stand up again, you can signal with words that your contraction is over. No need to move yet. Stay put and communicate when you can. You'll want to stay completely relaxed and draped over your partner. Your partner can then easily and safely give you a ride back up by "walking" their hands—i.e., pushing down into their thighs—as they slowly stand upright. Using their arms to help carry weight will protect and support their back. They'll want to really push into their thighs to transfer the weight. As your partner gets more upright, more of your own weight will be dropping down into your feet, giving you a free ride up to vertical! This conscientious attention to how you stand back up will reduce the possibility of either person straining their muscles.

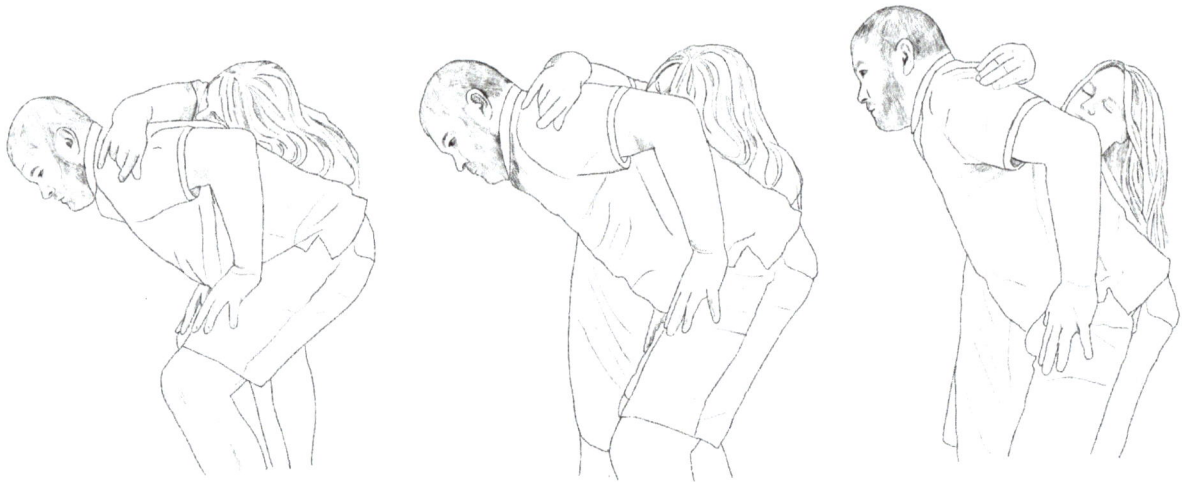

—Pause to practice the *Drape: Standing Variations* and *Partner Drape*—

Sitting

I love the simplicity of this labor position. However, if you do not honor it now as a worthy labor position, then you might not think to try it as a labor-coping destination in birth.

Sit on a chair (preferably one without arms, so that there is more room for the legs to be wide). Relax your feet flat on the ground. If your feet do not reach the ground easily, place two equal-sized stacks of books, or some other stable object, under each of your feet. You want the entire bottoms your feet to make full contact with something solid. This helps ground a birthing person. You may also want to use a rolled towel or small pillow to place behind yourself, in order to support the lumbar curve of your spine.

Let your hips open comfortably. Allow the backrest to support you as you sit upright with a comfortably elongated spine. Close your eyes if you're comfortable doing so. Settle yourself into stillness. Take some nice full breaths.

A chair with a hard bottom can be a very effective place to labor. They really seem to bring on good, strong working contractions. When your sit-bones connect with the hard chair or ground, you can release the weight of your skull and torso down through your spine into your pelvis and then directly into the hard surface. It's your bony structure that transfers weight down and allows for less strain on your muscles as you maintain your upright posture. Your leg muscles can let go. Some people find it quite soothing to sit and rock in a rocking chair. Sitting on the floor may be productive, too. And, occasionally, switching to a soft bottom, like sitting on a yoga ball, pillows, or your bed, is also good.

—Pause to practice the *Sitting* position, sitting for several eye-closed breaths—

When you sit with the intention to be still you can focus on being present in your thoughts. You can devise a game plan if you need one. When you sit still you can attempt to face your truth with mindfulness. But what does it mean to "face your truth with mindfulness?" Take time to explore this. Think about it. Think about what it means to surrender to and survive your sensations, to be in that exact moment to get through that exact moment. If intellectually you can focus on the fact that your body will survive the sensation, then you can look to your heart to seek courage; you'll need stamina to endure the hard moments. While it is not useful to try to run away from your sensations, it is also not helpful to hold onto them. Feel them and then release their energy: yield, melt, scream, cry, settle, open, let go.

Please acknowledge that being productive in labor can be hard to handle, oftentimes because the contractions are so strong. Your response to hard work may be to try and minimize what's happening, but you will need to get through your hard work for it to be done. Maybe it's time to dig deep into yourself to find the courage to ask your uterus to bring it on. Are you ready to do your work? If the answer is no, ask yourself honestly: "what do I need now to help me feel ready?" Give yourself a concrete, attainable answer, and then get to it! Ultimately, be compassionate with yourself because the work is coming whether you're ready or not. And you will work through it. Remember: you will not be pregnant forever. The baby is going to come out.

Seated with a supported forward bend

Sit on a chair while leaning your head and upper torso over something—e.g., a large ball on another chair in front of you, the back of another chair, or even just by resting your forearms on your own thighs. Try opening your legs out to the sides while you lean forward with your upper body. Get creative and allow your head and shoulders to yield.

I spent a good portion of Arlo's birth on the toilet. In this same bathroom, as is the norm at our house, there was a big basket of dirty clothes. Julian, my partner, dragged the basket of clothes over to the toilet where I was seated and then placed the birth ball on top. I was able to sit on the toilet and relax my upper body and arms over the ball, which was now nestled in the dirty clothes. That worked really well for me, and I was able to get quite a lot of work done in this position.

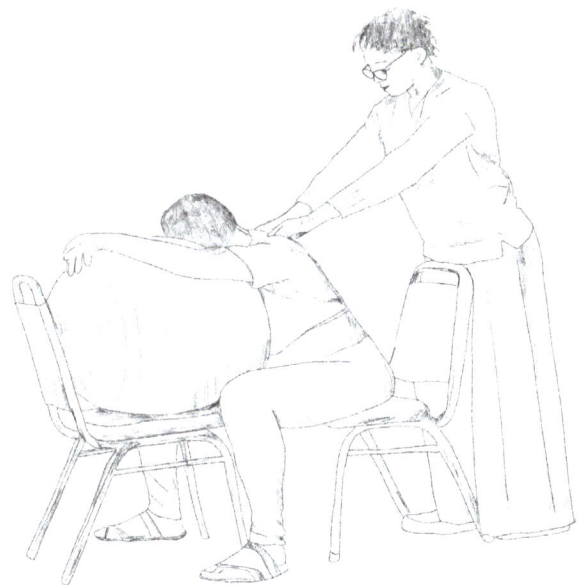

—Pause to practice the *Seated with a Supported Forward Bend* position—

The Toilet

As I alluded to above, I believe one of the best places to sit during labor is on the toilet. You have rehearsed and practiced and trained your whole life with this exercise! You are already good at the muscle memory of sitting down on a toilet, exhaling and opening up, releasing your various openings. When you sit on the toilet in labor you can use this training to your advantage. You can again open and let go, and if by chance you are leaking amniotic fluid, or you have some bloody show, or you need to pee or poop, you are already in a great place. So just exhale and let go.

Another benefit of sitting on the toilet in labor is that it creates an opportunity for privacy, especially if you are in a hospital room. A complaint I hear a lot from people who have hospital births is that they feel like they were constantly pestered by people walking in the room. Jen, a Bradley Method® graduate, related that "it felt like every few minutes someone wanted to take my temperature or blood pressure or ask me more questions or get me on the external fetal monitor." Consequently, many people have shared that they wished they'd had time alone or alone with their partners. Indeed, privacy helps get birth-work done. So go to the bathroom!

The bathroom can become a kind of temporary sanctuary. It's a funny thing about hospitals. The staff is typically ready to interrupt you like crazy while you are in the labor room, but step into the bathroom and, "Oh the bathroom, ok, you must need some privacy, we can wait… ." And just like that you buy yourself some time to tune in and focus on your process and grab a moment alone with your partner.

I encourage you to invite your partner into the bathroom and close the door. Partners, please don't be shy about going into the bathroom at the hospital with the birthing person. Once there, you can take your time. If the nurse calls in to you, one of you can call out, "Yup, we're fine."

Sitting on the toilet is often so effective for labor that, like sitting on a hard chair, it can be perceived by birthing people as too intense and therefore frightening. If it feels really intense for you, too, I encourage you to try to stay put through the contraction anyway. Calm your mind, you will be safe. You are experiencing a physical sensation. What exactly do you feel? Is something wrong or is this the feeling of the labor progressing? What does your intuition tell you? Your nerves are being stretched and pressed and molded. Allow yourself to feel this, keep breathing. It will be over soon, and you will be okay. *Release into the storm.*

—Pause to practice *The Toilet* position—

Straddling a Chair/Toilet

Another terrific variation of sitting is to try straddling an armless chair backwards. When you straddle a chair, you get a great amount of opening in the hips, plus you make your back and legs available for massage. As you lean forward over the back of the chair, your belly will naturally hang forward and down. You can place one or two or more pillows on top of the chair back so that you can drape over the pillow rather than the hard back of the chair. The more pillows you add, the more upright you will be. Your preference for your degree of uprightness will likely change throughout the labor. When straddling a chair, you will probably have to scoot all the way back, with your butt closest to the front edge of the chair, in order to have enough room for your belly to hang down.

A lot of hospitals do not have chairs without arms, at least not in their labor rooms, so you might have to look around once you get there. Better yet, try to locate one when you are on a tour, prior to the birth and ask hospital staff to put one in your room when you arrive. I had one couple who found a good chair in one of the waiting areas, so they dragged it down the hall to their labor room when the time came.

You can, of course, also straddle the toilet seat. Although if your house is anything like mine, you may want to do some advance cleaning to address the area behind the tank! Some people might enjoy having a blanket or pillow on top of the toilet tank to lean against, and others may like the coolness of leaning against the porcelain directly.

—Pause to experiment with *Straddling a Chair/Toilet* positions—

Sitting on a Birth-Ball

Another sitting alternative is to sit on a large birth-ball or yoga ball. Many hospitals have balls you can use, so be sure to inquire ahead of time if this is where you plan to labor. This will help you to get further down in space, lower to the ground. The softness of the ball can encourage you to release your pelvic floor, and it is a wonderful contrast to a hard chair. If you have access to both, switching back and forth might be very useful.

Sit on the ball with your legs open wide, with your feet and knees pointing out at 45° angles. You should feel stable while also achieving a large amount of opening in the hips. With your feet firmly planted, rock your pelvis front to back, side to side, and swivel your hips in full, gyrating circles. Try both directions for your hip circles.

Remember that the baby will fit through your pelvis, but you might have to jiggle her down and around a bit to help her find the right path. Hip circles will encourage your pelvic bones to shift and open. Let's face it, there is not a lot of extra room for this baby, so any movement you provide, such as swaying and making circles, getting up and down, or climbing steps, will encourage the bones to shift. This should help to facilitate the baby's journey.

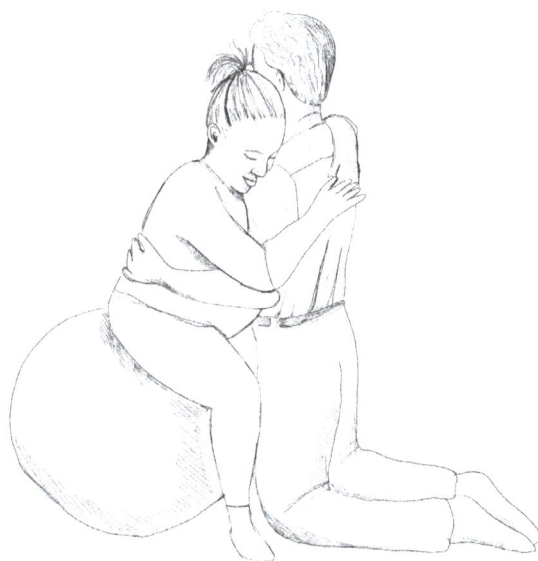

I personally love the Reverend Al Green's love songs and I think his tempos, rhythms and romantic subject matter are fabulous for the work of birth. Is there any music you might like to listen to while you practice your birth positions? Please consider that the energy that helped get the baby in there (or the energy that helped you decide to have the baby) is likely similar to the energy that will help you to get her out. You were probably physically loose and open when you got pregnant. Remember, when you're in labor, be loose and open to get your baby out. Even if you didn't have sex to get pregnant, you can still think about sex as a reference point. Sitting on the birth ball and letting your hips rock and swivel to some of your favorite music is one way to get there. Try tensing and releasing your vagina and pelvic floor muscles while sitting on the ball. Try to feel the increased blood flow that comes to the muscles each time you release them.

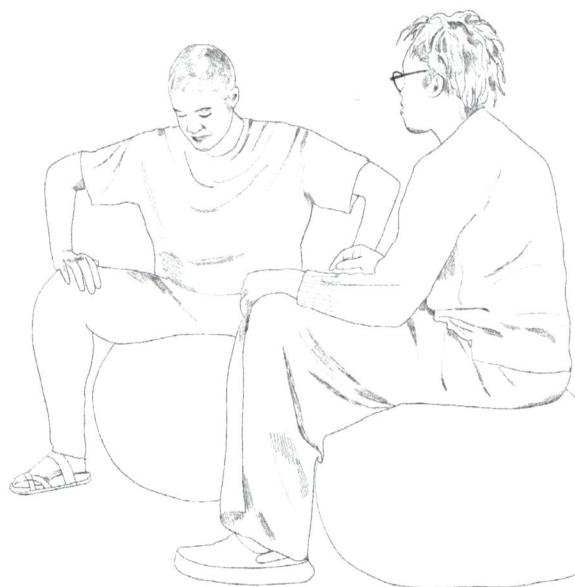

—Pause to practice *Sitting* variations—

Hands and Knees

The second-to-lowest level down in space is on your hands and knees. If you are prone to sore knees, use a pillow or gardening pad, or kneel on a bed or couch. As I have mentioned before, it's better to be proactive and try to keep your knees from getting sore, than to cope with such soreness after it occurs. So please use these props from the start of your practice.

Getting onto your hands and knees is excellent for any stage of labor. In this position, rock and roll your hips again and wag your tail. Can you make some more space for your baby? Will music help? Will kissing help? Will mindfulness help? How will you open so wide? Try being on your knees and draping over a birth ball, ottoman, big stack of pillows, a chair, or your partner. If you are going to a hospital, you can try raising the head of the hospital bed all the way up and then turning to face the head of the bed while draping your upper body over the raised portion.

While on your knees, please explore a variety of heights and angles for your upper body. It's quite reasonable to expect that as the birth progresses you will prefer your upper body to get lower and lower down to the earth.

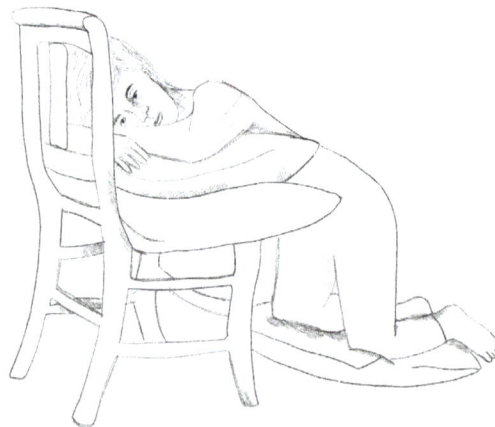

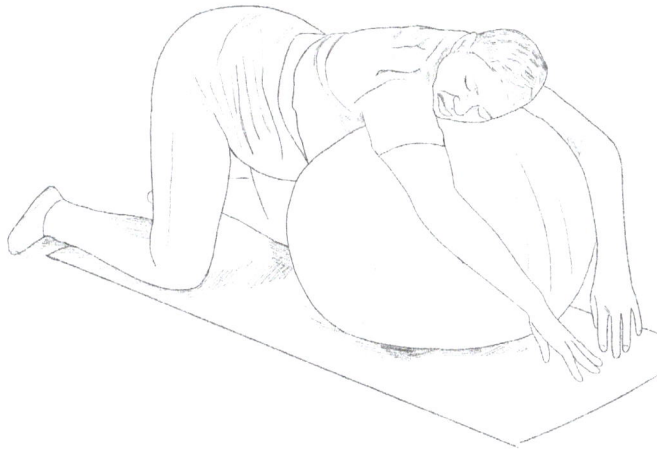

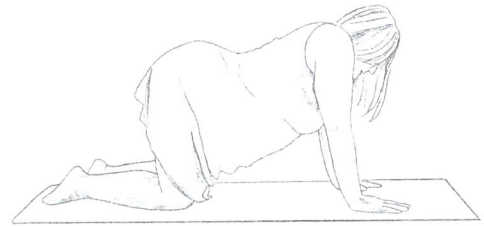

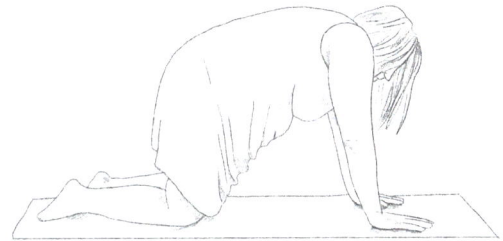

During the second stage in my home birth, I felt like there was an incredible gravitational force that was pulling me down to the ground. It really felt like this force was coming from the center of the earth to the center of my body, pulling me down and pulling the baby out. Although I have witnessed many people birth in many different positions, my experience was so strong, I always feel that muscle memory of being drawn down to the floor.

—Pause to practice a variety of *Hands and Knees* positions—

The Emergency Position

In the unlikely event that you find you have a prolapsed (falling out) umbilical cord or a hand or foot starting to emerge from your vagina: First grab the phone, call 911, and consider if you'll have to unlock or open a door. Immediately after that, get down onto your hands and knees. Lower your chest to the floor and support yourself on your chest or forearms. Hopefully, you are not alone and someone else can take care of the phone call and the door. Stack your palms on top of each other and rest your forehead on top of your hands. You'll want your torso as angled as possible, your chest as low as it goes, and your butt as high as it goes. This position uses gravity to slow the downward force on your body and baby. While you practice, see if you can feel how the baby's progress might be slowed in this position.

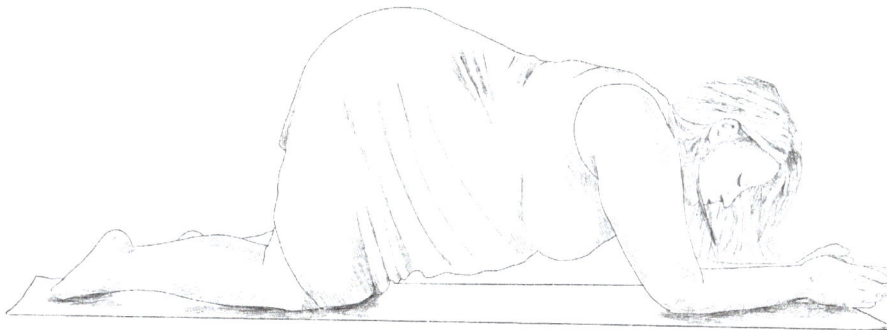

The above emergency circumstance is very rare. Please try not to fret over or dwell on these potential experiences. Rather, acknowledge that you have another tool available to you, should you need it. Try to place the information in your mind's filing system: out of sight and out of mind, but accessible in case of emergency.

When you are in good health and something unforeseen happens, you can count on your stress hormones to be there to support you when you need them. In an emergency your body will discharge chemicals that will give you increased strength, including the ability to do that which seems impossible.

Note: A baby's head coming out unexpectedly, if you are at term or close to it, does not usually constitute a medical emergency. It's just a surprise! In the event of such a surprise, catch the baby and keep yourselves warm, with skin-to-skin contact, until help arrives.

—Pause to practice *Emergency Position*—

Lying Down

This position represents you being at your lowest plane in space. The side relaxation position can be the foundation of this position and of a restful labor. This calm position allows a person to be the ultimate "multi-task master" by allowing them to simultaneously rest and work. The side relaxation position is a place where a person can most easily relax all the muscles that don't directly help to squeeze the baby out. (Review the side relaxation position in Week 2).

Partners: once you have helped the pregnant person get comfortable, lie down next to them and take a few moments to listen to each other's breathing. You may wish to set a timer so that you can really relax for the agreed upon amount of time.

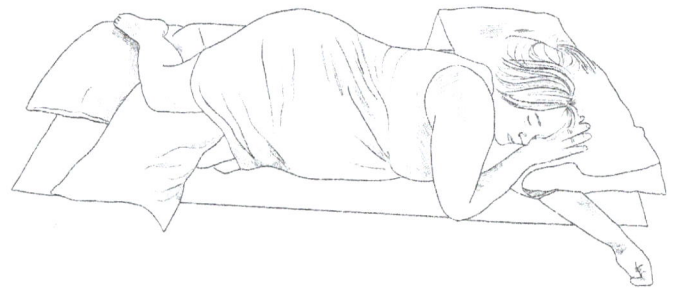

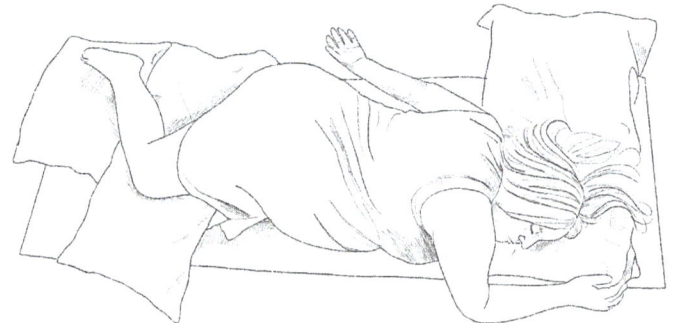

—Pause to practice the *Lying Down (side relaxation)* position—

That concludes my offering for first stage labor positions. I hope you have had fun trying them all on and that you are setting your intention to continue to practice them. Of course, coping with labor is not about isolated shapes or moments; it's helpful to connect the dots and allow the shapes and moments to flow. So onward we go...

Practice your labor dance

As a dancer learns dances, they study and practice sequences of movement. Connect your birth positions with fluidity and intention to make a birth dance. (But don't get stuck on any one choreography! Improvise and stay curious.) A birth dance can help your body open and give you the time to steady your mind.

By connecting different birth positions to each other, you can explore them in a variety of locations around your living space and make your labor experience your own. Reminder to the pregnant person: As you arrive in each position, focus on a long, slow exhalation. Hold onto positive and constructive thoughts. Think about relaxing the tongue in your mouth and relaxing your vagina and pelvic floor. Let your abdominal muscles go slack. Try to connect with your baby and, if you have one, your partner. Think about what you want *your* coping mechanisms during birth to include. Imagine. Use your creative powers in order to create the vision with which you can face your birth—with courage, pride, fierce stamina, and love.

Practice *all* of the above positions, even the ones that you don't necessarily like now. Try to refrain from making judgments about usefulness. Also be sure to acknowledge and discuss your favorites with your labor companion. Not every position will work in every part of every labor. This is why your birth dance should be as improvisational as the birth will be! It's impossible to know now what will really help until your time comes. Sometimes a position that doesn't make sense now is extremely helpful when you're actually in labor. Sometimes it's the reverse: something you like now doesn't work then. I expect that any position will only work intermittently during labor anyway; it's such a dynamic process, and you want to keep the baby moving. Because we can't know what will work ahead of time, it's important to practice everything you can now. If you write off a position or technique now, then you're likely to forget it during birth. You don't want to miss something that might have been helpful. Practice these positions now and increase your movement vocabulary. See what you can make up on your own. What other good positions for labor come to your mind?

Make your nests at home

Here is perhaps one of the most important homework assignments I have to offer you. *Make labor nests in your home*, like a cat that creates her own cozy birth space. Even if your plan is to transport to another birth location, you will undoubtedly have some time laboring while at home. If you have your labor nests worked out ahead of time, then you can revisit them in labor like an old friend and thus find some comfort to be able to leave for your birth location because you feel ready, not because you are unnerved and uncomfortable at home. Experiment as you explore the different environments around your living space. Where will you dance your birth? Are some spots conducive to certain positions? If you can labor in a bathroom, maybe you'll sit on a toilet, lean over a sink, or climb into a shower or tub? Try out several positions.

In keeping with the bathroom example: What's your bathroom like? Will you want to clean behind the toilet tank? Or do you want to make sure there is a pillow, blanket, or towel nearby to make you more comfortable? What colors will you see? What will you notice as you practice and prepare? For example, maybe as you drape over your partner's back, you will notice a crack in the baseboard paint that is in the shape of a lightning bolt. If you see that lightning bolt during labor, you may think "Oh yeah, I've been here, I know that." It's a crazy little thing, but somehow it reminds you that you did prepare, you did practice, you do have options, and you can cope; you are ready for this process. Think back to those affirming notes I mentioned, the ones that some women placed around their bathroom or other labor-nest spaces, in order to bring them comfort and remind them they are ready.

You'll absolutely want to feel comfortable having a contraction in your kitchen. What if you get hungry or want some tea? Whatever brings you into your kitchen, you'll be comforted to know ahead of time that you have a nest area or a position that works there, too. I encourage you to think about where else in your living space you can labor—maybe on a staircase, if you have one, or in another room or area that appeals to you, inside or outside. I also want to encourage you to find six or seven variations of positions in, on, and around your bed. Babies do like to arrive at night!

In preparation for her birth, one of my clients talked about her favorite chair by a big sunny window. She had imagined she would like to utilize this chair in labor, and then she did. She found several positions in, on, and around the chair that helped her to cope with her contractions. She especially loved the sun coming through the window, warming her while she sat. She laughed as she told me how she pushed and dragged this big heavy chair around the room, bit by bit as the day wore on, so that she might stay in the sunlight. She said that when they returned home from the hospital with the baby, it was funny and surreal to see her chair all the way across the room.

It is also important to note that returning home after a hospital birth can trigger many emotions and birth memories. While the above story recalls a humorous experience, I recently spoke to a woman in tears because she had planned a home birth but ended up needing transport to the hospital for a cesarean section. She and her baby both survived well, and she felt very good about the care she had received. But when she walked into her home after being discharged from the hospital, she was overwhelmed with emotion from her memories of labor. The fear, pain and frustration she had felt prior to her surgery all seemed to come crashing down on her as she walked through her front door. So she picked up the phone and called a trusted birth support person to touch base with (me). She had a good cry as she shared her experiences with me, and this act of sharing advanced her process of acceptance and healing.

Loss of control? Yes, please!

You can't control your birth so try to give up fighting that urge as soon as you can. The sooner you can make peace with the fact that the shit's about to get real, and this crazy-ass-large thing is happening, and a baby is going to come out of your vagina, the better it's likely to go. Releasing tension can actively help to reduce the intensity of your experience. That doesn't mean you won't feel giant, powerful sensations. You will definitely feel the biggest sensations of your life. This is going to be huge! But it all goes better when you can slow yourself down and try to yield into what you feel with courage. The sensations aren't going to kill you, you just need to feel them, ride them out, and give yourself up to the enormity of it all.

These sensations will pass. Use your mental powers to control your breathing and focus your thoughts. Let go wherever you can in your body and accept the tension you cannot release without judgement. When a birthing person can bravely follow and yield to their sensations, they often describe a feeling that they have somehow transported to another place in their perceptions. Many people call this new place "Labor Land." When someone is in "Labor Land" they can appear to be almost in a trance-like state. This is generally a very focused and productive time—the birth—when the birthing person is really allowing the work to unfold without the conflicts of trying to control what is ultimately beyond our mental control.

Most of us spend the majority of our days thinking and functioning on a very cerebral level: our universe exists from the neck up. Our brains are very busy. We live with a lot of mind chatter, and a kind of head superiority. Our thinking brain frequently overrides our physical consciousness. We often override physical signals, such as fatigue or thirst or lust, for example. In birth, by contrast, we want that thinking brain to settle down. We want the mind to yield to the body. Imagine that you can "think" from your belly, vagina, and butt. Let your primal-self take over.

Cast off your inhibitions and revel in your animal instincts. Let the farts fly! The more you can follow your animal instincts, the better you will understand and facilitate your process. Growl if you want to... it might actually help.

Congratulations on finishing Week 8's content. You are taking your pregnancy and education seriously. Thank you for your determination. You are having an empowered pregnancy, and that leads to a conscientious birth. You are doing it! You are becoming a more educated parent! Have a practice-filled and compassionate week!

HOMEWORK:

A) Review all labor positions

Make yourself a practice schedule, with your partner if you have one, and then practice. Remember to warm your body up first. Also take some time to acknowledge all the hard work you are doing now, in preparation for the hard work you will do when the baby comes.

B) Make your nests

When your practice schedule begins, use the nest areas that you designated around your home to work through each labor position outlined above. Likewise, identify several variations of all the positions you try and practice those.

C) Continue to develop your self-care routines

Make your best diet and exercise choices, and allow yourself the room to discuss your fears, hopes, and dreams. Practice relaxation techniques and focused breathing exercises—even just a couple of minutes a day can yield great results. Look for ways to express your creativity. Continue to interview your care providers, research in-person birth classes in your area, and have some fun!

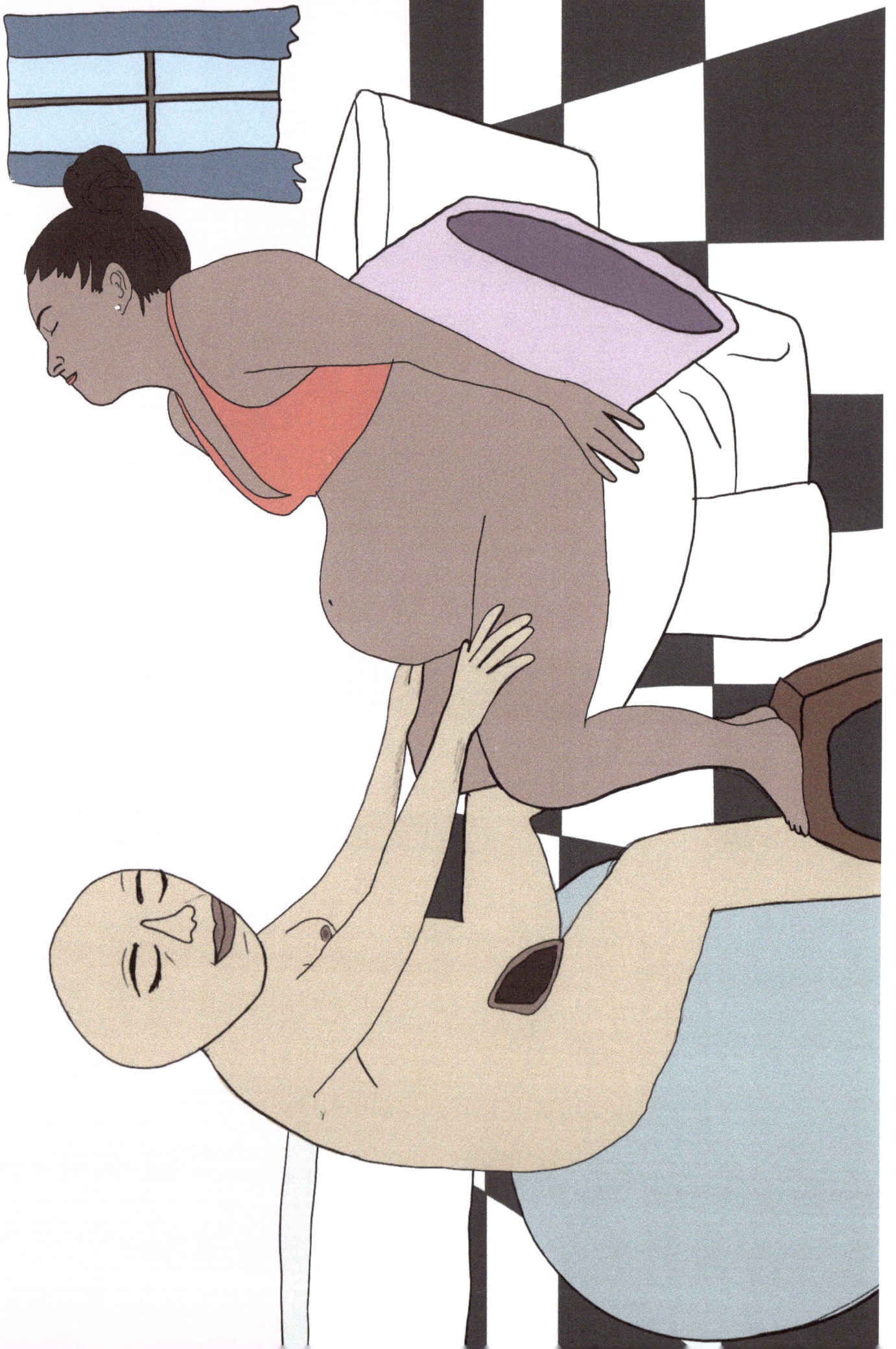

WEEK 9

Second & Third Stages of Birth

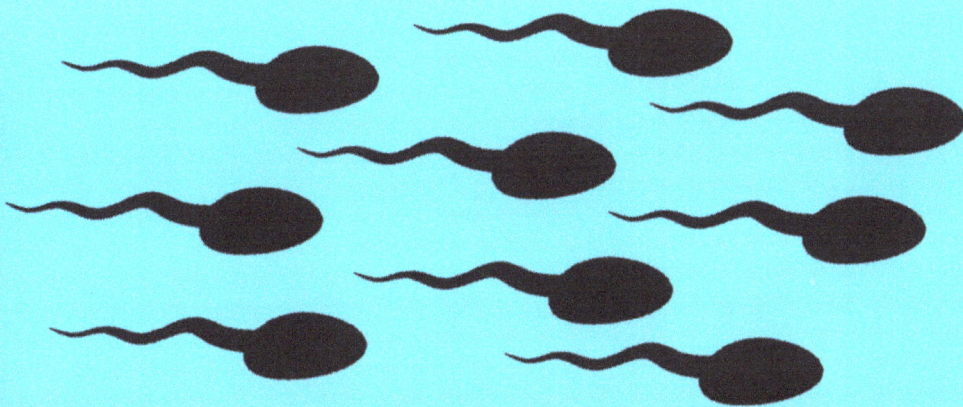

Chapter contents:

O *Second stage labor*

O *Second stage positions*

O *Third stage labor*

O *Third stage decisions*

THIS SPACE IS FOR YOUR NOTES AND DRAWINGS

Hello again. I hope you have been feeling productive in these passing weeks, and that you continue to make time for your medical consumerism homework. For example, have you researched any in-person birth classes yet? (Whenever possible, collect phone numbers and try to speak with a potential instructor to get a feel for the class.) Have you identified any labor nests or experimented with any first stage positions from last week? If not, what are you waiting for? Your baby is on the way! Regardless of homework assignments, I hope you are nurturing yourself with good food, positive social interactions, and adequate rest. How has your sleep been? If you can think of anything that might help you improve your sleep routines, I support you in trying to implement those practices. You want to continue your work toward managing stress.

Take a moment now to close your eyes, take a few deep breaths, and give yourself credit for a few of the things you were able to do this past week to care for yourself and your growing baby. Vocalize these things out loud. If you are unable to see some positive actions from the week, try to identify where your challenges are and then consider asking a friend to help you see your strengths. This week I will begin with describing how the baby actually gets out of your body.

—Pause for breaths and an accountability check in—

The baby's journey out

The baby spins her way down through the pregnant person's body, sliding two steps down, one step back. In medical language, this dance down and out through the vagina is called the Cardinal Movements. It is described through seven distinct fetal movements: engagement, descent, flexion, internal rotation, extension, external rotation or restitution, and expulsion.[157] First, baby's head goes into the pelvis, next the shoulders rotate, then her head turns, then her shoulders rotate again, she extends her head, twists again, and begins to emerge. Babies actively help, as much as they can. They reach out with their heads and they push their feet against the uterus as it bears down upon them. Sometimes babies' faces get a bruise or two as they navigate their bony head through your bony pelvis. That's okay, they can take it. Babies, like you, are pretty darn tough!

The Cardinal Movements, with their gentle back-tracking, allow for a gentler opening of the gestational parent's body together with giving the bones of the baby's skull time to mold. Head molding happens when the baby's not-yet-fused skull plates (bones) shift to help her fit through the bony pelvis.[158] A potentially startling effect of this head molding is when a baby is born with a pointy head. This can look weird, unsettling, and even scary, but rest assured this is not atypical. There are even some baby's heads that point off to one side, with asymmetrical head molding. This, too, is not atypical. If your baby is born with a pointy head, have no worries. It will ease back into place over the first few days of life, as the head molding continues to resolve. Marvel at your resilient baby! If you ever feel fearful and think you have to birth all alone, remember that your baby is actually helping—it's a duet! Your baby's job is to find their way out, and your job is to open wide!

But *how* does a vagina open so wide?

Increased blood flow to the genitals is how genitals get big. With arousal a penis grows erect. Vaginas get bigger for sex, too, and bigger still for birth. Starting early on in pregnancy gestational people experience increased blood flow to the genitals.[159] Then, when the uterus contracts during labor, blood flow to the tissue is first constricted and reduced, the muscle relaxes, and then blood flow returns.[160] With multiple contractions and releases, just like during sex, overall blood amount will increase to the area.[161] Passionate kissing, nipple stimulation, direct genital stimulation, and happy loving feelings are excellent ways to get big and open for birth; these actions all encourage blood flow to the genitals.[162] Likewise, for both birth and sex, negative thoughts or chronic tensions can impact how your body works, not only on a hormonal level, but also where and how your blood flows. This, in turn, can impact how open you can get. In order to relax enough to get our blood good and flowing into our genitals, most of us need to feel some privacy and to feel free from interruption and fear.

During birth, including second stage, the work is to follow your instincts and allow your body to do what it wants/needs to do. Having a plan helps to support this work and keep you focused. Consider, therefore, the sequence of a second stage plan going something like this:

1. Pick a position for your contraction. In this position, round your spine and wrap your upper torso over your baby. (Rounding your back increases intra-abdominal pressure.)

2. Breathe fully and try to let your breath soften and slow. Try making long slow "Sssssss" sounds as you exhale. Also, feel free to let out any sounds that come. Explore the power in your volume.

3. While contracting, use muscle strength as needed by pulling your belly in tight toward your spine (engage the transversus abdominus). The "Sssssss" breath helps with this muscle action.

4. In between contractions deeply relax abs, vagina, and butt.

5. Remind yourself that you will survive the sensations.

It's always a good strategy in birth (and in life) to try to slow down and elongate your exhales and to relax your body, especially through any chronic spots of holding tension.

Toss the word "push"

As I discussed in Week 3, to understand the physical action of second stage it is helpful to imagine getting the last bits out from a tube of toothpaste. You squeeze your way down toward the cap, so that by taking away the space inside, you force the contents down and out the only exit available. By engaging abdominal strength, primarily of the transversus abdominis muscle, you can support the work of the uterus contracting while keeping the vagina open. The word "push" is the common vernacular, but the action of birthing your baby is more like *squeezing in* your abdominals than it is like pushing something out.

To further help you anticipate some of the feelings—and better understand the mechanics—of your process, here is an exercise for this coming week. It returns you to the analogy between birthing and pooping!

This bathroom observation exercise will make it easier to understand the choices you might face during an expulsive contraction. *You can add force during a contraction by engaging the abdominal muscles or you can open by softening the abdominals, thus enabling the uterus to work on its own.* Of course, depending on the nature of your labor, each aspect of this process may feel completely involuntary. If that is the case, then just yield, soften, and surrender. In any case, you will be well served by focusing on slowing and deepening your breath, relaxing the pelvic floor, and visualizing your vagina melting open wide during each contraction. In between contractions rest and relax deeply, sip some water, and give yourself credit for being courageous enough to get through this. Again, you will be safe in your wild sensations.

A client testimonial: Dr. Wendy's story (Yes, even MDs take birth classes!)

By 12:10pm I knew that I was ready and wanted to start pushing. Actually, I didn't have much choice in the matter: the pressure was so intense that there wasn't any other option than to help squeeze the baby out. I "pushed" through 5 or 6 contractions and it was such an amazing experience to feel the baby's head crown and rotate. I looked down and saw my daughter entering the world... it was a girl. They placed her on my chest and she picked up her head and looked right at me.

Notes from Emily's vaginal birth:

My strongest body-memory of my own second stage labor is that I had to be on hands and knees in an all-fours position. It felt like I was being pulled down to the ground from the center of the earth.

I was overcome by my urges to expel. My providers had suggested—urged, really—that I try to slow things down, but I needed to yield to my sensations and shoot that baby out. I had no inclination or ability to slow down. I did experience a small tear requiring two sutures. The sutures never gave me a problem, and I healed up well without issue.

My own experience aside, I do encourage everyone (else!) to try to slow down and gently breathe through the actual crowning, sometimes referred to as a "ring of fire." You may or may not feel like you have any control at that juncture, so ultimately go with it and do whatever you need to. In the meantime, practice untucking your tailbone and hanging out in the squat position to increase the flexibility of your perineum, hips and legs. This preparation will aid you in second stage. If, like me, you cannot or choose not to slow the process down, advance squat conditioning will enable you to release your baby with the least amount of damage.

EXERCISE: TOOTHPASTE TUBE

Note: your support partner should read the following exercise aloud, as you try it. If you are solo, please read through it once in its entirety and then try it, and/or record it on your phone.

To get started, sit upright on a chair with your feet making full contact with the ground. If your full foot cannot reach comfortably down and flat against the floor, then please either sit on something lower or place something under your feet, like a foot stool or two relatively equal-sized stacks of books, blocks, or anything solid.

"Close your eyes. Keep them closed for the duration of the exercise. Exhale deeply. Begin to listen to and feel your breath. Encourage yourself to breath easily, invite your breath to slow."

—Reader pause—

"With your next inhale, visualize that you can relax deeply into your vagina."

—Reader pause for several breaths—

"Soften, release, and open up deep into your vagina as you inhale. As you exhale, invite the vaginal muscles to gently engage. Again inhale, open and soften your vagina, relaxing from top to bottom in succession. Exhale and gently contract. Inhale and release. Exhale and contract. Notice if you can feel blood flow increase as you soften and release deeply in your muscles. (Because we're humans, and not toothpaste tubes, we can use breath to open.)"

—Reader pause—

"Allow your attention to shift now and begin to visualize the bottom circumference of your ribcage. While keeping your eyes closed, feel the full 360 degrees of your ribcage. Reach your hands around your back and feel the back of your lower ribcage or that general area, if it's too hard to reach, or feel the bones. Starting there, trace your lower ribs, or approximate where they are located, with your fingers. Feel along your sides, all the way to your front center chest. Make contact with the full perimeter of your torso "tube" as best you can given your size and flexibility."

—Reader pause—

"Now relax your arms back down by your sides, with hands resting in your lap. Take a settling breath and try to sense the 360-degree tube-ness of your body. Can you feel reverberations from your hands outlining your shape? Connect to the feelings in your upper abdominal muscles. Visualize your abs as a corset of muscle surrounding your "tube." Breathe in,

opening the corset "laces," softening your abs as you melt open to receive the air. As you exhale, allow the muscles to gently return to an easy resting state of engagement from the upper abs down to your vagina, with a final bit of contraction pulling your clitoris down towards your tailbone, then release. As you breathe in again, soften, open, and release deeply to fill your entire abdominal and pelvic space. Let your shape respond to your breath."

—Reader pause for several breaths—

"Soften and open your body to fill with air. As you exhale, allow the air out from top to bottom. Follow the exhale with your attention: from the top of your "toothpaste tube," through your midsection, and down through the lowest abs at the top of the pelvis; squeeze in with the natural muscle action of the abs sinking towards the spine from all sides. Contract your transversus abdominis."

—Reader pause—

"Observe your pelvic floor muscles. Notice your tendencies. Can you feel the muscles ebb and flow with your breath? Imagine opening your vagina for birth. Breathe in and yield to open. As you exhale, imagine your abdominal muscles squeezing your baby out."

—Reader pause —

"Now, to end our exercise, as you exhale, focus your attention on being able to contract with strength in your vagina from the top of the vagina down to the bottom of your vagina."

—Reader pause —

"You'll open your eyes in a moment. But first, think about your upcoming week. Try to visualize that you can find some quiet moments to practice these breath and muscle observations.
Give your fingers and toes a little wiggle, stretch anyway you want to, then open your eyes."

Make time to practice this exercise from now until baby is born.

If you would like a bit more of a warm-up before we get into some second stage positions, please take a few moments now to move your body in any way that feels good and promotes circulation. Take a sip of water and use the bathroom, if there is need.

Second stage positions

In all second stage positions, during the contractions, the birthing person should round their spine and keep their chin down towards their chest. I did mention this earlier in this chapter but this information bears repeating. This will help to increase the intra-abdominal pressure and, in turn, help to move the baby down. Review the abdominal bracing exercises from Week 3, in order to coordinate breathing and engage the deepest abdominal muscles to squeeze the baby down and out. You also want to be sure that you retain your focus on keeping your vagina and pelvic floor muscles open. In all positions please also explore the differences you can feel in whether your hips are rotated in (knees point toward each other) or out (your knees point away from each other). There is anecdotal evidence that rotating the hips in, at their ball and socket joint, can help to open the pelvic outlet.[163] I encourage people to try the following positions with the hips turned in, out, and neutral (knees face straight ahead); see what you can feel in your pelvis and what makes the most sense for your body.

Squatting

Squatting is a spectacular way to move the baby down. When you squat, you open your pelvic outlet, utilize gravity, and remain in control of your own body weight with your feet firmly connected to the ground (or the bed). That sense of grounding helps many people through their second stage. Many hospitals have "squat bars," which are stabilizing bars that attach to the bed to allow a person to hang on while squatting on the bed. A person can also squat on the floor or in a tub of water. (To review the basics of how to squat, please revisit Week 3.)

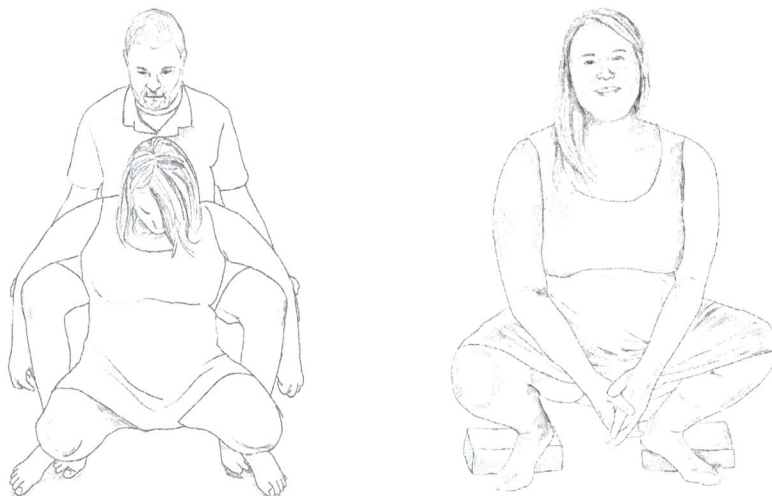

—Pause to practice—

Supported Squatting

There are many ways to support a squatting person. One can hold them under the arm pits from behind or kneel next to them and hold them under one shoulder. Alternatively, two people can kneel on either side of the squatting person, each supporting a shoulder. In my experience, the most useful way to support a person in a squatting position is while seated in a chair (or seated on the side of a break-away hospital bed, with the lowest section lowered all the way). A partner can sit on a chair with their own butt securely, but just barely, on the chair, with their knees well out and away from the chair. Then, the pregnant person, who is facing the same direction as the seated partner, can squat in the space between the partner's knees and drape their arms over their partner's thighs. This usually provides a great deal of comfort and support to the birthing person and should be simple and stress-free for the partner. Please give this a try now.

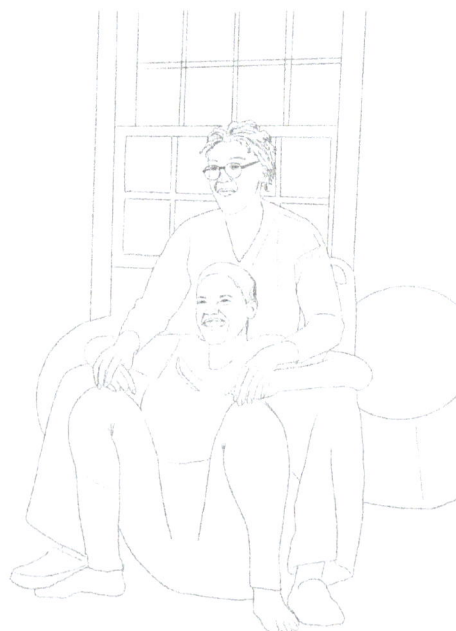

—Pause to practice—

Asymmetric Standing or Kneeling

Stand on one foot with the other foot up on a stool, chair, or ottoman. The raised knee and foot should be in alignment and over at a 45-degree angle. Likewise, when kneeling on the floor, the raised knee in alignment with the foot should be positioned open to the side. These positions can give you the ability to catch your own baby, as it empowers you to help wiggle them down and out. Standing or being on one knee can sometimes feel a bit wobbly, in which case you may appreciate having a partner nearby for physical support, especially in any standing variations.

—Pause to practice—

Kneeling Drape

The kneeling drape works well in a hospital bed. Raise the back of the hospital bed upright and get on your knees, facing the back of the bed. Then you can drape your head and arms over the raised back of the bed. At home, this position could be used by kneeling on the floor while draping over a chair, couch, birth-ball, or bed. Sometimes the usefulness of this position comes from the fact that the torso can remain fairly upright with no pressure on the sacrum and minimal pressure on the legs. Other times the benefit is that the arms and upper body can relax deeply. Also, as the urges dictate, the torso can become more horizontal by draping over a lower object.

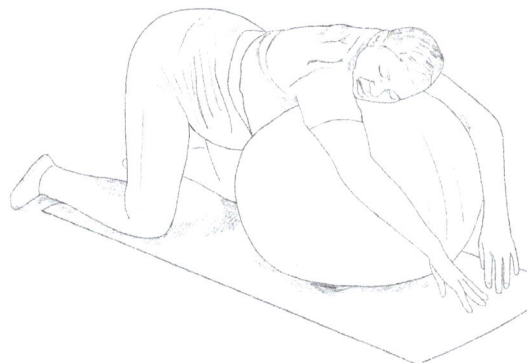

—Pause to practice—

Hands and Knees

Hands and knees (or, the all-fours position) is an extremely versatile and useful position to consider for second stage. You can do it on the bed or on the floor. It's very stable, with no pressure on the sacrum, and you can easily wiggle your pelvis as needed. If your knees are prone to getting sore while in this position on the floor, then please start off with a pillow or gardening mat under your knees to help prevent soreness. Wrist circles during your breaks can also help to ease any tension that may accumulate there while weight bearing.

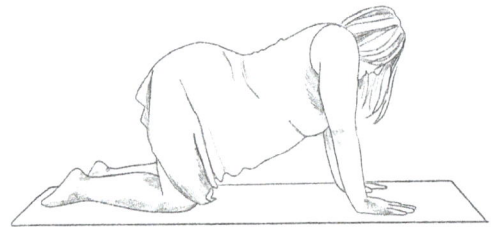

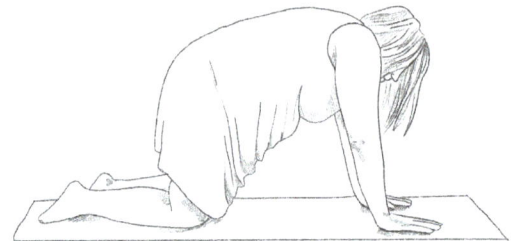

—Pause to practice—

Standing with Support

Standing with two feet on the floor, with a slight bend in the knees, while facing and leaning against a wall, or in the shower, can work well. Be mindful of the fact that in order to remain upright, this position does take some effort. A partner can help to steady you.

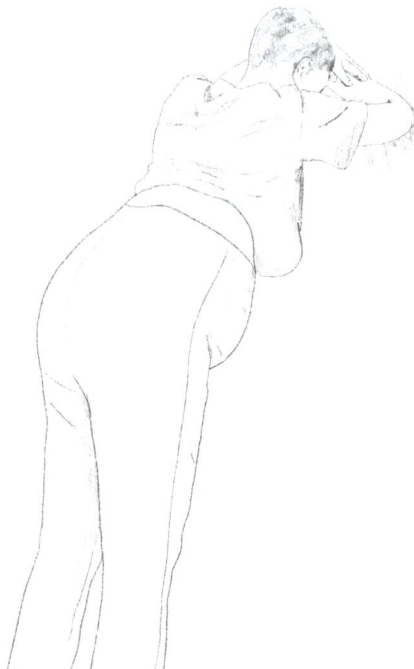

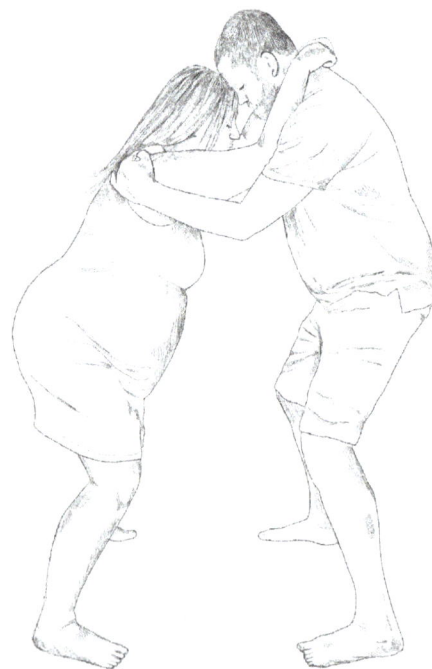

—Pause to practice—

Side-lying

Lying in bed on your side, with your top leg held up, can be a very effective position, especially for a person that is feeling exhausted. If you are at a hospital you can use the adjustable tray table with a pillow on it to support the raised leg. If your partner is supporting your raised leg, it is best if they are behind you, so that they are not leaning too far over while trying to hold the weight of your leg. Likewise, you can hold your own leg up with your top arm. Some people describe this as empowering and others say it's too much work. Try it out and see what you think.

—Pause to practice—

Side-lying with a peanut-shaped exercise ball

Peanut balls are relatively new on the birth scene. They are like smaller yoga balls that are cinched in the middle. They look like giant peanuts, hence the name. A birthing person can put one between their legs, comfortably resting the entire lower leg. In some cases, the use of a peanut ball while on an epidural can decrease the length of second stage labor and reduce the need for a cesarean section.[164] But a peanut ball is a wonderful option for any birthing person, epidural or not. The peanut helps to keep the pelvis open and the leg and hip well supported while side lying. If you or your hospital or your midwife have a peanut ball, I definitely encourage you to consider its use.

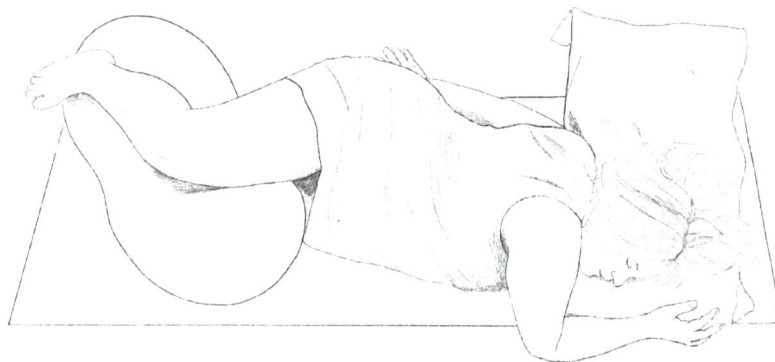

—Pause to practice (a stack of pillows is a good substitution for a peanut ball)—

Please continue over the next days and weeks to try all of these second stage positions described above and explore which ones seem to make sense to your body. One of my personal birth heroes, the late author Sheila Kitzinger, suggested getting a grapefruit to hold between your legs as you experiment with different second stage positions. It is comparable in size to a baby's head; plus, once you have figured out what position(s) make sense to you, you're left with a tasty and nutritious snack in the house!

When considering which birth positions might work for you, also think through the details of the baby's journey. And consider, for example, what you know about removing a tampon; it works well to put your foot up on a stool or the side of the tub, and to slightly bend your legs. Imagine opening to retrieve a tampon... or a baby! Maybe your midwife or birth location has a birthing stool. This is a small, kidney-shaped stool that you can use to approximate a squatting position. These variations can also be useful positions for getting baby out.

With all of this, the standard of care in hospital births remains for a person to be on their back or in a semi-reclining, sitting-on-the-sacrum position on the bed. Rebecca Dekker at Evidence Based Birth found that "most people who give birth vaginally in U.S. hospitals report that they push and give birth lying on their backs (68%) or in a semi-sitting/lying position with the head of the bed raised up (23%)."[165] These numbers add up to 91% of people in hospitals giving birth with their weight on their sacrum, effectively making their pelvic outlet smaller. This, in turn, forces the baby to go up and over the coccyx. But yes, babies can and do come out this way. In my educated speculation, the statistics cited above are as big as they are because people feel disempowered in their process and are undereducated as to the pros and cons of different positions. They don't speak up... don't know that they can... or don't know the options if they did. Now you know. So plan well and speak up!

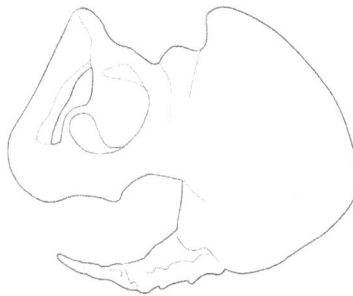

Pelvis in reclining position

Midwives usually have the skills and training to safely care for a pregnant person through their entire birth process, regardless of the positions they may move through as they labor and birth. Vaginal exams, fetal heart rate monitoring, maternal blood pressure monitoring, and catching babies can all be done from just about any position a person can get themself into, assuming the provider has been well-trained in midwifery skills. Doctors don't usually have this training. As a result, most obstetricians try to insist that you "deliver" on the bed, on your back or semi-reclining. Doctors don't generally care about where you labor during first stage, in part because they are not usually there with you. However, once you start your expulsive phase, they expect you on the bed and on your sacrum. It is generally the nurse's job to get you into position before the doctor arrives. That is where these such providers are trained to "deliver." Moreover, it's more comfortable for them because they can sit on a stool at the foot of the bed, which adds the additional benefit of proper positioning should they need to perform medical/surgical procedures, like an episiotomy.

During first stage labor picking your best labor positions is an entirely improvisational dance. During second stage, however, changing position becomes more challenging, so developing a plan now (like a more set choreography) can really support your having a more empowered journey. If your second stage is progressing well, aside from resting between contractions, there may be no need or desire to shift positions. But if a labor does not seem to be progressing well, a change in position should be first on the list of considerations. Many birthing humans do benefit from positional shifts in between contractions, for rest and/or to aid the baby—i.e., to jiggle her through the birth canal. *If second stage progress is unusually slow or stalls, it is important to change positions more assertively*. The baby might be poorly aligned and need help adjusting. It is important, therefore, for the birthing person to have knowledgeable physical support during this phase. Of course, a person can give birth by themself, but knowledgeable support makes it easier, safer, and generally more comforting.

Providers usually expect to do a vaginal exam when you start your expulsive, second stage. If you consent, you'll get on the bed (if you're not already there) and recline with your knees splayed open. This can be a tough, maybe even too hard a position to get out of on your own during birth. But tough or too hard doesn't have to mean impossible. You will be able to move yourself, and you can definitely speak up and ask for help too! (You do have the legal right to change your position.) Your plan—a good plan—may include that, after a vaginal exam, you will roll to one side and push yourself up with your arms to get into whatever position you want. Part of your goal now, therefore, is to form plans that will make your life easier during labor.

To be proactive and protective during birth pick a second stage position now, tell your support people what the position is, and ask them to plan to help you get into it at the start of your second stage (immediately following a vaginal exam should you consent to one). Picking the position now that you think will make the most sense to *you* while laboring through second stage can help you to organize/generate/release your maximum power when it's needed. First, "try on" several different second stage positions. Then be bold and pick the one in which you will begin your second stage. Commit to it. Tell you partner, tell your doula, tell your provider. It should be an easy commitment, because you can also change your mind in the moment of your birth!

If you do your homework now, then your birth partner, armed with this information, can ask (for example), "We discussed you pushing on all fours. Can I help you get up into that position now?" It will be easier to say, "No," than to ask for what one needs without any prompting. If you don't want to move from your back that is fine, of course. Just say no. You will still benefit from the homework, since now the subject is open for discussion. Someone else brought your attention to your positioning and invited you to participate in what happens next. This makes it much easier to follow your instincts and find the next position that works best. Having a plan for your team ensures (or at least maximizes) that your plan gets a fair chance. Note to the support partner: this post-vaginal exam check-in is best done as an active offer of assistance. An "active offer" is made by standing up and being physically ready to assist. It can be disempowering to feel like you can't move easily. Support people can help ease any shame or embarrassment when they actively, and kindly, offer their physical support.

Second stage rhythm

Contractions towards the end of first stage are usually fast and furious, leaving little time to catch your breath or regroup emotionally in between. For some people this fast, breathless pace continues all the way through the second stage. More frequently, however, contractions are spaced farther apart during second stage. Yet while the pace may slow, the effort, pressure, and intensity of sensation increase.

If you get extra time between contractions, again: use it to rest. Find a comfortable-ish position (nothing may be that comfortable), close your eyes, invite stillness, and breathe with concentration while you try to remind yourself that you will be okay. You will survive. Trust that if you just try (and try again) to relax your body, it will all work out. The time between contractions may grow to five or more minutes apart. This time creates opportunity to build strength through rest. You may be able to lie down or even sleep after each contraction. Even if you don't think that's possible, try it. You'll get more rest than if you don't try. And, if you want to stand or squat for second stage, remember that this doesn't mean you have to continuously stand or squat the whole time. You can assume a position for the duration of one contraction at a time. Don't forget to tell your support people ahead of time that they are to assist you changing positions during second stage should you want or need to move.

Medical consumerism tips

If you do not yet know your current provider's training and practices regarding second stage positioning, please investigate these now. Remember to ask your questions in an open-ended manner without leading your preferred answers. Be sure to clarify that you are asking about your position options for second stage, including the actual moments of birth. If you only ask, for example, if you can "labor in any position," then the answer will usually be "yes." Instead, you'll want to specify that you are asking about second stage and including "delivery."

Unless you are under the influence of narcotics or alcohol, or medically diagnosed with a psychological disorder or other legally defined incapacitated state, no one can make you stay in bed.[166] You are the boss of your body! But, if your current provider holds firm that you "must" birth while in bed on your sacrum, then you may want to discuss your constitutional rights and/or try to interview other birth practitioners. At the very least, it will help you to know what you are up against in advance of labor so that you are not caught by surprise when the time comes.

Make plans. Make plans. Make plans. You can let go of these plans, should you choose or need to do so. Trust yourself to think in the moment, on the fly, especially after doing all the good work of learning about your options. I trust in you! I always recommend that you emotionally prepare for the fact that in labor we can only loosely attach to plans. If your provider asks you to semi-recline for your contractions to progress the birth, you can certainly ask why they want you to do that and then say no or yes, as you see fit. It is fine to give any position a whirl. Babies do obviously come out from people in the supine position. Ultimately, just be sure someone is tasked with *creating a chance for change*. Again, if second stage seems to be progressing very slowly or seems stalled or there are any less-than-assuring fetal heart tones observed, shifting positions should be your first line of defense.

"Coached pushing" and why you'll want to say, "No, thank you"

In a hospital, nurses and doctors typically instruct a birthing parent to hold their breath and bear down as hard as they can for as long as they can through each contraction. A nurse directs her patient in a loud and authoritative voice. The nurse may count to 10 or longer to keep the person holding their breath and pushing longer and harder. It's difficult to hear your own body's sensations when someone is telling you what to do. Imagine you are in the bathroom voiding your bowels and I walk in and start firmly directing, "Puuuuuush! 1! 2! 3! 4! 5! 6!" I don't know about you, but if this happened to me, I might not be able to void my bowels all day and maybe not all week! Or, I might develop hemorrhoids from trying to force my body to expel. Directing a person to push interferes with one's ability to follow one's own sensations, and this can be harmful. When you direct "pushing," you increase chances of damage to the pelvic floor.[167]

In hospital, beware the cheering crowds

Let's think about labor from the hospital staff's perspective: first stage labor can be boring, as there's not so much to see. But when second stage arrives... Wow! A baby is going to come out! A whole new patient arrives for more staff to keep track of (and bill). The labor room typically gets more populated, with a definite increase in hustle and bustle. (This is not usually an issue during homebirth where the number of people attending is predetermined.) Depending on hospital protocol and circumstances throughout the labor, a pediatric nurse or a doctor shows up, and/or a new resident, or anyone else in training who happens to be on the floor. People want to see the amazing sight of a person releasing their baby, plus there are evaluations to be made, procedures to be considered, and information to be documented. As if the crowd alone weren't distracting enough, add to this the coaching technique I just mentioned and it's easy to imagine this phase turning into a sporting event complete with audience participation: "Push! Push! Push!"

For comparison, consider this: Most of us don't have locks or use locks on the interior doors of our home—with one important exception: the bathroom door. When it comes to opening our sphincters, we tend to work better with privacy. Again, our sphincters are shy. Voiding our bowels or our babies works best when we trust our environment to be calm and free from interruption.

Once again, you can protect yourself from the circus of folks chanting "Push!" with advance dialogue and planning. Of course, you can't control everything, especially what people around you might say. Thus, should you have a nurse or resident start encouraging you to hold your breath while they count, a partner can always whisper a counter-response: "Thank you, we have learned about that technique and maybe we'll try it later, but first my partner would like some quiet so that they may concentrate on their own sensations. We do appreciate your help and we'll try that way later if we need something different." It might take courage for the partner to interrupt the uniformed birth attendant, but be brave. Question hospital norms with kindness and respect. Critical thinking is important. If your questioning brings resistance, stand firm on the U.S. Constitution and ask if they have any kind of Patient's Bill of Rights (it varies by state) or a patient advocate you can speak with.

There could be poop!

If there is fecal material in your rectum when your baby passes by then, yes, the baby will squeeze the poop out of you with the pressure from her head. (Remember the image of the baby's head rolling down that tube of toothpaste?)

Maria, a former client, asks, "Is there any way to avoid having a bowel movement during the birth?" Some people naturally void quite completely at the onset of labor (remember that a lot of loose stool can be a sign of labor arriving).[168] Thirty and more years ago it was standard routine to give people an enema upon arrival at the hospital when in labor. This practice has been discontinued because the gestational parent's poop doesn't cause a threat to the baby. Additionally, most birthing parents and most nurses would prefer not to have a nurse administer an enema. Legend has it that Dr. Bradley only recommended an enema if a person was so concerned about pooping on the bed that they feared they wouldn't be able to fully release into their sensations. He understood it's not useful to hold back from any birthing sensations.

The truth of the matter is: you might poop just before the arrival of your baby. If that is too uncomfortable to think about, focus on the fact that loss of modesty is a sign of transition in labor. No matter how awkward it is now to think about pooping in front of your partner, nurse, midwife, doctor, and whomever else may be in the room, when the time comes you are not likely to care because there is a baby about to come out of your vagina! At the moment of birth, you are really *really* only going to care about getting the baby out—one singular, compelling thought. Plus, there is a good chance you won't even notice that you're pooping. So ask yourself, why dwell on it now?

All that being said, if you still anticipate being self-conscious enough that you'll attempt to hold your baby in so you don't poop during birth, then you might well want to discuss the use of an enema with your provider ahead of time. It might be just the added support you need to allow yourself to really let go.

Oh my gosh! You did it! The baby is out! My oh my what a monumental moment that will be. Later in this book I discuss what it might be like to meet your baby face to face, but let's not get ahead of ourselves. First we must finish the birth.

The third stage of labor

After what is sure to have felt like a billion hours of hard work, the baby is out. (Phew!) This is when the uterine muscle fibers step into the spotlight and show off their super-powers. When ordinary muscles contract, they get shorter; when they relax, they get longer. By contrast, when the uterine muscle fibers contract, if they can get shorter, they will. The amazing part is that, once shortened, they will *stay shortened in their relaxed state.* From there they will contract again and get smaller still, relax there, contract again, and get smaller still—all the way until the uterus returns to a pre-pregnant size. This can take about six weeks. This special uterine super-power is called "Retraction."

Retraction has three important jobs: 1) to expel the placenta; 2) to control the gestational person's bleeding; and 3) to return the uterus to its smaller size. During pregnancy a uterus cannot get any smaller because the baby, placenta, and amniotic fluid take up so much room. After the baby comes out, however, the uterine job of retraction becomes the birthing person's highest priority. With the baby out of the way, the next order of business is to expel the placenta. When the uterus can get smaller, it will, and this action begins to reduce the surface area where the placenta has been attached. Without enough surface area, the placenta begins to separate from the uterine wall. Once fully separated, the placenta easily slips down and out.

"When does the placenta get out and does that hurt?" I was taught the placenta should come out sometime between 5 and 45 minutes after the baby.[169] And, no, generally it does not hurt to birth the placenta.

From early in pregnancy the placenta modifies the gestational person's vascular system, enlarging blood vessels and diverting blood to feed the placenta and baby.[170] I once heard a doctor explain that, by term (meaning, when the baby is ready to be born), the blood vessels that feed the placenta are as large as fingers. That is huge for a blood vessel, and hence makes the time after the placenta comes out the most dangerous part of the process for a gestational parent. Nature has safely accounted for this threat by running the birthing parent's blood vessels through the uterine wall, functionally allowing retraction to clamp down the gestational parent's blood vessels, which in turn controls their bleeding.

> The uterine blood vessels that supply the placental site traverse a weave of myometrial [uterine muscle] fibers. As these fibers contract following delivery, myometrial retraction occurs. Retraction is the unique characteristic of the uterine muscle to maintain its shortened length following each successive contraction. The blood vessels are compressed and kinked by this crisscross latticework, and normally blood flow is quickly occluded [stopped]."[171]

This action of retraction is critical until internal clots can form and the birthing parent heals up. This is why the greatest risk for postpartum hemorrhage (PPH) occurs within the first 24 hours. However, the risk of PPH related to the placental site continues for up to 12 weeks.[172] In short, healing takes time, with the uterus continuing to play an important role. After the placenta is birthed there is always going to be some blood loss. But a well-nourished parent has likely already increased their blood volume 50% by term, making an average amount of blood loss a low risk (assuming the uterus is contracting well).[173]

If a gestational parent has not been well nourished, or their uterus is not contracting well, what should be a calm and happy period of time can become a medical horror story. The majority of postpartum hemorrhages result from what doctors call uterine "atony," which means the uterus has a lack of tone and is not contracting.[174] Why wouldn't a uterus contract? In order for the uterus to contract successfully, it needs an adequate supply of oxytocin as well as adequate uterine receptors open to receiving the oxytocin.[175] A lack in either of these elements could impede retraction and increase the risk of PPH. In third stage labor, ample amounts of naturally produced oxytocin helps to prevent hemorrhaging from the large blood vessels that had been feeding the placenta. On the flip side, if artificial oxytocin is administered in a continuous drip dose (for an induction or for third stage care), then this can flood the uterine receptors and render them unavailable.[176] Using Pitocin to induce or augment labor, for example, carries a significant increase in risk for PPH.[177]

Oxytocin works in concert with prolactin (another naturally produced hormone) to protect against hemorrhage, support emotional bonding, and benefit breastfeeding. Following a healthy, non-medicated birth, the birthing parent is typically elated that the birth is over and the baby is finally here. These happy feelings, in a calm environment, with parent and baby together, cared for as one, promotes optimum physiological functioning. It's calming for birthing parent and baby to be together. When they are together, the baby's nuzzling at the breast stimulates the release of plenty of natural oxytocin and prolactin.[178] If stress becomes an added factor directly after the birth, it can impede these hormonal releases, which in turn can further disrupt the uterus from contracting as it should.[179] During third stage labor a trained birth attendant should be watching the gestational parent closely, with periodic manual checks to feel for uterine tone and visual checks to gauge quantity of blood loss. Of course, this is all ideally done while not disturbing the parent and infant bonding or adding undue stress.

Third stage decisions

Now that you understand some basics about third stage labor, I want you to think about your own conditioned thinking about what happens after the baby is born. In other words, when you were growing up, what did you think happened after the baby came out? I grew up, for example, learning that the doctor takes the baby out of the parent's body, hangs the baby upside down, smacks it on the bottom to illicit a good cry, and hands the baby off to a nurse who will then weigh and wash the baby, and possibly hand the baby off again for a pediatric assessment and administration of vaccines—all before the baby is swaddled and finally returned to the mother. Thankfully, some of this may seem unknown or archaic to you dear readers, as you are likely a lot younger than me! But all of these historical practices post-birth create stress for the gestational parent and rob them of the natural hormonal support associated with a baby at their breast.

Please take a moment now to write down what you expect to happen to your baby immediately following the birth. And, if you don't know what your provider's routines are for the immediate postpartum, please ask them. Comparing their responses to what you've written below can help you in your planning and decision making.

What I will now have describe is the physiological care management of third stage. The gestational person and baby are kept together, with baby skin to skin on their chest, and the umbilical cord and placenta left alone. The placenta comes when it does, and once it does, an attendant periodically checks the gestational person's uterine tone and assesses blood loss quantity and their demeanor (how the gestational parent appears to be feeling). Physiological management is to respect and support the natural process. However, in the early 2000s medical research found that physiological management produces more blood loss and takes more time for the placenta to come out. As a result of those findings protocols began to change and now most in-hospital providers practice what is termed "active management."

Active management in third stage labor means that as soon as the baby is out traction is applied to the umbilical cord and the gestational parent is given the medication Pitocin (artificial oxytocin). "To prevent postpartum hemorrhage, medical evidence suggests that all women should have uterine stimulating drugs, umbilical cord traction, and early clamping of the cord."[180] This research was hard for me to accept: how could ALL birthing people need artificial hormones? This was also challenging for me to understand because for decades I had it drummed into my education that it was very dangerous to pull on the cord. As it turns out, this information is correct: cord pulling, if done incorrectly, can indeed cause the uterus to collapse in on itself ("inversion"), which can lead to excessive blood loss, hysterectomy, or even death.[181] I believe it is because of these associated risks that the homebirth midwives in my area still do not practice active management. Nevertheless, applying traction to the umbilical cord is a medically approved method for third stage labor.

Another concern about the routine use of Pitocin was raised by a labor and delivery nurse I know. She wondered if, as more staff become reliant on Pitocin to control bleeding, then physical observations from nursing staff could grow lax, which could in turn put some people in danger.

While the bulk of recent medical research gives active care management more weight than physiological care management, a 2019 review of available research also reveals that there may not be enough quality research on this, and that, subsequently, low-risk gestational people should be given access to information on both.[182] Given this, I want to look just a bit closer at this topic as you work toward making your own decisions. Please examine the wording in the following excerpt carefully: "The frequency of PPH [Postpartum Hemorrhage] is related to the management of third stage of labor. This is the period from the completed delivery of the baby until the completed delivery of the placenta." [183] The first sentence here presents an interesting statement because it implies, rightfully, that the occurrence of PPH depends, at least in part, on the provider (your maternity care "manager"). This is true, especially when your doctor doesn't spend time to talk with you about nutrition early on in the pregnancy and/or you suffer from malnourishment due to poverty, lack of education, or by adhering to self-imposed diet restrictions. Your care provider may have no idea of your nutritional status beyond the factor of weight gain. (Note that you can gain weight from poor sources of nutrition, too.) Think of how many of us, pregnant or not, aren't sure what to believe when it comes to how much of this or that to eat. As of 2011 in the U.S., for example, anemia in pregnancy was recorded for nearly 17% of pregnant women.[184] Statistically, that number represents a lot of women suffering from at least some form of malnutrition. If you are anemic, then typically you have not been able to build an optimal blood supply.[185] Now add stress as a compounding factor to this scenario. If babies are routinely separated from their gestational parent immediately following birth, we are causing negative stress with our medical practices. This stress decreases a gestational parent's chances of optimal functioning as I mentioned above. Not only that, but birthing people are stressed in labor from many things, including sometimes being cared for by hospital staff who are themselves stressed or just emotionally unavailable to lend support to a new and nervous parent.

These third stage decisions (and more) should be discussed with your provider and placed into the contexts of what your diet has been like (whether or not you are anemic) and what your plans are for the immediate postpartum period—with regard to parent-infant separation. For decades the routine here has been to separate the parent-baby couple for newborn evaluation and to administer a variety of newborn "routine treatments." (Some of these may currently be state mandated, such as Vitamin K injections and erythromycin ointment being required in NY State at the time of this writing.[186]) Thankfully, the importance of keeping parent and baby together and the benefits of skin-to-skin contact are starting to be better understood:

> Mother-infant SSC [skin-to-skin contact] is physiologically, psychologically, and clinically beneficial for mother and her baby. During SSC, contact, heat, and olfactory receptors which have strong vagus nerve stimulants can lead to the release of maternal oxytocin. Oxytocin is one of the most important uterotonic factors and plays an important role in uterus contraction, acceleration of the third stage of labor and controlling postpartum hemorrhage.[187]

Gestational parent and baby belong together and should be cared for as a unit. Removing a baby from her parent is sure to cause stress for each of them. Interruption of bonding and breastfeeding exploration makes it harder for the gestational person to have healthy uterine contractions, which in turn can impact their ability to control bleeding and initiate breastfeeding.

Another way that leaving parent and baby skin to skin helps is from the physical uterine stimulation. In other words, "when the baby is placed in skin contact with mother, the movements of the baby's feet on the mother's abdomen acts like uterine massage which can stimulate the uterine contractions and accelerates separation and exit of placenta and ultimately reduces postpartum hemorrhage."[188] Therefore, I again encourage you to discuss the immediate postpartum moments and consider requesting any initial assessment of baby's vitals be done while baby is getting as much skin-to-skin contact as possible on the gestational parent's body, and with minimal interruption.

Most healthy people experience strong enough contractions to control their bleeding even if the baby isn't nursing, as long as baby is skin to skin on their chest. When postpartum contractions do need a bit more oomph, offering the baby your breast is the most natural way to stimulate hormonal release. Nipple stimulation that mimics breastfeeding, such as pulling and rolling and squeezing the nipples, can help too. Nurses will perform what's called uterine "massage" to help stimulate contractions and control bleeding.[189] (I placed "massage" in quotes because most people find it rather uncomfortable.)

During my second pregnancy I was receiving dual care from an obstetrician and a homebirth midwife. I had some routine blood work done at the start of my third trimester (28 weeks). Both providers required the blood work to see my iron levels, even though I had been taking a prenatal vitamin with an iron supplement. (Please keep in mind: too much iron can also be a bad thing.) My doctor reviewed my test results and said everything looked fine. However, when my midwife reviewed the results, she was quite concerned that my iron was too low. She strongly urged more diet charting and she recommended that I switch to an iron supplement that would be more absorbable. I believe the obstetrician was completely unconcerned because he had a solution in mind; he figured he'd give me a blood transfusion if there were a problem. My midwife, by contrast, wanted me to get proactive to improve my overall health in order to reduce the chances of trouble developing in the first place. My midwife was adamant that I take the time early on to understand risks, and to take action to optimize my health and thus prevent whatever risk I could. I followed her advice. I started taking a new prenatal vitamin without iron, and started taking the plant-based iron supplement my midwife recommended. I continued to focus my diet choices on getting the nutrients I needed. I grew a healthy baby and had minimal postpartum bleeding and

I felt very well throughout. I wasn't retested, however, so perhaps it was just coincidence. But I was confident in my choice. You need to make your own choices!

To help reduce instances of PPH, it is my opinion that our healthcare system should be educating people on nutrition and treating even marginal anemia early on through education, diet counseling, and supplementation, where necessary. In addition, this same healthcare system should address and try to reduce birthing people's stress while working to avoid induction drugs for labor. I believe everyone needs and deserves a supported, well-monitored third stage, one that emphasizes the creation of a calm environment with undisturbed skin-to-skin time for gestational parent and baby. This is the gold standard of the midwifery model of care (although not every midwife practices this way). Just knowing this information can help you to improve your outcomes, regardless of your provider and environment.

I know that PPH is scary to think about, but if you are taking good care of your health now and making plans to have an undisturbed postpartum period, you can decrease your worry. For further reading, I highly recommend anything written by Dr. Sarah J. Buckley.[190] She writes well on the hormones of labor and on how to support naturally all parts of birth, including third stage.

If you do have anemia, or are borderline low, you should make eating iron-rich foods a very high priority all the way through your pregnancy and beyond. Cook in cast iron pans. Eat vitamin C-rich foods along with your dark greens for better iron absorption.[191] Disguise them if you have to! If you hate dark greens, then get super creative with spices or try hiding them in soups, mashed potatoes, wrapped in dough, or mixed into fruit smoothies. When you responsibly utilize prenatal care and have a birth attendant at your birth and try your best to eat well and get rest, in tandem with education, *and* you have undisturbed contact with your newborn, you give yourself the best chance of safely sailing through third stage labor.

If you do not have access to knowledgeable providers who treat you with respect, which is, sadly, the case for many people, then it is more imperative that you do your homework now.[192] I believe that with education all birthing people can learn to support their own optimal outcome. Remember: birth is a healthy human function. No one needs to make perfect choices at every meal or have their dream provider. With education you can advocate for the best care practices. Again: just trying to do what you know—and learn—to be good is usually plenty good enough. So take a few breaths... express any concerns and make a plan to pick up this book for your next week's lesson.

Congratulations on another chapter read. Give yourself credit for all the hard work this represents and try to appreciate how awesome you are. I am wishing you a wonderful week. Practice mindfulness and please continue to actively approach your relaxation training.

HOMEWORK:

A) Bathroom observation exercise

Mindfully observe how you void: what sensations do you get, how do you respond to them, and does your breathing change?

B) Pick a position for second stage

Try out several second stage positions. Experiment with both contracting and deeply relaxing your deepest abdominals, vagina, and butt. Try positions with hips rotated in and out. Focus on breathing all the while. Be curious about how the pelvic floor and diaphragm work together. After exploration, choose a second stage position that feels like it makes the most sense to you. It might be a clear and simple decision for you or it might feel like a guess. It is a guess regardless, but still make that guess. Once you have made a decision, talk to your partner and provider about it. Enlist their help to assure that you won't remain on your back out of neglect or coercion. And rest assured that if, at the time of your actual birth, the position you picked now seems like a really bad idea, you will simply say, "Nope," and then get into the position that is more appropriate.

C) Ask your provider about second stage positions. Here are some questions to consider:

- ○ "In your opinion, is there a best position to give birth in? And if so, why?"
- ○ "What is the most common birth position for clients (or patients) that you attend?"
- ○ "Are there any positions that you consider unacceptable for your clients to adopt during the second stage of birth?" "
- ○ "Do you ask your clients to stay on the bed?"
- ○ "Have you ever caught a baby from a client who wasn't on a bed?"
- ○ "What are the most unique positions you've seen gestational people adopt for their delivery?"

D) Ask your provider about third stage protocols. Following are some sample questions:

- ○ "Please explain your routines for managing third stage labor. What is typically done and what routinely gets monitored?"
- ○ "Do you think there is anything I can do now to help prevent postpartum hemorrhage?"
- ○ "Please describe immediate newborn care practices to me."
- ○ "What are the pros and cons of giving a woman Pitocin after her baby comes out?"

Remember to keep your questions open-ended and your attitude positive. Be eager to learn about your process and your provider's expectations and practices. Once you leave the appointment you can decide how you feel about the answers, and what to do if there are any points of conflict between your provider's practices and what makes sense to you.

THIS SPACE IS FOR YOUR NOTES AND DRAWINGS

THIS SPACE IS FOR YOUR NOTES AND DRAWINGS

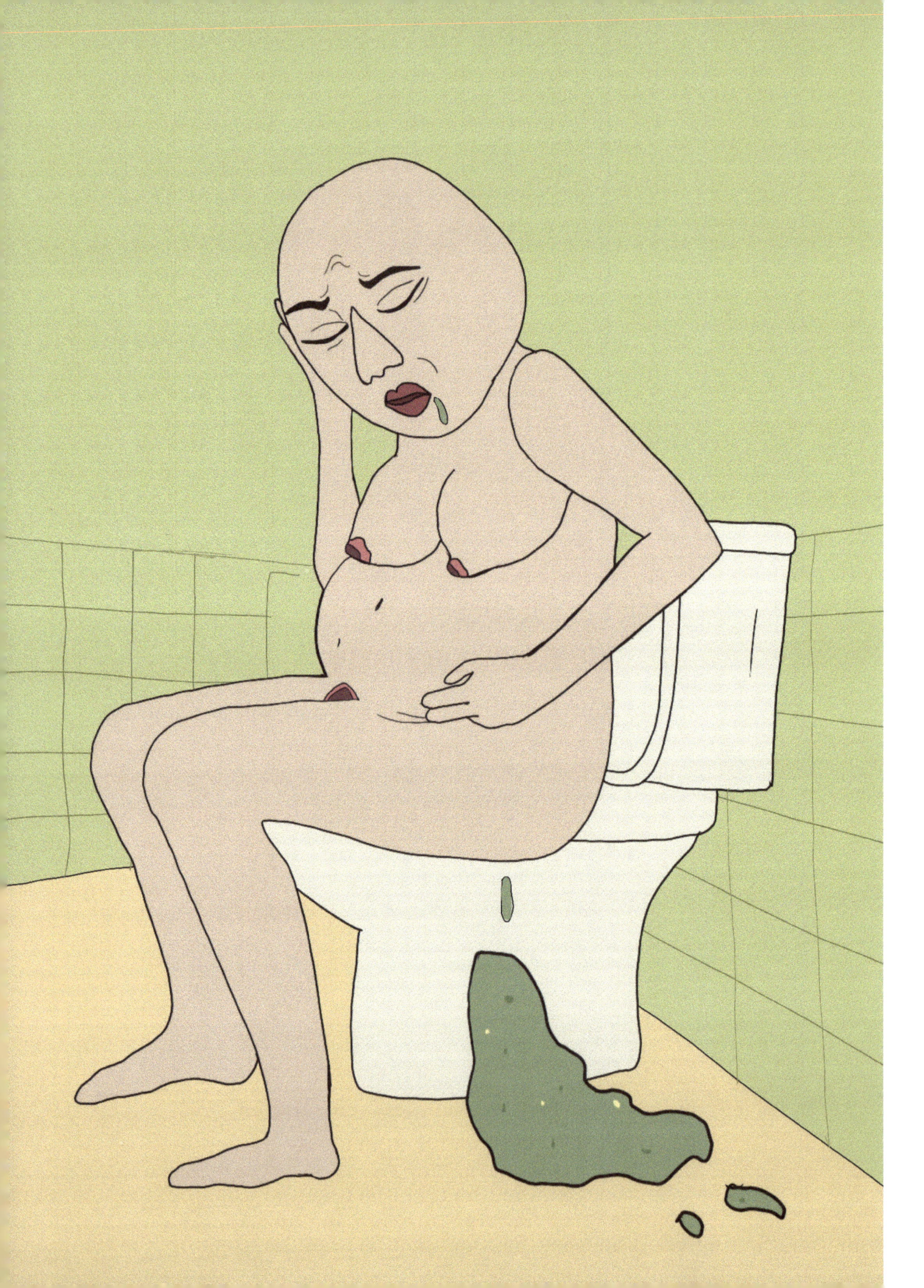

WEEK 10

Expressions of Birth

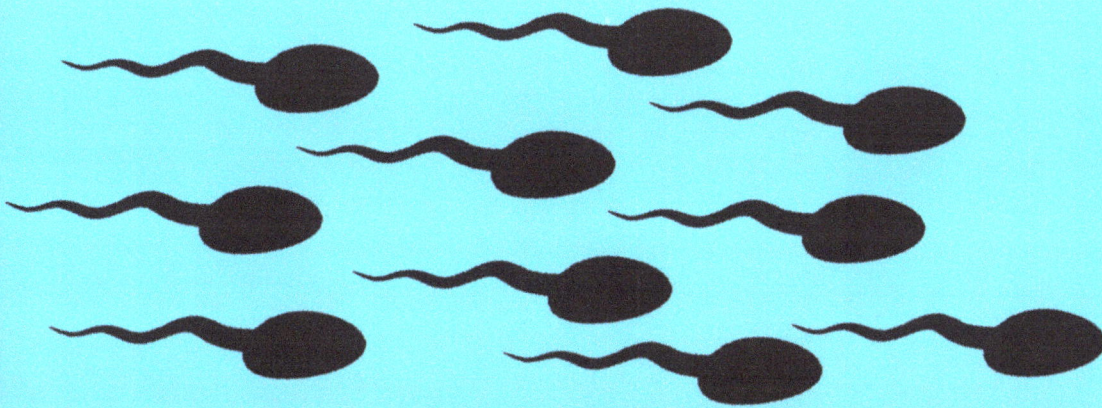

Chapter contents:

- ○ *Emotional and physical experiences during labor*
- ○ *Labor interruptions*
- ○ *The vaginal exam*

THIS SPACE IS FOR YOUR NOTES AND DRAWINGS

Welcome back! How is everything going? How are you doing? I hope this week finds you building courage and confidence with each passing lesson. How are you managing stress and your needs for self-care? What about second stage positions: have you investigated those and identified your preferred position in which to begin second stage?

Remember: doing this now, investigating and identifying your preferred position for second stage and then communicating that position to your birth team, will help you to attain an empowered birth, one that utilizes the positions that make the most sense to you.

Stop now to reflect, tune into your baby, and honor however it is you are feeling in this moment.

—Pause—

During this week's offering I explore some aspects of the whole birth process, from the perspective of what it might feel like or how the different stages may be expressed. But first let's get even a little more grounded in our breath and our experiences of self-care.

Self-care accountability

I want to check in on your diet and exercise. To do so, I have included some example conversations from my classes throughout what follows. While it is always important to make time to reflect on your choices, it is also important to acknowledge the feelings that may inform these choices. With this in mind, I have peppered the discussion below with some sample responses to the general question of, "how did you do this past week?"

> **Marta:** "I am doing pretty well with food, though the heart burn is getting to me. And exercise, that's not going so well. I should be doing more."
>
> **Emily (instructor):** "What do you think your exercise obstacles are?"
>
> **Marta:** "Working. I am just so tired."
>
> *After saying this, Marta launched into a tirade of what she should be doing. She was clearly feeling inadequate and overwhelmed.*

If you are tired, you may need more rest. Or, you may need more exercise. Exercise can give us energy, even if it feels exhausting just thinking about it![193] Try to closely evaluate your circumstances and look for opportunities to make positive changes—even a small shift can make a big impact. Sometimes feeling burdened by all the "should's" in life makes it more difficult for us to act. If you are burdened or overwhelmed with a long list of things you *should* be doing but aren't getting done, try boldly taking some things off your list. Assess what you *have* been getting done and give yourself some love for your worthy accomplishments. Give yourself permission to *not do* something extraneous on the list, even if this is just a temporary fix. You won't be pregnant forever. In time, when you are healed from the birth and acclimated to parenthood, you will eventually be able to take on all the responsibility that comes screaming at you in the years ahead! Right now, however, you need to reduce your expectations of what you can push yourself through and recognize the strength in what you *are* accomplishing.

Allow yourself to be humbled by the magnitude of the experience of building a baby. It bears repeating, again and again: you won't be pregnant forever. If you can make your to-do list smaller, the tasks that remain may be less overwhelming and your time spent pregnant may well be more enjoyable. If you haven't been getting a lot of exercise done, try thinking of exercise instead as a smaller task. Try to encourage yourself to do a few small stretches, or a couple of short bursts of physical activity—even short intervals can support your healthy goals.[194] When "exercising" feels too huge, look for short opportunities to be active instead. Can you dance to two songs? Maybe three? Can you do that once or twice a day? Or maybe you would prefer to walk in-place while watching a favorite show, or take a walk around the block. The minutes add up. Several short sessions of moving your body can positively impact your feelings, especially if you include a few moments of conscientious breathing. One of the great things about moving our bodies is that movement usually inspires more movement. The more you do, the more you feel like doing! Little changes are often more effective than trying to reinvent yourself with great big ones, especially during pregnancy.

Importantly, if you are feeling run down, then please re-evaluate your sleep habits and diet, in addition to your workload. You may want to revisit diet charting and track your food intake for the week. Determine if you are still reaching or getting near to your target goals, especially for protein, dark greens, and water. Also, see if you can go to sleep one hour earlier each night, that can often help you to feel a bit rejuvenated.

> **Lisa:** "I am feeling better and eating better. I have been doing the pelvic rocks and pelvic floor exercises... The pelvic rocks really help with the pain I get in my hips. But I am not getting much cardiovascular work done."

In our culture people are often (usually!) forced into pitting self-care against economic survival. Priorities have to be made, even if these priorities are competing at the same level: it's a question of individual health vs. finances for food and rent, for example. We have to work hard in our professional lives at the same time that we must take care of our own health (and maybe the health of other family/friends) plus the pregnancy. In the end, addressing health problems that have set in can be far more expensive (in time, money and energy) than working proactively to prevent them. Your baby is depending on you. You are going to need strength and stamina to birth and for parenthood. If you go into birth run down and exhausted, you will have much greater challenges, with increased need for intervention. Being rested and strong will help you to handle the challenges that are coming. I am not wanting to add undue pressure here. Work or health, it's an unjust choice. So we do what we can, when we can, and how we can. The lessons in this book are meant to bolster your ability to do this! Plus, as parent to a new life, you are adding more hope to the future. Maybe your baby will grow up to be a powerful change-maker, making these kinds of unjust circumstances a thing of the past.

> **Jean:** "I'm really eating more protein and feeling better. I have much more energy than I had a few weeks ago. I think having more eggs in the morning and just in general paying more attention to my protein has been good. I am getting to exercise. I was good at it before the pregnancy and I enjoy it, but I do sometimes get frustrated that I can't do what I used to."

Everything is changing. Listening to your body's signals is so important. Accepting all the change and learning to yield is challenging, but it does facilitate growth.

> **Evelyn:** "I am doing okay. Some days are definitely better than others. I've really switched to grazing. If I eat a big meal, then I'm more likely to get heartburn. So I find that I am nibbling throughout the day and evening. It's kind of a challenge to keep track of everything that way, but I seem to feel better. I feel like I am eating constantly."

Remember: as your baby grows, so does the pressure on your stomach. This is again why many people find that eating small bits of food throughout the day and night is more comfortable as their pregnant bellies get bigger. Nevertheless, this may feel weird, like you are indeed "eating constantly." Pregnancy is hard work. When it comes to any food and exercise obstacles, please be compassionate with yourself. Each new day brings a chance to make a new good choice. How are you feeling about the diet and exercise choices you've made this past week? And what are some goals for the coming week?

The experience of birth

We are all unique individuals. How we express the feelings we feel, the magnitude of our feelings, and the amount of time that we feel them is as unique as we are. Despite these individual differences, there appears to be a common emotional progression in labor. As the Bradley Method® teaches, the emotional developments of birth are as follows:

At the beginning of birth:

O   Excitement: joy and/or uncertainty

For the bulk of first stage:

O   Acceptance/serious concentration/capable

At the end of first stage:

O   Self-doubt/disorientation/a moment of pause or complete road block at the juncture of letting go

Second stage:
- ○ Determination/sometimes frustration
- ○ Re-focused concentration
- ○ Renewed energy

Third stage:
- ○ Relief that the birth is over and curiosity about the baby

When I first started my training in the Bradley Method® I learned the above progression as the "Emotional Sign-Posts of Labor." I must admit, at first I didn't quite believe the premise of the curriculum. It seemed unlikely that there would be clearly expressed emotions correlating with each stage of labor. I had heard of such different birth experiences, ranging from the sublime to the nightmarish, with births lasting from minutes to many days. How could there be a common progression of emotions?

Through additional sources, I went on to learn about the work of Dr. Kubler-Ross, which showed that when people are dying or grieving they also move through a fairly dependable order of emotions.[195] This isn't true for every person, of course, but the majority of us do experience at least some of the five phases of grief in the order that Kubler-Ross outlined: "Denial," "Anger," "Bargaining," "Depression," "Acceptance." Learning these ideas about grief helped me to remain open to the possibility that in birth people might also sequence through a fairly dependable series of emotions. Birth and death are similarly sized major life transitions. What, then, can we learn about where a person is in their birth process if we listen to their feelings and observe their behaviors? As it turns out: a lot!

(Early and mid) first stage emotions

At the onset of labor, you are likely to feel revved up. "Is this REALLY it?" "What was *that sensation*?" For some it may feel like freak-out stress more than excited-happy energy, but both are energized states. You and your partner will do well to try to calm and conserve this energy. Aim to feel the surge pass through you; allow it to pass by and try not to burn it up in action. You need to reserve some of that buzz for the work to come. This early expression of excitement will last a few minutes or a few hours, or it will be intermittent over several days, maybe even weeks. Each pregnant person will express and react to their excitement—or heightened state of arousal—in their own way.

Once the reality sinks in that labor has really begun, excitement begins to fade and you'll head into a state of acceptance. No longer wide-eyed and wondering, you are now busy working—you are *doing* the work. For most of first stage, pregnant people tend to maintain this acceptance with a serious sense of resolution. When given a little bit of cheerful, kind and confident support, you will feel capable of coping with your contractions. You may or may not feel happy about the work, but you'll be getting through it either way. Think about how you are currently anticipating your birth. Are you happy about it or dreading it? Or somewhere in between? There is no right or wrong answer. This is not a time for judgement. It's an opportunity for reflection and to put words, images, melodies or movements to your thoughts and emotions.

—Pause here and discuss in whatever form you are moved to do so—

During most of first stage labor, in between contractions, the answer to the question, "How are you *right now?*" will likely be that you are okay and able to continue. This place of acceptance, of just *doing*, is likely to be where you will spend the most time in your labor. "Acceptance" is the longest emotional phase of labor for most birthing people. You'll eat, drink, rest, poop, pee, change positions, and rest some more. You will focus on your breath. You will try moving and swaying, rocking and rolling, kissing and singing, showers and tubs, walking and resting—all to help yourself open and encourage that baby to come down.

Slowly, or not so slowly, the work will start to escalate. In birth, it generally takes more time for the first five centimeters of the cervix to open than it does for the last five. This can make for a steep ascent to the top of your proverbial mountain at the end of first stage. This is not an absolute rule, just a common phenomenon.

Physical expressions of first stage

As I have mentioned in Week 5, a contraction often feels like a tightening or squeezing through the entire uterine/abdominal area. But the exact sensations are hard to predict, you may or may not feel sensation in the low back, the vagina, the anus, the hips, and even the thighs. Generally, a contraction follows a wave-like pattern: it starts slowly and builds until it reaches its apex, then it begins to wane. Of course, sometimes contractions can feel like they go from zero to 100 in an instant. The wave can vary from a gentle ripple to a full-fledged tsunami.

Some people describe contractions as stretching or pulling sensations, rather than squeezing or tightening. Contractions can start anywhere on the continuum, from mild to profoundly powerful, requiring maximum concentration. Contractions can begin with a regular or irregular pattern of duration and frequency. Most people do eventually get into a pretty regular pattern of contractions, but some never quite organize the way we expect, and these people still manage to get their work done.

Most people start labor with contractions that are mild, short and farther apart. As the birth progresses, the contractions get stronger, longer and closer together. By the same token, many healthy births also include starts and stops that require a variety of effort all the way through.

Remember that in early labor many people exhibit a physical restlessness that corresponds with increased emotional excitement. If you, the birth partner, come home and find that your pregnant partner has gotten more housework done in the last couple of hours than they have in the last few weeks, you should take notice! For example, if they have just washed all the baby clothes, rearranged some of the baby's furniture, and are now energetically scrubbing something, beware of the change in their activity level. It's often a sign of labor arriving or advancing. By contrast, labor might bring with it a noticeable decrease in activity/productivity. It's the *changes* in behavior that are the biggest clues.

Full, slow, and steady breathing and a focus on softening the body helps to support the work of birth. Remember: a person in labor may or may not want to be touched or spoken to during a contraction. They may need to sway their body, rock their hips, and/or hang their upper body. Having their eyes closed frequently supports their efforts to tune into their process and concentrate on being present and calm. But calm may be impossible especially at the end of first stage.

Transition (late first stage) emotions

For many people, this steep part of the climb towards full dilation creates a fairly reliable emotional stress point—transition. Although, as I have mentioned (see Week 5 for review), this is not identified as an actual medical phase of labor, transition is a well-known term that refers to a time during birth when certain qualities emerge that fairly consistently correlate to the last few centimeters of dilation. In other words, there are both emotional and physical characteristics common to the transition between first and second stage.

In transition a person has to release their deepest inhibitions to let go. Similarly, during sex, one must let go of inhibitions to have an orgasm. In short, we have to release control and let our babies out. For most of us in labor, there are moments of balking at this release. We question our abilities. We worry about what will come once we open. But eventually, most of us in sex and in birth, get to a place where we are so fully consumed with our process that we experience a total loss of modesty and we can completely yield to our instincts and feelings. This happens best when we feel safe, private, and free from interruption.

People who have survived sexual abuse or other forms of violence are uniquely vulnerable to having extra tough challenges at this juncture in the birth. Feelings of fear or anger, even flashbacks, can all intrude. If you are a survivor, finding supportive places to talk about the upcoming birth process and your past should be helpful. When you explore concerns at hand, you are well on your way to steering through potential emotional roadblocks.

After years of uncomfortably teaching people that transition was full of such negatives as those outlined earlier (self-doubt, distress, fear, anger, disorientation), I began to ask myself questions: If birth is a part of our sexual function, then can I learn something about birth by thinking about sex? You bet! During transition, the contractions come one on top of another and there is less of a break between them. During sex, the contractions also build until they are coming one on top of another. And, wait a minute. That's not usually a bad thing. It's good! Very, very good! Usually we don't want our contractions to slow or stop during sex. During sex, faster is (eventually!) *much* better. The same goes for labor. Contractions tend to get faster and that is good. And yes, it is also certainly challenging to cope with.

During transition, a birthing person might be so internally focused, in their own "labor land," that they may feel a bit disoriented. They may wonder, "When did the sun come up?" Or, "What day is this?" This happens during consensual sex, too! Have you ever thought or heard the expression, "I fucked my brains out?" Maybe you've "come to" after sex and been surprised to find yourself all turned around on the bed, or even across the room? (Where is my shirt? My pants? Tee hee.) This disorientation isn't necessarily bad. On the contrary, it's the result of a very engaged process. Likewise, for many people during consensual sex, a moment of pause may be reached, a juncture at which the choice needs to be made to try to delay or stop what is happening or to open and release into the powers of sensation. This is all true in birth as well.

Remember from past lessons in this book: the words we use color and define our expectations and in turn influence what's possible. The emotional signs of transition do often include a sense of trepidation about what comes next. Phrases such as "Make it stop!" or "I am too scared!" or "I can't do this anymore, I need drugs" often get thrown around. Instead of deploying this language of self-doubt, there is an alternative way to acknowledge that labor will include a reliable stress point at the precipice of letting go and rely on language full of acceptance, promise, and strength. For example, "I am safe in these big feelings" or "I can yield and let go, staying focused on my breathing" can still help. "My body evolved for this process" or "I will survive! I can do it! I can do it! I can do it!" are also great thoughts and mantras. Many of us hit a place in the free fall of birth where we wonder if we'll make it to the other side. Being able to acknowledge the positive power within yourself will help to get you through.

For some pregnant people, knowing in advance what other people have gone through in these emotional terms can help. It may allow them to recognize and work with their own feelings if/when they develop. I am not suggesting here that you go looking for negative feelings. Please do not expect to doubt yourself. It is entirely possible that you will find ecstasy in your sensations and yield with ease into your process as it unfolds. But, if you do start to doubt yourself, then remember that you're in equally good company. Centuries of birthing people before you have faced this challenge and come through to the other side. Together with the support of all of humanity you will survive the toughest moments and triumphantly transport your baby earth-side. The cheerleader inside yourself can say, "Yes this work is hard, but I have come this far! I am getting my work done! There *is* a light at the end of the tunnel!" And if that sounds like a bunch of cheery bullshit, remember: people endure far worse experiences and under more severe circumstances—and they survive. You can too. You are having a baby. And while, yes, this is hard, it is also wonderful and amazing. When in doubt, let go, give in and let it happen.

Physical expressions of transition

In transition the contractions tend to get very close together. The strength of the contractions starts to peak, making this activity quite intense. The work may also affect the digestive tract. Nausea and vomiting are common physical symptoms of transition. However, some people vomit during early first stage and then continue frequently throughout first stage and into or through transition. For them, vomiting is not a sign of transition; instead, it's clearly a tough labor, and one in which they need to work hard at staying hydrated. For feelings and physical developments to help us read—or map—a labor, we need to see development. In other words, for vomiting to be a sign of transition it first needs to arrive after hours of first stage work.

Shaking and trembling are other physical behaviors occasionally seen during transition. This shaky feeling can be subtle or quite dramatic. If the shaking comes on strong it can be frightening, as you might think you are (or they are) having some kind of neurological meltdown. Rest assured, it can be a normal part of birth.[196] (People can also get strong shakes and trembles directly following the birth. I had a great deal of shaking throughout my cesarean section, too. But more on that later.) A brisk rubbing or stroking massage can help to calm the nervous system of a trembling birthing person. By creating an overload of intentional sensations, we can sometimes distract the shaky nervous system. Warm blankets and aromatherapy are other things to try. Inhaling the scent of some essential frankincense or lavender oil, for example, may provide a soothing way to calm a shaky nervous system.

Most labor contractions follow a wave-like pattern. They start slow, build to a climax, and then fade. But some people in transition have what we call a double peak contraction. (Is this like being able to have multiple orgasms?) A double peak contraction is when, just as the contraction starts to wane, it peaks again. This may be hard to get through, but you can. You will survive. (Remember: Your body has evolved to do this work.)

In transition you may experience dramatic temperature changes, such as freezing cold or sweating or maybe cold feet with a hot head (any variation is possible). Ice packs, heat packs, extra blankets, opening a window, and even stepping outdoors for fresh air are all possible comforts for a person experiencing big temperature changes.

I once looked over at my client at a birth, during her transition, and saw that she was mildly flushed. I turned away for a brief moment to take a note and when I looked back she was drenched in sweat. A thousand beads of sweat covered her face, yet outwardly she hadn't moved a muscle. That's proof of a lot of metabolic work! By the time you're in labor you've been pregnant for a long time. The process started with these little itty-bitty cells and now you have this gigantic baby and a placenta and your entire circulatory system is intermeshed with another person's and your endocrine system is in hyper drive and you are just about to be "un-pregnant" in one big, gigantic surge of activity. Wow, ow, grrr... and it's over. It is only logical that your nervous system would be keyed up as you make these preparations and adjustments. Even if your labor is a whole day or a whole week, it's still a relatively short time for such a big change to take place.

Second stage emotions

Usually the arrival of second stage is marked by a refreshed sense of clarity and a renewed surge of energy; a second wind for second stage. When a person senses development in their progress it can be deeply motivating. For some, second stage work brings a relief from the more passive (opening) work of first stage. Now the birthing person can use their force and the results are often quite direct. They can feel the baby moving down, which can really boost their determination.

Nevertheless, very different experiences in second stage can occur. Some people describe that the work of second stage was not to push or bear down or use force, but to let go further and continue to allow the process to happen to them. While some people really and truly find relief, leaving them to greatly prefer second stage to first, others find second stage their biggest challenge. Some people say their sensations were so strong and burning during second stage that they had to work harder than they ever imagined possible. These people say that to move the baby down took unfathomable amounts of muscle strength and that they endured outrageous amounts of pain. I have heard second stage described as if trying to give yourself a shot or to cut yourself. It's hard to lean into the work with great amounts of muscle force when you expect the work to bring strong, painful sensation—which it does.

You won't know for sure how you will feel about your own second stage until after you've had your baby. Regardless, I do expect that when your time comes you will have an increase in energy and a strong motivation to get your baby out.

Physical expressions of second stage

During one of my potluck dinners for sharing birth stories, a client related: "As they wheeled me down the hallway to my room, I kept telling anyone that would listen that I would be okay if I could just take an enormous dump." Her partner laughed and quipped: "Yeah, an enormous 8 pounder!" We all erupted in laughter, and the other new mothers nodded in agreement.

One of the most common harbingers of second stage is indeed when a person expresses an urge to move their bowels. When this happens, it is because the baby has gotten low enough to apply pressure to the gestational person's rectum, giving them a sensation that they recognize as the urge to poop. (As I briefly discussed in Week 7, many people also get loose stool at the early onset of labor; nature's way of cleaning you out and making room. So if you haven't already completed your Bathroom Observation homework from Week 9, plan to get it done this week!) On a daily basis, we get the urge to move our bowels when the rectum is full. When poop pushes against the rectum wall it creates a pressure sensation that communicates to the brain that it's time to void. In labor pressure on the rectum from the baby's head (or butt or other presenting body part) also tells the brain to expel the contents responsible for creating the pressure. This external, rather than internal pressure on the rectum wall results in the sensation of needing to void. All this is to say, you already know something about what it will feel like when you get the urge to void your baby! Sure, the baby is bigger than the typical poop and the sensations may be much more intense, but the anatomical feedback system is essentially the same.

Other ways people attending a birth know a person is beginning their second stage include changes in the behavior and breathing sounds of the gestational parent. In first stage, when they exhale, the out-breaths tend to be long and open (with or without sound). But in second stage their breath often starts to sound caught and interrupted, and sometimes they begin to grunt. Their grunts may start gently or arrive at full-force. It depends on the nature of each particular birth. Moreover, a birth partner or provider might also see the birthing person getting low to the ground (if they have been encouraged to move around and find their own positions) and/or noticeably *not* moving as much as they were earlier. A person entering their second stage may even growl.

Third stage emotions

Once the baby is out there is immense relief that the birth is over. Many feel great joy that they've come through alive. Some people feel pretty rocked by their experiences. It's normal to have a variety of emotions about the birth immediately following—not to mention mixed emotions about the newborn, including curiosity, concern, love, uncertainty, amazement, and disbelief. Some people feel connected to their baby right away and others don't feel very connected at all. Bonding and getting to know each other can sometimes take time. Many a new parent has thought or said, "Where did this baby come from?"

In anticipation of the moments directly following your birth, please prepare to be accepting and forgiving of yourself. When you meet your baby, you may feel instantly in love or you may not. It's not a measure of your ability to parent. Your first feelings and reactions to your baby are in no way a referendum on your parenting or even the slightest glimpse into what is to come. When your birth is over you will need to process and recover from what just happened. Your hormone levels and emotions will be in flux. You may have a swollen or sore vagina, or you may still be on the operating table with your c/section being closed up. You will need to drink fluids, eat something, and sleep. (The Bradley Method® recommends orange juice immediately following birth to replenish fluids, potassium, and natural sugars. If you like OJ, go for it. If you don't like OJ, pick something else nutritious that you like and plan for that.)

How you feel when your baby first comes out is just that: it's how you feel *at that moment in time*. Nothing more. When we can feel our feelings without making harsh judgments, then we can process them, release them, and move on. When we are intolerant of our own feelings, then we give ourselves emotional hurdles that must be cleared before we can move on. So please prepare to be compassionate with yourself. You have a lot of new experiences ahead of you.

Physical expressions of third stage

People are usually elated, relieved and physically exhausted once the baby is out. They often forget that there is a placenta still to come. The contractions that follow the baby's birth are rarely difficult. As I mentioned previously, the placenta typically follows the baby out in 5 to 45 minutes. It's warm, soft, and usually falls right out requiring little to no effort from the gestational parent. Postpartum contractions, or "after pains" as they are sometimes called, will continue for several weeks, until the uterus has returned to its pre-pregnancy size. These after-pains are usually not painful for a first-time parent. But they can be challenging for a person after their second or subsequent births. After a second, third, or fourth birth it takes more work for the uterus to return to its non-pregnant size.[197] I was totally taken aback by the contraction intensity for the first three days after my second child was born. Every time I would start to nurse, I would get these incredibly strong uterine contractions that hurt like hell. I remember really having to focus on my breathing and my baby to get through them. My after-pains didn't last long into each nursing session, just the first few moments, but I definitely dug into my conscientious breathing to help me cope. Again, if this is your first birth, you are likely to hardly notice these pains at all.

For the first hour and a half immediately following a birth, the gestational parent and baby are usually wide awake and extremely interested in each other. After that they'll both be ready for some sleep.

This concludes my descriptions for the physical expressions and emotions of the various stages of labor. I will now go on to explain some ways to help support a challenging transition. Because it is such a reliably hard part of the birth, it deserves some further attention.

Support tips for transition, or any tough time

A birthing person who is doubting themself needs calm, optimistic encouragement. It's important to realize that the same coping techniques that had been working earlier may still work for you now. You'll likely do well if you—with the help of your support person, perhaps—can coax yourself to shift your focus back to the basics of *closing eyes, tuning into breath, conserving energy* and *surrendering to—softening into— the feelings*. Remember that releasing body tension where you can, in the parts of you that don't directly work to birth, can help you to get through this.

Relaxing deeply is one way to productively cope with the toughest moments. But if that is not working, another coping tool is to release the feelings with sound—wailing, moaning, singing, crying. If you're feeling doubtful, or your partner suspects you are, then together you can muster some positive and compassionate energy to help carry you through. If the support person meets your panic with calm certainty and a steadfast belief in your amazing abilities to survive this, you will get back on track. You can do this.

For the support person: you can generate energetic love, from your heart to theirs. You can beam your energy into them to give them strength. Beam them some confidence, too. Offer them positive, warm encouragement. Love them and share that you know they are strong enough and that birth is safe enough. Give them that and they will grow stronger.

Here is an example:

> **Person in labor:** "I can do this, I can do this... I cannot! No! Now I can't do this!"

> **Partner/support person:** "Yes, you can, you *are* doing it. You *are* birthing. And you are doing it perfectly well, as great as anyone ever has. I understand you may feel totally overwhelmed. This is completely overwhelming. So let go completely and let this process happen to you. Surrender to the process. This is happening. And you are strong, you will survive. Go with it; let your birth

happen. You are going to get through this and your baby is going to be out and this birth craziness will really and truly be over. You are safe and your baby is safe. You are doing an amazing job. I am in awe of your birthing abilities."

Please consider for a moment what it feels like to be truly *overwhelmed*:

Over-whelm
:upset, overthrow
:to cover completely; submerge

That's intense. It's a real or metaphorical drowning and that's got great potential to have moments that really suck. Giving birth is huge and some of it can be so *so* painful. As a support person, be sure to let the birthing person know you understand that and that you still believe they will survive. Remind them that you are right there with them and that you know they're doing an amazing job. Say to them, "Yes you can, yes you can, yes you *are* doing it, *you are doing it*, yes you can. You're handling it like a pro. No one has ever done it better. Ever. This is miserably hard. Cry, scream, or go quiet. But you can survive, do it, and know you are doing it perfectly right. You are strong enough. Carry on Super Hero! I am here if you need me. Have a sip of water. I love you!"

> **A plausible response to that positive support:** "Oh, okay. I guess I can try. I guess it's my only choice, really. Maybe I can survive just a little longer. I have to get this baby out. And the baby seems okay. So okay, I can. Yes I can, yes I can. I'll go on a little further."

Of course, there will be times when a person will answer, "Nope. I know you think I can survive this, but you are wrong. I'm done. I cannot endure this any longer. I want to try pain medication *now*. I am telling you right now that your job as my partner is to get me some pain medication, now!" And this steers our discussion here into an important, if quick side note: transition is, in my experience, the most common time laboring people request pain medications.

Partners are not gatekeepers for pain medication. Your response to the above request should be, "I will go right now and get someone to help you get pain medication." Then do it!

An educated person can make educated choices as they need to. It's unethical to deny a person pain drugs when they want them, but it's also unethical to deny them a complete education of the risks they'll introduce with the use of pain meds—and this, in my experience, happens a lot. People should be taught during their pregnancy about the types of medications available, the risks that are associated with them, and also that a person should ask for pain medication during labor if they want it. (And this would be in addition to practical birth coping and support education, such as is included in this book!) Plenty of evidence-based information is available on the risks and benefits associated with the drugs; however, most providers (at least in my area) scantly address the subject, if they mention it at all.

Most prenatal visits cover the brief essentials of screening for hypertension and monitoring weight gain. Then, during labor, providers want to be compassionate problem solvers, so they offer medication. At this point they will hastily go over a few brief and incomplete points about some associated risks. But this is unfair to people in labor. The hard work has already begun. Their concentration is elsewhere. Therefore, in order to make a truly informed decision about pain medication during childbirth, one really needs to collect information prior to the onset of birth. Learning enough to make an informed decision takes energy and attention to be able to process the information.

People in labor don't have either and so it's arguably not truly an informed consent, especially when the drugs offered were initially presented by the professional as being a viable solution to a perceived problem. (More on offering pain medications, and their risks and benefits, coming later in this book, so please keep reading! Yay you, you are working hard to be a great parent! Your baby and I appreciate your efforts.)

The support partner can bring comfort during transition by being happy, calm and proud. The support partner can also use facts to help ease the birthing person's insecurity:

- "This fearful feeling you're sharing sounds like it might be that you've arrived at transition. If that's the case, you will soon be feeling the urge to push the baby out."

- "The baby's heart tones have been strong and healthy. That baby can't wait to get out here and meet you."

- The pressure in your butt that you are describing is because the baby has gotten so low in your body. This is good, the baby has to get low to get out."

- "You are healthy and strong."

Make these the facts of the support you provide. Let the birthing person know that they look beautiful, that you're impressed with their courage, and that you trust and are in awe of their process. When the partner and care providers are calm and confident, a birthing person can feel safe enough to meet their own fears, and then push on to birth their baby. If they need something, anything, they can ask. If you, the support person, have been sitting down, stand up and show them you are there, ready and able. Both of you need courage now more than ever. Remember: courage doesn't mean you are not scared. Courage means you acknowledge your fears and move forward. Stay focused on your most basic coping mechanisms during transition and you will eventually get to the arrival of second stage.

If you do hit a place of self-doubt or fear during birth, what do you want to happen? For example: "I don't want medication offered, I want emotional support. I want my partner to believe in me, hold me and love me. I want them to tell me I can continue, and that it is all okay, and that I am amazing and healthy and safe and beautiful." Once you figure out what is possible, identify what you want. Then you can work on trying to get it. Learning how to manage doubt and fear are important tools for navigating labor and the maternity care system alike.

Fears (yours or your provider's) can trigger interventions. As I have been trying to illustrate, the hospital-based maternity care system in the United States is built on the economics of fear, and it's a very lucrative business. It's no wonder that we, as a nation, are doing so poorly in maternity care compared to other developed and developing countries. So many people in this country are left doubting their abilities and feeling betrayed by their bodies. Put what you are learning in this book to good use. Evaluate and reevaluate your plans for support and your attitudes toward giving birth. The goal here is that you believe your birth to be a privilege earned through good health, love, support, and informed practices, rather than something to dread or that you just have to endure.

On *offering* pain meds to a "patient" (Don't!)

When a medical professional offers pain medications in labor the message that translates is that this set of experienced and objective eyes (the birth professional) sees a person who can't do this on their own. In other words, this person is in need of assistance. We understand that the provider sees a kind of deficiency, or that the "patient" would somehow benefit from something external. Their birth is a problem and they'll benefit from medical support. This is an unfortunate, albeit common interpretation.

Additionally, most of us think that if a doctor, nurse, or midwife is offering us something, then it must be safe and approved. We look to our medical care providers to know what is best in stressful situations. And we often allow their confidence to stand in for our own. In other words, the offer of pain medication during labor can imply to the person in labor that their body isn't strong or capable or healthy enough to handle the birthing process at that time. Consequently, we internalize that the drugs are something we should take, that they will help us, and that we'll be better for their use. Likewise, we assume that whatever risk may be attached will not be a big deal. While all of the above may turn out to be true, please also remember that a medical care provider may also offer drugs because they can satisfy two key issues for *themself*: 1) they believe they have given you enough information to make an informed decision and 2) they can feel good about themself for being compassionate.

When a person in labor, through their own process, thinks about using pain medications, those are their private thoughts. They may or may not speak up about them. If/when they do, their request should be honored. By the same token, I hear from many people that they had tough moments during birth when they considered asking for drugs, but didn't. They got on with the work at hand and birthed their baby. I also hear from people about their medicated birth stories. It's a common thread: if these people weren't the ones to initiate a request for pain medication, once someone, usually a birth professional, had offered said pain medications, the choice became a focal point for their thinking. It seems that once someone, particularly an experienced birth professional, has planted the seed of drugs, it becomes particularly hard to get over the implicit message of deficiency and our innate desire for approval.

For these reasons, I counsel my clients to discuss the topic of medication ahead of time, and to make a request that they do not want anyone external to offer pain medication during labor (providers or partners!). This does amend the standard of practice for giving informed consent and informed refusal, which includes a provider communicating options and risks *at the time a decision needs to be made*—i.e., during birth. (Further discussion of informed consent/refusal comes in Week 11.) To be clear, I am not suggesting that your medical provider abandon the legal dictates of informed consent and informed refusal. But because childbirth is, biologically, a healthy human function, with predictable stress points, I am suggesting that pain medications be discussed *beforehand,* rather than during birth, so that the decision not only to use pain medication (or not), but also to think about the option of pain medication in labor is left truly to the birthing person.

My clients generally ask their providers to document in their chart that they have discussed the available methods of pain management and their associated risks and are requesting that all members of the birth team be informed to trust that the person will ask for the pain medication if they want it. No one is to offer them pain medication. Many clients report that even after these conversations, people at the hospital do still offer drugs. It's a habit borne out of repetition, to be sure. But at least the birthing person knows they tried to protect themself from this intrusion. And this is an important moment of self-empowerment.

You may have a terrific group of people attending you, professionals and loved ones who completely understand that you are capable of making the pain medication decision all by yourself. But if you really don't want anyone to offer you pain meds in labor, let them know ahead of time and think about making homemade signs to tape outside your labor room door to remind all those who enter *not* to offer you pain medication. If you are offered the drugs, it will take a bit of effort to get beyond it, but you can. Now that you understand the power differential at play here, I believe that this will give you more strength to honestly assess your own needs, resist temptations put forth, and move beyond unwanted recommendations. This isn't about the pros or cons of drug use; this is an issue of owning one's own experience. Keep learning through your pregnancy so you don't need to task yourself with sorting out your feelings during your labor.

On interruptions during labor

Interruptions influence our release. Think about the last time you took a dump or were making love. What would have happened if I walked in on you? (Your response should itself interrupt your reading of this lesson—hopefully it brought out a laugh!)

Modern birth is saturated with interruptions that most folks take completely for granted. Even minor interruptions have a direct effect. For those planning a home birth, avoiding interruptions is sometimes part of a deciding factor for picking their birth location. For those planning a hospital birth, traveling to the hospital is an interruption of process, but that's just the beginning. Filling out insurance, privacy, and consent forms; waiting for an elevator; answering the nurse's long list of questions; and submitting to (or even just the decision to consent to) a vaginal exam, electronic fetal monitoring, an IV needle stick, blood pressure and temperature monitoring—this is all just in a routine, healthy person's birth experience. Talking through all of these elements beforehand can help you to prepare emotionally and to make practical plans to get back on track during the actual birth. It is easier to cope with interruptions if you can see them as such because then you can proceed to get yourself emotionally back into your birth.

So I'll amend my previous question and ask it this way: How would you get back on track if I walked in on you during sex and you wanted to resume your love making?

A practical plan to resume labor might be to take a shower as soon as you can. You can largely dictate when you need a shower, but you might as well get through all the admitting stuff first so that once you do get into the shower, you are done with the bulk of routine interruptions. At this point you can use the privacy and the soothing water to help you regain your birth groove. (With regard to this shower example: if you do consent to IV fluids, then you will need to cover the IV site in plastic or refrain from getting into water altogether, because the IV needs to remain dry. So take this into consideration, too.)

There is variation in admitting procedures from hospital to hospital and group to group. Ask your provider ahead of time what to expect. Most providers will have standing orders in place that cover general admitting practices for people in labor. Electronic fetal monitoring for 20 minutes is a standard of care, for example. There are some providers around the country that don't automatically do 20-minute electronic fetal monitor strips. Instead, they use a hand-held Doppler ultrasound device, and they listen during and directly after a contraction or two. Keep in mind that contractions are demanding, so it may be tough to really allow your process to unfold while simultaneously trying to be a good patient. This is especially challenging if the staff seem stressed, rushed, bored, distant, judgmental, or doubtful about the birth process. Tense people beget tense care.

It's no secret by this point in the book that my general view of the industry of hospital maternity care is one that is built on the self-perpetuating foundation of doubt in a birthing person's abilities. When professional experts say things like, "Oh dear, you do look so tired," or, "Everything is okay now, but it might not be later," it's hard to avoid doubting yourself. So please consider that you don't need to succumb to this systemic institutional doubt. You don't have to take on someone else's doubt. Doubt is different than facts. If a provider presents you with facts, you may well want to act with interventions. You can insulate yourself with information about birth and a plan for continuous support from an educated partner, friend, relative, and/or a doula. Research the routine practices and outcome-statistics of your prospective care providers and go to a variety of hospitals to see if you detect differences. Be picky, if you can. Try to control the ideas and images that you focus on for birth preparation and during labor. Acknowledge that there will be interruptions and devise your own best plans to cope with them. You can create a safe place in your mind that can protect you in your process, regardless of where you are or how much you are interrupted.

I imagine you are starting to see that it may be hard to settle back into your birth work once it begins in earnest. Again, knowing this all ahead of time, can really help you to devise plans to account for the challenges. It becomes less about the actual interruptions and more about your preparations for their inevitability. Having a game plan will help you to find the courage to release into this new experience. Just seeing the interruptions for what they are will support your being able to stay on course and adapt as needed. And, of course, there do exist amazing fleets of incredible care providers that practice in hospitals and homes across the country. These providers understand birth and have deep compassion. There are thousands of loving people that protect laboring people and gently usher them through with minimal interruption and maximum respect and kindness. Birth works. History and its generations of birthing people are on your side. Keeping this close to mind can help counterbalance whatever doubt may creep in from those maternity care providers who may not be as compassionate and respectful as you had expected.

The role of the vaginal exam in pregnancy and birth

The vaginal exam is a medical test. A test is a tool; it's not good or bad. It's a means to collecting information. And you have the right to consent, refuse or postpone any medical test you choose. You also have the right to rescind your consent no matter what you have previously said or even signed: informed consent and informed refusal—your legal protections—include the right to withdraw consent previously agreed to. (Again, I will go into more detail about Informed Consent and Informed Refusal in next week's lesson.) Therefore, before you agree to a vaginal exam or any medical test, you should understand what data will be collected and whether the data will be actionable. Remember: "actionable" means that you or your support partner or your care provider can do something with the information. Will you do something differently based on the test results? Likewise, you will also want to know how accurate the test is and to find out if the test is likely to lead to further testing. And what are the concerns if you do *not* take the test. Are there any alternatives to the test? What risks are associated with taking or not taking this test? It is only with a good understanding of the answers to such questions that you can then make an informed decision.

Vaginal exams are called by many names: vaginal exam, internal exam, pelvic exam, cervical exam, bi-manual exam (two hands), and digital exam (done with fingers). These all refer to someone putting their gloved and lubricated fingers deep into your vagina to feel around for your cervix and whatever else the exam is meant to discover. The test can be performed by a midwife in an office or home setting, or by a resident, nurse practitioner, physician's assistant, midwife, or doctor in an office or hospital.

Someone performing a vaginal exam will first instruct you to lie down on your back, or in a semi-reclining position, with your knees opened wide. (I have witnessed a midwife perform a vaginal exam on a woman who was on her hands and knees, but most providers in my area won't consider the hands and knees position as an option, likely because they wouldn't trust what they were feeling in this varied position.) Regardless of position, the attendant will lead off with the pointer and middle fingers. They will aim their fingers in, back, and up, in an attempt to find and feel your cervix. The provider will use their other hand to feel for the uterine fundus (the top of your uterus) and sometimes they will want to apply some force down from the fundus (creating "fundal pressure") to see if they can move the baby down to better feel more of the baby from the inside hand. What the provider focuses on in the exam will depend on where you are in the pregnancy or birth process.

The most common times that a low-risk pregnant person will get offered a vaginal exam are once at the start of a pregnancy and then again at the onset of labor. Initially, providers use the vaginal exam to check for normalcy of the anatomy: cervix, bony structure, and vaginal walls.[198] The vaginal exam then usually only happens again when labor

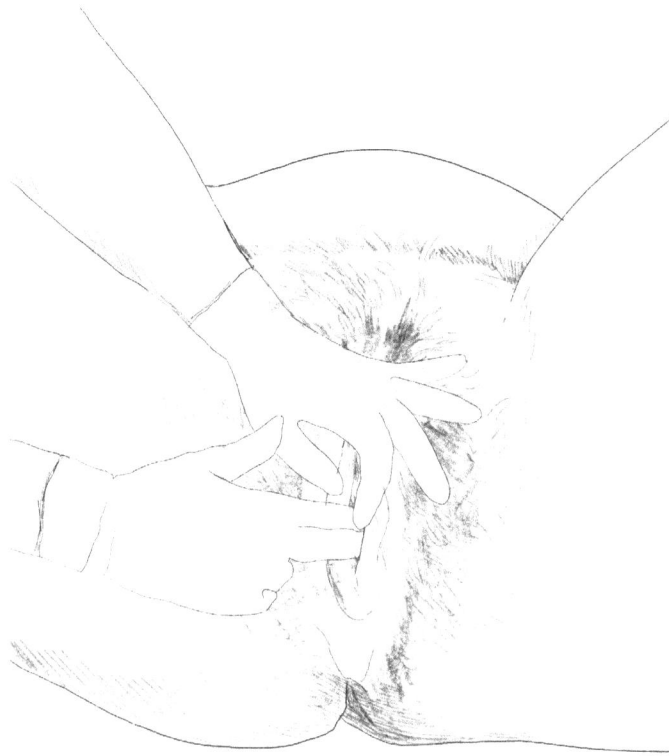

arrives to help determine progress. However, some providers will do another exam during the end of the pregnancy. And some practices, like many in my area, even suggest giving weekly exams from week 36 on, until labor begins.

Once labor begins there is more consensus across the spectrum of providers for the test to be commonly utilized—be it by a midwife or hospital medical staff. (Note that more consensus amongst providers still doesn't mean it is necessarily appropriate for you and your care. The choice remains yours to make.) After this initial in-labor exam, its use is again varied; some providers ask to perform the test every couple of hours, others seem not even to ask but just assume that they will perform multiple exams, while still others do not consider the test again until second stage arrives or something seems to deviate from a healthy normal process. Once birth-signs point to second stage labor arriving, there is more, but not complete, consensus and many providers suggest or expect a vaginal exam. The frequency of vaginal exams during second stage depends on how quickly the baby is moving down.

The vaginal exam can be used to try to understand four things related to measuring what, if any physical labor changes have begun or, if clearly started, how far the pregnant person appears to have come through the process: cervical "**dilation**" (if or how much the cervix has begun to open); cervical "**effacement**" (if or how much the cervix has softened and shortened); "**station**" (how far down, if at all, the baby has moved into the pelvic bowl); and "**presentation**" (what part of the baby seems to be set to come out first). Based on these measurements, educated, best-guestimates are made about how much more labor is left to go.

While the vaginal exam is a very common medical test, it is my opinion that it has a very limited role in helping to safely navigate the birth process. Moreover, due to the extremely intimate way the information is collected—i.e., fingers being inserted into your vagina—I believe it requires thorough consideration prior to consent. Therefore, as you consider the vaginal exam, keep in mind that this exam is a snapshot of a moment in time. The information collected is old as soon as it's collected, and thus what it might mean about the future of your pregnancy, or the start of your labor, is a guess at best—even when an educated one. In short, **the vaginal exam is not predictive.** And yet, how can you not react to the resulting information from such a test?

One of my former clients had planned a romantic getaway, just a couple of hours away from her home, before the labor was due to arrive. Then, after consenting to a vaginal exam, she was informed that she was already almost two centimeters dilated at 37 weeks. She and her partner cancelled their weekend rendezvous. They went home and excitedly packed their bags and sat by the door waiting for labor. Days and days and days went by. Mama was anxiously examining each twinge the entire time. It was exhausting, and ultimately all for naught. She didn't go into labor until a couple of *weeks* later. By contrast, I had another client, also at 37 weeks, who let her husband get on a train to go out of town for a few days, because they had just had an exam that showed no changes in her cervix. Of course, later that same day, her labor began—full steam ahead. Her partner missed the first few hours as he frantically tried to get back home. An hour or two from *now* you could be in a drastically different place in your journey. We don't know for sure when or how your birth will start or progress and there are no medical tests that can tell us that (yet). You can be dilated to varying degrees for weeks before your actual onset of labor, or you might not begin to open until labor arrives. You might take many many *many* hours of hard work to dilate two or three centimeters, or you might go from two centimeters to ten in 30 or 40 minutes.

Remember: we are not machines. We have bodies that perform biological functions subject to environmental, physiological, and emotional variables. How long does it take you to poop? Is that rate useful to measure against everyone else's rate of defecation? Or against your own rate, across a single week? I have seen healthy people, free from pathology, dilate from two centimeters to 10 centimeters in less than one hour, or over 20 hours, or longer. Even assessing the baby's position prior to the onset of birth disregards the fact that babies continue to move and shift. The vaginal exam tells us nothing about your health in the process; we rely on your blood pressure and other vital signs for information about how you are coping physically. Nor does a vaginal exam give us any information about how the baby is tolerating the uterine environment. What we get from the test is a glimpse at some part of what has or has not happened physically so far.

From my perspective, your most important work to do, with regard to understanding the usefulness of this exam, is to discuss with your provider (or potential provider) the role of the vaginal exam in their maternity care protocols and how they see it being useful or not during your care. In what follows, I share my own thoughts around when I think the test can be helpful, some drawbacks to consider before consenting, and some risks associated with the test to help you evaluate and perhaps expand upon whatever else your provider tells you.

When might the vaginal exam be useful?

Some birthing people are quite eager to know what is going on with their cervix at the end of pregnancy, or when they first see their provider after labor has begun. Getting that information can feel like a critical bit of mental support that helps you to understand your process. Although this information may not be directly actionable, if it satisfies a burning need to know, then great (as long as you have first done your homework and considered the test thoroughly beforehand, including explored any potential risks). Another instance in which the vaginal exam may be a good choice is if you are traveling to the hospital during labor. The results of this exam may weigh into your decision about *staying* at the hospital or returning home.

Sometimes people laboring at home start to get antsy about whether or not everything is going okay with the labor. They may want to get some reassurance by checking in on their vital signs (fetal heart tones and parent's blood pressure). If at this juncture baby and parent are deemed healthy, and if from an interpretation of the vaginal exam it appears that they still have a lot of work left ahead, then they may choose to leave and go home feeling assured. Many people I have worked with get to the hospital only to realize that they appear early in the process. At this point, they have vital signs checked and if all is well they leave to get more work done in their own private space. In my classes I council that upon arrival at your birth location, if you are found to be less than four centimeters dilated, and your travel time home is one half hour or less, then you may consider returning home. There are no guarantees that you will have time to go home before things pick up speed, so you'll also have to weigh what else is happening, such as the timing of the contractions, how the gestational parent is feeling about going or staying, and what emotional signposts have been expressed so far. If you do live more than 30 minutes away from your planned birth location, you may want to retreat to a hotel close to the hospital. (If you are more than 30 minutes away from your planned birth location, and if you can, start saving money now for this potential expense.)

Finally, the vaginal exam can have a positive role during a slow-to-progress second stage. If a baby makes no progress down over several hours, and the gestational parent has tried several different positions, and still no progress has been made, there may be a reason for medical intervention. Although it can take a very long time to push out a baby, it's important to note some progress being made. A baby who is moving down, be it ever so slowly, is likely fine. But a baby that is not coming at all might really need some help, and so a vaginal exam could yield actionable test results.

Risks associated with a vaginal exam

The first, most clear risk involved with a vaginal exam is positioning. Simply having a laboring person get into a bed on their back can sometimes cause problems for the baby. The weight of the baby on the gestational parent's major blood vessels, as they recline on their back, can reduce the parent's blood flow, which can in turn stress the baby. If the baby is stressed by the parent's position, which is ostensibly meant to help them, a catch-22 situation can result. Consider this: you are laying down on your back for a routine vaginal exam. Perhaps the baby is bothered by the position and "complains" with disconcerting heart tones. The doctor becomes fearful and so decides to try to "control" the situation. To do so, this doctor must rely on emergency training, training that requires that the patient remain on their back. The doctor's, the parent's, and the baby's stress levels continue to rise, potentially causing complications that began as an elective test to measure progress.

Data interpretation is another area of risk. Once a vaginal exam is complete, the data collected will be interpreted. Data interpretation is even more subjective than the physical measurements. These so-called measurements of a vaginal exam are done with fingers not rulers. Consequently, there is ample room for different providers with different sized fingers to make different measurements of the same cervix. Data misinterpretation can lead to wildly misunderstanding what's going on. In a rare but real example, I heard a story once in which a resident did a vaginal exam and declared the woman was only one centimeter dilated. This seemed illogical to the woman and her partner (she had been getting a tremendous amount of birth work done over many, many hours prior to their arrival at the hospital). As they were discussing what her options were, she began to grunt. It turns out that she was fully dilated and the baby was in a breech position. The young resident had mistakenly measured the dilation of the baby's anus, not the mother's cervical opening.

Extreme misreads aside, it is also important to note that an observation of anomaly early in the pregnancy, in an otherwise healthy person, may be completely inconsequential for the continuation of a healthy pregnancy and birth. But having this information may leave a sense of doubt and mistrust about the person's abilities to birth, for both the pregnant person and their provider. This is especially true if the provider has commented on the size of the person's pelvis.[199] These doubts can have a powerful influence on what unfolds.

Timing, coupled to a misinterpretation of data, presents another potential risk. Once in labor, an initial vaginal exam can be used on a pregnant person to create a baseline for labor progress over time. Doing so, however, can have unintended consequences, such as adding to a person's stress for not doing their birth work fast enough for the provider's schedule. The most conservative of doctors might write or leave standing orders to check your cervix once every hour or two. These doctors have been trained to understand that a cervix should be dilating between 1.2 and 1.5 centimeters per hour.[200] Therefore, if you are not progressing at this rate, your provider could diagnose your labor as "dysfunctional," "failing to progress," "stalled," "prodromal", or they might say you have a "protraction disorder." Each of these medical terms bring with it a negative connotation (and possible medical intervention), which could in turn increase your stress around the birthing process, without necessarily revealing an actual problem.

Infection is of course another risk associated with a vaginal exam. When you put something, anything into the vagina, there is the potential risk of infection. This risk becomes magnified once your amniotic sac has ruptured. Likewise, the physical maneuvers of a vaginal exam can cause cervical bleeding, which can certainly contribute to stress levels rising and a provider's interest in more testing.

"Stripping the membranes" is a procedure, as described on the Mayo Clinic's website, when "your health care provider inserts his or her gloved finger beyond the cervical opening and rotates it to separate the amniotic sac from the wall of your uterus." The Mayo Clinic reveals that "you might experience intense cramping and spotting. If bleeding becomes heavier than a normal menstrual period, contact your health care provider."[201] Within the uterus, small connective tissues help to support the amniotic sac. When a provider is feeling the cervix in a vaginal exam the membranes can be stripped either on purpose or by accident. Whether the membranes are stripped on purpose or by accident, this can be painful and may lead to bleeding. The hope is that, when this is done as an intentional action, it will help to stimulate labor by irritating or nudging on the thinning process.[202] The goal here would be to shorten a pregnancy (and bring on the labor), which is another decision *you* would need to make *with* your care provider. Membrane stripping should require specific medical consent. Nevertheless, it can happen accidently. And I have had clients whose doctor seemed to think that consenting to the vaginal exam also gave permission to strip the membranes. Based on those experiences, I recommend that if you consent to a vaginal exam, you engage in discussion with your provider about membrane stripping *prior to any exam*. This conversation can help you and your provider to identify your preferences and set clear expectations.

Another risk that I want you to consider here, as a result of the vaginal exam, is that you might feel demoralized if it is found that you are not as far along as you hoped. This disappointment can cause stress and weigh down your spirits. This stress can impact your self-esteem and drain your strength, energy and courage to continue. How might you feel if, after you had been working with contractions all night (let's say, 12 or 15 hours of hard work) and then, when you arrived at the hospital or your midwife arrives at your home, you were told you were only two centimeters dilated? (You had been thinking-praying-wishing that you were almost done!) I know I would feel pretty knocked down, perhaps forgetting to remind myself that this test score doesn't necessarily gauge how much labor time is left. And it certainly doesn't reveal my goodness and ability as a birthing person. As I will continue to say throughout these lessons: be compassionate with yourself. Remind yourself of the incredible hard work you are accomplishing, regardless of exam results.

Some labor work is harder to measure

In addition to the benefits and risks discussed above, and when it comes to assessing progress, I think the vaginal exam warrants other unique considerations. Some healthy labors can stall, for example. Meaning, someone's cervical dilation doesn't change yet contractions continue. What causes a stall, and how impactful it might be to the health of the birth process and the baby is not well understood by science (yet). But my thinking is that during this time, it is likely that the contractions are getting other work done. For example, maybe a baby is trying to adjust their position and so there isn't yet really a need to open the door? Maybe for some humans it may take them longer to transfer their immunities into their colostrum (the first breast milk). (Immunoglobulins, antibodies in a pregnant parent's milk that help to build the baby's immune system, are found in highest concentration directly after birth.[203]) Other possibilities may include the fact that a birthing parent isn't opening their doorway yet because perhaps the baby needs more physical stimulation to get their lungs or nervous system ready for independence; or perhaps the parent is not quite emotionally ready to release their baby. Science has yet to uncover many of the unanswered questions regarding the birth process. I do love to think about how much more your children will know by the time they are expecting children of their own. In the meantime, what follows are still more situations I think can be helpful to think through ahead of needing to consent to or refuse a vaginal exam.

The vaginal exam on the cusp of second stage

Person at the start of second stage: "Grunt! I have to poop! Grunt, grunt, grrrr."

Provider: "Hey, that sounds like you're pushing. Let me check you. Lie back please."

[**Or, Nurse:** "Hang on, don't push! Let me get the doctor/midwife to check you!"]

If a vaginal exam were to be done at this point a person would be found in one of two states: still in the process of dilating or fully open. Rarely, another option could be diagnosed: a third state called a "cervical lip." This scenario is when the cervix has not dilated evenly, which results in a small section of the cervix that has yet to open. A cervical lip can detain the baby's descent, but it is soft tissue and eventually your baby is going to get past it. If in the past you have had any surgical procedures that have left scar tissue on your cervix, you may be more prone to a cervical lip in that area. If diagnosed with a cervical lip, you can try side lying, especially if you can lie on the side that has the lip. This added pressure can help to thin the tissue from the weight of the baby's head. (Please note: this can be extra painful.) Also, if a cervical lip is diagnosed, it is worth trying to lie on your *back* (yes, here it can be helpful). You then want to pull your belly up toward your chest, as I explained in the belly lift technique for back labor (see Week 7). This lifting can sometimes help a baby get around the lip. Some providers will offer to try to manually move the lip around the baby. This, too, can be effective, but also quite painful. Finally, some midwives argue that a cervical lip should be ignored completely based on the idea that we shouldn't know about it in the first place because of the unnecessary nature of the vaginal exam at this stage.[204] Eventually, whether you know about a cervical lip or not, it will open. I do encourage you to discuss this possibility with your care provider, as it makes an excellent interview question: "What will you recommend if I develop a cervical lip while I am dilating?"

Cervical lips aside, a vaginal exam can reveal that you're still not fully dilated, but you have an urge to expel! In this situation, the concern expressed by some providers is that if a person "pushes" before they're fully dilated, the baby's head might damage the cervix. Some providers explain that pushing before you're fully dilated might cause swelling and even tearing of the cervix. Well, yes; however, this is of special concern when people are instructed to hold their breath and bear down as hard as they can—a misguided pushing technique that many doctors and nurses still support. Consequently, the birthing parent is warned: "Do not push yet!" (And cue the scary music.)

Being told not to push when you are having an urge to void can be hell, because most of us just can't stop. The stress builds because people care about their babies. People will do *anything* for their babies. People want to be good patients so that they can be good parents. At the same time, they can't control the urge to push, so they feel like they are terrible people doing something damaging. For perspective, imagine being sick with diarrhea and someone stands in front of the bathroom door and won't let you in, saying, "You can't go." You know what's happening is out of your control; it's just a matter of whether you get to the toilet or you poop in your pants. I've heard countless stories from people who have expressed that they felt fear, pain, and frustration because they couldn't do what they were being asked, i.e., to not push in spite of strong expulsive sensations. To instruct a person to fight their birth sensations, and try to keep the baby inside, is both stressful and potentially bad for the baby. I have had several prospective clients seek out a Bradley® class singularly motivated by this past birth experience. These people were fiercely determined to try and avoid such a situation again. This subject too provides interesting interview material as there are differing opinions. Some providers, most often midwives, hold the following perspective: if a person lets their body do what it needs to do, with their mental attention focused on relaxation, *and* their birth attendants provide a calm and supportive environment, then they won't force anything. These trust-your-instinct providers believe that a person should be encouraged to follow their own sensations and listen to their body.

As I've already discussed, you, as the birthing person, do not necessarily need to add abdominal force to your expulsive contractions. If you should have strong urges to "push" and yet you've been found not to be completely dilated, instead of using force, focus on relaxing your abdominals as best you can while visualizing the soft tissue of your cervix melting open. This is extra hard work, to be sure, as you'll need to keep your mind focused on melting into this release. A person in labor cannot stop their strong sensations. If the birthing person's and the baby's vitals are stable, then there's no medical necessity to intervene (even with a cervical lip). Keep doing the hard work!

So, what about the opposite scenario: when a vaginal exam reveals that you are fully dilated but you don't have an urge to expel? Again, the immediate health of gestational parent and baby should be considered first. Does everything still seem fine with assuring vital signs? If the answer is yes, and the only issue is that the gestational parent is fully dilated but doesn't yet have an urge to expel the baby, then the support partner and/or care provider should ask them to explain what they do feel. Frequently in this (often infrequent!) scenario, a person says that they are tired. At this point, if they can rest, they should. There is no immediate medical need to get the baby out. Nevertheless, the common solution here is to tell the person to push. And this can work. Sometimes you can actually nudge the baby down just low enough that you start to feel pressure on your rectum and gain clear sensations to void. But imagine trying to poop with no real urges; it can go nowhere quickly. Trying to void without urges can be ineffective and exhausting. My pal Madge slept for two solid hours at 10 centimeters, and so did her husband, and her midwife! It was great that they got that rest because she went on to push for four solid hours (hard work!) before delivering her beautiful baby. So if you are found to be fully dilated but don't yet feel any new urges, ask yourself what you do feel and then consider the pros and cons of following those instincts.

A vaginal exam at the onset of second stage has some other unique challenges to consider. As was mentioned above, sometimes the baby doesn't like the supine position. But what about the gestational parent's experience of reclining back at this late stage of labor? Many people report that it is uncomfortable to recline on their back from the end of pregnancy all the way through birth. And yet typically, after a vaginal exam, the provider leaves the birthing parent on their back, hopefully with the good news that they can begin pushing. But this position can have a negative impact on the gestational parent, the labor, and the baby. If the birthing person has been making progress in an upright position and then they are counseled to recline on their back for an exam, it's possible to lose some progress. The baby could float up and out of the pelvis a bit, away from the cervix. Perhaps more importantly, however, is the fact that when placed on their backs, birthing people often report that they felt stranded, like that beached whale or a turtle on their back.

It is very hard to move your body when the baby's head is getting low in your pelvis. Most mammals don't move around much during the expulsive phase of birth; humans are generally no exception. At this point the birthing person is extremely preoccupied with the process, so they won't easily ask for help to move. On the one hand, coping with the contractions doesn't leave much energy to ask for help. On the other hand, the birthing person might not realize how a position shift could help. To ask for help is difficult. Even on the best of days, under the best of circumstances it can be tough to identify what you need. Under the duress of childbirth it's going to be even more challenging, especially if what you need is the most basic self-care, such as rolling over or sitting up. Simply asking can require great emotional effort. And it might feel like you need 10 people plus a crane to move you. I've had many clients, regardless of their weight, share that they felt too big to move, which led to their feeling embarrassed by their need for help.

Further complicating this issue is the fact that many obstetricians will restrict a person from adopting the more physiological upright or all-fours positioning during second stage. Moreover, even if a provider would "allow" one to birth in a non-reclining position, they may not fully estimate their power to influence positioning choices. If our healthcare provider tells us to get into a particular position, for example, we may be hard pressed to disagree. As a result, from a provider's perspective, they may not think to have you change position or even ask if you want/need to. In my opinion, what they don't understand is that we, as patients, seek approval and are taught that being good patients means waiting for and following instructions.

I have heard many stories of people who, as they pushed their babies out in the supine position, were thinking some variation of, "What the heck am I doing on my back?" After the vaginal exam, people often stay on their backs, even if it feels totally wrong, simply because it's hard to move or because they were told to get into that position. And then they wait to be told what to do next, which can be an elusive direction that may never come. **You can avoid this common pitfall in your own birth by bringing your attention to the issue now during pregnancy and choosing a second stage position** *before* **birth arrives.**

There are a few more vaginal exam considerations to explore, but first it's time for a mindfulness break!

—Pause. Get up. Stretch your body in anyway(s) that feel good. Tune into your breathing—

I hope you were able to find some comfort in your stretches. I am happy you have picked the book back up. Please forge ahead, you are so near to the end of this week's reading!

Final thoughts on the vaginal exam

Should you decide to consent to a vaginal exam (and prior to the beginning of the test), I believe it empowering and protective to clarify two key things with your provider: 1) If during the exam you ask them to stop mid-exam, that they will promptly do that and remove their fingers immediately. (Think of it like the conversation that is often had at the dentist's office before they begin to drill. Most dentists remind the patients that if they raise a hand or even just grunt, the dentist will stop immediately.) And 2) please clarify your preferences with your provider, or ask any remaining questions about stripping your membranes.

Sadly, a client once reported to me that, during her labor, not only did her midwife not ask permission to strip her membranes; the midwife didn't stop the first few times the woman called out for her to stop. In fact, this client had to scream "STOP!" several times before the midwife ultimately did. This led my client to file a complaint with the state, as a case of sexual abuse. Sadly, the state belittled her complaint by claiming that vaginal exams are an obstetric standard of care. This shocked both my client and myself; effectively, the state did not respect her right to say no. Ultimately, simply filing the complaint became a useful processing step toward her own healing, even with the unsatisfying outcome. While she contemplated further action, she decided to walk away and focus her remaining maternity leave on her baby.

Please take a deep breath and exhale any fear that story may have churned up. You can feel confident that by learning to have an advance conversation you will be protecting yourself to the best of your ability. A vaginal exam, like any other medical test, has its place. Birth interventions are not good or bad, they are tools. Sometimes they are used appropriately and sometimes they are not. Please ask your care provider to teach you about their routines. It is helpful to know when and why they will suggest vaginal exams for you and how the information measured might be actionable or not. Then and only then can you make informed decisions when the time comes.

As of today, with what you are thinking and feeling right now, explore any thoughts or remaining questions you have about a vaginal exam below.

Truly participating in your care decisions is easy to give lip service to, it may even feel easy to plan for, but in real life it can take great fortitude to go against the expected norms. In-hospital vaginal exams rarely involve providers obtaining true *informed* consent. Many providers assume that consent is implied for routine standards of care. There are enraging stories I have read of providers not asking permission before inserting their fingers into someone's vagina. While most providers will verbally ask first, they neither rarely, if ever give you any real space to refuse or postpone nor do they mention any risks or provide any alternatives. Instead, the in-hospital vaginal exam, once you are in labor, is approached as if it is a basic necessity.

In my experiences and practice, I have found it very uncommon for a person to feel empowered enough to question or refuse a vaginal exam; I know I wasn't. We are culturally educated to accept the provider's authority. In this case, it means to lie down and submit to vaginal probing without clear evidence of improved outcomes. If only I had a dollar for each time I heard a person say *with surprise*, "You mean I don't have to have a vaginal exam?!" Time after time I have answered, "No. Of course you don't *have* to have a vaginal exam. You don't have to have *anything*. *You* get to choose what care, if any, you receive. No one should put fingers into your vagina without your consent. And before you give consent for someone to put fingers into your vagina, or administer any other test, you should be clear about how you and the baby will benefit from consenting. For truly informed consent or refusal (which again I will discuss at greater length in Week 11) you will need to make in-the-moment decisions based on what is actually happening. So be prepared to have these conversations more than once! Then in labor, based on the best available information, combined with your preferences, you can make your own best decisions.

Okay, that's it for this week. Hooray! Another week read! You are rocking this parenting work! Please read your homework assignments below and take good care of yourself throughout the week. Next week we'll dive into some more medical decisions that may be coming your way. I wish you a great week!

HOMEWORK

A) Research vaginal exams

Ask your potential provider(s): "When and why do you generally recommend vaginal exams/membrane stripping during pregnancy and during labor?"

B) Research your providers' skills for emotional support

Interview your providers about their ability to provide emotional support should you begin to doubt yourself.

C) Stick with your self-care

Please continue to practice conscientious breathing and relaxation techniques, remain or get active, respect and express your feelings, and eat your best nutrition.

THIS SPACE IS FOR YOUR NOTES AND DRAWINGS

THIS SPACE IS FOR YOUR NOTES AND DRAWINGS

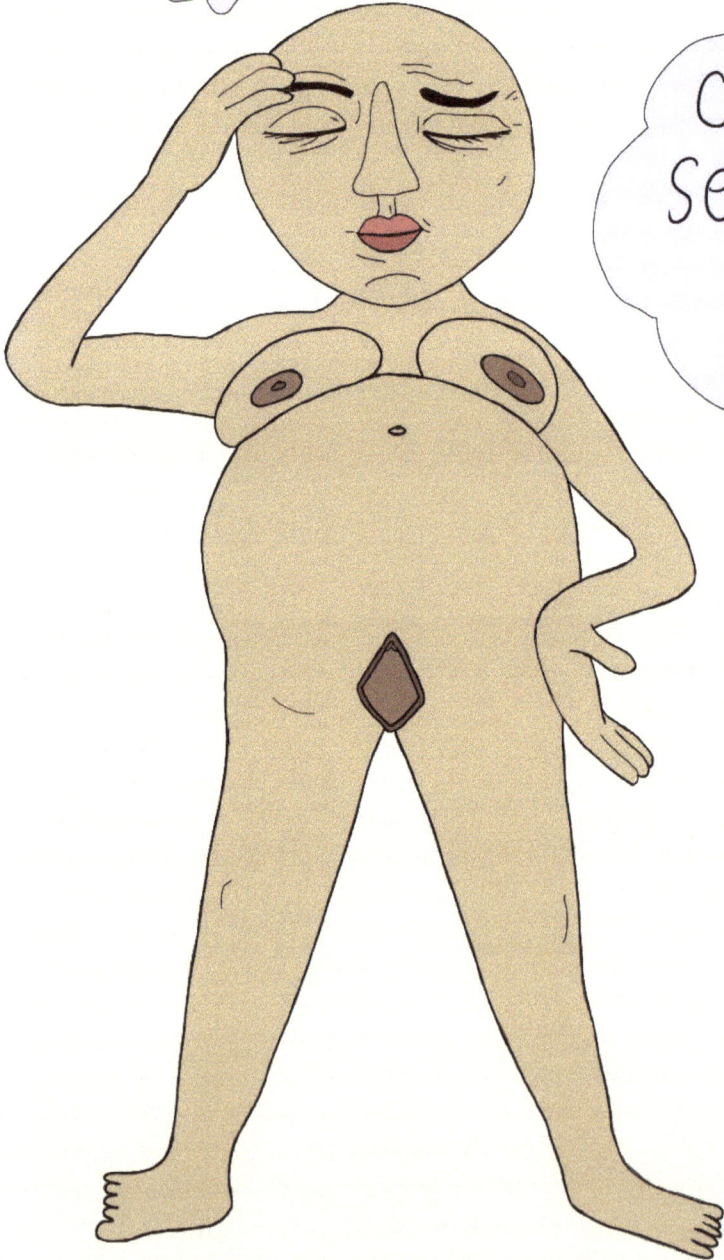

WEEK 11

Inquire and Decide

Chapter contents:

O *Medical decision making*

O *Informed consent/ Informed refusal*

O *Birth plans*

O *Common routines upon hospital admission*

THIS SPACE IS FOR YOUR NOTES AND DRAWINGS

Hello hello! I hope this past week was positive, restful, and productive. Of course, I know you're living a real life, so if this was a tough week, I hope you found the strength to work through whatever stressful turmoil came your way. Pregnancy can add so many physical challenges to an already very full life. A good cry can be a great release, and help to reset your focus. So can reading a good book! Let's reset and reinforce your focus as you settle in to read this new week's lesson: Take a deep breath and release what you don't need to carry. Take another breath and say "Hi" to your heart as you exhale. Tune into how you are feeling and then say "Hi!" to your baby. Tune in to how your baby is feeling. Take a few more check-in breaths with eyes closed before continuing on.

—Pause—

Have you been able to eat well and move your body? Was there any space to practice breath awareness, relaxation, and visualization skills throughout the past week? If you did not practice one or more of these recently, oh well. Let it go. No shame, guilt, or fear. If it was a hard week, consider that breath and relaxation exercises can help in a variety of stressful moments other than birth. This coming week, should you choose, you get to try again. Any time is a good time to practice, whether it's in the midst of a stressful moment or as soon after as possible, when you are going to sleep, just waking up, sitting in traffic, sitting on the toilet, etc.

Your food, rest, and exercise choices continue to be vital to you and your baby. If your belly is starting to get huge and you think that means it's now okay to slack on your nutrition, you're wrong. Fetal brain development, for example, picks up speed in the last trimester; the "baby's brain roughly triples in weight during the last 13 weeks of gestation, growing from about 3.5 ounces at the end of the second trimester to almost 10.6 ounces at term."[205] It makes good sense, therefore, to keep trying to eat well. By giving yourself the best nutrition and learning how to manage your stress and calm yourself when needed, you can increase your chances of raising a person healthier over their lifetime. Let last week go. Let's dive into this week's content now and look to the bright future for you and your baby.

Navigating your options

Your birth, like your pregnancy, puts you in the driver's seat to answer many important questions about your care. In this week's lesson I will elaborate on making medical decisions in response to getting your questions answered. I also further discuss your rights and responsibilities as a patient. My job here in this chapter—and peppered throughout this book—is to inspire you to investigate your legal rights and protect yourself.

Your provider's job is to present information and suggest a course of action where one is warranted. Your job is to make informed decisions. Because you will live with the outcome of these decisions, it stands to reason that you should have the final say. And you do, albeit with some critical exceptions. Fetal rights remain one prominent and volatile example within the United States that, in some instances and in some states, (currently) override gestational people's individual rights. In the United States there are (supposed to be) legal guidelines established to help you understand what information you need to make your medical decisions and to help you navigate the doctor/patient relationship with regard to the decision-making process.[206] In maternity care, in particular, it behooves you to stay actively involved in the decision-making process by demanding (politely, at first) that your providers refrain from coercion and give you adequate information to make educated choices. It is worth keeping close to mind that the United States are poorly represented internationally with regard to maternal and infant mortality. Simply going with the status quo may therefore not be in your best interest.[207] It will be useful for your maternity care now, as well as for all your future interactions with the medical system, to work towards being a person who makes their own medical decisions (ideally in cooperation with your providers) and to therefore get a solid handle on this important process.

You are your own best advocate when it comes to medical decision making. Getting and staying involved in the process is crucial. So let's review how the decision process should go. Ideally: First, your provider will make an assessment by collecting data (clinical exam, blood tests, medical history, etc.). Next, they will put forth a possible course of action. Your job is to respond to this *proposed* course of action and *decide* if you want to follow some or all of what it contains, as well as to inquire about possible alternative actions—including no action. As I've mentioned several times before, you will need to determine if the benefits outweigh any potential risks. And to do this you will need accurate information. In my experience, and what has been set by the legal precedence of informed consent and informed refusal for medical decisions, you should always pair the evidence-based facts that are communicated to you with what your instinct and intuition are telling you. What you want and how you feel both matter. Cultural and/or religious beliefs matter. It's your body, your life, and the life of your baby. I therefore urge you to weigh the circumstances of your situation, including your provider's experience and information, with what your gut is telling you. Then, make your informed medical decisions.

No one can predict the future. All you can ask of yourself is to try to make your best and most informed decisions in the moment when you must make choices. For the healthy human function of childbirth, when you gather facts ahead of time and build trust with your provider, the process can feel smooth and straightforward. During birth the only decisions you will ideally need to make are ones like what position to try next; to drink some water or juice or have a snack; to rest or to move; to go outdoors or to stay in; to listen to music or enjoy the silence. Nonetheless, some home births and most hospital births often carry myriad "routine" interventions that need not be accepted as "optimal" before your questions are answered and a satisfactory conversation has been had.

I don't know about you, but I did not grow up learning to participate in my healthcare decisions. I didn't know that it was my responsibility to question providers and then make my own, informed decisions. My experience has taught me that we have been culturally educated to assume that if a provider suggests a course of action, then it has already been proven to be in our best interest. To refuse a recommended course of action is to breach the power structure of doctor-knows-best. In other words, saying "no" to your medical professional requires one to put on your critical-thinking cap and take on significant responsibility for your physical outcomes. It also puts you at odds with cultural norms, leaving aside that it is a legal mandate for your providers to engage you in the decision process. During my first pregnancy, I didn't understand any of this. I certainly didn't know what factual information I needed to navigate my own healthcare. But the following information on informed consent and informed refusal can help you.

State laws and court decisions vary regarding informed consent, but the trend is clearly toward more disclosure rather than less. Informed consent is required not only in life-or-death situations but also in clinic and outpatient settings as well. A healthcare provider must first present information regarding risks, alternatives, and success rates. The information must be presented in language the patient can understand and typically should include the following:

○ A description of the recommended treatment or procedure;

○ A description of the risks and benefits—particularly exploring the risk of serious bodily disability or death;

○ A description of alternative treatments and the risks and benefits of alternatives;

○ The probable results if no treatment is undertaken;

○ The probability of success and a definition of what the doctor means by success;

○ Length and challenges of recuperation; and

○ Any other information generally provided to patients in this situation by other qualified physicians[208]

In sum, your doctor has a legal obligation to inform you of your diagnosis ("identification of illness") and your prognosis ("opinion on course of disease") in language you can understand. Your doctor is (supposed to be) obligated to describe what your options of treatment are, including alternative treatments, the option of delayed treatment, and the option of no treatment. Ultimately, with few exceptions (as stated earlier), you make the final decision, even if your provider doesn't agree or think it's your best decision. Moreover, if doctors are trained to see disease and yet birth and pregnancy are healthy functions, then it is likely useful to ask yourself and your provider: "Could what's happening now be a healthy variation?"

Consider the following questions, use them as a "cheat sheet" when speaking with your provider, and satisfy your own responsibility to make an informed consent, postponement, or refusal:

○ Why are you worried that my baby and I aren't healthy? What is the medical concern at this moment? (Diagnosis)

○ What is the provider's prediction of outcome as it relates to the current circumstances? (Prognosis)

○ What is the course(s) of action—medication, test, or procedure—that the provider is proposing?

○ What are my potential risks and benefits associated with this proposed plan of action?

○ What is the expected outcome of this course of action? How likely is the plan to work?

○ Does this drug, test, or procedure frequently lead to other drugs, tests, or procedures?

○ Are there alternatives to this plan of action, including *not* doing something right now? (Note: each alternative plan should also have its associated risks explained.)

○ Could this—whatever is happening now—be a healthy variation of the childbirth process?

○ How much time are you comfortable giving me to make my decision?

This last question can help you to measure your provider's concern level. The more time they are willing to leave you alone to make your decision(s), the more this correlates with less concern over any immediate issue. If your provider is going to send you home or walk away from your side for a couple of hours, for example, then that demonstrates a lower level of worry than an insistence that a decision be made while they stand at your bedside. Use this information to calm or center yourself should you feel stress—assuming, of course, that you yourself feel comfortable waiting! If you are uncomfortable about something being wrong, but your provider seems uninterested, please be insistent and demand medical attention. Again, your intuition matters! (Consider also that a provider *should* have your best interests in mind while also not wanting to risk their livelihood through malpractice.)

Assuming you do have some time to make your decisions, I encourage you to clear the room of all hired healthcare attendants, such as doctors, midwives, nurses, and doulas. (Importantly, however, doulas should be the last to leave the room, as this would give the doula and client [you] time to address any questions or concerns that remain. But if the doula is your singular support, then they should remain with you at all times. If you are partnered with a co-parent, you'll want to look to the doula for guidance but still ultimately have a few moments alone with just you and your partner. Creating space for the primary parents to have alone time to discuss the decision also provides some breathing room should the couple have any concerns about the doula, which can happen.) As a general rule, I believe the folks who will live with the consequences of their decisions should have a moment or more together for making their own birth intervention decisions. Clearing the space should also include any additional friends or family that may be in attendance.

Bear with me here as we continue to dive deeper into medical decision making. As I've mentioned in previous lessons, your doctor or midwife has a legal responsibility to obtain informed consent or refusal. Additionally, you (are supposed to) have further legal protections afforded by the U.S. Constitution. If someone touches you without permission, for example, then they should be held accountable by law: "A Battery is any physical contact with another person, to which that other person has not consented. An Assault is an attempt to commit a battery."[209] Loopholes and legalese notwithstanding, your body is your property. No one can touch you without your consent. With regard to your maternity care, this includes your nurse, midwife, doctor, husband, sister, mother, *anyone* who has been asked to stop or told "no" before or during any practice or procedure.

I lament that teaching medical decision-making tools is not a routine part of all healthcare, especially in maternity care. In my experience, these legal rights, with their inherent patient responsibilities, are rarely, if ever fully explained to the patient. How different our healthcare system might look if informed, medical decision-making were explained at the start of each new provider/client relationship. According to *A History and Theory of Informed Consent,* by Ruth R. Faden, Tom L. Beauchamp, and Nancy M. P. King, a provider is not supposed to coerce your decisions through fear or other tactics.[210] Your provider is not supposed to minimize known risks or inflate possible outcomes for any proposed treatment or condition. Your healthcare provider is not supposed to perform any tests or procedures or to administer any medications without your explicit informed consent. And yet, these things happen. I have witnessed risks being minimized, coercion being used, and outcomes inflated—including, as I described in the introduction of this book, a surgical incision made without discussion. I believe that by reading this book, and learning to ask useful questions during pregnancy and birth, you can help to protect yourself and, by extension, your baby.

The informed consent/informed refusal responsibility and accompanying legal arguments stem from past malpractice cases in the U.S. that have focused on whether a doctor has committed battery by doing something bad or without consent, or if negligence can be proven due to inaction or a failure to explain a practice, procedure, medication, risk, etc. before its administering. While I am not an attorney, the legal waters appear murky. The doctor's rights, the mother's rights, the concept of fetal rights, monetary pressure, and the obligations of corporate powers (not to mention the fear of lawsuits), all currently collide in a very messy intersection.

What consent forms are you signing when you enter the hospital for exams, to give birth, etc.? Does one broad consent form really get your provider off the hook for excluding you from decision-making processes? These are no simple questions to answer. But **educating yourself** and **speaking up** remain two of your most powerful tools to navigate the healthcare system and your own decision-making process. You can and should bring whatever conversations you want to the table during your prenatal visits. Likewise, and just as important, if you have already consented to something, you can change your mind and postpone or withdraw your consent at any time.

I do believe that one should enter the provider/client relationship with the assumption that our healthcare providers are good people who want to help and are trying their best to do what is right. Sadly, however, real life in healthcare reveals people frequently being coerced into compliance. Our healthcare providers in the U.S. are under a lot of economic and legal pressure; they can't always see or enact the empathetic or ethical perspective. For example, a woman shared with me that her doctor said to her in labor, "I have to rupture your membranes or the baby can't come out." This is a false statement. Babies can be and are born without artificial rupture of membranes. It unsettles me equally to consider that a doctor wouldn't have cared or that she wouldn't have known that she was making a false statement. In other words, did she knowingly mislead her patient because she wanted to rupture the membranes, in the hope that the birth could be sped up (and thus obtaining consent might be easier if the patient thought it were necessary)? Or, is our medical education so woefully inadequate that the doctor did not understand this basic fact of birth? Either scenario is disconcerting and underscores my strong recommendation for patients to educate themselves as healthcare consumers.

In fact, if you'll permit this quick, but illustrative digression, with amniotomy (the artificial rupture of membranes), once the membranes are ruptured, the risk of infection is increased. Additionally, if the baby is still up high in the pelvis when an amniotomy is performed, then there is an increased risk for a prolapsed umbilical cord (when the umbilical cord comes out of the vagina before the baby does.) This is dangerous and likely leads to emergency surgery, which adds numerous unexpected, rapid decision-making factors to the birth process. Meanwhile, although rupturing the membranes may or may not work to speed up a labor, many maternal healthcare providers maintain strict time limits during labor, which in turn can lead to a cascade of interventions from the moment of membrane rupture: 1) IV fluids; 2) antibiotics; 3) Pitocin, which will in turn come with continuous electronic fetal monitoring, restricted diet, and then possibly a fourth intervention: cesarean section.[211]

To return to the aforementioned example of the patient-doctor interaction, no risks or alternatives were presented to the patient in combination with the announcement. In fact, the doctor did not even ask her for consent; rather, she abruptly informed her patient of what will happen. Clearly, being lied to infringes upon a patient's right to make an informed decision. In this case, the woman who shared this story with me had not covered informed decision-making, amniotomy, or birth-in-the-caul (i.e., being born within an intact amniotic sac) in her birth class. If she had, as you are now, she might have been better able to call out her doctor on the false statement and engage in a productive conversation about alternatives.

Prior to pregnancy many expectant people are young, healthy, and have had very little interaction with the medical system and its complicated legal, ethical, and financial networks. This lack of experience and education leaves people vulnerable to potential civil rights infringements. Additionally, poverty and racial discrimination, the usual suspects for civil rights infringements, further add to the risk of maternity rights abuses and bodily harm. (Of note: babies of Color treated by physicians of Color are statistically more likely to survive compared to non-White babies being cared for by White providers.[212] The same may well be true for the gestational parent.)

To protect yourself, start by asking your care provider for information and stand firm on your need to be educated and respected and to participate in your healthcare decisions. For example: What is your provider's and your local hospital's protocol in relation to consent forms and informed medical decision-making? As I see time and again, a person will enter the hospital in labor and then be given vaginal exams, IV fluids, and electronic fetal monitoring. They will be denied food and they may even have their membranes stripped or undergo an episiotomy, all ostensibly under the general consent forms signed at the start. It is understood by hospital staff that the initial consent that was signed covers everything, which effectively takes away any need for the hospital staff to discuss your care options with you. This, in turn, makes it much more difficult to question individual routines. If you find yourself in this situation, remember: *you can retract your consent at any time*, for any given procedure, drug, test, or practice, and you can also choose to postpone consent until a later time. If you need more information, such as research that proves improved outcome, ask for it!

Over the years I have had clients report that they were made to feel that routine IVs, electronic monitoring, vaginal exams, and being denied food were procedures to which they *must* submit—as if the word "routine" were synonymous with "have to." It's not. My clients generally start off believing that the use of these routines has been scientifically proven to improve the safety of gestational parent and baby. But as I have already begun to explore (and will continue to demonstrate in what follows), interventions come with known associated risks. None of these seemingly normalized standards of care, e.g., IV fluids, electronic fetal monitoring, denial of food, and frequent vaginal exams, are actively improving fetal or maternal outcome in the United States. If they did, we might very well rank much higher in international standings.

So where does this information on informed consent leave you? You have some important homework to do:

- Talk to your providers and talk to other providers specifically about informed consent and informed refusal and standard care practices.
- Take hospital tours. Even if you are planning a home birth it is good to see where you would transport, if needed.
- Ask questions.
- Discuss decision-making expectations.
- Ask if there is a Patient's Bill of Rights and any consent forms ahead of time.
- Discuss routines and your rights to refuse or postpone them.

During birth is not the time to try to focus on paperwork or to question standards of care. Use your pregnancy wisely and build a confident and trusting relationship with your care provider(s) early on.

Birth Plans

What are they? As I have witnessed, over the last three decades, people interested in natural birth have been writing documents that outline what routines they would like to avoid and what coping measures they would like to implement. The intent of this document is to help people influence the care they receive. Typically, a person writes the document and then discusses it with their doctor or midwife. Once agreement is reached the final version of the document is added to the birthing person's medical chart. This addition to the chart then alerts the hospital staff that your provider has seen and approved these guidelines as acceptable. "Birth plan," therefore, is the common vernacular for a document that a gestational person (and their partner, if they have one) can write and share with their provider to clarify their desires for care during birth. Generally, people planning a hospital birth are the ones who write birth plans, because those planning home births assume that individualized care is inherent in the homebirth model. A birth plan, by definition, aims to foster individualized care. Some people planning homebirths do still write birth plans, in the event that they transfer to hospital.

There are real limitations to a birth plan. Although it presents a set of guidelines, your birth plan is not legally binding. It does not lay out medical directives. Instead, it articulates the wishes of the patient should the birth process go "according to plan." With this in mind, some care providers are very receptive to such documents while others feel disdain. Providers who like them know that involving the patient in shared medical decision-making improves patient satisfaction and reduces lawsuits. Providers who dislike such birth documents generally feel defensive, insulted, undervalued, and burdened.

We do need to ask ourselves: is it wise to give directions to medical professionals? The answer, in my experience, leaves room for interpretation: no, yes, and maybe! It depends on your providers, what they are suggesting, and your relationship with them. It also depends on your level of childbirth education. As you think about whether or not you want to write a document for your medical chart, consider this additional insight: Some nurses and their superiors make the stereotypical judgment that anyone with a birth plan is a control freak and doomed to a cesarean section. Yikes! But let's look at it from their point of view. Imagine that I show up at your job and make suggestions about how you should do your work. How might you feel? How many births have you been to? This is why I consistently recommend talking with your provider ahead of time about their planning and preparations and their feelings toward birth plans. If they say a birth plan is a good idea, ask them what elements they like to include (and not include) and why. If they say a birth plan is a bad idea, ask them to explain thoroughly why this is so. If you don't love their answers in either case, you may want to consider interviewing other providers.

Are birth plans well named? Another issue to consider (again) is that you cannot plan a birth. Trying to plan how your labor will unfold is like nailing Jell-O® to the wall; it's a lesson in futility. We cannot control the birth process any more than we can ultimately control our providers and hospital staff (and, eventually, our children). In other words, a birth plan is not a script. Nevertheless, a birth plan can help you to clarify your own expectations for your own care. It can act as another support tool as you navigate through the hospital-care machine. Finding agreement on your birth plan between you and your provider, well ahead of your actual birth, can help you to build a foundation of trust and open communication. It can create a positive and strong foundation on which to perform the amazing improvisation that will be your labor and your baby's birth. For these reasons, I much prefer the idea and title of a "birth values statement" or "expectations for care" in place of "birth plan." Words matter, as I've stated before. However, in this case, "birth plan" remains the less wordy and more readily known articulation industry-wide, so it's probably best to stick with it—knowing all that it can and can't accomplish. (If you can think of a better document title, please use it and pass it on!)

Should you write a birth plan? I once had one couple write a birth plan that was a single block paragraph that articulated their understanding of their own legal rights to informed consent and refusal. This presents more of an exceptional example to the typical birth plans I've seen, which look to reduce the use of unnecessary medical intervention, facilitate continuous contact (including rooming in) with the baby after birth, and to communicate the gestational parent's wants/needs. A birth plan therefore often includes the birthing person's support requests, such as music, water, dim lights, food, massage, positive words, large birth balls, extra pillows, etc., as well as (for example) their desire for their baby to be exclusively breastfed and whether or not to delay routine newborn tests and procedures, like a newborn bath or eye drops. Ask yourself now if you would benefit from writing a birth plan and what you might include in it.

For an important perspective *against* writing a birth plan, check out Pam England's *Birthing from Within*.[213] England argues that writing a birth plan demonstrates that you do not fully trust or agree with the practices of those who will be attending you, and that you likewise do not fully accept the standards associated with the location (hospital) you have chosen. As a result, she suggests that, instead of writing a birth plan, the more productive work would be to seek out providers and a location that you truly do trust. Or, rather than working on a document that attempts to control or dictate care, perhaps your time would be better spent strengthening your ability to advocate for yourself, and working through whatever fears and other emotions are related to your surrendering to the birth process and your new responsibilities of parenthood.

Writing a document can expose you. It can expose your level of education, your concerns, and maybe even your attempt at control. At the same time, however, I believe that a birth plan or other such document can be a useful tool for making some unnecessary routines go away, such as IV fluids or a newborn bath soon after childbirth. It can demonstrate to your hospital staff that you do understand the birth process and that your choices are your responsibility and well within your legal rights. In short, a birth plan may be the most useful as a communication tool, revealing that you have discussed the issues contained therein with your provider and that you wish these guidelines to be followed by all care providers who work with you during your birth process.

If you determine that you do want to write a birth plan, then the next step is to continue to learn about the routine hospital and provider practices to which you will be exposed. Knowing the difference between when something is ordered/offered because it is simply a routine or because it is indicated for your specific care can be extremely helpful as you navigate the choices that await you in birth. It will also be helpful to examine and prioritize your feelings about each of the possible interventions.

Please also keep in mind that many hospitals now offer a birth plan template, a form letter that includes pre-populated choices with check boxes. If your hospital uses such a template, I suggest taking it as a starting point and then writing your own document with your priorities highlighted at the top of the page.

As I have mentioned, you'll want to communicate comfort measures and coping strategies that you anticipate being helpful, because this will enable you to better direct your care. Including what you want, and not only focusing on routines to avoid, can help you to set a positive course. The work of envisioning your best possible birth can be an effective guide for you. If you can dream it, does that help you get there? I think, yes. I would argue that establishing what you value about your birth process is different than trying to control your birth. Your only real control is in the choice of who will support you, what location you pick, and how you care for yourself—including what messages you give to yourself about your birth process. Additionally, it is important to remember that how much you learn and what you prioritize remain within your control. Educating yourself on healthy birth, hospital routines, and common interventions is paramount to communicating effectively with your team. All of these factors will impact your ability to open your vagina wide and let your baby out.

A typical birth plan creation process might go something like this:

1. Figure out how you plan to cope with the challenges of birth.

2. Learn about your provider's and your hospital's routines.

3. Evaluate the evidence that supports these routines and how you feel about each routine.

4. Prioritize your desires and concerns.

5. Write up a first draft.

I encourage people to start with something that resembles a grocery list of things you want to happen and things you don't want to happen, and then go from there. Use the space below to take some additional notes:

Once you have something written you'll want to share it with your provider at an upcoming appointment. Let your practice know ahead of time that you would like dedicated time to review your birth plan document. Be mindful that it may be better for them to make a separate appointment for this discussion. That is the respectful way to ensure that you and your provider can have the necessary time to focus on this specific element. (If your talk time occurs during an appointment that includes a physical exam, please make sure you are fully clothed for your discussion. This can help provide an added level of comfort and confidence.) It is common in this discussion that some expectations will need clarification and that some differences in perspective may need to be hashed out. Hopefully you can find agreement and you can proceed to the final draft. If you really cannot find a place where everyone feels comfortable, then it's time—if options exist—to interview other practitioners. I am always in favor of second opinions, if you can obtain them.

When the final draft of your birth statement is ready, it should be reviewed by your provider and then become a formal part of your medical chart. Many people have also found it helpful to bring extra paper copies of their birth plan with them to the hospital, for added comfort and just in case the document somehow went missing from their chart. Some providers will sign the document and others will not. It's not legally binding one way or the other, but a signature can help to assure the nursing staff that you have your provider's support.

When writing your document please pay close attention to the tone and language you use. The words you choose will be your personal introduction to the staff. It is fine to be bold and strong. It is also fine to be brief or extremely wordy. It is *not* necessary to ask permission for what you want. You are making a statement that expresses your understanding about how best to support you, your values and expectations. So say whatever you want to say, how you want to say it. This is to be your personal document and it is not anyone's job to tell you what to include. All that being said, there are some specifics you may want to be sure to include. For example, I recommend employing a respectful, strong tone, rather than a controlling one. I also suggest that if you don't want pain medications, include that you don't want anyone to *offer* you the pain medications. The hospital has drugs, if you want them you can ask for them. Meanwhile, as I've discussed previously (in Week 10), having the medications offered to you can potentially undermine your confidence. Therefore, if one of your goals includes not using pain meds, then it is imperative to be bold and forceful with your language: **Do not offer pain medications.**

I recently had a woman report that during her labor, after she had told her nurse that she did not want to take any pain medication, the nurse left the room. Moments later the anesthesiologist came in to find out *why* the patient didn't want any pain medications. In my opinion, the explanation was unnecessary in the first place and the doctor's insistence on its discovery could feel akin to coercion (as it did for the woman who shared her account), or at the very least make the patient second-guess their decision while in labor. I am lingering on the particular suggestion around including a "no pain meds" statement in your birth plan because the pro-pain-medication force in healthcare is strong, *very* strong.

There is a general culture of anesthesia that does not include the question, "Do you want medication?" Any such question is more likely to be articulated or implied as, "Are you ready for your medication?" As an example, take a look at the obstetric anesthesiology webpage from the NYU Medical Center, a large teaching hospital in New York City.[214] As of 2022, it states that, "Each year, nearly 6,000 women give birth at Tisch Hospital, and more than 80 percent receive epidural pain relief for labor. Among first-time mothers, more than 90 percent choose epidurals."[215] Teaching hospitals, in particular, do have a unique culture of their own, but they help set the broader cultural tone with their teachings. If you want to take ownership in your decision to medicate or not, ask yourself how you might react by an offer of drugs and/or knowing that most first-time mothers apparently "choose epidurals." It is helpful, if planning a hospital birth, to look into the culture of your hospital.

Another important factor to consider in this discussion is the real presence of racial disparity in pain management. From a 2020 article by the American Association of Medical Colleges, Janice A. Sabin, Ph.D., M.S.W, writes:

> False ideas about Black peoples' experience of pain can lead to worrisome treatment disparities. In the 2016 study [published in the *Proceedings of the National Academies of Science*], for example, [medical] trainees who believed that Black people are not as sensitive to pain as White people were less likely to treat Black people's pain appropriately.[216]

If you, dear reader, are a person of Color, then it is also imperative for you to have a discussion with your provider in advance of your birth about how best to access any pain medications should you desire them during your labor. Then include this discussion in your birth plan.

Choosing to use or reject pain medications

Your study of pain medications begins with you. Your feelings, intuition, and preferences are the foundation of any sound medical decision. Figuring out how you feel about pain medication (before labor begins) is a critical exploration if you are planning a hospital birth. Pain medications are generally unavailable for homebirths. However, it is still useful if you are planning a homebirth, because one can never be sure they won't need or want to transfer to a hospital.

In my classes and here in this book, I choose to delve into the feelings around pain medications before we get to the facts: specific options, routes of administration, risks and benefits; that's all coming next week.

But first, it's time to see where you are at now. Do you have any biases, fears or pressures about pain medications that weigh on you?

What do you already think about how drugs affect you?

Are you comfortable or uncomfortable with altered mental states that can come from pain medications, alcohol, or cannabis (for example)?

From past experiences do you think you are very susceptible to the affects or do you think of yourself as having a high tolerance?

Do you have judgements—good or bad—about the use of pain medications in labor?

If there is a primary partner, what are their feelings about the use of pain medications for labor?

Share with yourself and your partner (out loud or on paper) what you anticipate it might feel like for you to tell your birth story to your family or friends. Set the hypothetical scene by visualizing yourself after birth, holding your healthy baby while you share the details of how the birth unfolded. And then you get to the part of the story where you share that you made the decision to get an epidural. Can you anticipate how that part of the story might feel? As of today, right now, knowing as little or as much as you may know about the specifics, please try to answer this hypothetical question: *If you were sharing your birth story, holding your baby, how do you anticipate feeling about your use of pain medication?*

Over my 28 years of teaching (and counting!), I have heard a variety of responses to the above question. Generally, however, the answers fall into two categories:

1. Some people anticipate feeling fine about their decision. They usually express confidence that if their story turns out to include pain medications it was because all else had been tried first, but further support was deemed necessary.

2. Others describe anticipated challenges in that scenario. For those who imagine that it would be a hard story to tell, they speak of disappointment. They describe a sense of loss, akin to a feeling of not having achieved a goal. Many of these people answer that they think they would judge themselves harshly, that they wouldn't have been strong, capable, or brave enough to follow through without pain medication. For some who anticipate disappointment, they expect that their negative feelings would be because of their own inadequacy. For others they anticipate that their disappointment would be directed toward their care provider and/or the failure of the hospital to provide adequate care. And a small percentage of people have said that they could anticipate feeling a sense of shame and failure so great that they wouldn't even want to share their story if they do end up using medications.

Admittedly, these last responses break my heart. I do not see the use of pain medication as any kind of failure. I understand that each of us is trying to make our own best choices, given whatever circumstances we face, at the moment that we have to decide. I decided to write this book *because* I want people to be able to feel good about making their best-informed choices. If you have done your homework, which you are indeed doing, in part, by simply reading this book (and which you can build upon with an in-person class near you, if you choose), then I am confident that you will have many good approaches and tips to try for natural coping techniques and a good decision-making process. I am also confident that you will not only be able to endure your birth, but that you may also even find pleasure in it—with or without medications.

For those of you who know that you want to use pain medications, please also practice non-medicated pain relief techniques. In the event your medications do not work (which can happen) or your anesthesiologist is delayed in getting to you, these techniques can be helpful to try. Overall, it's good to have options. And we should be conscientious in our decision making, for it is each of us that will live with the consequences of our choices.

What follows are questions useful to explore prior to birth, and then again in labor, in order to help you make conscientious decisions around medication use:

○ How does the gestational parent feel prior to birth and about their own use of pain meds during birth? (Although it is the pregnant person who makes the final decision, it is also useful to discover and consider a primary partner's feelings and attitudes in response to this question, as well as if/how those feelings contribute to the decision-making process.)

○ What is available? (What types of drugs are available and what are their routes of administration?)

○ What are the known risks associated with what's available?

○ Are there benefits to using pain medications? If so, what are they?

○ Are pain medications ever medically necessary? If so, when?

If you, the pregnant person, knows prior to birth that you don't want to use pain meds, but then once in labor you change your mind, ask yourself (or discuss with a support person in advance to ask you): why now? What is it about what is going on right now, physically and emotionally, that is making me change my mind? Am I comfortable with my caretakers? How am I feeling about the emotional, physical and mental support I'm receiving or not receiving? What, specifically, are my physical sensations? Where am I with my emotions? Am I feeling strong or weak, determined or unsure, capable or overwhelmed? Am I feeling pain, exhaustion, low confidence, frustration, anger, or fear? Am I hoping to medicate something going on right now? Or am I more concerned about what I'm expecting up ahead? Addressing some of these questions may lead to support solutions that don't call for medication. Answers to the above questions can also help a support person redirect or reframe the birthing person's thinking and help them to find stamina. And, certainly, sometimes by exploring these questions the answer becomes without-a-doubt clear: it is *now*, now is the time for medication! Teasing out your feelings is your best clue to identifying and receiving the most appropriate form(s) of support. Knowing your feelings prior to birth and then being conscientious in your decision process can help to empower you in the moment and preserve confidence for your birth memories.

To more fully understand the thoughts, values, influences, and circumstances that weigh on your decision to use or not to use pain meds, it is helpful to consider them in the context of where they primarily exist: the hospital. In what follows I am going to walk you through an imagined hospital door and guide you through an exploration of some of the most common hospital procedures that you are likely to encounter as admissions routines (read: standards of care for everyone with the same diagnosis, such as a healthy person in labor) as well as some potential concerns surrounding the use of these routines. This information is also important to you, dear reader, even if you are planning a homebirth because as I mentioned, you never know if you might end up transferring to a hospital mid labor.

In next week's lesson, Week 12, we will take a deeper dive into the nuts and bolts of pain medications, bolstered by this broader perspective through which to think about your choices.

EXERCISE: STRETCH BREAK

If you've been sitting or reclining in bed while reading, consider first stretching out through your fingers and toes and then rotate your ankles a few times. Then stand up and do some whole-body stretching. Open up the sides, front, and back of your body. Include deep breaths in and out, and tune into your breathing rhythm. Feel your body. Feel your feelings. How are you right now? Please try not to judge your feelings, just tap into them, notice them, feel them, and accept that this is how you are feeling *right now*. Nothing more, nothing less.

—Pause to move and breathe—

Walking in the hospital door

When planning for a hospital birth, it's helpful to prepare to cope with myriad standard interruptions and interventions. So much stuff happens once you walk through that hospital door: hallways and elevators full of other people, insurance questions, medical history, blood work, fetal monitoring, changing into the hospital gown, IV access, vaginal exam, etc. All of this includes needing to interact with several different people, multiple times, the "routine" of which can pose significant interruption to the natural-physiological birth process.

As early in your pregnancy as you can, I encourage you to find out exactly what will be expected of you at your planned birth location. (Again, even if you are planning a home birth, it is still important to understand what goes on in the hospital because there are no guarantees that a planned home birth wouldn't have to transfer to a hospital. Therefore, having an awareness of hospital routines and culture prior to your birth is just good preparation.) Once you gather these expectations, consider closely what your best options are, or if there are any other choices that need to or can be made.

If you have any doubts about where you are planning to birth and you do have (or at least think you have) alternatives, then I *always* encourage you to investigate your other options as fully as possible before you make any final decisions. This work helps you feel good about walking in the door. You can change your mind more than once if you need to. If you don't have any alternatives accessible, use your time to strategize ways to minimize the impact of the parts that you don't like. Of course, if, after your investigation, you are feeling good about your birth location—excellent! But still look to mitigate interruptions and any "extra" work from your admission process. Is there paperwork you can take care of in advance? Do they have a refrigerator you can use for your snacks? Knowing what to expect when you walk in the door helps you to walk in with confidence. It comes down to doing your homework. As I've said before (and will say again!): this will all help you to make your birth experience as comfortable and empowering as you can for yourself and your baby.

The hospital gown (or, as it's sometimes called, "Johnny")

It's called a "Johnny," at least in part, because it provides for easier toileting on "the john" (a once-common name for "toilet"). The hospital gown is a rarely questioned—if even noticed—intervention, which is precisely why I'm going to take a moment here to discuss it! I think it's best to plan to wear your own clothes in labor. Hospital gowns are what sick people wear. And who really knows how they are meant to be worn? (Are you supposed to leave the open part in the back or the front? Different medical practices have different preferences, which can also change according to procedure.) At the time of the baby's final descent you are likely to end up completely naked, because birthing is hot-sweaty-hard work and you can't have any underpants on or the baby will be held in. But earlier in the labor, when you are likely still to be dressed to at least some degree, I highly recommend that you skip the gown and wear your own clothes. Speak up. What you're wearing can influence your mood. Pick colors you love and go for comfort, practicality, and good (even sexy) feelings.

Intravenous (IV) fluids

IV fluids are prescribed for hydration, in order to maintain fluid levels or to replace lost fluids.[217] IV fluid is made up of water with salts added (sodium and potassium). Dextrose (sugar) can be added depending on medical circumstances and the managing providers' orders. The fluids are administered through a plastic catheter inserted into your vein that is generally placed either on the inside of the forearm or through the back of the hand.[218] The catheter is inserted by needle, taped down, and attached to tubing that hooks up to a bag that holds the fluids. The bag often hangs from a pole that is on a stand on wheels. The amount of fluid given is controlled by a flow monitor (usually computerized) attached to the tubing. Other medications can be added directly into the same tubing and vein access, should they become useful.

Administration of IV fluids is typically one of the first medical interventions given to a person who shows up at the hospital in labor. The routine order for IV fluids has, for generations, also meant that a person would be restricted from eating food or drinking liquid. ("NPO," which stands for Non-Per-Os, which translates to "nothing by mouth.") Thankfully, this unfounded and potentially dangerous policy of food and liquid restriction is changing.

The fear has been that if there is food in your belly and the doctor needs to put you under a general anesthesia (for an emergency c/section, for example), then you could potentially vomit and inhale the vomit; this would be very dangerous indeed. However, people with food in their stomachs do get emergency surgery if they need it. In recent years, anesthesiologists have admitted that there is no basis for them to deny healthy gestational people food or drink in labor.[219] If you are hungry, you should eat. If you are thirsty, you should drink. Yes, you may throw up. But remember that the act of vomiting might actually help your birth progress.

If IV fluids are a routine intervention, and, as we have previously discussed, an intervention is a tool, then your educational goals should help you to determine when such a tool is helpful and when it might cause trouble. If you are low on fluids when you arrive at the hospital, or if you become dehydrated at any time, then you will feel and function so much better once you get some fluid into you. But if you are managing to drink oral fluids and haven't been vomiting a lot, then you may choose to refuse an IV, unless or until some other circumstances develop that could change your decision (such as becoming dehydrated or if you choose to take pain medications, which are delivered intravenously). Note that refusing an IV upon admittance to the hospital does not mean that you cannot get one later if you need one. What it does do is change the routine practice of IV application to one based on how you are developing through the circumstances of your labor.

IV fluids appropriately used are a great use of science. IV fluids, used in conjunction with the patient being allowed to drink additional fluids by mouth, have been shown to decrease the actual length of labor by about 25 minutes. Clearly, being hydrated is important. By the same token, it is also important to note that there have been no studies that look specifically at IV vs. no IV use in labor. Existing studies looked only at IV fluids *with* additional fluids by mouth vs. IV fluids *without* additional fluids by mouth. And interestingly (but not surprisingly), current studies also have not included any measure for patient satisfaction.[220]

Provider-client conversations about routine orders, such as IV fluids, are best held well ahead of actual labor and then again during labor, as necessary. If disagreements exist, seek second opinions and do further research. If you receive push back from a nurse or a resident while you are in labor, politely ask to speak to your provider or the attending provider directly.

To help you think through your decision to accept or deny routine IV fluids upon arrival at the hospital in labor, ask yourself this: Are you generally capable of keeping yourself hydrated? Yes, of course you are. Will that automatically change once you get to the hospital? If your answer is no, that doesn't have to change, then please commit to continue to keep yourself consistently hydrated. You will also want to think about this: In addition to fluids, an IV line provides easy access for medications to be added, such as antibiotics, narcotics, and oxytocic drugs (drugs that stimulate contractions.) Also keep in mind that an IV can be administered at any point when other interventions become needed. And, IV fluids are a required intervention when an epidural is going to be used. In this case, the IV is used to help stabilize your blood pressure, which the epidural might cause to destabilize. Plus, if an emergency arises, an IV can be placed quickly. Emergency surgery, for example, is done all the time on people with no previous IV in place. It is my opinion that if a person needs an IV, then they should get one at the time that they need one.

IV's sometimes hurt, not just at the moment they are inserted but with a constant dull ache at the needle location. IV's can also complicate a person's ability to move freely, and this can be a factor to complicate labor. As we discussed and practiced in previous weeks' lessons, babies generally benefit from a birthing parent's positional changes. But the gestational person is less likely to move around and accommodate their own sensations if they are tethered by an IV attached to an IV stand. As a result, many people report feeling stress due to the IV application itself (maybe you also have a fear of needles?)—and we know that excess stress can interfere with the person's birth hormones and distort their natural process. At the same time, some people report feeling comfort from getting an

IV because it gives them a sense of protection and a feeling that hospital staff are contributing to their safety. How do you think you might feel to have an IV in your arm? Should you feel that a routine IV might be useful for you, please engage in a conversation with your provider about how much IV fluids might be beneficial and how much might be too much, and what too much might mean. "There is no consensus on acceptable maternal oral intake or need for intravenous fluids during an uncomplicated labor."[221] In sum, different obstetric practices may prescribe different amounts of fluid over different periods of time for a gestational parent (and their baby) to receive during labor, so it is important to open this discussion early.

If too much fluid is given (overhydration) it can cause severe swelling for the gestational parent and an artificially high birth weight for the newborn. Inflated birth weight for the infant can cause a cascade of problems. Typically, a newborn loses weight over their first day of life outside the womb.[222] Pediatricians acknowledge that a newborn can lose up to 10% of her birth weight and be considered healthy and normal. However, if a baby has absorbed too much IV fluid from her gestational parent, then her birth weight will be elevated and the normal weight loss can seem larger than expected.[223] An unexpectedly high newborn weight loss can result in an admission to the neonatal intensive care unit (NICU), which may also include the administration of formula. These "fixes" to the iatrogenic problem (caused by too much IV fluid) will surely cause excess stress, which will in turn impede the gestational parent's endocrine system from releasing the oxytocin and prolactin they need to control their own bleeding, retract their uterus, and increase their milk production—and all of this is stressful for the baby, too, which complicates bonding.

Another concern with the use of an IV is that it can reduce the amount of emotional support a birthing person may receive. Many a partner can be squeamish or insecure about hugging a birthing person for fear of getting caught on the IV and causing harm. In addition, the psychology of the association between IVs and illness can mean that the people who are caring for a laboring person with an IV may confuse the fact that they are a healthy person birthing and not sick. The IV can also confuse the laboring person themself about the fact that they are not sick.

One more aspect to consider: the option of an "IV port." This is a procedure that places an IV catheter into your arm and then caps off the entrance port, leaving it ready to use at a later time. (This is also called a heparin lock, heparin well, hep lock, or hep port.) An IV port is frequently offered to a birthing person who resists routine IV fluids.[224] The IV port may not restrict movement like a full IV because the person is not tethered to the tubing, bag of fluid, and pole on a stand with wheels. Nevertheless, it can be equally uncomfortable, discourage mobility, reduce emotional support, and relate a sense of illness or impending danger. In one of my classes, a student spoke up: "But my doctor said if I were to rapidly go into shock my veins could collapse and then they wouldn't be able to get an IV in." A paramedic in the class replied, "If someone needs access, we gain access. I don't want to gross you out, but we get IV access in dead people." In a true emergency, if any healthcare provider is having trouble getting an IV started, then they will "call a code" over the hospital loudspeaker (or call an ambulance) and emergency staff swoops in to help. Depending on their training, an emergency healthcare provider will either get the IV into the arm or they will insert what's called "a central line" or "central venous catheter," gaining access through the jugular vein in your neck. Still more, the provider can consider another procedure that goes directly into your bone, called Intraosseous (IO) Cannulation: "Establishing an IO route for vascular access allows medications and fluids to enter the central circulation within seconds."[225]

Our country's emergency personnel are, for the most part, very well trained. Hospitals are where the emergency staff are continuously ready for action. Every day, across the country, people who have been seriously injured, become acutely sick, or suffer from chronic conditions are saved and/or administered supportive care by people who know how to get an IV access in when they have to.

While big bleeding emergencies might be scary to think about, it is also important to understand that healthy people in labor don't just rapidly or unexpectedly go into shock. They would have to have suffered some sort of trauma or have some underlying pathology or suffer from serious malnutrition. If you experience unexpected bleeding, or any significant blood pressure changes, dizziness, headache, or other medical development, including vomiting more than once or twice, and especially if you are also having diarrhea, then, of course, seek medical attention immediately. You will likely—and you should—get an IV. By the same token, if a gestational parent has fears about living through their birth, then it's possible that the administration of an IV port or IV fluids may be exactly the intervention to reduce their anxiety.

Take some breaths and check in with yourself: Do you have any of the fears related to IVs or emergency care?

Fetal monitoring in labor

During labor the baby's heart tones are routinely monitored to try and prevent problems related to oxygen deprivation and stillbirth. For decades it has been believed that oxygen deprivation during birth caused cerebral palsy (CP); thus, if providers could monitor enough, then they could prevent that harm. Now scientists understand that the majority of cases of CP happen before birth begins, are likely the result of a congenital abnormality, and that monitoring with cardiotocography (CTG)—first called electronic fetal monitoring (EFM)—has a false-positive rate for CP that is 99.8%.[226] This exceedingly high false-positive rate leads to an increase in operative births (cesarean section, forceps, and vacuum extractions). It also appears that this monitoring does not reduce stillbirths, admission to NICUs, or lower Apgar scores. (Some researchers feel that the relationship between stillbirth and monitoring is at best inconclusive and needing more research.[227]) There are no studies that have looked at monitoring vs. not monitoring. The research thus far has all been on the use of CTG vs. intermittent auscultation (IC), which is hand-held monitoring done with a doppler ultrasound or a fetoscope (a modified non-electric stethoscope). My takeaway on this subject is that we are clearly not saving enough babies with this technology or the evidence would be more evident. Meanwhile, the standard of care in hospital continues to be CTG, likely because it helps a provider or hospital protect themselves should they be sued.[228]

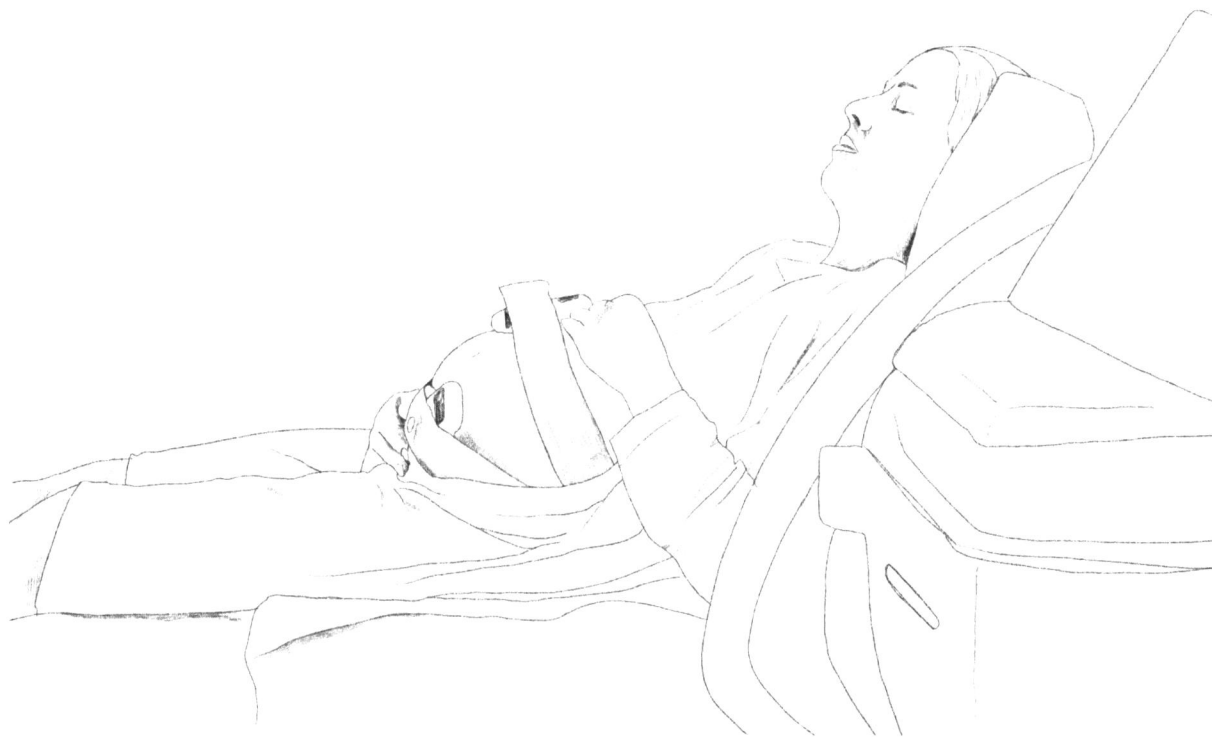

In home births, providers use a variety of hand-held devices, including fetoscopes or doppler ultrasound. In hospital, providers *can* choose from a variety of tools for fetal monitoring, but the standard of care is cardiotocography.: "cardio" means "heart," "toco" relates to "contractions," and "graphy" means to "record". CTG therefore spells out what the device does: it measures and records the fetal heart tones (FHT) and the uterine contractions and provides a paper tracing of the recorded information allowing one to see what the fetal heart rate is before, during, and after a contraction. CTG provides for a more specific definition than EFM (electronic fetal monitoring), which could be interpreted to mean any device that uses electricity. In practice, the label EFM is still used regularly, and you may find the terms being used interchangeably with your provider and occasionally here in this book. As described in Week 1, the CTG machine itself consists of a computer base and two hockey-puck like sensors. The puck-sensors get placed on the pregnant person's belly, the sensors are held in place with straps, or occasionally taped down to the belly or held in place by a tube-top-type stretchy band placed over the abdomen. The sensors can be hand-held as well, but that is rare because it requires so much nursing time. One puck relies on ultrasound waves to read the baby's heart tones and the other is a pressure gauge that reads the strength and duration of the uterine contractions. The pucks are attached by cables to the computer base that can display, record digitally, and provide a paper print out of the image of the two lines of data next to each other. This is the data used by the provider to determine what the heart tones are doing in relationship to the contractions.

Knowing (read: interpreting) exactly how the fetus is responding to the contractions is an approach that was supposed to improve outcomes; however, the monitoring has not been shown to improve outcomes as scientists had hoped. In fact, the only clear reduction in harm that CTG is associated with is a reduction in fetal seizures. While seizure disorders are very rare, if you are worried about a seizure disorder (perhaps you have a medical history that includes seizure disorder, for example), then it may be very appropriate to your care. But given that use of CTG is the standard of care in hospital for *all* pregnant people, we have a case where the standard may not be appropriate for the majority. As I point out in my birth classes, if the United States was leading the world in maternity care outcomes, then we might joyfully embrace such standards of care. But given our track record, it is imperative that we question all care routines and make sure they place our needs front and center. Your care should be appropriate to your individual health history and your values. From her review on the evidence of routine EFM (CTG) Rebecca Dekker highlights this important reality:

> Standard of care does not mean best practice, and it also does not necessarily mean evidence-based practice. This catches doctors, nurses, and midwives in a catch-22: the use of EFM is not best practice for many women. However, if the baby has a bad health outcome, failure to produce an EFM strip as "proof" for the court can be seen as failure to meet the standard of care. The lack of an EFM recording increases the chance that the hospital will lose the lawsuit or have to settle the lawsuit, losing a large amount of money either way. EFM is a great example of how care that protects the interests of the care provider does not always protect the laboring person's best interests.[229]

This can understandably become so overwhelming to think about. To know what's going on in any instant seems like it could help improve our outcomes. But knowing isn't always actionable in positive ways. CTG/ EFM doesn't address the causes of fetal seizures; it also doesn't tell us anything about the impact of those seizures. What we do know about EFM/CTG is that it has a high false-positive rate for trouble, and this false-positive rate leads to a great number of cesarean sections, which are, in and of themselves, a very serious major abdominal surgery that presents increased risk for gestational parent and baby. (More on cesarean sections coming up in Week 13.) Research from the National Institute of Health in 2019, published by Health Services Research, found that the effectiveness of the monitoring technology in protecting babies remains an unanswered question:

> Despite this widespread use of EFM, particularly in the Western world, the efficacy of this technology remains controversial. This is particularly the case for our understanding of the impact of EFM on decreasing the risk of fetal death and fetal asphyxia…What is clear [is] that the use of EFM has led to an increase in the cesarean delivery rate since being introduced as a tool to assess fetal status at any point in time.[230]

While being monitored many people report that they felt stressed by not being able to move or change position for fear of dislodging one or both of the sensors. Others have mentioned that their care takers seemed more focused on the monitor than on them, the birthing person. And I once witnessed a woman looking to the monitor to see if the contraction she was having was a "big one" or not. I felt like I was witnessing a massive disconnect for that woman; a mind and body split as she deferred to the technology over her own immediate sensations. One concern I have is that because most pregnant people don't feel comfortable on their backs and most monitoring forces pregnant people onto their backs, the baby is essentially placed in the exact position that can cause pressure on the parent's major blood vessels—and this in turn could affect the monitoring that is occurring. Could the act of placing a pregnant person on their back, for example, create a situation that causes a "less than reassuring" fetal heart tone?

An alternative to using CTG would be to use Intermittent Auscultation (IA), with either a fetoscope or a handheld Doppler ultrasound device. As I mentioned previously, scientists do not yet fully understand if IA improves outcomes because there are no studies (yet) that look at monitoring vs. no monitoring. With IA there is no pressure gauge and no paper trace; one is just listening—typically during and immediately following a contraction—to determine how the baby recovers from the contraction.[231] This type of hand-held auscultation requires more time from the nursing staff.

> With hands-on listening, the nurse, midwife, or doctor actually has to be at the bedside of the laboring person every 15-30 minutes during the active phase of the first stage of labor and every 5-15 minutes during the pushing phase of the second stage of labor. Each time they use hands-on listening, they must take a minute to listen to the heart rate while palpating the mother's abdomen with their hand to feel for a contraction.[232]

While this extra time can be burdensome for the staff, it can be a plus for the laboring person. Hands-on listening provides for more freedom of movement in positioning. In addition, more regular connection with a birth attendant can help build a relationship and provide a more continuous and personal feeling of being cared for. Hands on listening is a more intimate experience. This intimacy can soothe and build trust between birthing person and birth attendant. When birthing people feel cared for and comfortable with the people around them, it is easier for them to cope with their physical experience. In other words, continuity of care not only feels better but improves outcome:

> Research shows that continuous support during childbirth is linked to a 25% decrease in the risk of Cesarean, an 8% increase in the likelihood of spontaneous vaginal birth, a 10% decrease in the use of any medications for pain relief, shorter labors by 41 minutes on average, and a 38% decrease in the baby's risk of a low five-minute Apgar score. One unexpected benefit of hands-on listening is that it requires caregivers to spend more time with the laboring mother—and their more frequent physical presence may actually lower pain and increase satisfaction for their patients.[233]

Of course, in real life, hospital staff are tasked with many responsibilities that take time and attention away from one-on-one caring. And training is another factor contributing to whether or not IA is available as an option for your care. As I have discussed with a variety of providers, many feel insecure about their listening skills as they have been reliant on the CTG technology for so many years. Like with all of your upcoming choices, you have your work cut out for you to evaluate what options you actually have and how you feel about their impact on your birth. The topic of CTG/EFM provides a good opportunity for you to engage in prenatal discussion with any prospective providers. If you have a provider insistent on CTG, or any other intervention, always feel empowered to ask them to provide you with the research in support of their recommendation.

> To make a fully informed choice, laboring people need to understand the potential risks and benefits of the different approaches to fetal monitoring. Evidence supports hands-on listening—a low-tech, high-touch approach—for people giving birth without known complications. Practice guidelines encourage the use of hands-on listening with low-risk people. However, hands-on listening is still not easily available in most hospitals. In many birth settings, low-risk people are still told that EFM (either continuous or intermittent) is required during labor. The reality is that there are system pressures in hospitals that limit doctors, midwives, and nurses from truly supporting birthing people. Too few nurses and increased computer duties (frequent charting for medical, legal, and insurance reasons) limit nurses' ability to perform hands-on listening.[234]

Please remember that you can (are supposed to be able to) consent, refuse, or postpone any care that you don't feel comfortable consenting to in the moment. It is also important to understand that with the use of any pain medications, as well as Pitocin or any other contraction-stimulating medications, continuous monitoring is indicated. Once you add drugs into the pregnant parent's body, it is necessary to watch for the fetal reactions; they don't always tolerate these drugs well and so then we need to watch closely and respond accordingly.

Now, take a deep breath in and exhale completely. Take a moment to remember that you have a strong and capable being growing inside you. Birth complications are tough things to think about. Take another deep breath in, and as you exhale focus on releasing negative stress and tuning into your growing baby. Imagine your baby happy and healthy. If we dwell on the worst things that can possibly happen it will be very hard to even get out of bed in the morning. Use the lessons you learn throughout this book as motivation to make thoughtful decisions. Control what you can control: good diet, adequate rest, exercise, etc. Seek out social support and maternity care providers that are respectful and honest. Try to grow a positive attitude. (Practice makes perfect!) Work to let go of what you can't control or don't need. Take another deep breath in... and exhale.

Your feelings, your circumstances, and your perspectives really matter. As you continue to learn and grow through your pregnancy you are likely to feel a variety of emotions in anticipation of your birth. Please honor your feelings, acknowledge them and work toward acceptance if you are not already there. When you can express your feelings through discussion, journaling, art, dance, sex, etc. you can know them better. Becoming better acquainted with your feelings can help you to release them, which, in turn, can help you to make room for the new feelings yet to come.

What possibilities lurk in the future for you? Maybe your birth can be pleasurable? Some people use the terms "ecstatic" and "orgasmic" to describe their birth experiences. Is the pain associated with labor a medical problem waiting to be fixed? Or part of the natural process? Do fears infect or worsen physical feelings? These are just some questions to linger on as you grow. Notice as you learn. Do your feelings change? Do new questions arise?

Congratulations on coming to the completion of another chapter. When you first put the book down, take some time to stretch and review labor positions. Take deep breaths and the time to settle into each position. When you are done, give yourself some love for taking these steps to care for yourself and your baby. Take good care this week: eat well, rest well, be active, and try to include some time in nature, even a teeny city park or a city roof top can help you to connect to the natural world around you. Try to tune into your feelings about medication and be compassionate with yourself and the people around you. Please give yourself a pat on the back, you are doing the great work of pregnancy! Hooray for getting this far.

Eat well, rest well, be active, and know that I am wishing you a great week!

HOMEWORK:

A) Birth Plans

Discuss written documents/birth plans with potential care providers.

B) Research your provider's routines

Further investigate your local provider's routine procedures, and if planning a hospital birth include research into that hospital's routine protocols for labor and delivery.

C) Examine your feelings about the use of pain medications for your birth

Further investigate your emotional responses to using or not using pain medications. Examine not only what your feelings are but also look at the messages you may be receiving from your family, friends, co-workers, and providers or from your culture.

THIS SPACE IS FOR YOUR NOTES AND DRAWINGS

THIS SPACE IS FOR YOUR NOTES AND DRAWINGS

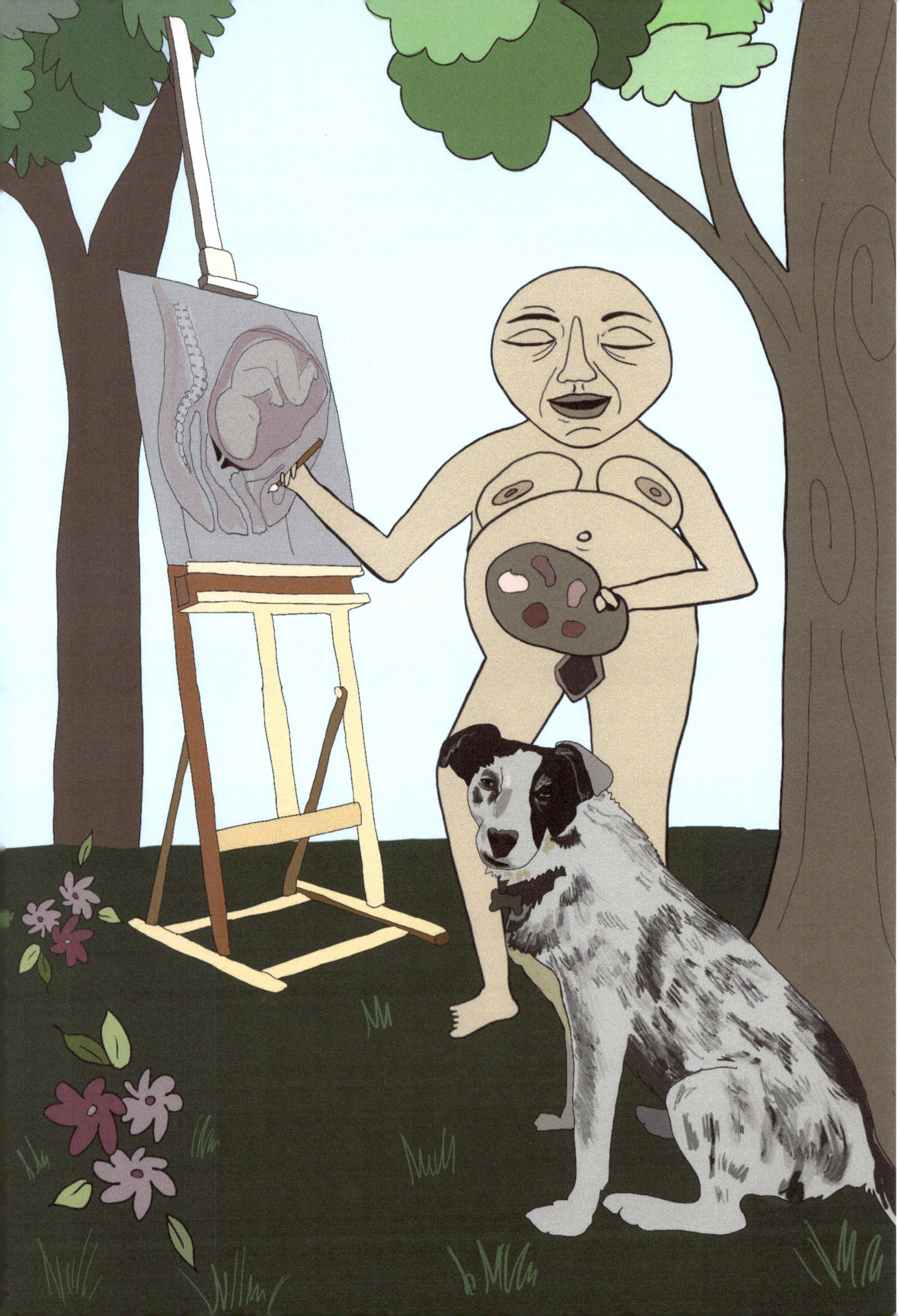

WEEK 12

Science and Your Nature

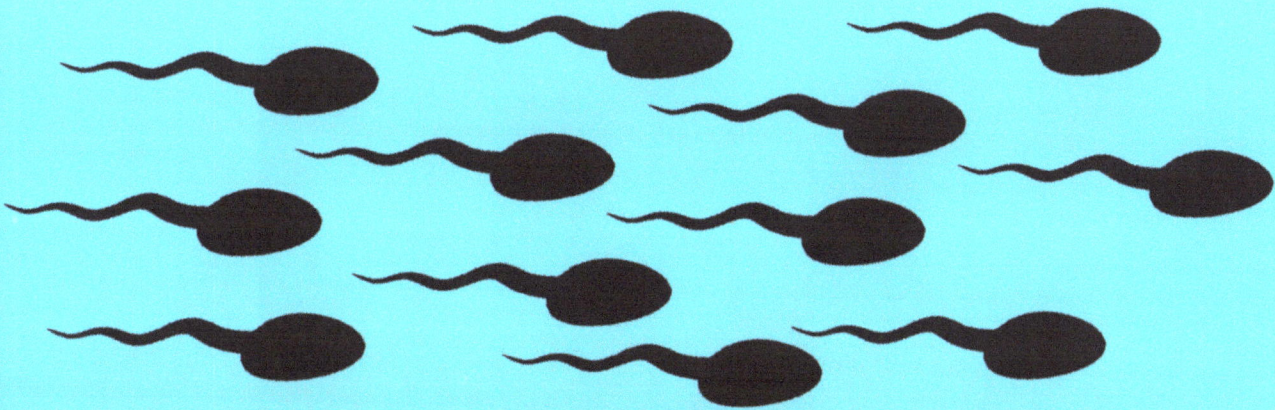

Chapter contents:

- *Analgesics and anesthesia*
- *Length of gestation*
- *Induction methods*
- *Induction decisions*

325

THIS SPACE IS FOR YOUR NOTES AND DRAWINGS

Welcome back, I hope your week has been a good one. If you were stressed, were you able to consider the stress as an opportunity to practice a relaxation response? If it didn't work out that way, that's okay. Continue to be compassionate with yourselves. At present, there remains now, later, and tomorrow to practice. Eventually, of course, you will run out of time before birth, so do make this practice a priority now. Practice will improve the effectiveness of conscientious relaxation, and relaxation will make your labor seem less painful.[235] Congratulations on picking this book back up, that is a great kind of self-care, too.

Given that last week's content included an exploration of feelings about pain meds, it is now time to learn about the evidence-based details of your options for medications and their associated risks. For it is only once you have sorted out your feelings and gathered all your facts, that you can make your best decisions.

What types of drugs will be available to you?

Exactly which drugs or combination of drugs will be available to you during your birth depends both on the hospital you go to and on individual provider preference. Because a lot of variation exists in this arena, not every drug option can be covered here. And the details of drug selection and mixing of these drugs likewise goes beyond the scope of this book. What this chapter focuses on are some of the most prevalent drugs that you are likely to encounter/be offered if you are in labor in a hospital. At the same time, this chapter will provide you with appropriate contextualizing information to increase your confidence and question-asking skills. No matter the specific drugs or combination of drugs, be sure to ask your maternity care provider to clarify their prescribing habits for pain management and to explain their relationship with the anesthesia department's prescribing practices. You may also want to research the possibility of having a consultation with an anesthesiologist early on in your pregnancy, even if you don't intend to use medications for pain. (Note: if you do have health insurance, this mid-pregnancy anesthesia consultation might be covered, with a bit of a push.) Your opinions and emotions may shift as you read. Remember you cannot really plan a birth. Continue to process your opinions and emotions as you forge ahead through your reading.

There are two broad categories of pain medications: **analgesics** and **anesthetics**. Analgesics are defined as "any drug that relieves pain selectively without blocking the conduction of nerve impulses, markedly altering sensory perception, or affecting consciousness."[236] Analgesics can be given by mouth, injection, or added by IV. The medication travels through your blood, including through your placenta.[237] Analgesics numb or cloud your perception of the pain. You still feel your contractions, but these types of drugs can turn down the volume of sensation or "soften the edge" of your feelings. Acetaminophen (Tylenol®) or a couple of martinis, for example, can have an analgesic affect, although neither of these come without their own risks. (I mention them here simply for means of comparison and illustration.) Some frequently prescribed analgesics include: Butorphanol (common brand name Stadol®) and Fentanyl. Analgesics can be, and frequently are, added to an epidural.[238] However, typically an epidural uses anesthesia (see below for this definition and explanation).

> **An anesthetic** is defined as:
> any agent that produces a local or general loss of sensation, including pain. Anesthetics achieve this
> effect by acting on the brain or peripheral nervous system to suppress responses to sensory stimula-

tion. The unresponsive state thus induced is known as anesthesia. General anesthesia involves loss of consciousness, usually for the purpose of relieving the pain of surgery. Local anesthesia involves loss of sensation in one area of the body by the blockage of conduction in nerves.[239]

Local anesthesia is what I will focus on in this book, as the need for a general anesthesia in labor would be for the rarest outlying emergencies only. Local anesthesia does not produce loss of consciousness or even a foggy mental effect. Anesthesia blocks nerve transmission, which means that no pain is communicated to the brain and no sensation is felt by the nerves, or area of nerves, that have been targeted. Bupivacaine, for example, is a commonly prescribed anesthetic.

Local anesthesia is administered as a "spinal" or an "epidural." The difference between the two is that a spinal is a onetime injection into your spinal column, whereas an epidural involves a catheter that is left in place to continuously administer medication over time.[240] For a spinal, the needle is inserted into the center of your spinal column, medication is deposited, and the needle is removed—again, no apparatus is left in place. In an epidural, a needle is inserted into the Dura, a thin space surrounding the spinal column, and a plastic catheter (several centimeters long) is inserted. The needle is then removed, but the catheter stays in place in your back.[241] This catheter is then taped down on your back, in order to help hold it in place, and attached to tubing that is connected to a bag of medication hung from an IV stand. The epidural tubing is finally attached to a computerized flow monitor, which allows providers to control the amount of drug given.

A spinal is easier to administer because it consists of a single injection and no catheter has to be placed.[242] Keep in mind, however, that with this spinal a provider does have to gauge how long pain relief is needed and use medications that can satisfy that duration of time. Spinals are usually preferable for cesarean section, for example, because the duration of this surgery is generally predictable. For comfort in labor, the time frame is harder to predict, and so epidurals are often used to provide longer term relief. To be clear: the words "spinal" and "epidural" refer to the route of administration, not a particular drug.

I would now like to give you an overview of some commonly prescribed obstetric drugs and risks that are associated with them. (Note: the information that follows is not exhaustive. Rather, it is meant to provide you with a foundation from which to do your own research and decision making.)

Common obstetric analgesics

Fentanyl
Fentanyl has many side effects, including: drowsiness, lightheadedness, weakness and fatigue, feelings of elation (euphoria), dry mouth, difficulty urinating, difficulty breathing, constipation (which may be severe) and skin reactions, such as irritation, itching, or hives.[243]

Stadol®
The most common side effect is drowsiness. More infrequent side effects include: abnormally low blood pressure, dizziness, lightheadedness, depressed appetite, headache, nausea, reduced urination from kidney complications. And rare side effects can include: depression, tinnitus (ringing in the ears), high blood pressure, slowed heart rate, vocal cord swelling, itching, larynx spasm, decreased lung function, area of collapsed lung, bronchospasm, itching, rash, hives, fast heartbeat, hallucination, confusion, nightmares, blurred or double vision, dry mouth, irritation of stomach and bowls, nervousness.[244]

<u>Nubain® (Nalbuphine hydrochloride)</u>

Nov. 30, 2005 — The U.S. Food and Drug Administration (FDA) approved in the August safety labeling revisions to advise that use of nalbuphine HCl [Nubain] injection during labor and delivery is associated with a risk for serious fetal and neonatal adverse events...

On Aug. 23 [2005], the FDA approved safety labeling revisions for nalbuphine injection (Nubain, made by Endo Pharmaceuticals, Inc.) to warn of the risk for serious fetal and neonatal adverse events associated with its use during labor and delivery.

The placental transfer of nalbuphine is high, rapid, and variable, with a maternal to fetal ratio ranging from 1:0.37 to 1:6. Fetal and neonatal adverse events have included reports of fetal bradycardia, respiratory depression at birth, apnea, cyanosis, and hypotonia. Some of these events have been life-threatening.

Although maternal administration of naloxone during labor has normalized these effects in some cases, severe prolonged fetal bradycardia has occurred, and in some cases, resulted in permanent neurologic damage. Nalbuphine has also been linked to reports of sinusoidal fetal heart pattern.

The FDA advises that nalbuphine be used during labor and delivery only if clearly indicated and the potential benefit outweighs the risk to the infant. Newborns exposed to maternal nalbuphine should be monitored for respiratory depression, apnea, bradycardia, and arrhythmias.

Nalbuphine injection is indicated for the relief of moderate to severe pain.[245]

Although the FDA changed the label to warn of the concerns about the use of Nubain for labor pain relief, as late as 2021, while I was working at a birth as a doula, one of my client's was offered Nubain for pain relief—with no discussion of the fact that the FDA still says that Nubain is contraindicated for labor, unless other medications have failed to work.[246] There were no other choices offered to her and no information that using Nubain is now considered an off-label use. It is surely important to do your homework before labor begins!

<u>Demerol® (Meperidine)</u>

According to RxList.com, "Meperidine crosses the placental barrier and can produce depression of respiration and psychophysiological functions in the newborn. Resuscitation may be required. Therefore, meperidine is not recommended during labor."[247]

Obstetric anesthesia

<u>Bupivacaine</u>

Bupivacaine Pregnancy Warnings:

Bupivacaine has been assigned to pregnancy category C by the FDA. Animal studies have revealed evidence of embryolethality [toxicity that kills the embryo] at doses exceeding the maximum recommended daily human dose and developmental toxicity when administered subcutaneously [under the skin] at clinically relevant doses. There are no controlled data in human pregnancy. Bupivacaine is only recommended for use during pregnancy when benefit outweighs risk. This recommendation does not exclude the use of bupivacaine at term for obstetrical anesthesia or analgesia.

Local anesthetics [like Bupivacaine] rapidly cross the placenta. Adverse reactions in the mother and/or neonate are dependent upon the route of administration, procedure, and amount of drug used. Toxic reactions may include alterations in the central nervous system, peripheral vascular tone, and cardiac function. Maternal hypotension [low blood pressure] during obstetrical procedures has occurred during regional anesthesia. Elevating the patient's legs and positioning on the left side will help to prevent this effect. The fetal heart rate should be continuously monitored.

Bupivacaine Breastfeeding Warnings:

Bupivacaine is excreted into human milk. The manufacturer recommends that due to the potential for serious adverse reactions in nursing infants, a decision should be made to discontinue nursing or not administer the drug, taking into account the importance of the drug to the mother.[248]

I continue below to discuss some additional risks to consider before you decide to use an epidural, spinal, or analgesic by injection or IV or inhalation. Epidurals, for example, increase your chances of spiking a fever during labor. Although scientists do not yet fully understand why or how epidurals cause fevers,

epidural analgesia is associated with a more than four-fold increased rate of maternal fever in randomized trials... without corresponding increases in neonatal infection. Although expert review suggests that epidural fever is not infectious in etiology, no clinical or laboratory criteria accurately distinguish between chorioamnionitis [infection in the amniotic sac] and epidural fever.[249]

When a gestational parent on an epidural does spike a fever during their labor, they are typically okay and not terribly bothered by the fever. However, because it remains unclear if the fever is from the epidural or from infection, neonatologists and pediatricians must actively consider the danger of sepsis (a toxic infection). An infection can be life threatening for a newborn, so if you spike a fever in labor, even when it is likely a result of your epidural (assuming you have no reason to suspect illness), your baby will probably be sent to the NICU for prophylactic antibiotics immediately following birth.[250] Having your baby sent to the NICU for prophylactic antibiotics could add significant negative stress, including an increase in the challenges to establish breastfeeding and the birth parent's recovery. Additionally, overuse of antibiotics is cause for public concern as the dangers of drug resistance and super bugs are real. As scientists learn more about the development of a newborn's microbiome (the inner world of beneficial bacteria) we may learn even more reasons to try to avoid the need for antibiotics during birth and for the newborn.

Another potential problem that might stem from an epidural is reduced mobility and its ripple effect. A pregnant person who is unable to shift positions, because they can't feel their lower torso and legs, likewise cannot aid the baby in their journey down and out. Note that some people on an epidural are able to have some movement and sensation possible. Anesthesiologists have made remarkable progress in being able to target which nerves get numb. Years ago, if you had an epidural, you were always made completely numb from the point of injection downward, with no urge to push and no ability to feel anything in your legs.[251] That can and will still happen; but now I also hear people describe that they could in fact move their legs and feel themselves contracting due to careful epidural placement. Additionally, I have heard nurse's stories about non-obstetric patients on epidurals who were helped to change position including standing on two feet, with assistance.

In a recent conversation I had with an anesthesiologist I asked him about such mobility with epidural use. He said there was no reason that a laboring person could not be helped to move, at least a little bit, while on an epidural. He said it often doesn't happen "because women don't ask." By contrast, I have had clients ask and be rejected. In fact, the same nurse who first told me about her experiences of helping to move non-maternity epidural patients on another floor in the hospital told me that, when she herself was in labor and on an epidural, her own (informed) request to shift positions was flatly rejected. Clearly, I mention all this to encourage you to ask your providers about the possibility of moving, including supported standing, while on an epidural. Because now you know that if a pregnant person can shift their position, then it will reduce the chances that the baby gets stuck in its own difficult position.

Highlighted below are some additional medication risks to be considered, gathered from Gilbert Grant's "Adverse Effects of Neuraxial Analgesia and Anesthesia for Obstetrics," from May 2020.[252]

- Systemic Toxicity: Poisoned by the drug in a bad reaction, or from too much drug, or from too much put in the wrong place.

- High Spinal: When the drugs make you numb higher on your body than the level the drugs were injected. The most serious risk associated with a high spinal is that the diaphragm could become immobile and you might have to be put on a ventilator until the drugs wore off.

- Inadequate or Failed Block: The drugs don't work at all, or work everywhere except for a part of your body that hurts and still has full sensation.

- Pneumocephalus: When air gets introduced into the cerebrospinal fluid it can cause a rapid onset of an extreme headache.

- Spinal Epidural Hematoma: Bleeding into the spinal column from a vascular structure punctured by needle or catheter. The pressure from the blood can cause nerves to be compressed, resulting in pain and/or loss of sensory, motor, bladder, and/or bowel function. Immediate surgery to relieve the pressure is necessary to try to avoid permanent nerve damage.

- Uterine hyperactivity or increased uterine tone, which can cause increased blood loss and can cause complications for the baby or for the placenta to descend.

- Maternal hypotension: Gestational parent's low blood pressure, which reduces the amount of blood profusion through the placenta and can be of particular concern for the baby.

- Fetal Bradycardia: Slow heart rate, which may result from uterine hyperactivity or increased uterine tone.

- Fetal respiratory depression at birth secondary to opioid use.

Keeping in mind all of the above potential risks, make no mistake: popular opinion still falls on the side of the relative safety of pain medications during labor. Take, for example, this 2020 headline on a webpage from the University of Missouri health care system: "All About Epidurals: A Safe Pain Management Option During Labor."[253]

Nurses and doctors and even some hospital-based midwives often promote the use of medication, directly or indirectly, by failing to provide adequate emotional support or by failing to truly inform pregnant people about the risks incurred with the use of pain medications. There are still more risks to consider than what I have mentioned. Again, this chapter is not and cannot be exhaustive. The last such risk factor I will mention, therefore, is the fact that epidural drugs need to be produced in a sterile environment. Mass producing sterile substances raises concerns relating to the toll of corporate penny pinching at the labs where drugs are made. Are you sure that everything is going to be sterile and that no contamination has occurred at each of the steps in the process until it's in your spine? Sadly, contamination like this did occur in 2013, at a compounding lab (where drugs are made) in New England. Hundreds of cases of meningitis were ultimately traced back to medications that were produced in this lab, which had bacteria contamination.[254]

Nitrous oxide

In 2018, some hospitals in my area started offering nitrous oxide as an option for labor pain management. It has been used in England for labor pain for decades and dentists in the U.S. and elsewhere have been using it for generations as well, to help relax and anesthetize their patients.

Nitrous oxide is an anesthetic "that rapidly crosses the placenta."[255] As a labor pain medication it is highly effective at reducing the tension and anxiety that often comes with the big sensations of labor, but it isn't so great at actually taking away pain. (It works more like an analgesic than an anesthetic.) Any reduction in negative stress can tremendously improve a person's experience even when they can still feel discomfort. Some folks report feeling a very pleasurable and relaxed feeling from its effects, and as a bonus, it doesn't take long to work. The effects are usually felt within the first minute of use. That is quicker relief than just about any other pharmacological pain relief option. Another benefit is that, in labor, use of nitrous oxide is patient controlled, meaning that the laboring person places the mask over their own face to inhale when they want a dose. This self-administration can be empowering, which can also help to improve a person's experience. The use of nitrous oxide doesn't restrict one's ability to move or change position, although it can leave one a little wobbly and warnings do include not to operate machinery under its influence. These positives lead to a high level of satisfaction reported by those who have used nitrous oxide for labor pain.

Because nitrous oxide has been used in dentistry for over 100 years in the U.S., and in labor abroad for decades, it is generally considered to carry very low risk and be an effective labor pain management medication because we don't see evidence of harm. The general thinking, therefore, based on the lack of harm observed, is that the amount and concentration used for labor pain does not appear to present risks beyond the possibility of nausea, headache, dizziness, sleepiness, or disassociation (i.e., the feeling that you are somehow detached from what is happening).[256] But scientists understand that nitrous oxide does impact certain cell functioning for the gestational parent as well as the fetus, and that more research is needed to fully understand these cellular changes and their implications. For example, nitrous oxide has been shown to interfere with certain cell receptors that result, in part, in lowering vitamin B12 levels while raising homocysteine levels.[257]

> Homocysteine is an amino acid. Vitamins B12, B6 and folate break down homocysteine to create other chemicals your body needs. High homocysteine levels may mean you have a vitamin deficiency. Without treatment, elevated homocysteine increases your risks for dementia, heart disease and stroke.[258]

What does this mean to you and your baby if you use nitrous oxide? Based on observed use it appears not to mean much. However, in a review of the pros and cons of nitrous oxide for labor pain one reviewer mentions that nitrous oxide might not be an appropriate choice for pregnant people with low vitamin B12 levels.[259] Scientists also have remaining questions about the potential of gene alterations for the fetus.

> Nitrous oxide may decrease serum vitamin B12 and folate acutely. Prolonged Vitamin B12 and folate shortage was associated with epigenetic changes [changes that impact how genes work] including altered cardiometabolic risk factors in human offspring. [Cardio = heart function and metabolic = how your cells make energy.] Nitrous oxide generates ROS [Reactive oxygen species] which are known to cause DNA damage or epigenetic modifications.[260]

Another area of concern is that there is a potential for the hospital staff to be exposed to high levels of nitrous oxide, from day-in and day-out patient use. Hospitals can use equipment to reduce the amount of ambient nitrous oxide in a room where it is being used. However, the gas continues to pose some threat to those workers tasked with processing the used gas. And finally, it is considered to be a detrimental greenhouse gas, meaning it negatively contributes to climate change, albeit in a very small way.[261]

As I think about what I have learned about nitrous oxide, I find it deeply reaffirming of the meditative techniques I offer you throughout this book. When we can relax deeply, even when the sensation is intense, we can manage the labor and any pain that comes with it. If you take your relaxation, breath awareness and visualization skill building seriously you will have tools that can help you try to manage your sensations without any potential risks. As I have pointed out earlier, and it bears repeating, meditation skills are associated with all kinds of positive health benefits and the skills are useful well beyond the work of birth.

Okay, but which drug might be best for me?

At present, there isn't much agreement across the country as to the best drug or dosage for labor pain management. To provide some context to this, I've included below some excerpts from an obstetric nurse online chat room, from 2020.[262] I found the lack of agreement in their responses enlightening, in that they allow for you to build your own confidence through research and investigative questions to your care providers. This particular chat thread began when a Registered Nurse posted the following question, with the subject line, "Fentanyl for Labor Pain?":

> Hello Everyone,
>
> We don't routinely give IV Fentanyl here for labor pain. A physician recently wanted one of our staff members to give this to her patient. The staff is not comfortable giving this to labor patients. Does your facility use Fentanyl IV for labor pain? If so, is there a protocol that involves placing the patient on a cardiac and SaO2 monitor? I would appreciate any input. Thank you!

What follows is a cross section of the variation of opinions:

> We don't give fentanyl iv (and wouldn't). We do give nubain and I routinely gave stadol at another facility. Both facilities use fentanyl and bipivicaine as epidural ingredients...

> We give Fentanyl all the time for labor pain. We usually give 100mcg/hr prn for early labor pain. We don't have any special monitoring; it is a narcotic and we use all the usual precautions that we do with any narcotic. We have had good luck with it.

> It is among the several choices for labor pain among nubain and stadol. We give anywhere from 25-100 mcg q 1 h for labor pain, via slow IV. Like with any narcotic, as ... said above, you need to watch its effects on mom and baby and understand the more it is used, the less the effects are felt.

> We give it to women who we consider too far along to be able to take meperedine [DEMEROL]. Only women less than 3 cm are allowed meperedine, but they can have fentanyl up to 7 cm because it's [sic] effects wear off faster. We don't place them on cardiac or oxygen sat monitoring.

We pretty much stopped using demerol in any form on our floors (even in PCA), quite some time ago. It is implicated causing seizure activity in some people, I have read in several journals. And they are finding fentanyl and morphine much more effective, especially in post-surgical pain control, with fewer side effects. Go figure?

I gave Fentanyl quite a bit at the first facility where I did L&D. I also got some when I was in labor with my first, but it only helped through about 2 contractions. I went from 0/100% to delivered baby in about 2 1/2 hours. I don't think much would have helped. Now, if I could have gotten that intrathecal that I wanted that the anes. resident wouldn't give me since I was a primip... [Primip is short for primiparas, which in medical speak means producing a first child, or having only had one child.]

Fentanyl is supposedly bound up more in the placental villi, resulting in less getting to the fetus... sorry, no documentation other than the word of a reputable OB and a reputable anesthesiologist! Anyone else ever heard of this?

I have heard that too as well, one facility I worked at, fentanyl was used exclusively, 100mcg every hour up to 3 doses, no matter how far they were dilated. another facility ONLY uses demerol/ phenergan which I think is useless 90% of the time, and another used stadol or nubaine, I've had good luck with nubaine. Interesting how different places can be!

As you can see from the sampling above, which drugs and doses really are the best is difficult to determine: "Interesting how different places can be!" The lack of understanding and agreement creates challenges for choosing optimal care for the client and staff alike. All these drugs are still being used today, in varying doses. New drugs do enter the market, which may provide you with additional available options by the time you go into labor. And sometimes doctors rethink older drugs, such as with Nubain and nitrous oxide (laughing gas) mentioned above.

"Safe" is a relative term

I know every one of us desperately wants safety. But what does "safe" really mean? The Merriam-Webster dictionary defines "safe" as "free from harm or risk: unhurt." In the context of striving for a safe birth, "safe" means to reduce usage of things that increase risk factors while also increasing support with emotional warmth, confidence, encouragement, and respect. *Natural birth education is therefore the most powerful tool you can have at your disposal.*

Education and self-advocacy and self-care take practice. There isn't a simple pill to take to make it all okay, although I once read a midwife's candid remarks in which she suggested that acetaminophen (known more commonly by the commercial name of Tylenol®) was a reasonable drug to consider for childbirth. I was surprised I hadn't come across this seemingly simpler approach before. But simpler isn't always simple. Acetaminophen is not risk free, and there is mounting evidence that its use during pregnancy may be linked to autism in the children who were exposed to it during gestation.[263] (It appears that these risks of acetaminophen may be worsened with the addition of the common antibiotics Amoxicillin® or Augmentin®, and/or exposure to glyphosate® Roundup® a popular herbicide.[264]) Be sure to talk to your provider and do your own research before taking any over the counter medications, or combinations of medicines! There are so many ways pain meds can have a negative impact, in the midst of whatever positive effects they were created to achieve. So I encourage you again to put your energy and stamina into practicing relaxation and breathing techniques. As you practice working inward, you are supporting your natural process. Listening to (tuning into) your breath and your sensations of body, and having the ability to focus your thoughts on a singular task or image can build confidence. This, in turn, can help you to reframe birth into a manageable experience. *Confidence is a big part of creating an empowering and transformative birth.*

"When *are* the risks of pain meds worth it?"

Quick and absolute answer: When the person in labor wants them.

As much as I believe in preparing for an unmedicated birth, I just as fundamentally believe that anytime a laboring person asks for pain medication they should get it. I will always stand behind my belief that all people deserve the right to agency over their own body. In this context, then, birthing people deserve respectful and compassionate care with thorough information, including an honest assessment of options, risks, and alternatives, to support their process. During birth, pain meds attempt to provide a kind of support. If a person needs more support than they're able to give to themselves and receive from the people around them, then they should feel comfortable to try whatever is available. In my opinion, to deny a person the opportunity to make their own informed choice is cruel. But it happens every day in labor rooms across the country, especially if you are a person who is marginalized by the dominant culture. Documentation has shown that providers, in practical terms, consider women, people in poverty, and people of Color to be less reliable to report their own pain than wealthy White men. If you are a woman, a transgender, gender non-conforming person, a person of Color, and/or a person living in poverty, then it is particularly imperative that you discuss pain management options and medical decision making well in advance of your birth. You also want to gain a clear understanding of your legal rights with regard to your medical care. I repeat: anyone who wants the medications should have access. But because our rights and our access are not universal, it remains paramount to do your research, communicate clearly, and hold firm to making your own best decisions.

Like one of my past clients did: She went into labor on the rebound from a stomach flu, which had included needing IV fluids and an overnight in the hospital. She was still weak from illness when her birth arrived two days later. She had no energy reserve. She took an epidural and slept deeply for several long hours. She woke refreshed and fiercely determined to birth her baby. Against her doctor's advice she chose to have the epidural removed. Her doctor worried that if she wanted another epidural later in the process, he would not be able to safely provide one. But she was clear: she asked for the drugs to help her sleep. Now that she had gained the rest she needed, she wanted to birth without the drugs. She gave birth to a beautiful (and giant!) baby girl, through many hours of magnificent hard work and without the need for further medical intervention.

Once you take control of the decision-making through informed conversation with your healthcare providers and support team, there is still a lot to unpack around the choice to medicate your birth. It may surprise you to learn that this decision is as personal and intimate as it is political. For example, people who are tired are, in general, more predisposed to take pain medications than those who feel rested. The CDC estimates that as many as 1 in 3 adults are getting inadequate amounts of sleep.[265] Translation: many Americans are chronically tired. Add to this that few people have the luxury, education, or the patience to focus *prenatally* on resting, and this results in many, many people starting off their labor already very tired. (Are you feeling tired right now?) The good news is, no matter how tired you are you will get through your birth. Humans can face great exhaustion under grueling circumstances and still carry on. Another past client's support partner was a soldier, and in class he talked of the unbearable exhaustion he faced routinely in war. Through his Bradley® class he then heard hospital birth stories in which birthing people were often offered medication for exhaustion. He was shocked at how quickly and frequently this happened. He saw it as undermining the confidence of the birthing person. Actually, he was outraged. He told our class that if he could go a week or longer carrying heavy weaponry with no real sleep in a war zone, then surely a healthy person given fluids, snacks, pillows, and kind words can get though several tough, long days of birth. While the comparison may be apt, and can help you to tune into your own strengths during labor, especially when you are feeling more tired than perhaps you've ever felt before, it is also important to keep in mind that each person's circumstances, determinations, and thresholds are different. Again, build up and have faith in your own strength (you're not likely to see more than a day or two of labor), but also continue to be compassionate with yourself.

To repeat: advocate for your own choices as best you can in the moment that you must make your decisions. This is a personal act. But as I alluded to above, even such a personal act can be influenced by political, sociocultural, and even economic pressures. It is impossible to ponder pain medications, for instance, without also addressing our fee-for-service healthcare system in the United States. Consider that the financial outlook is better for hospitals if pregnant people medicate, or "medicalize" their births. Hospitals are in a constant battle to stay ahead of the rising costs of doing business. The ripple effect of increased costs from supplies, tests, related procedures, and personnel directly equates with billable dollars. With each additional intervention, warranted or not, more billable dollars are generated.

Consider also that nurses, doctors, and other healthcare providers have a lot on their plates. Most hospitals are functioning understaffed, under-slept, and over stressed by a million stressors that erupt in a hospital each day (and this was the state of operations *before* the coronavirus pandemic, so imagine this same state exponentially worse now)—not to mention the burdens they shoulder in their own private lives. Healthcare providers are spinning all of this while caring for you. And caring for you means, in large part, documentation, which equals time spent with their face in a computer screen. It's understandable, therefore, that hospital staff, as kind and supportive as they may or may not be, are not necessarily motivated to help you find alternatives to drugs. Pain drugs can help a harried staff member feel that they are helping to calm and quiet you with a minimum of actual input on their part. It's rare (but possible) to find healthcare providers that have the potent combination of time, motivation, and useful midwifery-based knowledge to help support you through your birthing journey.

There are of course pockets of amazing birth communities across the country where hospital staff are outstanding from bottom to top. But even nursing shift changes, for example, can be tough on nurses and birthing people alike. When the relationship is going well a shift change can leave a birthing person feeling abandoned. If the next nurse on duty has a very different energy—which they more than likely will—it can create extra burden on the birth. While I have heard multiple stories of great nurses that stayed past the end of their shift to help maintain continuity of care and see a person through their birth, your job now is to try to make your best plans for your birth—and that kind of extraordinary care is impossible to plan for from a nurse. By contrast, a doula, friend, or relative can provide a more reliable, planned-in-advance opportunity for such continuity. (More on doulas coming in Week 15.) Moreover, nurses, as a primary example, can have a tremendous impact on what a person perceives as their own choice. During healthy birth, even a gentle and well-meaning nurse can be directive, perhaps in ways completely unintended. These interjected directions can have a positive effect or a negative one and can result in steering a person off their own birthing plans or course, especially because these directions come from a perceived authority. I have witnessed nurses exclaim, "don't have the baby yet!", because the midwife or doctor was not nearby when the woman had been sitting on the toilet or on all fours on the floor. (Note: To refrain from releasing your baby can create risk for baby. Follow your urges and let your baby out. The toilet or on all fours on the floor are perfectly reasonable places to catch a baby.) Nurses truly are heroes in our healthcare system, and birthing people often appreciate direction, so there is no one best description of good care. *But sensitive collaboration is imperative for optimal outcome.*

I once arrived at the hospital with a mom who had already been in labor close to 36 hours. She was strong and doing remarkably well and had not mentioned any interest in medications. She was ready to be admitted because she knew the birth was getting near. But once we were in the labor room, we had to work hard to avoid the insensitive comments of the nurse on duty. This nurse exclaimed, "Oh my gosh! How long have you been in labor? Without an epidural?! I never would have done that! I have a 9-month-old at home. I got an epidural in my birth, but then I had to get a c-section!" She went on to make a joke about wanting a zipper for future births, but by then I was ushering my client away and into the bathroom so she could get back on her own track. My client was confused by the comments, and I suspected if I hadn't been there as doula, and if the primary partner hadn't been well educated to support birth, these comments could have undermined her confidence. The nurse was trying to be kind, and she was clearly still processing her own birth, but these were insensitive comments to share in that moment, especially given her role as an authority in the room. The laboring person should not be tasked with needing to process the choices that this medical professional made for her own birth and was now selling as the better choice (noting, too, the clear distinction between my client's naturally progressing birth and this nurse's birth that concluded with surgery). Again, my client was strong, but that comment created an unnecessary hurdle at 36 hours into what ended up being a triumphant and uncomplicated birth at a total of 42 hours.

Over the years, I have heard many stories of nurses directly suggesting pain meds are a good idea, complete with emotional pressure and with no mention of any increased risks. Likewise, many other stories exist of nurses who provide spot-on support, complete with a respectful and protective attitude and an assortment of emotional and physical coping tools that are not medication-based. But which nurse you get when you arrive at the hospital remains the luck of the draw—and these stakes really are too high of a gamble. Therefore, the more you are aware of and understand these potential hurdles now, the more you can prepare appropriately and respond with confidence.

Keep in mind that medication has been normalized as the fix for the so-called "medical problem" that is childbirth. Labor pain management drugs are not necessarily a medical "must" for the patient's health (contrary to if a patient needs insulin because their pancreas isn't making any or medication is necessary to control high blood pressure); rather, these drugs can bring another element of compassion into the birthing process. So I repeat: when a person asks for the drugs, they should get them. One way or another, a gestational parent must find a way to work with their body to get the baby out. Reducing negative emotional stress is key to completing the birth process. Stress-induced prolonged labor can lead to fetal distress. A very tense or hysterical reaction to a difficult birth process, or to the people in the room, can render a person unable to calm themselves—even if they have the good fortune to have excellent support from their caretakers. When a person finds no other way to yield to their process, drugs that attempt to relax them can sometimes help the process to continue.

Embracing birth and willfully surrendering into the power of the contractions can help a person to escape the need for interventions, such as pain medication. But the challenge of softening into surrender, and trusting that birth is tough work—albeit manageable work—can seem impossibly hard work in a tense, doubting, or busy environment, especially when one may already be exhausted before labor even begins. This is why doing your research now and deciding how you feel about the possible risks and side effects from pain medications is as important as the self-care skills, breathing practices, and mindfulness techniques you are building each day. (Not practicing? Let that go and start tonight!)

— (This is your teaser practice for your longer session later tonight.)
Pause to take a few breaths with eyes closed.
Notice how your body feels from the top of your head down to the tips of your toes—

To continue to help you make your best plans, and grapple with the range of possible birth experiences, think about birth as if it were sex. Sex can occur through a range of experiences, from violent rape and coerced-through-threat rape to consensual sex that is ultimately painful, to sex that doesn't hurt but isn't satisfying, sex that is only mildly satisfying, sex that is pleasurable and joyful, sex that is so tender and profound that you weep, or sex that is universe-rocking ecstasy. Sex can also be sober or under the influence of alcohol or drugs. If I left out any categories on this spectrum, feel free to update or amend as you see fit; this comparison is for you to consider in what follows.

Now think about the range of experiences possible in birth... the spectrum of choices should look similar. If a person feels terrified, violated, directly or indirectly threatened, humiliated, embarrassed, interrupted, ignored, judged, rushed, abandoned—physically or emotionally, then they are not going to have a good birth any more than they would have good sex (fetishes aside). Likewise, when a person feels safe, free from interruption, emotionally connected, supported, and in sync with their rhythms, the potential for ecstasy is much improved—in birth as in sex. With this comparison firmly in mind, think about what some of the possibilities are for your birth. Ask yourself, in the context of this section's focus: when would drugs for pain be a good idea? In my opinion, it's still as straightforward as when you say so. My deep and only hope is that a birthing person has access to genuine knowledgeable support and birth education, including birth physiology and practical skills like the labor positions and other coping tools taught in this book, prior to any decision point.

I'll say it again: people in labor are particularly vulnerable to the messages they are given. The more exhausted one is, the more susceptible one is to the opinions of those around them. If everyone, especially the hospital staff, is telling a person that they are too tired and that the drugs will be good, then it's hard not to believe them and easy to be swayed. By the same token, if birth attendants express a strong belief that one is capable and amply equipped to handle the birth challenges without medication, then the birthing person will likely be able to tap previously unknown powers.

Unfortunately, if/when you talk about wanting an unmedicated birth, you may find that you get a lot of push back from the people around you. Many a Bradley® student reports that they are mocked or forewarned by family, friends, and coworkers. "Don't be a martyr" is a common directive given to a pregnant person when they discuss an unmedicated birth. Or, the ever-ominous, "Yeah, you think you're so strong now, just you wait!" My antidote for these naysayers is to turn the conversation back on them. With genuine interest (and hopefully a degree of real warmth), try to respond with, "Oh, have you had an epidural? Did your partner? Tell me about it. What happened? How did you arrive at that decision and how did it work for you?" By shifting the conversation away from you and your choices and back to them, you can shed light on what happened and help to contextualize the comments. If someone has a strong interest in pushing you to take pain meds, it's possible that they have some unsettled feelings about their own or their partner's birth. Sometimes people take comfort from knowing that other people will make the same choices they made—or make the choice they wish they had made. Regardless of why someone is urging you to take drugs for your labor pain, there will certainly be things to learn from their stories and concerns and to utilize as part of your decision-making processes. At the very least, shifting the focus back to them relieves you of being the focus of unsolicited direction.

Believe it or not, to the majority of the people I meet who are already pregnant, birth is thought to be unimaginable, impossibly hard, and kind of gross! It's no surprise then that negative stress can come from our own internal battles and assumptions as much as from outside influences. You can use the mindfulness techniques I've been discussing throughout this book to quiet your mind and explore how you are really feeling. Promise yourself now, for example, that you will try to become an expert in *rest* and in *focusing your attention*. Genuinely apply yourself to the self-care of deep relaxation and sleep. Rest like your life depends on it by lying down and closing your eyes, with no phones, no screen time, no reading, and no music or TV, in a dark room or with as low light as possible, with no body movement or with as little as possible. Explore your breathing to quiet your mind enough to listen. With prenatal practice, as well as continued practice during labor, you can improve your ability to notice, redirect and reduce destructive thinking. I find walking is also helpful as a meditative practice—no headphones, no talking, just walking and listening to my breath.

When considering what pharmacological options are currently available I can make an educated guess that there are drugs and procedures in use today that will be deemed unsafe in 25 years or so, when your kids are ready to have kids. Just like we can look back 25 or 30 years (or more) and see practices that we no longer find acceptable today. There is still much to learn and appreciate about human gestation and birth. Meanwhile, a lot of trial and error continues, including experimentation with using drugs "off label," which means for treatment of a diagnosis different than for what the drug was initially approved. Experience shows that it's not just researchers alone; it's also up to doctors to figure out how best to use their tools: Is this drug good, at this dose, for this patient with this condition? The research looks good, it smells good, and so it *should* be good. The pharmaceutical company that makes and pushes the drug says it's good, the U.S. Food and Drug Administration (FDA) says it's not proven bad, and there is a market for it. Thus time marches on through experience and expanding knowledge. Some drugs come on and stay on the market. Some drugs are taken off. Your task now is to do further research, consider what your options are, and to understand the broader impact those choices may have. Then you can make your own, best-informed decisions.

Now it's time to let the information on pain medication settle and to tune into another area of challenging pregnancy decision points. Should one induce labor?

How long should your pregnancy last?

It's hard to know for sure. In the 2013 article, "Length of Human Pregnancy and Contributors to Its Natural Variation," published in *Human Reproduction Oxford Journals,* A.M. Jukic et al. state that "among natural conceptions where the date of conception (ovulation) is known, the variation in pregnancy length spanned 37 days, even after excluding women with complications or preterm births."[266] In other words, researchers found that when they knew the date of conception, healthy babies varied in gestational age anywhere between 1 and 37 days. This variation suggests that it is a largely impossible task to predict exactly when your baby is ready to be born. The only one who knows for sure is your baby—and she isn't likely to tell you this information ahead of time. (In fact, I'm fairly confident that this won't be the last time your child withholds information from you! The challenge of waiting for the baby to arrive is an embedded parenting lesson in learning to accept our children's independence.) It may be hard to cope with, but we just can't predict the perfect birth date.

Keep in mind, too, that the last days of prenatal development are quite important to the newborn. The rate of brain growth in the last trimester is extraordinary. From week 35 to week 39/40 a baby's brain grows by 75%.[267] These last weeks of gestation are clearly not a time to skimp on your nutrition, nor are they a time to shorten gestation unnecessarily. Time in the womb matters.

Neuroscientists have found that some neural development may not ever happen at all outside of the gestational person's body. It seems that the unique sensory environment of the womb enables certain kinds of neural connections (the network in the brain) to be formed in the fetal brain that do not seem to happen at all once your child is born. In studies that followed preemies into adulthood, researchers were surprised to find both how prevalent neural development deficits were and how the deficits presented. Although the earliest-born preemies had the worst and highest level of developmental problems, 44% of older, stronger preemies were found to grow into adults with developmental deficits. As Alison Abbott revealed, in her 2015 article, "Neuroscience: The Brain, Interrupted," published in *Nature*, "the effects seem to continue into adulthood... most of those who experienced problems had short attention spans, and as a group they tended to underachieve academically and career-wise."[268] This same article goes on to suggest that the developmental problems may stem from the introduction of strong stimulations, such as the change in gravity, visual stimulation, cold air, and other comparatively harsh nervous system stimulations that are experienced by a baby born prematurely. This research suggests that the early introduction of these new sensations can cause the baby to interrupt their process of laying down key foundational pathways that are formed in the sensory-protected womb environment.

To put the question of human gestation into further context, consider other examples of gestational variation in nature: Some apple trees mature their fruit earlier in the season than other species of apple tree, just as some apples ripen earlier than their counterparts sharing the same tree. Likewise, some babies arrive early, while others take more time. In addition, if you had a natural conception, can you know the absolute day that you conceived? The answer is a resounding no. There is a six-day window during which conception can take place. Even when people menstruate regularly, there can be differences in when ovulation occurs from month to month.[269] And this is to say nothing of that 37-day variation within healthy human gestation discussed above. A former client and support partner, Malik, once asked, "With so much variation in the length of gestation, how will we know if my partner should induce or not?" Great question. Let's discuss an answer.

The most important step in this decision-making process is to first *anticipate that you might have to make this decision*. Once again, early research helps you to think about this ahead of when you may need to make any actual decisions. If, however, you are there right now (late term), then take a deep breath and exhale some of the fear you may be feeling. Focus on connecting into your baby emotionally and physically and follow your gut and your heart. Ask your providers to explain what their criteria are for deciding to induce as well as their preferred induction methods. Your provider can give you a date that they believe induction of labor is indicated. That's what having a medical protocol means: "If such and such thing happens, then we do such and such. If, for example, you get to three months from next Tuesday still pregnant, then I'll suggest X, Y or Z (such as testing, then medication and/or a procedure, and then possibly more testing)." Some providers seem to rely primarily on dates for induction proposal, while others will want first to take and interpret tests, such as the "Non-Stress Test," or Cardiotocography (CTG), also called electronic fetal monitoring (EFM), and the Biophysical Profile (an ultrasound scan).

The Non-Stress Test (often parents think it should be called "the stress test") is conducted with the same CTG that is used in labor.[270] The Biophysical Profile is an anatomical scan like the one many have early in pregnancy. Both the Non-Stress Test and the Biophysical Profile rely on ultrasound waves.[271] Based on the data collected and its interpretation, your provider may recommend induction—and hopefully they will also discuss honestly the risks and benefits of this induction. Unfortunately, some providers do act like they can insist on induction. I have heard too many stories of induction coercion based on threats and false pretense. Knowing your provider's induction habits, and their actual rates of induction early in their patients' pregnancies, can help you to think more clearly—and thus make your best decisions—about what you want to do should you get well past your due date.

In the absence of specific medical indications, such as high blood pressure, uncontrolled diabetes, or other medical conditions relating to baby or mother, the motivations for induction typically fall into two categories: 1) fear of a large baby getting stuck or injured during a vaginal birth or 2) fear of fetal death secondary to the placenta degrading beyond sustainability. Although fear of large babies is prevalent, obstetric guidelines *do not* recommend induction of labor before 42 weeks for healthy gestational people only under suspicion of a large baby.[272] Remember: there are no accurate ways to measure a baby's weight at term. Using ultrasound or physical assessment, providers can be off in their weight prediction, with the most common error showing that the baby is bigger than she actually is.[273] Not only is weight estimation (and what it might mean to your outcome) inaccurate, there is no consensus among providers as to what is considered too big—the range often falls to just under nine pounds to almost 10 pounds.

When a provider suspects a large baby, this suspicion alone can become a complicating diagnosis for the birthing person and their baby. Rebecca Dekker, from Evidence Based Birth, presents evidence that women who were *thought* to have big babies, but didn't actually end up having big babies, had more problems than women who didn't know to expect a big baby but birthed one anyway. While large babies can experience shoulder dystocia, small babies can get stuck, too. In fact, half of all shoulder dystocia cases happen to medium- or small-sized babies. In either case, a well-trained attendant can usually help prevent injury. A difficult birth for any baby can result in a broken clavicle (collar bone). But these injuries are not usually serious, not particularly common, and most don't require any treatment. It is generally agreed, for example, that the risks associated with induction are greater than the risk of a broken clavicle.[274]

If fear of a large baby doesn't ultimately hold up as a medical reason to induce before 42 weeks, then perhaps fear of fetal death should be the greater consideration. Placentas, like people, grow, mature, decline, and eventually stop functioning enough to support life. As they age, placentas can and will start to develop calcifications. These are hardened areas of tissue that reduce the amount of blood flow that can be filtered (perfused) in that area. If calcification starts early enough and progresses fast enough (which is more common in smokers and those with other health complications), then the baby may die. At the same time, 20 – 40% of healthy babies will be born without any complication at term with some degree of placental calcification.[275] If you get to 41+ weeks, you may choose to try to image the placenta with ultrasound, which can help to gauge blood flow through the umbilical cord vessels. The accuracy of this test is most useful with 3D ultrasound. Even with unanswered questions about the safety and efficacy of fetal ultrasound use, it may prove a good choice for you if you go past term.

To induce is rarely a simple or stress-free decision. In my pregnancies I sometimes would fret as I questioned various obstetric practices: Was I being selfish? Would I be jeopardizing my baby's wellbeing if I just kept deferring to nature? The answer is: maybe. More babies do die before 39 weeks and after 41 weeks.[276] The difference in inducing at 41 weeks versus 42 weeks appears to be the difference between one fetal death in every 2,986 pregnancies at 41 weeks versus nine fetal deaths out of every 2,953 pregnancies at 42 weeks.[277] It also appears that there are fewer cesarean sections associated with induction for late term than for deferring to nature. However, researchers have yet to study the long-term outcomes for these induced babies and admit that more research is needed to understand when exactly is a "best time" to choose induction.[278] With what is known (and with what isn't) we forge ahead with a great number of inductions in the U.S. "The rate of induction of labor in the U.S. has risen from 9.6% in 1990 to 25.7% in 2018, including 31.7% of first-time births."[279] As you digest this information I urge you to find compassion for yourself. Facing big decision points for you and your family are what I have found to be some of the hardest parts of growing up and growing into a parent.

Induction methods

Some providers begin the process of induction during an office visit, with the procedure called "membrane stripping" that I explained in Week 10 while discussing vaginal exams:

> Stripping or sweeping of membranes involves inserting the examiner's finger beyond the internal cervical os [cervical opening] and then rotating the finger circumferentially [in a circle] along the lower uterine segment to detach the fetal membrane [amniotic sac] from the decidua [lining of the uterus].[280]

There is evidence to support that membrane stripping can help to shorten the length of pregnancy. However, scientific questions remain as to the best timing and frequency of membrane stripping to gain an optimal outcome. I once heard a midwife say that, based on her personal anecdotal evidence, frequent gentle sweeps and nudges beyond the cervical opening are most effective. But, again, evidence-based medical research has yet to study this. You may find that your medical provider discusses membrane stripping once you approach 42 weeks. If possible, ask your provider about the risks and benefits of membrane stripping and their thoughts about it early in your pregnancy.

The experience of having your membranes stripped is varied. I have heard it described as "insanely painful" as well as "no big deal." This variation from excruciating to very mild depends on the ripeness of your cervix, your ability to relax under the circumstances, and the level of gentleness or roughness a provider brings to their technique. The cervix is rich with blood vessels, so some spotty bleeding may also occur as a result of this procedure, regardless of the pain factor. As I've stated before, I recommend that prior to consent you discuss use of an obvious safe-word, like "Stop" or "Ouch," with your provider. Ask your provider to verbally consent their agreement that, should you say, "Stop" or "Ouch," they will halt the procedure immediately and then check in with you for further consent and instructions. It doesn't matter that you initially said "yes" to the procedure. Remember: you can withdraw or postpone consent at any time; it's your legal right. Confirming this consent agreement is a smart practice for any procedure that involves something going into your vagina, including membrane stripping, vaginal exams, or a vaginal ultrasound wand.

If/when the agreed upon induction date arrives, hospital admission is generally in the evening. This is especially true if a gestational person is found to have an "unfavorable cervix," meaning they show no signs of effacement. Depending on this "favorability" of the person's cervix (for lack of less offensive terminology in common use), orders will be written. "Favorable" cervixes might skip a step and go directly to oxytocic drugs like Pitocin. For "unfavorable cervixes" orders are first written for synthetic prostaglandins, which will be applied and then reapplied throughout the night. Prostaglandins are hormones that soften and help thin the cervix.

The two prostaglandins generally considered to begin the process of cervical effacement are dinoprostone (brand name Cervadil®) and misoprostol (brand name Cytotek®.) Misoprostol is a drug with a controversial history.[281] In fact, the drug manufacturer and the FDA have stated that it is contraindicated for use during pregnancy. The drug was originally invented to treat ulcers and has also been used to initiate abortions.[282] Consequently, when misoprostol is used for labor induction it is being used "off label."[283] As we discussed previously, in all branches of medicine, doctors experiment with using drugs "off label," or for some other purpose than what they were first approved to treat.[284] While this has led to many useful discoveries and effective treatments, it has also led to some horrific tragedies. Using drugs off label can turn the patient into a test animal. *Born in the USA*, by the late Marsden Wagner, describes several maternal and fetal deaths from the 1990s related to the misuse of misoprostol (Cytotek®).[285] When given in high doses via IV, the drug caused hyper-stimulation of the uterus, which caused a variety of problems, including excessive bleeding, uterine ruptures, and maternal death.

Alternatively, when the misoprostol manufacturer and the FDA warned obstetricians not to use misoprostol on pregnant women, the ACOG (American College of Obstetricians and Gynecologists) was and remains unhappy about this restriction. They've continued to experiment with the drug, because they are confident that it is an excellent drug of choice for induction of labor. Doctors now understand that a small dose applied topically to the cervix is an effective ripening agent, and thus far has not produced evidence of the adverse outcomes seen with the high IV doses. Again, ask your provider about their preferred induction medications. Misoprostol may be the appropriate choice for you, but it's good to have some backstory and the thoughts and intentions of your medical care provider.

For synthetic prostaglandins, the current drug delivery system of choice is to get the medicine up onto or near to your cervix. One method uses a vaginal suppository (a tampon-type medicated pad on a string) that's inserted into the vagina, with the gestational person typically asked to remain in bed for some time afterwards (two hours is recommended) so that the medication stays in place. Another method used to help start an induction is called laminaria, or laminaria sticks, which are small cylinders of a dried seaweed product (they look like a small stack of toothpicks) that get inserted into the cervical opening. Sometimes laminaria are inserted in an office visit and the client is then set home for the night (but this practice is not standardized.) Once in place, the laminaria absorb moisture and expand like a sponge helping to open the cervix.

Once the induction has begun, fetal monitoring is indicated to make sure that the baby tolerates the medications. Additionally, IV fluids will be administered. And it's possible that your medical providers will want to restrict your diet. A nurse will monitor your vital signs throughout the night: heart rate, blood pressure, temperature. (An elevated temperature could signal infection.) If you are in this situation, it can be really hard to get a good night's sleep before the big day of labor, so try to rest as much as you can.

Assuming that gestational parent and baby have tolerated the medication well up to this point in induction, oxytocic drugs (remember: artificial uterine stimulating drugs) will be started in the morning. These synthetic hormones should cause the uterus to contract. Pitocin®, or "Pit" as it is frequently called, is typically the drug of choice. A low dose will be added to the IV, and then every half hour the dose will be increased until a "therapeutic level" is reached. Note that this "therapeutic level" is decided by the provider, so it is again recommended to discuss with your provider when this level would be reached and why before the actual induction.

Although oxytocic drugs like Pitocin® are administered by IV when providers want to start or augment (increase the strength of) the contractions, which would be done by increasing the overall amount of the drug in the bloodstream, scientists do understand that this is not the way nature works its magic. During pregnancy and also during labor, the number of oxytocin receptors within the uterine lining are increasing, i.e., more are switching on.[286] It is the increased number of turned-on receptor sites that increases sensitivity to the oxytocin, rather than the overall amount of hormone in a person's bloodstream. Scientists believe that in natural labor a person releases a flood of oxytocin about every 6 – 10 minutes. A route of synthetic administration that mimics the natural rhythmic release does exist but it is very expensive and not readily available to the general public. As I mentioned in Week 9, scientists now understand that an overall increase of artificial oxytocin can render the uterine receptors unavailable.[287] This likely explains why Pitocin® doesn't seem to work for all people and why there is an increased risk of postpartum hemorrhage associated with induction drugs.

Amniotomy

In addition to drugs, many doctors will also want to incorporate the procedure of amniotomy, the artificial rupturing of the amniotic sac. Amniotomy does appear to shorten the overall length of the induced birth by as much as 5 hours.[288] Providers use a tool called the "amnio-hook," which looks like a common crochet hook, only sharper. In order to have this procedure, a person must have at least some effacement and dilation.

Amniotomy risks include infection and prolapsed umbilical cord, a serious emergency requiring immediate surgery. Due to the risk of a prolapsed cord, amniotomy should only be performed if the baby's head is solidly against the cervix, as this reduces the chance of prolapse.

Once the membranes are ruptured most providers put time limits in place to complete the birth. If these limits aren't met, then antibiotics are started, labor augmentation with medication such as Pitocin® is discussed, and/or the birthing person is prepped for surgery (for a c/section).

Induction risks

Induction does not always work. Some people who receive Pitocin®, for example, do not then begin contractions. For others, Pitocin® works too well and causes many contractions closer together and sometimes stronger and longer than they would be normally. (This is the more common side effect.) This increase in activity can be stressful for birthing people and babies alike, but for different reasons.[289] At the height of a natural contraction babies experience decreased oxygenation. Evidence suggests, however, that they do not actually experience low oxygen levels; instead, babies seem to get better at utilizing the oxygen that is available. In other words, although contractions decrease overall oxygenation, the baby's oxygen levels stay about the same. More work needs to be done to better understand how and why this is.[290] In my mind, I imagine that the contractions are like a massive massage and that all of the baby's physiological systems receive a crazy amount of deep tissue work. However, under the effects of Pitocin®, some babies may not tolerate the increase in frequency, strength and duration of the contractions, which is why increased monitoring is essential.

I do think a lot about what labor is like for the babies. For instance, maybe physiological birth is like a meditative, massaged state of mind. Or, maybe the experience is super stressful for them. Regardless of the thoughts and feelings that babies experience during labor, it seems to me that the decrease in available oxygen must slow their processes down, which in turn might aid in the transition from in-utero to earth-side.

A healthy baby, of course, recovers easily between contractions (otherwise humans wouldn't still be around). But, when contractions are artificially close together, and potentially stronger and/or longer than they would be naturally, this takes away some of baby's recuperation time. This reduced recovery can cause fetal stress that can then grow into a serious state of fetal distress. This is super stressful for the birthing person, too, who aside from trying to cope with the news that their baby isn't tolerating the drugs well, is also trying to cope with their own considerable physical and emotional duress from the experience of the reduced recovery time. Consequently, inductions frequently go hand in hand with a desire for pain medications, which, as we previously discussed, introduces their own set of risks.

Pitocin® is a powerful, artificial hormone that our bodies utilize in myriad ways both known and not yet understood. The long-term effects on the baby from Pitocin® use in labor are still not fully understood, for example, with some specific questions remaining about its impact on epigenetic changes as well as breathing behaviors (including sucking and swallowing).[291] In my experience and research it appears that not just gestational people but also their babies seem to need additional help after providers attempt induction. Following is an excerpt from an ACOG news release on a study that finds a correlation between Pitocin® use and neonatal intensive care admissions:

> Researchers found that induction and augmentation of labor with [artificial] oxytocin was an independent risk factor for unexpected admission to the NICU lasting more than 24 hours for full-term infants. Augmentation also correlated with Apgar scores of fewer than seven at five minutes.[292]

Note that Apgar scores below 7 indicate that a baby will need at least some medical support at birth. Oxytocic drugs like Pitocin® or Cytotek® can therefore add additional risks for a birthing person, including an increased risk of uterine rupture for people who have had a previous uterine surgery, an introduced risk of premature birth, and, as was mentioned earlier in this book, an increased chance of postpartum hemorrhage.[293] Note, too, that the numbers of inductions, cesarean sections, and postpartum hemorrhages have been on the rise.[294] As a consequence, using induction drugs during your birth could also add risk to any future pregnancies.

—Pause, take a deep breath—

I know this is tough stuff to read and process. I offer it all here as further food-for-thought as you continue to create your birth plan and practice your decision-making thinking and approaches. Being informed is important, but it can be harsh to process. Remember that pregnancy is a time to process fears. Everyone has a fear of something. When learning new information, if it stirs up your fears, get curious. I find it helpful to get super specific; again, talk, write about, and/or draw your fears. These exploratory actions can yield information helpful for making plans and medical decisions during your birth process. *Have a goal of expressing fears as a path to releasing them.* If you ever find that you are dwelling on your fears, and that you cannot release one or more of them, please try to seek out a trusted and experienced friend or mentor and/or a mental healthcare professional.

Take another deep breath now. ... ... Try to let go of any physical tension you can tune into. Relaxing the mind helps to relax the body, just as relaxing the body helps to relax the mind. Take a short time right now to give your brain a rest from thinking. I want you to revisit and practice the following Buddhist observation exercise, repeated from Week 2:

EXERCISE: BREATHING WITH A MINDFULNESS PHRASE
(REVISITED FROM WEEK 2)

Try to slow down and sync up your silent words with your breathing action.

As you breathe in think, "I am breathing in."

As you breathe out think, "I am breathing out."

With your timer set, or by giving yourself an approximate time allotment, it's now time to practice. Remember to fill your inhale with inhale words and to fill your exhale action with the exhale words. Try this with eyes closed in any comfortable position.

Non-medicinal ways to try to induce labor

Endocrinologists know a lot about the hormones at play during birth and during sex. But science has not yet taken up the research to try to prove, with empirical standards, that sex is an effective method for inducing or augmenting birth. Nevertheless, I want to propose that the obvious may well be right in front of us: sex is a good tool for induction and augmentation. So let's consider more connections between sex and birth.

Just as medical inductions generally start with the administration of synthetic prostaglandins that soften or ripen the cervix, men's ejaculate (semen) contains natural prostaglandins. In addition, as was cited above, membrane stripping hastens the birth. During heterosexual sex, for example, penetration from a penis can stimulate the cervix in a way that is similar to the medical procedure of membrane stripping. (A dildo can do the same thing minus the natural prostaglandins, for those who might want an alternative to a penis for cervical stimulation.) Furthermore, although scientific proof does not yet exist to support that sexual intercourse helps, medical evidence does exist that breast and nipple stimulation can cause contractions in people with "favorable" cervixes, in which some effacement has begun naturally. Likewise, we already know that medical inductions work better once the cervix has started to efface.[295] Whether it's from self-pleasuring or sex play with a lover, or even through the use of a breast pump, nipple stimulation can help people go into labor (usually taking about three days). Moreover, research suggests that nipple stimulation appears to be protective for postpartum hemorrhage.[296] Rebecca Dekker, of Evidence Based Birth, writes:

The available evidence does support breast stimulation as a non-medicine or a non-pharmacological way to improve the ripening of your cervix, start labor and reduce rates of postpartum hemorrhage, and in the large, randomized trials, we did not see any adverse effects. However, there are some case reports that did warn of uterine hyperstimulation after breast stimulation and women should be counseled of this risk by their healthcare providers if their providers are recommending breast stimulation.[297]

The way I see it, with sex play you are priming the pump of your sex/birth hormones and getting blood flow to the genitals. Plus, since so much in life is better with sweet kissing, it shouldn't be a surprise that it can help with labor, too! Any pleasurable activity that helps get blood flowing to your genitals will help. And if you are lucky enough to have an orgasm, you'll flood yourself with all the right hormones and muscle activity to move things along even further. Sexy, happy—even if a bit awkward—sex can help release stress, build confidence, and move the birth process along. And please note: If for any reason intercourse or any other kind of sex play is not desirable to you, then of course such an act should not be entertained. You may find yourself taxed by your pregnancy in ways that render you too uncomfortable. In these instances, masturbation may be more tolerable and should be considered. However, if your amniotic sac is ruptured, *do not* insert anything into your vagina, be it a penis or dildo or fingers, etc., as this can introduce the risk of infection.

Acupuncture is another medication-free way to attempt to induce or augment a labor. As you may already suspect, there is not a lot of Western scientific research to support acupuncture being beneficial for induction. "One small study at the University of North Carolina found that women who got acupuncture were more likely to go into labor without a medical 'push.'"[298] Nevertheless, it has been used in Chinese medicine for thousands of years as a way to jump start labor. (In Week 14 I will share two acupressure points that may help to start or augment a labor, so keep reading!)

The decision

Regardless of what induction-method is used, the decision to induce is a big deal. Parenting is hard. You must now make life or death decisions in a new, real, and immediate way. The induction decision forces us to decide to do something that potentially could end up causing harm to a healthy process, or it could save the day by avoiding a potentially deadly biological mistake. Many of us, even on a good day, have a lot of churned up emotions about the onset of birth as we arrive *at term*. When you get to late term, it's not uncommon to have increased emotional agitation, especially around medical decisions. Knowing your provider's induction rates and methods well in advance can help you to build that trusting relationship, which in turn can help you to feel confidence in their guidance and in your own decision making if/when the time comes.

As you consider how you would make your choice, if the choice becomes necessary, it continues to be useful to assess (and reassess) any and all concerns or doubts that you or your provider may have about your ability to grow and birth a healthy baby. In other words, do you or your providers have any reason/fears to believe something is not healthy? If the answer is no, keep yourself focused there; you are healthy and you have every reason to believe your baby is healthy, too. If you or your providers do have reason to be concerned, then here is where your decision-making should dwell.

Here are two important things to remember from this week:

1. "Among natural conceptions where the date of conception (ovulation) is known, the variation in pregnancy length spanned 37 days, even after excluding women with complications or preterm births."[299]

2. If your care provider tells you, "if you haven't had the baby by X date, then you'll be induced," remember this: it is always your decision to be induced, not your provider's.

Be cognizant of not giving your provider the power to complicate your natural birth process by inserting deadlines. Take control of your last weeks of term by engaging in those conversations well ahead of time. And to help you engage in those conversations it is helpful to connect to your feelings now from this reading. As of today, can you imagine choosing to induce or choosing not to induce?

Please take a long stretch break now that you've finished this week's lesson. Include deep breaths and closed eyes to help you feel your feelings. Congratulate yourself for all your good work. Be proud of yourself. I am proud of you, too! I send you revitalizing wishes for a great week ahead.

HOMEWORK

A) Practice mindfulness

Try committing to two-minute sessions, 3x per day, of seated breath awareness this week (set an alarm). Also use this time to tune into your baby.

B) Discuss induction and augmentation with your provider

Investigate their preferred methods and timing of interventions.

C) Talk to other parents

Investigate stories of epidural use and induction.

D) Explore any worries that you or your circle of support may have

Assess possible circumstances or concerns that you, your provider, a support partner, family member(s), or friends may have of you not being able to grow and/or birth a healthy baby. We are vulnerable to the thoughts and ideas of those around us, so it is useful to bring these voices to the surface.

E) Have a good time where you can

Make time for self-care that includes fun.

THIS SPACE IS FOR YOUR NOTES AND DRAWINGS

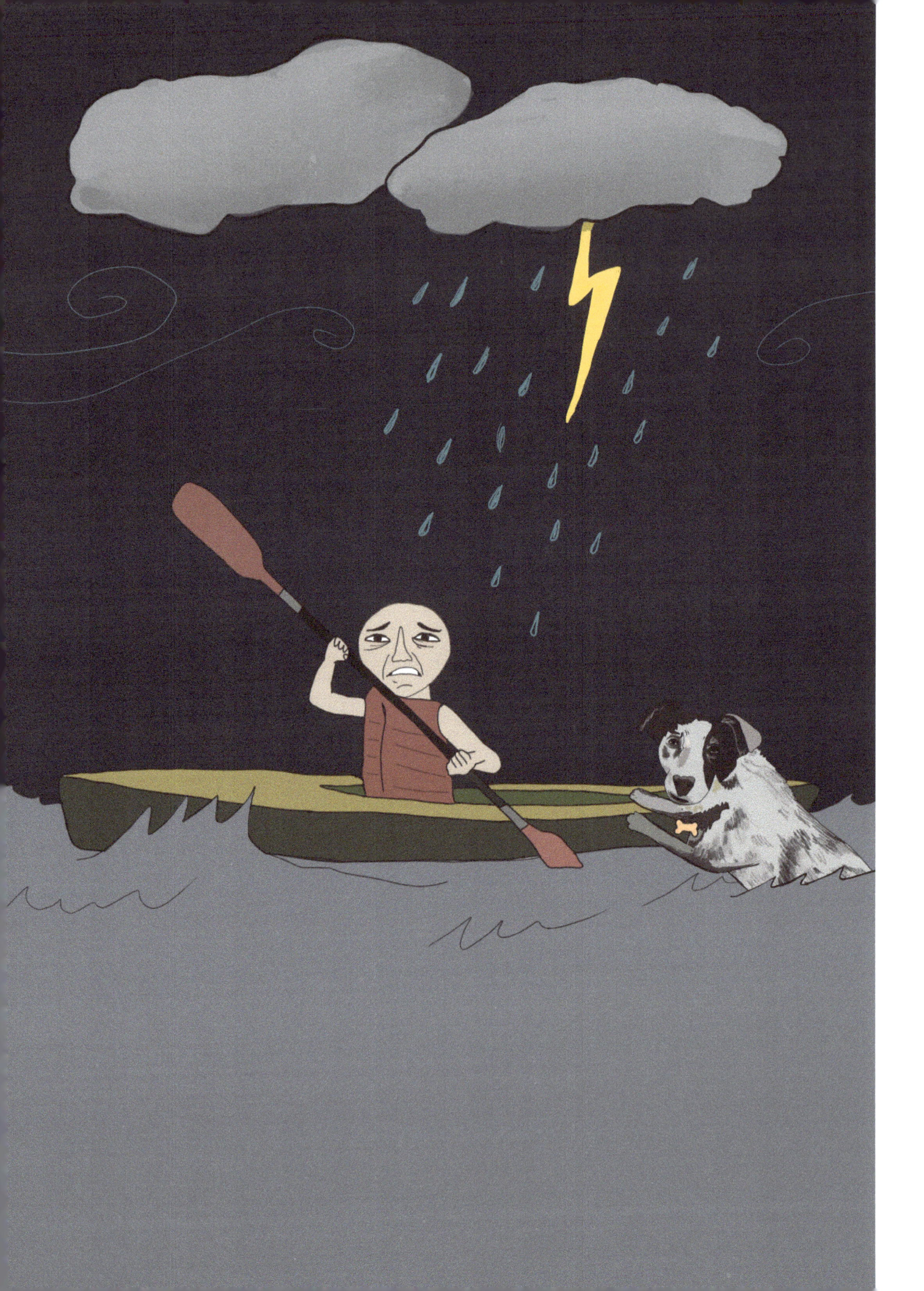

WEEK 13

Fear and Fortitude

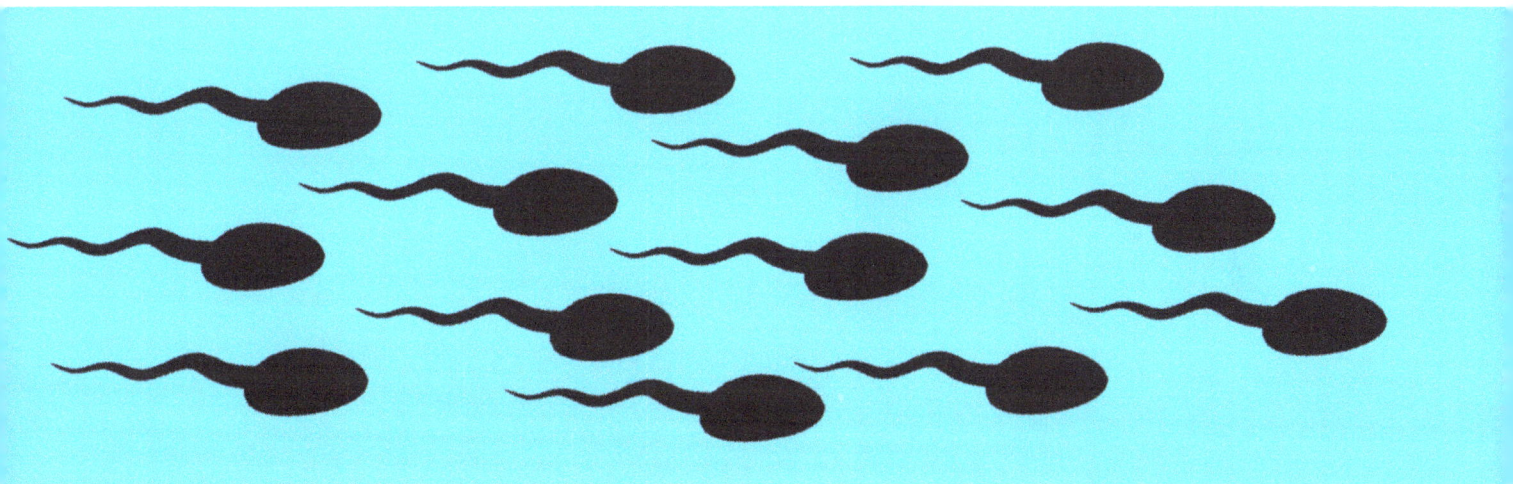

Chapter contents:

- O *Coping with dread*
- O *Surgical births*
- O *Loss*

THIS SPACE IS FOR YOUR NOTES AND DRAWINGS

How have you been this past week? I know last week's reading and exercises were heavy in their content: medications, induction, and making tough decisions. This week may feel heavier still as we work through the topic of fear contextualized through the subjects of cesarean section and stillbirth. I have included these topics together in this chapter *not* because one necessarily results in the other (it doesn't), but because both relate to and remind us immediately of our mortality and mortality itself is a common carrier of fear. As you read this week's lesson you'll naturally feel your emotions churn. It's okay to think—and read and write or draw—about worse-case scenarios. You can't make something bad happen by saying, "I don't think I can handle _____." Instead, by bringing your fears to the surface now, by articulating them directly, you can work through ways to cope and prepare yourself with strength and compassion.

Before we continue into this chapter, please stop now and think back over your past week. Close your eyes, take a few deep, conscientious breaths, and reflect. Try to identify a positive choice that you have made recently and give yourself well-due credit.

—Pause—

If identifying a positive choice was tough, identify a moment when you made a less-than-optimal decision and consider some alternate choices that you could have made. Be gentle and try to see what there is to learn going forward.

—Pause—

Now give yourself credit and feel strong for recognizing that your ability to make better choices is something you can develop—we're all working on it!

Feel your feelings

Confronting, even welcoming and embracing, your scary thoughts and emotions is one way to explore coping methods in a potential crisis. You want to be *in touch* with your feelings now so you can continue to process them productively in the moment of crisis and beyond. Anticipatory worry about unknowns can rattle us deeply, but when we stir up the worries from deep down in our belly (and we've all got them to some degree), we can better know them, and then we can devise more on-point coping strategies. Many have experienced that the way out of rough feelings is to go through them. The cliché is apt. To know our fears is not the same as to be deterred by our fears. The goal here is to figure out what's going on inside and then muster the courage to face the future undeterred.

Facing your fear can in turn help you to live in this moment, *your birthing moment*, as best as you can.

Ways to feel your feelings and acknowledge your fears can include such activities as talking, reading, writing, drawing, and dancing. (Writing[300] and drawing[301] in particular are both research-based methods to help you manage feelings of dread.) But this, of course, is not an exhaustive list (and the research might not matter to you). So think about what might work for *you*. Get creative and/or return to creature comforts. For myself, I find courage in the words of poet-artist-activist Audre Lorde: "When I dare to be powerful—to use my strength in the service of my vision—then it becomes less and less important whether I am afraid."[302]

Fear takes a physical toll. It releases stress hormones, which is exhausting in itself, and this leaves us in need of restoration.[303] If you are already living with a lot of fear, then you know well what I'm talking about. Now that you are expecting baby, you may have new fears directly related to the process of birth and/or parenting. But look at this from another perspective: new fears create the opportunity to find new courage. Courage for birth can be grown by arming yourself with information about how your body (or your partner's body) works. It can also be grown by devising strategies for coping with worst-case scenarios. Courage doesn't mean we are not scared; it means we *are* scared, but that we've identified the fear(s) and we move forward anyway. One way or another the baby is coming out and will be your responsibility. But you can decide, right here and now, to build your courage for birth and parenting. You can do this. This is completely in your control, and I am convinced that you have what it takes.

Please now describe, by saying out loud, something that is worrying you about the remainder of your pregnancy, the birth, and/or parenting. Next, please write down some notes about any concerns or fears that bubble to the surface in this moment. And think about how you might cope, should these fears materialize into reality.

Thank you for thinking about those concerns. Now, take a few breaths with your eyes closed, and give yourself permission to leave your fear on the page. Trust that it will be there if you need to return to it. But maybe you don't have to carry it with you. You don't need to fix or try to solve anything right now. Let the acknowledgement of the feelings settle, allow for some release, and look toward growth to germinate from the seeds you've planted. Take a few more breaths now and deeply exhale some of the physical stress out of your body.

—Pause for some releasing breaths—

We all experience loss. Loss comes in many ways. Loss of life, loss of ability, loss of health, loss of control, loss of dreams and expectations, loss of love. Facing life's challenges is what happens when we're alive, loving, and growing up. Just as much as life can create fear, it can inspire deep meaning and empowerment.

The question to keep asking yourself is: "Are the choices you've been making leading you to where you want to go?" If your fears are weighing too heavily and releasing them is going nowhere fast, consider taking a more direct and proactive approach. For one example, you can evaluate your selfcare routines and see if maybe one small tweak can make a positive influence towards making peace with your concerns or improving some particular health habit you think could use some attention. Maybe journaling as a self-care method can help you explore your thoughts and feelings. Maybe this creates space to support your best intentions with regard to practices that you feel could use some tweaking. Talking with a friend or another pregnant person can also bring comfort, and can help you hear your own voice. If you have concerning thoughts that are intrusive, or somehow make it harder to function the way that you would like to, professional counseling should be considered. And, of course, seeking out various kinds of education (which you've already begun, as you work through the lessons in this book!) is an excellent form of proactive support. If you are scared your baby might be born with a birth defect, for another example, you can seek out people who were born with birth defects, or people raising people with birth defects, and talk to them to see if there is anything they wish they had known earlier or they wish that their parents had known.

Pregnancy is a very vulnerable time. As you get bigger you can't even get up and run away from the mythological tiger in the room. Be compassionate with yourself, knowing that it is normal to have fears and concerns about the unknown journey ahead. And try to ask yourself the hard questions, explore difficult topics, and return to your coping strategies again and again. Individuals will likely be called to and comforted by a variety of coping techniques. Don't shy away from trying several different options and approaches. This is really all we can ask of ourselves in the face of our fears.

As you read about cesarean sections in the following section it's useful to keep in mind that a surgical birth is a birth, and it may be your birth. I didn't see it coming but it was my first birth, and in time I learned to see it with all of its unique wonder, loss, and joy.

Cesarean section: the ultimate obstetric intervention

A cesarean section (c/section or c-section) is major abdominal surgery. In brief: a local anesthesia by route of a spinal or an epidural (if one was already in place) is administered, only in the rarest of emergencies might a general anesthesia be used, and then a surgeon will cut open all the layers of the abdomen to access the uterus, with internal organs often being moved out of the way. Next the uterus itself will be cut open to allow for delivery of the baby and the placenta by manually pulling both out. Finally, everything is put back in order and the abdomen is sewn back up, layer by layer.

This surgery can be lifesaving for the birthing person and the baby, but it also carries with it many serious risks. For the birthing person the immediate risks include infection, hemorrhage, deep vein thrombosis (a blood clot), and pulmonary embolism (when a blood clot breaks loose and goes into the lungs.)[304] In addition, as I will explore shortly, once a person has had a cesarean section, in subsequent pregnancies there are new and serious risks for placental attachment complications.

As a birth educator, I value the byproducts of empowerment and satisfaction that my work supports. I work hard to inform my clients of their options, just as I am doing here through this book. The question is: when is it necessary—and when may it not be necessary—to have a c/section to birth your baby? In what follows below, I discuss several conditions, starting with those that would demand surgery.

Placenta previa is a rare condition in which the placenta grows in front of and blocks the cervical opening. With no doorway, there is no way out for the baby; surgery is required. Fortunately, this serious complication announces itself with cervical bleeding during the pregnancy.[305] Because this condition should be known in advance, looking for the cause of the bleeding presents a medical need for investigation. A fairly quick diagnosis can be made using ultrasound. A related condition is **low-lying placenta.** This is when the placenta lies very low and near the opening of the cervix, rather than directly in front of it. As the cervix begins to make changes at the start of labor, a low-lying placenta can introduce the risk of early separation of the placenta in the area near the shortening and thinning cervix. Remember that there are large blood vessels feeding the placenta. Therefore, as the cervix starts to open, there would be potential risk that a low-lying placenta could start to separate prematurely. A full placenta previa or a very low placenta at the end of the pregnancy, are both indications for a cesarean section.[306]

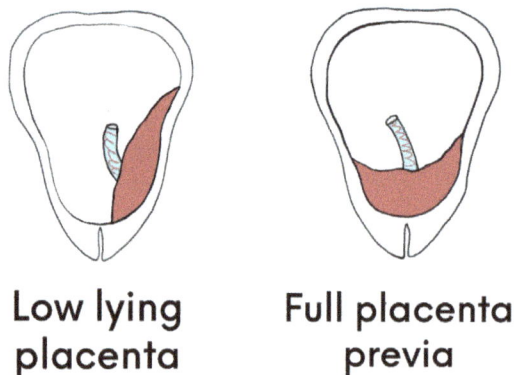

Low lying placenta   **Full placenta previa**

Important to note is the fact that many pregnancies start off with a low placenta and then, as the pregnancy continues, the placenta grows and the uterus grows so that for most people the placenta ends up away from the cervical opening. In other words, knowing the placental position early in the pregnancy is not an indication of where the placenta will be at term. In my opinion, if you have an early ultrasound that shows a low placenta, you do not need frequent ultrasounds to monitor, which is a common practice; instead, you need one more test when you get to term. Nevertheless, each person's circumstances are unique. So please be sure to discuss this topic with your provider.

Placental abruption is a rare, but very dangerous emergency scenario in which the placenta starts to separate before the baby is born. It is life threatening for the birthing person as well as the baby, making surgery a necessary emergency option. According to the Mayo Clinic, risk factors for this serious condition include abdominal trauma, very high blood pressure, having had a placental abruption before, drug addiction, and being pregnant after age 40.[307]

A **prolapsed cord** is when the cord comes out before the baby. This is also considered an emergency situation that requires surgery. (Prolapsed cord should always be considered as a risk resulting from an amniotomy, or the artificial rupture of the amniotic sac.)

A **transverse fetal position** at the start of labor is when the baby is completely sideways inside the uterus. Babies just can't come out sideways, making this scenario another clear indication for a surgical birth. However, there is a medical procedure called an "external cephalic version," during which a baby's position is manipulated from outside of the gestational person's abdomen, by the provider's hands.[308] Sometimes this external version works, sometimes it doesn't, or the baby flips right back into the transverse fetal position. Risks of the external version include fetal distress from cord compression, premature rupture of membranes, placental abruption, and the need for immediate emergency surgery. There are also age-old midwifery practices, such as the Central American rebozo techniques, that can help to adjust the baby's position. Rebozo work to adjust fetal position should only be performed by a culturally competent and well-trained birth attendant.[309] Another resource for improving fetal positioning is the website, SpinningBabies.com, which lists very helpful information on optimizing fetal positioning.[310] Regardless of the techniques used, if the baby remains in a transverse position, surgery will become necessary. (See Appendix for fetal positioning resources.)

Preeclampsia, a pregnancy complication associated with high blood pressure, may be able to be managed by induction (see Week 2 for review). If not, then surgery will be required, because it can become too dangerous to wait for birth. A pregnant person's platelet count is one of the barometers used to measure if it's time for surgery or not. Platelets help your blood to clot. In preeclampsia, a person's platelet count may start to drop.[311] If your platelet count starts to fall, the surgery must be done quickly.

If you have **genital herpes**, and there is an active lesion at your birth, then you will not want to risk the baby coming in contact with this virus. Surgical birth is therefore indicated.

Not all medical conditions present a clear "yes" response for undergoing a cesarean section. Conditions such as **diabetes, cephalic-pelvic disproportion (CPD), breech position**, and **fetal distress** fall into a grey area. If you are diabetic and have not been controlling your blood sugar levels well (because your providers cannot help you to figure out how to control your blood sugars and/or you're a non-compliant diabetes patient), you could grow a baby too big to deliver vaginally and would thus necessitate surgical intervention. By contrast, if your blood sugars have been well monitored and regulated, then you should continue to be a good candidate for a spontaneous vaginal birth.

In cephalic-pelvic disproportion (CPD) the baby's head is too big to fit through the mother's pelvis. The only way to accurately diagnose this is to encourage the birthing person to try different second stage positions and to give them time and encouragement. Although researchers are still studying prolonged second stage labor, it is currently understood that 1) first-time gestational people should be given at least three hours and 2) more time may be advisable, based on individual circumstances and progress.[312] I have had many clients report that their second stage labor lasted much longer than three hours, with the longest being 10 hours (and the midwife was comfortable about the progress being made—albeit slow). I have also heard of women getting a CPD diagnosis even before they are fully dilated. I had at least one client years ago who was given this diagnosis at 36 weeks because she was very large (fat), and so the doctor thought the baby would be too big to fit. How can you tell it won't work until you have tried? The birthing person's pelvic bones move. The baby's head plates will shift. How can you tell your baby won't fit *before* you are completely dilated and have been trying to squeeze that baby out? You cannot. If the baby is moving down, even in the smallest of increments, then a prolonged second stage is not necessarily an indication for surgery. But, if vaginal exams show that the baby is not making any progress *at all*, and the person has had good support to get into a variety of different positions over time, then something isn't right and medical intervention may very well be in order.

Breech is the word used to describe a baby who is head-up inside the uterus, with either her butt or her legs presenting first—rather than her head, as in the more common vertex (head-down) position. There are some added risks to catching a breech baby vaginally, as I discussed in Weeks 1 and 7. Thus your provider should have specific skills and understanding to safely navigate a breech birth. Unfortunately, as I previously mentioned, most U.S. trained medical doctors are no longer taught the art form of catching breech babies vaginally. A terrible gap in information exists, and what was once fairly standard care has now become a standard reason for surgery. Nevertheless some midwives and doctors do possess training and skill in breech delivery. So again, use this as another good interview topic in your search for care providers.

Fetal distress is an absolute indication for surgery, and yet this is also not without its grey area. If the baby seems to be in trouble, you want to go right in to get the baby out. The question, however, is *how* it is determined that the baby is in distress. As I discussed in Week 4, cardiotocography (CTG, also called EFM or electronic fetal monitor) can give us misleading or inconclusive information; it can be very hard to know if the baby is under the normal stress of labor or in true distress, and the technology, remember, brings a high rate of false positivity for cerebral palsy. I know this is hard to wrap your mind and heart around. It is for me, too. I wish I had simple answers and clear decision points to present in this scenario.

Elective or emergency cesarean section

It is important to understand that there are two classifications of cesarean section: elective and emergency. Elective will usually feel like an emergency to the person having it, but elective means there is time to discuss, decide, get consent, prepare, etc. An elective cesarean can be planned or unplanned, but there is no outstanding pressure to act *now*. In an emergency cesarean section there is no time; providers are afraid someone is dying. The staff will move as fast as possible to get the person into the operating room—no discussion, no partner, and no in-the-moment consent. This scenario is one potential outcome relating to why the hospital asks you to sign a general consent before being admitted.

The majority of surgical births are, in fact, elective. To further discuss this hypothetical birth scenario of an *elective* cesarean section, I will assume that the pregnant person is healthy, low risk, and has had no interventions used thus far (such as IVs, medications, etc.). This was the case for my first birth, in which everything was going along fine and then the baby flipped into a breech position while I was in labor. (This is unusual but can happen.) First things first, you'll want to ask your provider all your questions for informed consent: e.g., Why are you suggesting the surgery? What are the risks associated with the surgery? What are the risks of not doing the surgery? Are there any alternatives to doing the surgery? Could this be a normal and healthy variation of birth? How much time are you comfortable giving me to make my decision?

Once you have collected all your data, as I discussed in Week 11, I strongly encourage you to ask everyone to leave the room except for your primary partner or other most trusted confidant. Ideally, it's you and your partner or trusted pal—just the two of you—having a moment alone together to make this decision. You'll need to check in with each other, with limited to no distractions. You can ask each other, "Are you ok? Do you have any more questions? Are you ready to make this decision?" When the two of you are alone, it can feel much safer to express any reservations, or to admit that you don't fully understand something, or to figure out what questions still remain. We can usually ask the "stupid questions" more easily when we are alone with a primary or other trusted support partner. And even when the choice is completely obvious to you, you can still benefit from asking everyone to leave the room, giving you some quiet time to reflect. When your own answer is "yes" to the cesarean section, formal consent to the surgery follows.

The next series of events will be a whirlwind, so having that moment alone with your partner can help to ground you. The prep activity will likely be swift, busy, and surreal. And the next thing you know, the baby is here. Meaning, the next time that you will be alone with your partner, you won't be alone with your partner—your baby will be with you! In short, this moment of decision-making and reflection would be your last moment to touch base, be alone, and check in with each other. After you've done that, you can ask everyone to come back into the room and you can give them your decision.

Preparations and the procedure

Assuming you are already admitted to the hospital and in a labor room, the following procedures generally take place in that room: If you don't already have IV access in place, then an IV will be inserted and fluids will be administered. Medications, such as antibiotics, may be administered, too. You'll also be placed on the fetal monitor (CTG/EFM). The nurse will give you an antacid to calm your digestive activity (a small amount of sweet, goopy drink). Your nurse will shave your upper pubic hair and low belly. You will have an anesthesia consultation, which will include discussion to determine the best route of administration and drug options available for pain control during the surgery. If you already have an epidural in place, generally that will be left in place and utilized for the surgery. The anesthesiologist will also take another medical history. This may feel frustrating, as you have probably had to already give your history and you might assume that it must be written down somewhere in your chart. It has been recorded, yes, but the reality is if your anesthesiologist is now going to take responsibility for your life, they don't want to trust that your prior history was correct, or correctly noted. So they take a new one. After your consult with the anesthesiologist, your nurse will want to insert a Foley catheter into your urethra (the hole out of which pee comes). You can request to have the catheter insertion delayed until after anesthesia has been administered in the operating room (OR). Once all of the above has been done you are ready to go to the OR. At this point you are usually separated from your support person. You will be wheeled into the OR and anesthetized.

While this is happening, the nurse will typically take your partner aside, instruct them to scrub their hands, give them scrubs to cover their clothes, a clean mask, a cap for their head, and booties to go over their shoes. This will ready your partner to go into the sterile operating room in order to be with you during the surgery/birth.

Once in the OR you will receive the Foley catheter (if not already inserted), along with any additional medications, an automatic blood pressure cuff on your arm, possibly weighted arm restraints around the area of the wrists, and a pulse oximeter on one finger (to measure oxygen saturation levels). A paper curtain will also be hung from a bar that blocks your view of your abdomen.

After your spinal anesthesia takes effect, and you have become appropriately numb, your partner is brought into the room. (Note to your partner: when you first walk into an operating room, please don't touch anything surgical. You should touch your partner; squeeze their hand or arm, caress their face—any part not near the surgical field. Everything else in the room should be off limits to your hands.) The nurses usually put a stool by the head of the table for a partner to sit on, where their view is likewise shielded by the same paper curtain that shields yours. If you or your partner wants to watch the surgery, then you should both feel empowered to do so. Your partner can stand up and watch, and you can request a mirror to be held at an angle that allows you the view you want.

Before the first surgical cut is made, a nurse or anesthesiologist will do a pin prick test on you to make sure that the anesthesia is working correctly. The pin prick test, as the name would suggest, uses a sharp pin to determine if you have feeling from the soles of your feet, up your leg, and onto your abdomen. The medical staff needs to know that the medications are doing what they are supposed to do. Sometimes there are strange reactions to medication and because the anesthetic drugs don't always work, the pin prick test helps the staff to determine that the drugs are indeed working as expected. Once you are successfully numb, a surgical assistant will cover your abdomen with a sterilizing solution, such as Betadine®, and then the obstetrician is ready to make the first incision.

There were a few things I experienced during my own surgical birth that I have been sharing with my clients ever since. The encouraging feedback I've gained from this sharing has convinced me to include it here, as well. I had tremendous shivering and shaking in my upper body from the time I got my spinal anesthesia through to my time in the recovery room. I felt cold, so very cold. The shaking scared me and was uncomfortable; I thought I might shake right off the table. I asked the anesthesiologist if this shaking was a problem and received the short answer of "no." But the shaking was probably the worst part for me. I now know that my shivering is quite common and probably the result of a combination of being cold from the IV fluids, tired from laboring, and fear.

Overall my surgeon was kind and spoke to me frequently, giving me many reassurances that everything was going well throughout the surgery (although he never did address the shaking). I also heard surgical assistants counting. At first, I wasn't sure what that was and then I realized that someone was counting clamps, sponges, and other medical instruments that might be going into me so that they could then count what they were taking out of me. This helped to ensure that nothing got left behind inside the incision. At one point I also smelled smoke, like burning hair. I realized what was burning was me; someone on the surgical team was cauterizing my blood vessels to stop the bleeding. Although this can be unnerving to think about, it is a typical part of the procedure.

Even when you are numb and the anesthesia is really working, you will likely feel some tugging sensations as the doctor performs the surgery and removes your baby and placenta, both of which are pulled out manually. I describe my own experience this way: imagine that you have a tight bathing suit on or maybe a pair of tights and the section around your abdomen is all twisted up and you need to tug in small increments to get it moved around and straightened out. One of my clients recently described her tugging sensations as if someone were kneading dough on her belly. Being awake for your surgical birth is a crazy thing, and amazing in its own way. I was—and still am—grateful that we have gotten as good at modern medicine as we have! And, just as my experiences can be helpful to hear ahead of time, I encourage you to speak with friends and family members who have also gone through a cesarean birth.

Under most elective-surgery circumstances it takes about 15 minutes to get the baby out and then about 45 minutes to put the birthing person back together. (Under emergency circumstances doctors can usually get the baby out in much less time.) Putting a person back together is an important job; you don't want the surgeon to rush.

In my surgical birth the doctor said, "You have a big baby boy," and he pulled my son out and briefly held him up over the curtain for me to see. The baby was crying and so was I. They quickly dried him off, did a brief examination of him, wrapped him up in a blanket and handed him to my partner. I vividly remember looking up at baby and daddy and thinking, "Thank goodness my partner is here, I couldn't possibly hold my baby with my arms and upper body shaking so much." It was such an incredible comfort to know my baby was in his daddy's arms.

During that whole 45-minute period that you are being stitched back up, your support partner should be able to stay by your side, holding your baby. This is assuming, of course, that your baby is doing fine (because in this hypothetical we don't know what reasons caused you to have to have this elective surgery in the first place). Note to the partner: if you find yourself standing there in the OR holding your baby, try to remember to hold the baby up next to the birthing person's face. They will do well to smell each other and feel each other and see each other. Any connection is good, even if the birthing person is asleep!

Once the surgeon has finished stitching, stapling, and/or gluing you back together, you're wheeled into the recovery area. This is generally a curtained area outside of the operating room. You will likely stay in the recovery area for two to four hours, while the medical team monitors your vitals and makes sure that you have tolerated the surgery. If you and baby are both doing well, then it is entirely possible that the first breastfeeding can happen right there in the recovery area. Your support partner, a nurse, and a doula (if you have one) should help in any way needed. Note that doulas are sometimes allowed into the actual surgery, along with another primary support partner, but not always. By contrast, doulas are almost always allowed in the recovery room if the birthing person is stable. In recovery, you may or may not be able to hold the baby on your own, so your partner and/or doula can help get your baby up to your breast and allow the process of breastfeeding to begin. It is not so important that the baby get nutrition right then and there. Rather, it's helpful to start the learning process of breastfeeding as soon after the birth as possible. Perhaps your baby will just nuzzle at the breast. This is totally fine. Moreover, it is helpful for your healing because it encourages uterine contractions, just as it provides comfort for you and baby. Maybe your baby will latch right on and suckle like a pro. This is great, too. Our goal should be to follow through on as physiologically normal a progression as possible, from birth to baby at the birth parent's breast, regardless of the interventions that are needed along the way.

If you and your baby need to be separated after the birth, you'll want to work at getting re-accustomed to each other and to establish breastfeeding as soon as possible. Breastfeeding is ideally established immediately after birth, but the first concern must be that each person is stable. Once everyone is stable breastfeeding can be introduced. And don't worry, there is a plethora of breastfeeding success stories after several hours, days, or even weeks of separation. Also, please be aware that while it can take extra days for your milk to come in after a surgery compared to a vaginal birth, your colostrum will continue to provide adequate resources for your baby. Thus, there is no inherent need to supplement.

I was separated from my baby after my surgery. I was left alone in recovery while my baby and my partner went off so baby could have an X-ray. They didn't tell me at the time, but my baby had a deep indentation at the end of his spine, just above his butt, and they wanted to take an x-ray to make sure that it was in fact closed, and not a spinal column issue. I didn't know why I was alone, but I didn't know that it wasn't normal either. It was lonely and I was pretty freaked out from having to go through the surgery. Plus, it was the middle of the night. Plus, I was still shaking. And I was thirsty and had the worst dry mouth I could ever have imagined. I am sure this helped lead to some of the fear that I felt 18 months later while I was processing the experience. At the time, however, I trusted that I had just experienced a relatively normal surgical procedure. This is a very good example of why it is good to have a doula or extra helper with you at a birth. It would have been immensely comforting to me, and to my partner, to have had someone with me while he was with the baby. Several hours later, when they moved me out of recovery and into a room, my partner came in to see me. Soon after that they brought me my baby. It was a good three, maybe even four hours later that I got my baby to my breast. He latched on like a pro, and we had no trouble establishing breastfeeding.

Pain medication after a surgical birth

My advice: take your post-surgery pain meds early and as often as you need them. The key to a speedy recovery is to get you up and moving. If you refuse the meds, or try to limit yourself, you won't be as active. This can slow down your recovery and could result in a prolonged need for pain medication. The benefits for you heavily outweigh the risks to the baby. You will of course be observant of your baby, like noticing if your baby seems extra drowsy or is reacting to the meds in some other way. Then you can stop and try another medication and/or approach to recovery. There are emerging protocols for pain management that rely heavily on ibuprofen and acetaminophen that seem to significantly reduce opioid use.[313] But even for my clients that used opioids, I personally don't know anyone whose baby has had problems with their birth parent's post-surgical pain medications. The breasts do seem to filter a bit more than the placenta does.

There will be several days, maybe even a week or two or longer, after your c/section when you will need to have the baby handed to you for breastfeeding and then taken from you after breastfeeding. You should not be bending over and picking up your baby or placing her down until you are more healed. (Most providers will give you a weight limit for what you can pick up while healing. If your doctor doesn't mention it, please ask.) Remind yourself that your surgery cut you open at your core. Be compassionate and patient with yourself. Changing your position and moving around is going to be painful and difficult for a while. But you will heal.

If you haven't had a cesarean section, you may not realize its status as major abdominal surgery. So many of us have grown complacent in our thinking about cesarean sections. We talk about it as "the other way that babies are born," asking "how are you going to have your baby—vaginal or c/section?" As explained above, cesarean sections are serious surgical procedures and shouldn't be treated as if choosing between a chocolate or a vanilla milkshake. We sometimes forget that birthing people and babies can have serious complications from this procedure. The difference in healing time between a vaginal birth and a cesarean section can be tremendous. And this difference can also impact how a person orients to the new job of parenting.

Cesarean section risks for the birthing person

- Delayed initiation of breastfeeding (which is associated with less breastfeeding.)
- Deep Vein Thrombosis (blood clot)
- Pulmonary embolism (blockage in the lung from a blood clot)
- Hemorrhage
- Infection/Abscess formation

○ Dehiscence (separation of surgical incision, uterine or abdomen)

○ Surgical mistakes (such as a cut baby)

○ Nicked bowel

○ Placental attachment disorders in subsequent pregnancies

Because placenta attachment disorders create life threatening risk, they deserve further illumination here. Normally the placenta attaches to the inside of the uterine wall. But scar tissue (from a previous surgery, for example) is thinner than typical uterine tissue. This thinness can allow the placenta to grow abnormally deep into the uterine wall, causing placenta accreta, or even through it, resulting in placenta percreta.

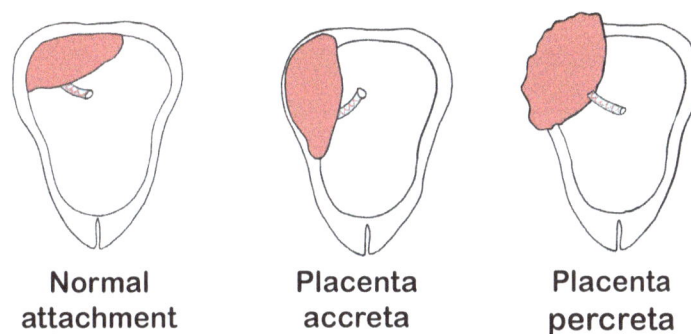

Normal attachment   **Placenta accreta**   **Placenta percreta**

These abnormal attachments create a life-threatening potential for hemorrhage immediately following birth during third stage labor, when the placenta should be detaching and can't. If a part of the placenta can't detach, the birthing person has no way to stem their bleeding. It is through the process of retraction that a person stops feeding the placenta with all of their blood. Remember that retraction is the word for when the uterus contracts and gets and stays smaller (because there is no longer a baby keeping it big). These contractions cause the uterus to shrink, which is what in turn crimps off the blood vessels that have been going from the birthing parent into the placenta through the uterine wall. Without the ability to crimp off those blood vessels, a person will hemorrhage from the enlarged vessels that have been feeding the placenta. When this happens, the birthing person's life must be saved via emergency surgery, usually including hysterectomy (the complete removal of the uterus). Note that ultrasound can be used during pregnancy to (sometimes) determine placental attachment abnormalities and location in relation to any scar tissue. Placental attachment complications, when known in advance, necessitate appropriate surgical birth plans to be made. But as you will soon read in an excerpt from an ACOG care-consensus paper, ultrasound isn't always a useful diagnostic tool for placental mal (bad) attachments. These dangerous complications are on the rise in the U.S. and are associated with both the increase in cesarean section for birth and the increase in maternal mortality rates.

I first became aware of the increase of cases of placental attachment complications around 2011:

> Once a rare event that affected 1 in 30,000 pregnant women in the 1950s and 1960s, placenta accreta now affects 1 in 2,500 pregnancies... In some hospitals, the number is as high as 1 in 522. And doctors say the main reason is the dramatic rise in the number of cesarean sections.[314]

It was clear to me then, and it is even more true today: birthing people and babies are facing substantial increases in risk that appear to connect directly to the normalized care practices that have led to upwards of a third of all babies being cut out. ACOG published the following in their obstetric care-consensus paper in 2018, and then reconfirmed it in 2021:

Rates of placenta accreta spectrum are increasing... A 2016 study conducted using the National Inpatient Sample found that the overall rate of placenta accreta in the United States was 1 in 272 for women who had a birth-related hospital discharge diagnosis, which is higher than any other published study. The increasing rate of placenta accreta over the past four decades is likely due to a change in risk factors, most notably the increased rate of cesarean delivery.[315]

The ACOG consensus paper continues:

Although ultrasound evaluation is important, the absence of ultrasound findings does not preclude a diagnosis of placenta accreta spectrum; thus, clinical risk factors remain equally important as predictors of placenta accreta spectrum by ultrasound findings. There are several risk factors for placenta accreta spectrum. The most common is a previous cesarean delivery, with the incidence of placenta accreta spectrum increasing with the number of prior cesarean deliveries. Antenatal diagnosis of placenta accreta spectrum is highly desirable because outcomes are optimized when delivery occurs at a level III or IV maternal care facility before the onset of labor or bleeding and with avoidance of placental disruption. The most generally accepted approach to placenta accreta spectrum is cesarean hysterectomy with the placenta left in situ after delivery of the fetus (attempts at placental removal are associated with significant risk of hemorrhage). Optimal management involves a standardized approach with a comprehensive multidisciplinary care team accustomed to management of placenta accreta spectrum. In addition, established infrastructure and strong nursing leadership accustomed to managing high-level postpartum hemorrhage should be in place, and access to a blood bank capable of employing massive transfusion protocols should help guide decisions about delivery location.[316]

Take a breath here and remember that through self-care and education you are doing an outstanding job of proactively protecting yourself from these complications. My intent is not to inundate you with fears but to help motivate you to keep going with the work of making your healthiest choices. One such choice: when you can safely avoid a primary cesarean section, it is in your best interest to do so, particularly if you may ever consider a subsequent pregnancy. Also consider that additional risks for the newborn can emerge.

Post-surgical complications for baby

- Delayed start to breastfeeding (can increase breastfeeding difficulties)
- Trouble breathing in first few days of life[317]
- Surgical injury (baby was cut)
- Asthma
- Allergies
- Obesity
- Inflammatory bowel disease[318]
- Microbiome deficient (baby doesn't get exposure to helpful bacteria in the vagina). This deficiency has been associated with the abovementioned asthma, allergies, and other immune disorders.[319]

The implications of a deficient microbiome are startling, far reaching and remain an area of emerging research.

> From birth, the gut microbiota are responsible for the activation and development of the immune system, the development of the central nervous system (CNS), and the digestion and metabolism of food. Early life is a critical period for microbial colonization, which not only affects the health of the infant, but also is profound to long-term health planning.[320]

To say that the microbiome is of critical import is an understatement. Learning about this import weighs on my own birthing history. Although my oldest was (mostly) an "A" student throughout his education, he has suffered with serious autoimmune illness. Over the years, I have often wondered if he was made more vulnerable to such disorders by his surgical birth and the impact this had on his microbiome. Knowing that the microbiome impacts the development of the nervous, immune and digestive systems should not only cause us pause in our standards of care that lead to so many surgical births; we should also closely examine our use of prophylactic antibiotics during labor and for the newborn. One of the ways scientists are looking to mitigate the risks associated with microbiome deficiency for the surgically born newborn is through the practice of "vaginal seeding." From ACOG:

> Vaginal seeding refers to the practice of inoculating a cotton gauze or a cotton swab with vaginal fluids to transfer the vaginal flora to the mouth, nose, or skin of a newborn infant. The intended purpose of vaginal seeding is to transfer maternal vaginal bacteria to the newborn. As the increase in the frequency of asthma, atopic disease, and immune disorders mirrors the increase in the rate of cesarean delivery, the theory of vaginal seeding is to allow for proper colonization of the fetal gut and, therefore, reduce the subsequent risk of asthma, atopic disease, and immune disorders. At this time, vaginal seeding should not be performed outside the context of an institutional review board-approved research protocol until adequate data regarding the safety and benefit of the process become available.[321]

There is also a move to make the birthing experience through cesarean section as natural as possible, with birthing person getting baby placed on their chest immediately following birth, for example, which would be comforting and aid bonding and breastfeeding initiation. But not all providers will accommodate such advances (again, be sure to ask your interview questions ahead of time). In the meantime, my advice is to continue to do what you can to avoid the need for a surgical birth, and to emotionally let go of what you cannot control. As I mentioned before, try to pick a provider and location with low rates of surgical birth, eat well, exercise, and educate yourself—like you are doing now. You are well on your way.

If you do end up needing a surgical birth, please keep in mind that a lot of variation exists in how people recover from a cesarean section. Some people seem to bounce back rather quickly, in days. But for most people it takes several weeks to feel comfortable being up and around. It takes time to build strength and stamina and physical confidence. Some people feel that it takes months to feel recovered. Seeing a good physical therapist, one who specializes in pregnancy and the pelvic floor (including postpartum and surgical issues, such as scar manipulation) can help to fast track your recovery. It is excellent birth preparation to locate such a provider now, should you need one later.

For me, the emotional healing took longer than the physical. About a year and a half after my cesarean section, while my son took a nap one afternoon, I took some time out to read. I was working through my reading requirements for the Bradley Method® teacher training. That day I was reading about cesarean sections when I was overcome with a physical reaction. I started to cry and shake and shiver. I couldn't control it. I was trembling and I felt cold and so scared. Right as this was happening, my partner happened to come home. He was alarmed to find me in such a state and wanted to know what was going on. When I could finally calm down enough to speak, I told him that, in fact, I had been really scared during my c/section. For 18 months I hadn't realized it—I hadn't been able to feel how scared I had been of the surgery. I hadn't allowed myself to feel my fear, as fear, until that day. 18 months later, while reading about the procedure, it all came flooding back and I was able to relive and acknowledge and work through my fear.

I thought I might die, and I was so very cold, but at the time of the actual surgery, my overwhelming feeling was that I needed to do this and therefore it was ok. As I recovered from the surgery, and I was learning to parent and breastfeed, my feelings about the surgery centered twofold on feelings of gratitude that everything turned out ok and on sad feelings about not being able to push my baby out. Again, it had taken me 18 months to be able to process this fear. Yes, I was very afraid of the surgery, and probably also afraid of becoming a mother. And here in a different apartment in a different city, 18 months later, I was safe enough and ready to feel what I had had to stuff down at the time.

That was me. You will be different. Nevertheless, all of us will need time to process our experiences and learn from our births. Surgical births and other major interventions can provide a lot of additional issues to process and to learn from. Now I look back at my birth and I can understand my participation. I can feel the triumph and the pride and the courage of my birth. I understand much of what I learned, and I have made peace with my sadness and the sense of loss that I felt. I have healed from my surgery, physically as well as emotionally.

Express yourself

In the early days and weeks of my surgical recovery, while I was trying to process what had happened, friends and family would occasionally say to me, "Don't be sad, hurt, or angry over your birth… look at your beautiful baby!" The comment would make me mad, really mad. It took me a while to figure out why, but here is my understanding now: As humans we are totally capable of, and entirely entitled to have, different feelings about what happened to us in birth—from how we feel about our babies to our becoming parents. If I said something negative about my birth experience and someone answered with, "but look at your beautiful baby," it felt like they were misinterpreting my comments about my birth. I heard such comments not as being about my baby, but about my being a mother. This misinterpretation would bring out my angry-mama-bear attributes. (Look out, here come the claws!) The fact is most people have feelings about their birth process that are very different than their feelings about their babies or parenthood, and they need room to express them all. For the partners, it is very important that you understand this. It will be quite helpful to you both if, as you listen to and witness feelings about the birth process, you know that these feelings are likely quite different than the feelings felt about the transition to parenthood or feelings about the baby. (Reminder: if you are left with difficult feelings after your birth, expressive writing and drawing can help you heal.)

EXERCISE: STRETCH BREAK

Please read through the following stretching exercise, then try it. If you are with a partner, take turns reading it out loud as the other works through the exercise.

"Stand up. Take a few deep, slow breaths. Close your eyes and place your fingertips on your own shoulders, on the same side. Gently and slowly begin to make circles in the air with your elbows, encourage your chest and upper back area to open fully as you circle, first in one direction and then the other. Breathe fully. Gently engage the muscles between your shoulder blades.

As you continue to circle your arms, keeping your eyes closed and slowly changing direction when you want, bring your attention to the soles of your feet. Feel your connection to the earth. Feel gravity holding you. Now, let your arms rest down by your side. Keep your eyes closed. Visualize energy coming up from the center of the earth, through the center of your feet, up through your legs and torso, and then shooting out of the crown of your head. Maybe it's helpful to see the energy as a cobalt blue color. And then, from just above your head, feel the energy wash down over you, protecting you, renewing you, nourishing you. The energy comes from the center of the earth, through your feet, up through your body, out of the top of your head and then washes down around you."

—Reader pause—

"As this visualized energy showers down around you, try to visualize the energy first in cobalt blue and then in all your favorite colors. Feel the color shower as protective and comforting. Let the energy heal any parts of you that need healing. Use your imagination; it's a powerful tool."

—Reader pause—

"Keeping your eyes closed, let the image fade. Now bring your attention back to your breath. Observe your breath going in, observe your breath going out."

—Reader pause—

"Now let your attention shift and try to identify something you feel grateful for."

—Reader pause—

"Now open your eyes. Tune into your body and stretch or move any parts that need attention. Take a sip of water, and return to reading."

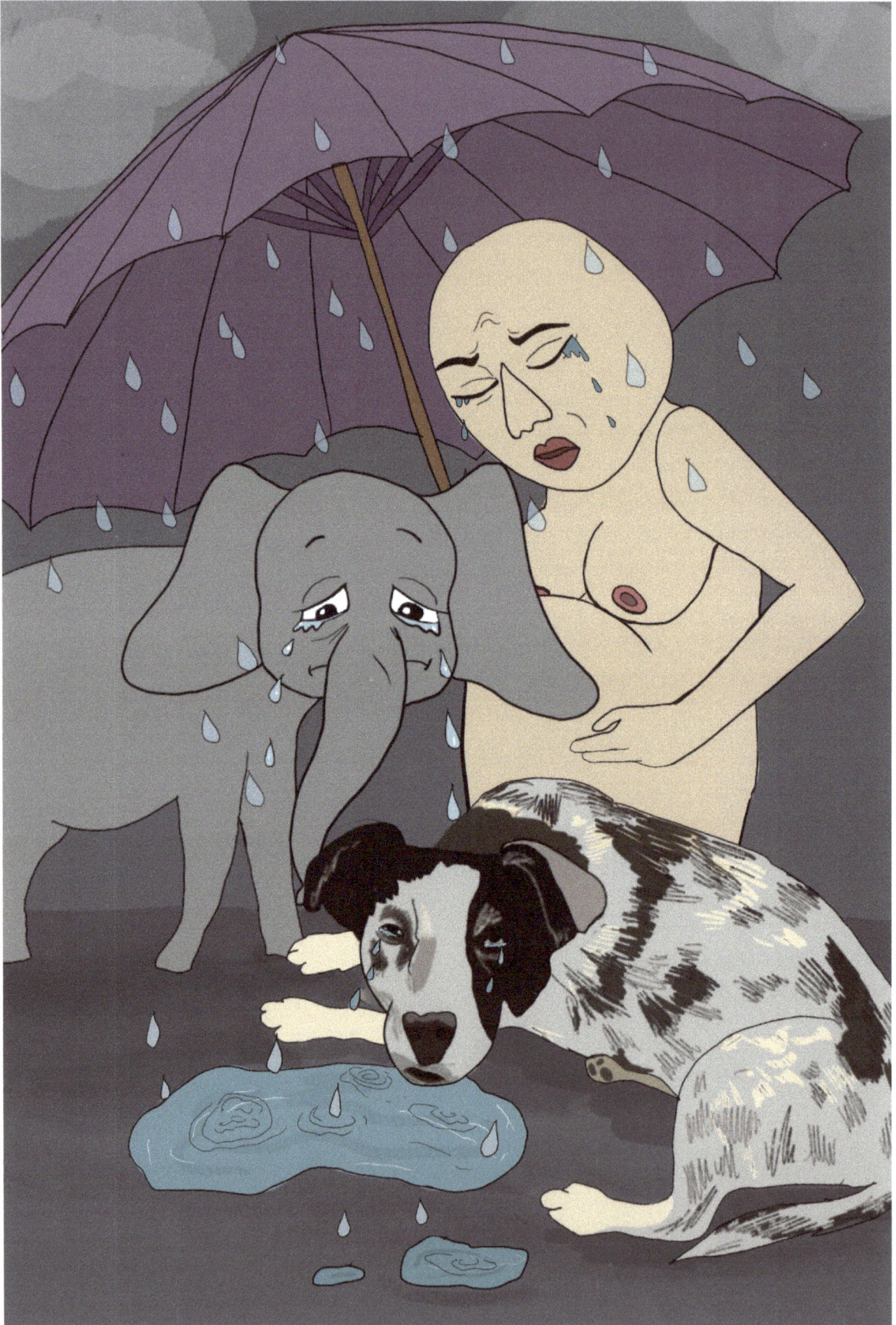

Trigger warning: A discussion of stillbirth experiences follows

This information may not be appropriate for every reader. I am aware that you and all readers bring a multitude of past experiences to this reading, and certainly some of you are trauma survivors. If this feels too much for today, give yourself that space and return to this section when you are ready. Or skip this section and continue on to the check mark ✅ shortly before the final section of this chapter: "Some observations of medical thinking." Either way, please be sure to conclude this week's reading with the offered relaxation exercise at chapter's end: "Relaxation through visualization."

⚠️ Coping with the unthinkable

This section is about when the reality of human nature slams you in the head and your heart shatters into a million pieces. The loss of a loved one leaves a hole in one's heart forever. I think it's no overstatement to say that most, if not all people during pregnancy have concerns about their baby's life, if not also their own. In this section, however, I am focusing solely on the loss of a baby. Stillbirth (a fetal death after 20 weeks of gestation) can and does happen. In research from 2018, published in the journal, *Bio Med Central Pregnancy and Childbirth*, the following were found to be risk factors for stillbirth: "Maternal factors, such as advanced maternal age, teenage pregnancies, maternal nutritional status, history of prior pregnancy losses, complicated pregnancies, and multiple pregnancies increase the risk of stillbirths. Poor socio-economic conditions have also been found to be associated with stillbirths."[322] There are roughly 24,000 Americans a year that experience this heartbreaking loss. Within this statistic it is estimated that as many as 1 in 4 of these deaths could be prevented if parents and providers were better educated and took more seriously the gestational parent's concerns about changes in their baby's activity level.[323] From the independent, nonprofit news source *ProPublica*:

> Federal agencies, state health departments, hospitals and doctors have also done a poor job of educating expectant parents about stillbirth or diligently counseling on fetal movement, despite research showing that patients who have had a stillbirth are more likely to have experienced abnormal fetal movements, including decreased activity...
>
> But federal agencies have not prioritized critical stillbirth-focused studies that could lead to fewer deaths. Nearly two decades ago, both the CDC and the National Institutes of Health launched key stillbirth tracking and research studies, but the agencies ended those projects within about a decade. The CDC never analyzed some of the data that was collected.[324]

So often these things stall due to politics and money, sadly. Even the American College of Obstetrics and Gynecology, in their latest practice guidelines, admit that there is not enough research concerning fetal movement and that parents should be listened to and included in decision making:

> There are insufficient data to make specific recommendations regarding fetal kick counts. Best practices regarding fetal kick counting seems to involve encouragement of awareness of fetal movement patterns, being attentive to the complaint of reduced fetal movements, addressing the complaint in a systematic way, and the use of shared decision making to employ interventions safely.[325]

My advice, as I repeat throughout this book, is still to listen to your baby and listen to and respect your feelings. If you are concerned about a decrease in fetal movements, be swift and resolute in seeking out medical attention. Do not worry about seeming like a worrier. In my opinion, you are the best fetal monitor there is. If you are concerned, you deserve to be taken seriously. Beyond that, it is also necessary to wrap your heart and mind around the fact that there are no preventative measures (beyond basic good selfcare) to be taken for the majority of the stillbirths that do occur. And so, learning about this rocky road and hearing stories of parental survival may help you to cope should you ever experience this tragedy of loss. Even something as fiercely sad as a child's devastating malformation or death can be lived through. A life with love and lightness can exist again, in concert with grief. Towards that goal, I am honored to be able to share the remarkably courageous and generous writings from two past clients of my Bradley® classes, each who experienced a stillbirth.

Rebeca's story

I was 39 and my husband 43 when we finally decided to try to have a child. After doing a fair amount of inner work, I was able to hold the beauty and love that surround us at the same time that I held the sadness and anger that I feel about our societal and environmental degradation. We were finally in a community that felt just right and welcomed us with open arms. I loved my life and wanted to share all this beauty with a child of our own, who might represent hope for the future. I felt I could face parenthood with joy and inner strength. We invited our child into our lives and conceived on our first try. Our journey as parents began.

I knew that miscarriages were common, if not talked about, and so we kept pregnancy quiet for the first trimester. I felt good, a bit tired at first, a bit of nausea, but otherwise wonderful. Nonetheless, I talked to my baby and told him that I trusted him to know if this was the right time and place to join us. If I miscarried, I would be sad, but I would be OK and accept that he/she was not meant to join us yet (we chose not to know the gender until birth). As part of our prenatal care we were offered non-invasive genetic screening, which we chose to pursue. If we had a child that had special needs, we wanted to know beforehand so we could prepare as best as possible.

It turned out our baby was highly (99.4%) likely to have Down syndrome. We chose not to have an amniocentesis to confirm the diagnosis. The risks were not worth it. We had eschewed ultrasounds up to that point but agreed to one post-screening. It was the first of many to come. We saw our baby on screen for the first time. The ultrasound confirmed several soft markers for Down syndrome. It was still too early to see if our baby would have some of the medical complications that often are present along with Trisomy 21, such as a heart defect or obstructed digestive system.

We also met with a genetic counselor who gave us lots of information about Down syndrome and resources that we could access in the area and nationally. As I read up on Down syndrome, I learned that there was a higher risk of miscarriage. I once again told my baby that I loved him and I wanted what was best for him and that he would know and I would accept whatever happened, but that I really wanted to be his mama.

Once our baby was big enough another ultrasound was scheduled to look at his heart. They detected a complete AV canal, which meant that his heart had an opening between the two upper chambers, an opening between the two lower chambers, and one valve, instead of two in the middle. This is a common defect in babies with DS. Fortunately, it is one that can be operated on a few weeks after birth with a very high success rate. We met wonderful pediatric cardiologists and had even more ultrasounds with them to check the development of the heart throughout the pregnancy. We also met with the NICU doctors anticipating a stay for observation after the birth.

We had started with a midwifery practice that attended births in a nearby hospital, but because of our baby's heart defect, the pregnancy was determined to be high risk and we had to transfer care to a big OBGYN practice at the area medical center an hour away from home. Nonetheless, and especially because we were determined to give our baby the best care we could so it would get a good start in life, we were on course for a natural, non-medicated vaginal birth.

We joined Emily's Bradley method class along with three other couples. We also hired a doula because we were now in a large practice where we did not know who would be the attending physician at our birth, and we wanted some continuity of care. We also anticipated meeting some resistance to our birth preferences and wanted back up should difficult decisions present themselves. As an added benefit, our doula happened to have an adult daughter with Down syndrome and was also a great support in that regard as we learned more about this new community that we now belonged to.

During one of our classes, Emily asked us to share a fear that we had with the rest of the class. I shared that I was afraid that our baby would die. I was not obsessed about it, but it was a real and present fear and I was trying to be accepting of it so that it would not become a problem during labor. I was trying to be compassionate with myself and this fear that I had. I accept that life and death go hand in hand and by choosing to bring about a life I had to accept that one day that life would end. It could be something related to my baby's heart, the increased chance of Leukemia due to DS, SIDS, a random accident... anything. It might happen during gestation, at birth, shortly after, it might not be for many years... I like to be prepared, but I didn't think there was anything that I would be able to do to prepare for that eventuality and I had to accept the possibility and let it go.

The pregnancy continued and I felt healthy and strong. As we got closer to our due date the doctors suggested that I be induced at 39 weeks due to an increased risk of stillbirth, because of my age (now 40) and my baby's Down syndrome diagnosis. My husband and I tried to be good health consumers and get them to tell us what exactly that increased risk was so we could compare it to the documented risks of medically induced labor. They were not able to provide data and I could not find it anywhere that I researched either. At each weekly ultrasound our baby seemed to be doing well and growing as expected. The placenta and cord looked healthy. We felt strongly that we wanted our baby to have the benefit of a full gestation both for the health/size of the heart, lung development, and anything else that we might not know about yet. We also did not want to expose our baby to medication or artificially stimulated contractions that might put extra stress on his heart during labor. I suggested increased monitoring and induction at 40 weeks if I had not gone into labor spontaneously. The practice agreed to this without resistance.

I asked my baby to give me a sign if I was doing the wrong thing, to let me know if he needed help coming out. I had a dream that I suddenly gave birth and held my baby. At first it didn't cry, but then it did and I thought with relief, "Oh, it's alive!" It was not a completely reassuring dream and I feared I might be misinterpreting it, but despite worries that I might be making the wrong choice, we continued on course for spontaneous labor. I tried acupuncture, massage, sex, and breast stimulation to try to induce naturally (or eliminate any obstacles to labor on my end) as we neared the due date.

I was scheduled for an induction at 40 weeks and 4 days, on the days that two doctors who were supportive of my birth plan would be on duty. The day after my due date was a busy day with lots of appointments. I last remember feeling my baby move around 12:30pm that day as we sat in a waiting room at my husband's doctor's office. Later that day, I started to feel contractions and later that evening figured out I was in labor. I had planned on laboring at home as long as possible with our doula there.

As we got the car packed for the hospital, contractions came harder and faster but very irregularly. I breathed through them as I did dishes, but I thought I had not felt the baby move in a long time and wondered if that was normal. We left a message for our doula and called Emily and the hospital. Emily and the doctor on call both said we should go in if I was concerned, and since I had not felt movement we decided to go to the hospital as soon as we could get ready. Our doula called back and said she would meet us at the hospital. On the drive over I listened to meditations in the back seat and tried to relax through the contractions. I tried not to worry about the lack of movement. We got to the hospital to find our doula waiting and we took some time to get to L&D [Labor and Delivery] as I worked through contractions with Eric by my side. We checked in and the doctor and nurse met us and took us to our room. The nurse checked for a heartbeat and could not find it. The resident got the ultrasound but could not find a heartbeat. The attending on call confirmed there was no heartbeat. I was in labor. My baby was going to be born. But he had already died.

Right then I wished I could be put to sleep and wake up once I had delivered. Thankfully, that was not an option. I would have to go through labor and the hospital staff would honor our birth plan. Labor demanded that we focus on the task at hand and so we did. It was a beautiful bonding experience between my husband and I. I felt empowered by the ability to focus and relax during contractions. As I labored, I had some of the most consciously relaxed moments I have ever experienced. Eric had taken the class very seriously and was well prepared. He supported me through contractions and anticipated my every need. He helped me stay relaxed during contractions. He made sure that conversations stopped while I was contracting so I could focus on that and not miss important information. He was the amazing partner I knew he would be. We were both strong and present.

At one point, I asked the doctor if we had to worry about how long labor took because of having a dead body inside me. He said there was no need to rush labor, that I was being monitored but that it should be fine. However, he warned that my baby's body would be starting to decompose and might be in rough shape when it was finally born. I knew I wanted to spend time with my baby after the birth and that the longer he was inside of my warm body, the worse shape he would be in, so my priorities for the kind of birth I had shifted. I was no longer concerned about the effects of medications on my baby and I was willing to accept the risks to myself. Eric checked in with me about each of these decisions as they still presented some risk to me and were not part of our original plan. Feeling that I was making these decisions in a coherent manner, he supported me through them.

After laboring for another day, I chose to take morphine the second night so I could have some rest. I chose to have some Pitocin the next morning and allowed them to break my waters later in the day to speed up labor. When the artificially induced contractions came without pause and I could no longer relax between them, I chose to have an epidural. I made all these decisions consciously and I felt good about them because I had done all the work previously.

That night I pushed for less than an hour and my baby was born. Eric cut the cord and told me we had a son. He was placed on my chest, skin to skin, as I had wanted, and I held his warm slippery body as I pushed out the placenta. We held him and kissed him and looked at his beautiful body. He had been ready to come out, perfectly positioned, so all the blood had gone to his head and his face looked bruised. The rest of his body was pale and bloodless, his skin saggy and delicate. It was not as gruesome as I had expected, and I easily saw past it. We named him Jackson Daniel Torres-Rose. Everyone in attendance was kind and respectful and gentle with Jackson. The staff took photos for us on their camera, and we took some as well. After a while our parents came in to meet him. My mother and mother-in-law and sister-in-law held him. We forgot to take pictures of that and I now wish we had thought to do so.

When everyone left for the night, we bathed him and marveled at his little body. We dressed him and read him a bedtime story. We went to sleep with him in my bed and Eric on the cot beside us. In the middle of the night I woke up with severe chills so we put Jackson in the bassinet for fear that I would hurt his delicate body in my uncontrolled shivering and not wanting to have the heated blankets that the nurse brought for me make his body any warmer.

The next day the bereavement nurses came and helped to make a memory box for him, with hand and footprints. I got to wash him between prints. The smell of the paint made me think of preschool. I was glad to have that smell associated with him and to have the chance to clean him again. His nose and mouth would bleed at times, and I was again glad to be able to gently wipe him clean, to care for him as I had so looked forward to doing. They made plaster casts of his hands and feet and took an imprint of his thumb to be made into a silver pendant for me to wear. The hospital staff were all so kind and respectful of him. They were really wonderful. All of this was free of charge and we took advantage of it all, not knowing what would mean the most to us later. We called family and Skyped with my father and brother, who live farther away, so they could meet him, too.

As the day progressed his skin got more and more delicate; even though we were all being as gentle as we could with him, it was tearing in a few places from all the handling. We knew it was time to say goodbye to his body and go home to our new reality. Nobody pressured us. In fact, the nurses and doctors kept telling us to take as much time as we needed, but we didn't want to hurt our little boy's body any more. We took a video with him, sang to him, and read him another story, then we undressed him. I wanted to keep the clothes that he wore and that smelled like him. We wrapped him up like a little burrito and placed him in a well-padded basket. Then we gently covered him with more blankets. We couldn't accompany him to the morgue, so the nurse on duty stayed past her shift to take him down for us. We said our last goodbye at the service elevator and then went home.

We had his body autopsied so that hopefully some new knowledge will come of his death that will help others in the future, but we do not know why his heart stopped. We don't know what mechanism failed at the last minute. As with most stillbirths, the cause of death is unknown.

We had his body cremated and we keep his ashes with us, with the plan that one day all of our ashes will be joined together. We will also be planting a tree in the community garden in his memory this spring. We will be inviting friends and family to join us in a number of memorial walks this year and plan on decorating a memorial Christmas tree in town for him this coming December around the time of his death and birth. We will hold an informal memorial in our home at that time.

We are incredibly fortunate to have a wonderful community who have rallied around us and given us the perfect mix of space and support as we navigate through our loss. Our doula's support during the pregnancy, birth and loss has been invaluable. I believe that is why we are coping as well as we are. Eric and I have made a commitment to honor each other's individual way of grieving, promising to support each other and ask for support when we need it. We also made a commitment to accept what support is offered to us: food, money, reiki sessions, massages, paid dinner at a local restaurant, you name it. We knew that just as it is important for us to accept the support of our community as we heal from our loss, it is an important part of healing for our community to be allowed to help us through this.

Honoring death and honoring life go hand in hand and we are not whole if we keep the one cloaked in silence. The work that I had done prior to the pregnancy that allowed me to hold joy and sadness side by side has continued to serve me, and self-compassion is an ongoing practice. My son's short life continues to be a gift and source of blessings. His death causes me great sorrow and I miss him terribly, but I feel his presence and believe that I will continue to do so all my life as long as I am open to it. It is hard not to wonder if different choices would have resulted in a different outcome. I know it is a pointless exercise and so I try to be gentle with myself when I feel guilty. I trust that he felt my love in the womb, knows how much I love him still, and that I tried to make the best decisions I could. I truly feel that my broken heart is more able to feel compassion and love for others and so that is a gift from my son, too.

I am thankful for everyone who pushes through the discomfort and tells me they are sorry for my loss instead of keeping silent. I am especially grateful to friends who were pregnant and close to their due dates at the time that Jackson died and I was in mourning, but who reached out to us nonetheless. I imagine that my experience might have frightened them. I worried I would be seen as a bad luck omen. I held my breath until each of their babies was safely born. They have let me hold their babies and be a part of their lives while still creating a space for my mourning and mourning the loss of Jackson along with me. I am thankful for all the friends and family members who continue to check in with me and keep Jackson in their thoughts and in our conversation. People say it takes a village to raise a child, but we have learned it also takes a village to mourn a child lost.

To aid you in the process of coping with such powerful emotions, it's beneficial to focus on your breathing.

As I read Rebeca's words, I am overcome with emotion from her story. Her strength and huge heart were apparent from the very first time I met her, midway through Jackson's gestation. She taught me repeatedly to be strong and compassionate in the face of the unknowns ahead. Joy and grief do live side by side. And I am grateful to Rebeca for her courage to share her experience. Please now be respectful of your own emotions after reading her story. Be mindful of the toll that reading about such sadness can take. No one feels strong enough to handle our saddest fears unless and until we have to, and then there is no (good) choice but to persevere. I ultimately chose to include this information because knowing some things ahead of time can support one's healing. And knowing that others have experienced such tragedy, endured and moved forward, is another important resource to keep in mind. For now, however, return to reading the remainder of this section if/when you are ready. What follows is another personal account of loss from a courageous mother, plus some additional related content.

Shennan's story

I always feel compelled to reassure people that this hasn't been all bad. While unimaginably painful and heart-wrenching, I have found gifts and blessings, overwhelming joy, peace, and growth as a result of this experience.

Pregnancy for me was the most joyful time in my life. I remember snuggling in bed with my partner, our puppy, and my huge belly completely enamored with my growing family. I said many times, "I don't know how I'm going to deal once the baby comes, my heart is going to burst! Just imagine when we have our baby laying right here," as I patted my partner's chest. I was so in love and so happy and relished in those moments.

But I was also waiting. Waiting for the next step. That next step when I could hold my baby in my arms, add him to our pile of bodies, limbs entangled under the sheets. I didn't realize at the time that that WAS our time. I WAS holding that baby and snuggling with him then. That WAS our family and that WAS our moment.

I lost my baby when I was 41 weeks pregnant. A cord issue. He was still in my womb when I learned he was no longer living. I had plans, of course, for the birth, though I told people (including myself) that I didn't have a birth plan. What

I meant was that I didn't have a formal, written birth plan. I was flexible in my ideas of how this birth would go. I didn't want to cling to unrealistic expectations. I had the dreams though, the fantasies. Laboring and birthing in my home with the comfort and support of my partner, midwives and their team, soft lighting, water, gentleness, quiet, peace. My mother's spirit watching over, ensuring our safety, bringing her wisdom from her own birthing experiences and all the births she had attended in her training to become a midwife.

I knew my fantasies could be thrown out the window. I knew labor and birth plans often are when it actually comes time. My biggest fear about deviating from the "plan" was because I had eaten a lot of sugar in pregnancy; I feared that I'd have a huge baby and wind up in the hospital with a C-section. I was terrified of going to the hospital.

The fantasies went out the window when I heard the words, "It's not good, they can't find a heartbeat." I heard these words from my partner. I'm still not sure if that helped ease the blow or if it made it worse knowing that he had to be the one to break the news to me after just hearing it himself.

The initial shock of learning that I would still have to labor and birth this child even though he was not living rattled me to my core. This felt like the worst possible thing anyone would ever have to do, and it ripped open even further the fresh wound of learning that my son had died. My body tingled, my soul trembled. I had been zapped with electricity, wet feet wading in shallow water. I didn't know how I would find the strength to birth this child. The news knocked me on my ass and I've been working to pick myself up ever since.

What I didn't realize was that the labor and birth of my son would still be amazingly beautiful. Something about death and birth occurring all at once, or rather, death occurring before birth, that shifts your perspective. There is so much beauty in both, yet so often we don't acknowledge the beauty in death. It is such a part of life, the natural world. I wanted a natural birth and that is exactly what I got. During my pregnancy I gave my son the space he needed to allow the natural progression to unfold. Like it or not, this was meant to be just as it was.

Though for labor I had to be induced with Pitocin, I declined all offers of pain meds and epidural. I knew that I needed to be clear and present for this experience. I couldn't allow space for drug-induced foggy memories or hangovers. I knew emotionally I would feel heavy enough and didn't want to aggravate that process.

Having the privilege of being clear and present for the birth of my son was the culmination of all of the anticipation surrounding birth in my world. Not only the anticipation during the 9 months of this pregnancy, but also the 31 years I spent wondering about mothering and childbirth and the more recent years I spent reading, educating myself, and talking to other moms who had given birth, the time I spent trying to soak up the experience, trying to know it. There is no amount of reading, education, or storytelling that can describe the beauty, rawness, and truth that is childbirth. Even when that experience also includes losing your child. For me, any fear that had sometimes overshadowed my excitement was completely shattered following Luca's death and birth. Had I not gone through the process of laboring and birthing my son I would still be filled with that fear and that wonder, and I am so thankful to have had that experience as part of my path to motherhood.

One of our midwives had encouraged us soon after we learned of Luca's death to hold our baby following the birth. Initially I thought this was a creepy and morbid practice and that I would never be able to hold a dead baby. Deep into labor I decided I had to hold this child and how thankful I am that I did. Once he came out, my midwife quickly wrapped him in a blanket and handed him to me. He felt so good in my arms, so perfect, as if he belonged there. His body was warm, not cold as I had imagined, and he settled into my chest as he would if he were alive. My partner and I were able to pick out features that we shared with him—most obvious were his lips, they were exactly like mine and I was so proud knowing we had grown this beautiful boy. We had a blanket from home so my partner swaddled him up in the fabric that smelled like home.

In the weeks afterward I spent time reading of other people who had experienced this type of loss and what their time was like with their children just after birth. Some bathed and dressed the baby, some invited family and friends to meet the baby, some took pictures, some spent hours upon hours with the baby in the hospital. Any number of these practices may have been helpful for me but, like holding him, I may have thought they were morbid and weird when the idea was first introduced. I would encourage parents in similar situations to take the time to do any and all of these things, even if it seems strange at first thought. Keep in mind that in most cases there is no rush, that you should take all the time you need with your baby and process the situation before saying your final goodbyes.

Following Luca's death and birth my partner and I decided to hold a ceremony honoring him. We would invite all our friends, family, and extended network of support, everyone with whom we had shared our experiences of pregnancy. Gentle guidance from our midwife led us to the Peace Pagoda, and a Japanese Buddhist ritual honoring Jizo, the protector of women and children, particularly children lost before birth. Fear overwhelmed me the morning of the ceremony as we walked up the path that leads to the temple and the pagoda and the indescribable beauty of the natural surroundings. We held the ceremony outside in front of the Jizo statue that greets you as you walk toward the pagoda. Subtle cues from our environment let us know that Luca shared that day with us, including a swarm of bees that opened the ceremony sending a loud hum through the atmosphere that seemed to settle and align the energy of the gathering. With very little planning, everything came together. The assembly of our wonderful community and the love that was showered upon us and throughout the group that day sent us home with our hearts refilled and bursting with radiant love. Since that day I have often wondered how can a heart be so broken yet so full? Perhaps that is just a part of motherhood.

If I could offer just one piece of advice to those parents who have lost a little one, or those experiencing any challenges, even parenting a living child, it would be to let your community hold you during those difficult times. Let people in. No matter what your religious or spiritual background is, accept the thoughts, prayers, and support of the people around you and let them lift you, don't hold back or isolate. I truly believe that it was the thoughts, prayers, and support of our community that carried us through Luca's death. We have had to walk through the grief ourselves, there is no getting around that, but having allowed the people in our lives to step in and carry us through the most difficult parts has helped more than I can say.

This journey has not been rosy, it has not been easy, it has not been fun. But it has been beautiful, nevertheless. And it still is.

Take some time now to tend to your heart. Feel your grief, your fear, and your love. Let your tears flow if, when, and wherever they arrive. To help you find solid ground, I again offer you the following breath counting meditation. Repetition builds familiarity, which in turn will help you to improve your concentration and to more easily utilize these techniques when under duress. And so, I urge you to again practice counting your breaths.

EXERCISE: COUNTING BREATHS
(REVISITED FROM WEEK 5 AND EARLIER IN THIS CHAPTER)

Read through this exercise and then set a timer for two to three minutes. Plan to use your fingers as a counting aid or not, as you choose.

Close your eyes and have the intention to allow your breath pattern to slow and deepen. You will want to observe your breath without forcing any changes to your rhythm.

After you breathe in and out, count quietly to yourself: "1."

After the next breath in and out count "2."

After the next breath in and out count "3."

Repeat this 3-count process until your timer goes off.

—Pause to explore this breath meditation. Get into a comfortable position,
turn your timer on, close your eyes and begin.—

I am personally and professionally indebted to Rebeca and Shennan for their courageous decisions to share their death and birth stories, and for their thoughtful and honest writing. Jackson's heart had some malformations. Shennan attributed Luca's passing to a cord complication, but after her piece was written she learned that there was an abnormality in the placenta and that her providers are not sure exactly what happened to Luca. Both deaths appear to be from biological pathology.

It is a rough transition from personal stories of loss to anything else. So let there be at least two general takeaways: the gentle reminder that we can live in the moment of our love right now and healing can happen. If you gather information on coping with loss now, you can then tuck it away in the folds of your brain. You will recall it if you need it. We can't control being human, but we can learn to put support into place. Pregnant or not we all live with the reality that you or someone you love might get very sick or die. When we are humans who love, we are assured of facing the pain of serious loss over the course of our lifetimes. But healing up around this loss can and does happen—and with it often comes new growth. Education coupled with love, along with compassion for yourself and social support, can help.

Many (maybe most?) people believe death should be fought at all costs. Perhaps you agree. I once did. But the older I get, coupled to my continuing years working with births, the more I find my agreement waning. I don't mean to diminish the sorrow of even one death. But death is integral to our natural process. Ultimately, your decisions to support life at all costs are yours to make. Questions of quality of life vs. quantity of life abound throughout our lives. Raising a child who has suffered from neurological or significant physical deficits, for example, can lead to an expansive, rewarding, joyous, and love-filled parenting experience. It can also be experienced as an emotionally draining, outrageously expensive, long-term haul through heartbreaking conditions. This is another one of the risks that we face as parents, as family, and as humans.

If your baby dies while you are still pregnant you will have some decisions to make. You don't have to decide anything ahead of time, but do keep in mind that you will still need to birth your baby. For future reference, please consider the following:

> Generally, it is medically safe for the mother to continue carrying her baby until labor begins, which is normally about 2 weeks after the baby has died. This lapse in time can have an effect on the baby's appearance at delivery and it is best to be prepared for this. Some women prefer to be induced as soon as possible because it is emotionally difficult for some women to think of carrying their deceased baby in the womb. If labor has not started after two weeks, induction would become necessary to avoid dangerous blood clotting. A cesarean is usually only recommended if complications arise during labor and delivery.[326]

Following a stillbirth, plan to spend time with your baby. This may seem morbid to you now, but it will be important to you eventually. You can amend your plans whenever you want or need to. While spending time with your baby's body, you'll want to take note of what you see, such as perfect little toes or well-formed ears. Can you find positive details? Give your baby a name. It's important to say goodbye and to acknowledge how different this is from what you expected. As Rebeca and Eric were able to do, consider engaging in some activities that help to let you touch base with a parenting experience, such as bathing and/or dressing your baby. You can take all the time that you need to say goodbye. Plan to take this time. Also, keep a memento of your baby: their little hat, a foot print, their ID band—something for you to have later on. It may feel unbearable at the time, but you will find comfort from a memento in the months and years ahead.

You will likely benefit from holding some kind of memorial service or funeral. The event can be as big or as small as feels right for you. From the first moments we learn of our pregnancy we start to dream and plan for that baby's full life. A ceremony to honor that life, and your own parenthood, as well as to say goodbye, can help you come to terms with what has happened.

Sleep and appetite disturbances after such a traumatic event are normal, but they will need attention. Drinking warm fluids, such as teas and broths, will be soothing to your body and a useful tonic for your broken heart.[327] You will benefit from reaching out for professional support. You and your partner will grieve differently, and those differences can cause a great deal of strain on the relationship. You both deserve professional support, and your caretakers should suggest it and help to facilitate getting the services you need. You will always have a sadness in your heart for that baby, but you can find some healing and happiness again. Volunteering to help other people can, eventually, be considered for its healing qualities in your recovery. Whether we love someone for a moment or a lifetime, it is our great joy and honor to have the time we do have. It is also our heavy burden to cope with grief when we experience loss. Healing—learning to live fully with our loss—can happen. This is worth repeating over and over again. Healing can happen.

------------------ **If you skip the section on loss, begin reading again below** ----------------

✅ Please take a moment here to honor the fact that if you are pregnant or intending to parent, or a partner who is intending to parent, then you are a parent right now. Parenting is not something that happens to you at birth, it's something that happens to you the minute you finalize your decision to be the parent. Please appreciate that you have this time together now, today, and with that, you have all the dreams and expectations you have for your future. You are a parent right now. Take a moment to tune into your little one.

It turns out that pregnancy not only brings dreams and expectations, it brings fetal cells to the gestational parent's body, cells—from the fetus—that appear, at least for some, to remain permanently in the gestational parent's body. Scientists have discovered that starting around 6 weeks of pregnancy, some fetal cells appear to migrate into the parent's body. These cells appear to be like stem cells, able to turn into a variety of other cells, and have been found dispersed throughout the gestational parent's body (brain, kidney, liver etc.). There is much for science still to learn about this "gift" from your baby that scientists call *fetal microchimerism*. Do the cells work for the baby aiding the process of lactation? Are the cells destructive or helpful to their host gestational body? And why does the gestational parent seem to kill off some of these cells directly after birth but other cells, in at least some bodies, are thought to survive for a lifetime? These are just a few of the questions that scientists continue to investigate.[328] Based on my own experiences, when I read about this research I couldn't help but wonder if the cells inside me, from my babies, were actually like little radio transmitters. My thinking is that maybe this helps explain why my "spidey-senses" always seem to light up when one of my kids is in need. Whether they were little ones asleep in another part of the house and had awoken sick, or whether they are, in adult formation, across the county and stuck on the side of the road with a flat tire, I frequently have felt, and continue to feel, a buzz of what, up until reading this research, I had referred to as my *long-distance umbilical connection*. Okay, maybe that's just me being weird; nevertheless, it brings me great pleasure to muse about all the ways that we are transformed through our pregnancies. And I get comfort knowing that I truly do always carry a bit of my babies inside me.

Some observations of medical thinking

Western culture often thinks of a doctor's job being one that fights death, at all costs. Doctors try to "manage the risks" by trying to control the situation. However, trying to take control of the natural birth process (which, again, is not an illness) can and almost undoubtedly will make the birth more stressful for the birthing person, which in turn makes the process more dangerous.[329] Increased stress increases risk for stalled birth and complications. Complications are met with more interventions, often creating more stress for both parents and providers, leading to more interventions still, creating what is often referred to as a cascade of interventions.[330] With interventions adding up, we can easily start to feel grateful to the medical team that tried to "fix" our broken selves, whose bodies are somehow not working. We tell ourselves, "the Doctor did all that she could. Thank god she was there."

From my experiences in the birth world and through my partner's medical career, there appears to be a common perspective that goes like this: if a doctor does something that causes a problem, but they can think of a way to try to fix it, then it is not that big of a deal. In other words, if the reasons are iatrogenic (doctor-caused) for what caused someone to experience a cascade of interventions and then this patient ends up needing surgery, but the doctor can do the surgery, then it's all okay. In our medical universe, with this logic, the doctor is not faulted for doing too much. In fact, providers are more likely to get blamed for not doing enough.

Cesarean section is the gold standard of "doing all we can." Please understand, cesarean section is a procedure that can and does save lives. Around the globe people are at risk when they don't have access to this surgery. Unnecessary surgical birth can be a nightmare indeed, but not having access to surgical birth when it *is* necessary is also a nightmare. The World Health Organization reports that between 5% and 10% of pregnant people and babies benefit from surgical birth. And yet, at a rate above 15%, the procedure appears to create harm.[331] While pregnant people outside of the United States, in poor and developing countries, are at risk from not having access to the surgeries they need, pregnant people in the United States undergo too many surgeries. This leaves me to wonder just how many surgeries in the U.S. are really the result of people being interrupted with early, considered-to-be-benign interventions, which then add up to so much disruption and a buildup of negative stress that the gestating person and baby really do get into trouble and really do need a surgical assist. We may know this for sure one day, but for now this is just my musing.

It is time now to let all this heaviness go. There is so much beyond our control. It's time to tune in to what we can control, such as what we are choosing to focus on right now. Please take another moment now to honor the fact that if you are pregnant or intending to parent, or a partner who is intending to parent, then you are a parent right now. Tune into your little one.

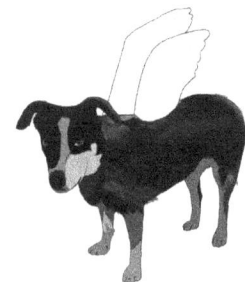

EXERCISE: PROGRESSIVE RELAXATION

If you are with a partner, one of you should read the following visualization while the other focuses on the relaxation it is meant to bring. Then switch roles. The resting person should now get into the side relaxation position. (Do you need a bathroom break or a sip of water first?)

"We have just worked through some very difficult information. You have done this now so that, in the event that you are faced with decisions about difficult interventions and/or the tragedy of loss, you will have some information to guide you.

Now it is time to let it all go. Allow yourself to file the information away in the recesses of your mind. Release what you don't need in this moment. Take in some full deep breaths, then exhale, relax your forehead, feel your brain settle in your skull. Allow your eyes to be heavy in their sockets. Let your jaw go. Let the tongue be heavy."

—Reader pause—

"Your breath can flow in and out easily, invite ease."

—Reader pause—

"Notice your sensations at your nostrils. Invite your head to settle into the pillow. Feel your shoulders, arms, and hands let go. Can you feel your blood flowing through them?"

—Reader pause—

"Let your muscles soften; let them sink into what's supporting you. Feel your chest and abdomen release, relax and settle into heaviness. Spread out. Soften. Let go. The air goes in and out easily, notice, and allow your shape to change in response."

—Reader pause—

"Breath is a refreshing and restorative gift."

—Reader pause—

"Let your belly really soften and widen. Imagine your low back spreading out and widening. Invite your hips and low back to let go, to soften and spread out. Invite release and softening in your pelvic floor, thighs, knees. Rest."

—Reader pause—

"Letting go should be easier than holding on. Release tension with your exhales. Let your lower legs, feet, and toes be heavy and soft and wide. Invite the soles of your feet to feel open and relaxed. Feel the legs lengthen as they let go. Release in your whole body, feel rest and warmth and comfort in this moment. Allow your breath to shift your shape. Allow your exhales to release what you don't need."

—Reader pause—

"Let go. Let your mind wander".

—Reader pause for several breaths (if not minutes!)—

"When you are ready to move, start with some gentle wiggling of the fingers and toes and gradually make your way up to a seated position. You've reached the end of this exercise."

Aimless relaxing allows you to process the information you have just consumed.[332] Focused relaxation and breath observation helps us develop coping skills for life. Progressive relaxation exercises, such as the one you just practiced, can both be meditative and help us release areas of our body that are holding on (perhaps unconsciously) to tension. I applaud your courage, your strength and your love. You are a wonderful parent and this baby is so lucky to have found you. I am wishing you a week full of good life.

HOMEWORK

Your homework this week is *no homework*. Reading this book is its own hard, beneficial labor. Please spend your time this week any way you want. You will undoubtedly need to continue to cope with the challenges of whatever else is on your life's plate, and you might want to catch up with any earlier assignments from this book that you have yet to get to. Or, truly, don't do anything! Time to rest and not *do* is also very important. This creates the time to love yourself and love your baby. Nurturing is an activity that takes time, attention, and practice. Please give yourself credit for tackling the challenges of parenthood head on and relish your downtime. Have a love filled week, and please take good care.

THIS SPACE IS FOR YOUR NOTES AND DRAWINGS

THIS SPACE IS FOR YOUR NOTES AND DRAWINGS

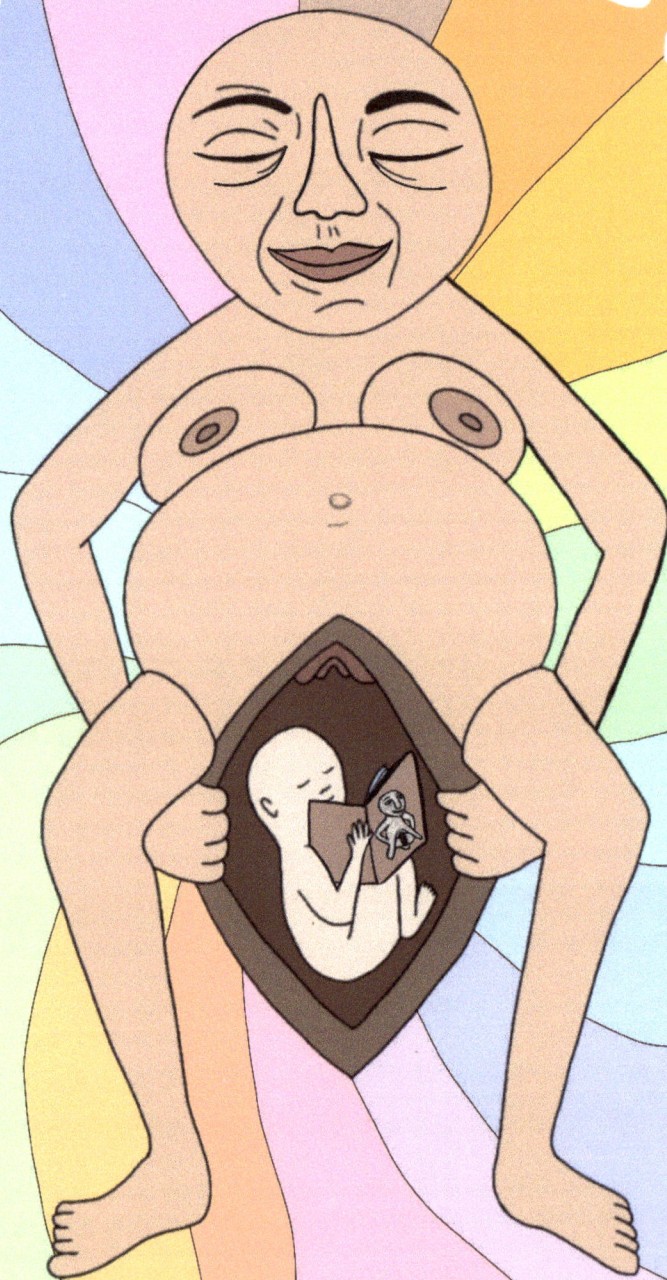

WEEK 14

Yes, You Can!

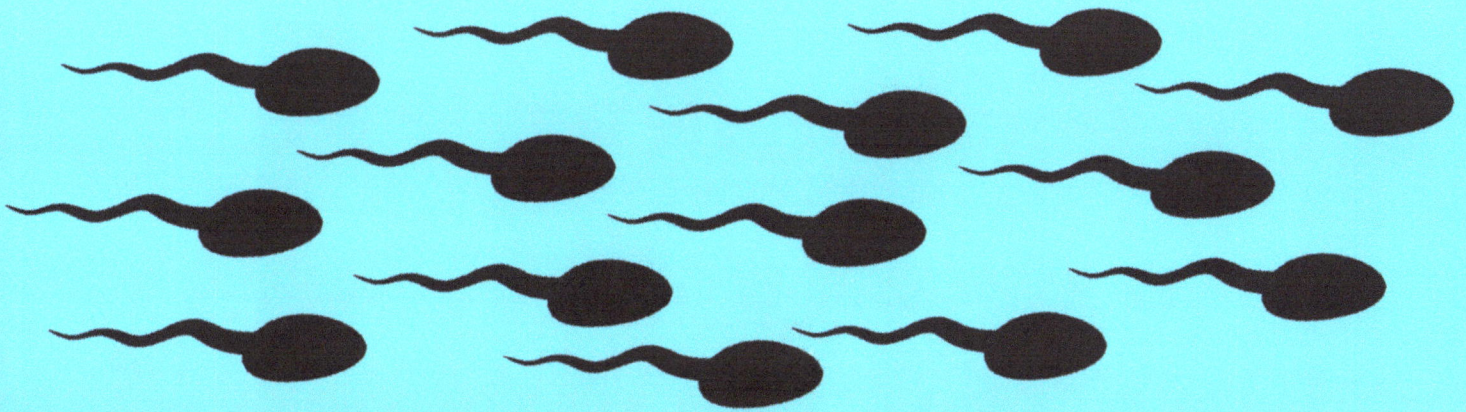

THIS SPACE IS FOR YOUR NOTES AND DRAWINGS

Welcome back. I hope your week was a healthy and forgiving one. I applaud you for coming back to class this week. I bet your belly is getting bigger. I hope you are getting enough sleep, enjoying your food, and taking some time for lightness and pleasure.

Last week's reading was intense, and the last few weeks have been serious with some frightening content. My heart aches with how hard it is to experience, or even think about loss. Having children is not just about raising children, it's also about raising ourselves—growing up. Growth takes time. It's time now, in this course, to bring your attention back to the phenomenal natural birth process. Let the emotionally heavy, brain-twisting medical information settle. The information is now there if you ever need it. Remind yourself that your body is amazing, you are healthy, and your baby is likely to be thriving inside.

Mindful breathing—it's a survival tool for birth and beyond. You really can feel profound benefits from just two short sessions of mindful breathing a day: once in the morning before you get out of bed and once in the evening before going to bed. If you haven't already adopted this practice into your everyday, now's the time.

Allow 2 – 3 minutes for this practice here today. Other times you can experiment with longer or shorter sessions.

EXERCISE: 3-PART YOGA BREATH

First get into the side relaxation position (or recline or sit comfortably) and close your eyes (after reading and setting a timer for a few minutes, or recording of course!)

"Start by tuning into your breath. Invite your low belly to fill with air as you breathe in, and then to empty and sink gently towards your spine as you exhale. Fill and empty your low belly with ease and comfort. Follow the rhythm of your breath. The belly gets big as you inhale. The belly settles and sinks as you exhale."

—Reader pause—

"Use your next inhalation to fill the low belly and then draw the air up into the midsection of your body, to about the level of your diaphragm. Then as you exhale, empty the midsection, and then empty the low belly. Repeat this two-part pattern: Fill the low belly, then fill the midsection, then empty your midsection, and empty your low belly. Again: Allow the air to fill your low belly, and then your midsection, and then allow the midsection to empty, and then empty the low belly."

—Reader pause—

"With your next breath, fill the low belly, fill the midsection, and then draw in still more air filling the top of your lungs—all the way up to your clavicle. Now empty the upper lungs, empty your midsection, and empty the low belly. Repeat: Fill the low belly, then fill the midsection, then fill the upper chest, then empty the upper chest, empty the midsection, and empty the low belly. Repeat this three-part breath for several more breaths or minutes, depending on your practice time. When you are finished, wiggle your fingers and toes and gently bring yourself back from your focused concentration."

—Pause to practice three-part yoga breath—

How was that? Do you notice any changes in your breath or how you are feeling?

On the topic of self-care, be sure to remember that it's not just what you eat or the amount of sleep or exercise you get. Create the space to listen to your breath. Building your social-support network remains another important element of self-care. Do you have friends that you can talk to? Being able to share your experiences and feelings and listening to your friends' stories can help build resiliency. Evidence shows that having friends to talk to can help you to improve your mood and be healthier.[333] Growing baby-friendly friendships now can help battle the isolation of parenthood later. Look to others who are expecting, new parents, and those with young children to make new connections.

While friends can be fun and protective, they can also be a drain. Do you have any relationships that are destructive, or so one-sided that they cost you energy with no return? Please reflect on your current social-support network. Take notes below on what is working, what isn't, and what may be missing.

Additional tactics for not only surviving, but loving your birth

Exhale

At the start of every contraction close your eyes and focus on a long, slow, and full exhalation of breath. This is so important I want to say it twice! *At the start of every contraction close your eyes and focus on a long, slow, and full exhalation of breath.* As you exhale, try also to relax your abdomen, vagina, and tailbone. As a bonus, if you can remind yourself that you are safe in your sensations, no matter how strong, you will be well on your way to rocking the challenges of your birth.

Value the contraction

I encourage you to think of each contraction as a gift. Contractions are not something to be dreaded; they are a cherished opportunity. I would love for you to think, "Thank goodness it's here, I can get this work done now. I hope it will be a strong contraction (maybe even a sexy contraction—should I try kissing?). Strong contractions get my work done. I want to move another step closer to my baby's arrival. I may be scared, but I can be courageous." The gift of the contractions is that this is how the baby comes out and makes this labor a memory.

As great as birth is, it's greater still to say: "I did that. I birthed my baby," past tense. But to get there the work to be done is being present, here and now, with the challenge of your sensations. And, where you can, you want to respect each contraction as a gift of opportunity.

Define "efficient," "tolerable," and "pleasurable"

Remember that the work of labor is about finding the courage to stay with the experiences you are feeling, to trust that you can live inside your sensations. That is how you can optimize the work that must be done to get the baby out—and that is your ultimate goal, right? We all want to get the most work done with the least amount of effort in the most efficient and/or tolerable, maybe even pleasurable manner imaginable. For each of you (and during each new birth), what defines "efficient", "tolerable," or "pleasurable" will be unique. Consider that your birth is a journey, an adventure to explore and create your own definitions for your own sensations during birth.

Let's take a moment now to think about how you are personally defining these words right now. What will it mean for you to be "efficient" during birth? Write your response below.

How will you define "tolerable" for your birth?

Can pleasure exist with pain? Try to imagine what "pleasurable" might look and feel like during your birth?

While in labor, seek out what is good. If you go looking for pleasure, you are likely to find it. Of course, "looking for pleasure" is very different than *expecting* pleasure or thinking that the contractions won't hurt. If you expect something other than hard work and fiercely overwhelming sensations, then you will be disappointed and more easily frustrated. *But hard work and pleasure are not mutually exclusive.*

Stay in the present tense (and probably, also, in your present position)

There's nowhere to run, so stay with and embrace your sensations. Suppose you feel a contraction coming on and you pick a position, but then as the contraction builds you think, "oops, wrong, this position sucks." Your first instinct will probably be to move, hoping to find something you like. But are you really going to "like" a position during a contraction? A past client shared the serious, yet comical story that during her second stage she almost fell off the bed as she kept scooting down it trying to run away from her own vagina.

What I am asking you now is to consider the fact that it *might* be good to try to stay put for the duration of that contraction. In other words, value the work you can do right then in that "wrong" position. Although changing positions and being active is often very helpful *between contractions*, as I discussed previously, constant movement (and constant thought about moving) *during contractions* does open the possibility to exhaust yourself outside of the work of the labor itself. If you are on an elusive goose chase to find that perfect position, the one where you can't feel any work being done, then you'll burn more energy than you need to. You don't want to be frivolous with your muscular or mental efforts. Try instead to channel your energy into the brain-power of coping.

Surrender to what is happening in the moment. A contraction requires a lot of metabolic effort, and that work becomes more tolerable if you can match the physical effort with mental effort to direct what you think about. Thoughts affect biology. Ideally, you'll want your uterus and baby to get first dibs on all your vital resources. You can achieve this by relaxing all the muscles in your body that do not directly help to birth the baby. And you can do this by being active in your thoughts. If you charge around in a desperate search for a place that doesn't exist, you will wear yourself down prematurely. When the going gets tough, remind yourself that what you are feeling is information from your nerves. You are safe and healthy and so is the baby. Birth is a healthy function with very big sensations.

I once witnessed a woman in labor decide to stand up and lean over a counter during her contraction. Once the contraction began, however, she started to grumble that she hated that position. Her partner and I both suggested she stay put and allow the contraction to do its work. We assured her we would help her find another position for the next contraction. So she stood through the contraction and grumbled, "Oh, I don't like this. Oh noooo, nooo. I don't want to be standing here. Oooooooohhhh." Although she complained, she ultimately chose not to move, leaning instead on our suggestion that she might want to finish the contraction before changing. Her complaining and moaning let us know that she was breathing fully; her eyes were closed and she appeared to be relatively calm and focused inside. She was allowing the uterus to be heavy and to do its work. When the contraction was over, she straightened up, we gave her a sip of water, and she decided to sit for a moment to consider what position she wanted to try next. Then, low and behold, as the next contraction began, she leapt up and returned to her position of standing and leaning over the counter! Again, she started to moan and complain that she hated that position. While she hadn't enjoyed it the first time, she knew on some level that she was getting good work done there. She ended up spending many contractions in that position, each time sitting or lying down to rest in-between. Her own body realized that although she herself might not have liked the position, the position was good for getting the work of labor done. Yes, it was difficult. But not getting the work done would have been even harder.

Practice your homework

Using relaxation and mental brain power to cope with strong and potentially painful sensations is a skill that—to be readily available in labor—should be developed over time. This isn't to say you can't or shouldn't try it anew in the midst of labor, but practice will undoubtedly help immensely. It will help you to prepare; it can be fun and feel good, like a warm shower or a giant hug or a massage or a bit of chocolate (yes, that kind of good!). Practicing will help to reduce your anxiety, because preparing for birth and family life is about cultivating love. If you are in a relationship or have a close support partner for labor, it's important to practice as a couple. The work will help bring you together and develop a confidence and connection from your shared base of information and strategy. Nurturing each other helps care for your relationship, and helps you model and prepare for nurturing your baby. What follows are some more exercises that get better with practice. (I will cue you to practice each one after you have read about them.)

Vocalizations!

For birth, don't be afraid to make noise. Cry, sing, moan, howl, curse, grunt, wail, or laugh. (And, of course, let the farts out, too!) Do whatever encourages you to release. Try to go where your energy takes you. The contractions of labor can be thought of as a huge surge of energy passing through you. This, again, is why some midwives call contractions "rushes": a contraction is a rush of energy that comes through a person. When it comes time to cope with these surges of energy many people find it useful to release the energy through sound. In fact, letting sounds out during labor, like big howling-moaning-open-wailing-sounds, is something that people do all over the world. In my birth classes I have been teaching and encouraging pregnant people and their partners to howl as an in-class exercise for many years. The benefits of practicing ahead of birth are plentiful and practice helps a partner (and siblings, if there are any) to become acclimated to large sounds. This reduces partner stress in labor and allows the birthing person a chance to face any feelings of inhibition ahead of time. In addition, the one doing the laboring can intentionally explore the different kinds of opening sounds (such as *ahhhs, oohhhs, wahhhhs,* and *ggrrraaarrrs*), which in turn makes the technique of releasing energy through sound more intentional and available. Think of and honor this practice of vocalizing as a potentially useful coping technique, one that is uniquely your own. You are creating your own birth song!

Some sounds promote opening, like the booming song of an opera singer, while other vocalizations can get very tense and tight, like those high-pitched, horror movie screams. To teach vocalizations, demonstration is always necessary. So please, "sing" along with me: First, pretend you are an opera singer. Open your mouth wide, arms outstretched, inhale deeply and fill your diaphragm, puffing out your chest, lifting your chin, and straightening your spine. Now exhale that great, big breath into a room-filling note: *Oohhhhhhh!* Second, pretend you are in a horror movie and you're running up the stairs to try to get away from whatever monster is pursuing you. You turn to see where that monster is, only to find it is right behind you! You scream—a short, quick, tight burst that squinches up your jaws, closes your eyes, and clenches your forehead in fear. If you are stymied by embarrassment doing these exercises, try to face your inhibitions with laughter and courage. Make some noise! (And maybe even warn family and neighbors that you're practicing.)

—Pause to practice vocalizing, try open and low-tone sounds
and have some fun with high shrill horror movie sounds too—

As you experiment with making sounds, I want you to imagine the arc of a contraction: it usually starts slowly and then it builds, climaxes, and wanes. Let your sounds start slower or softer and then build in volume to an apex. Then allow the sounds to diminish, like a wave that rolls back out to sea. As your sounds grow, open your mouth wide, like the opera singer. As the big sounds are flowing, try to relax your cheeks, the base of your tongue, and your throat. Allow the sound to generate deep down, low in your belly. Lower sounds can help keep the throat from tightening up. Try to make open sounds, like the opera singer, or like a yoga master saying *Ohhhhhhhhhhhhhhhhh-hhhhhhhmmmmmmmmmmmmm*, a cow *moooOOOOOOOOOooing*, or a wolf *hhhOOOOWWWWwwllling*. As you practice this, go for volume. Try to wake your neighbors up! Can you attain great volume without making your face and neck tight? Allow the sound to fill the room as you follow that arc of a contraction: again, start small, grow, peak, and fade. In birth it's the power of the contraction that will fuel the power of the sound, so in practice you will have to generate the energy for the sound. Be sure to practice the opera singer version and not the horror movie screams. Of course, it may be fun to experiment with both. Because in labor, if horror movie screams are what come out, just let loose with whatever you need to release. Let the sounds, and the contractions, pass through you.

Please try this exercise together, if you are with your support partner or have a friend, neighbor, or family member nearby. But don't be shy to try it alone, too. Remember that in labor the sounds may or may not come, practicing now simply makes vocalization a more available option—another tool—during birth. Vocalizing is an empowering way to work with your sensations. If you haven't tried the vocalization exercise yet, please try it now. If you just did it, do it again! Try it with your eyes open and closed. Which way feels better? Which way gives you more of a release?

—aaaaaaaaaaaaaaaaAAAAAAAAAAAAAHHHHHHHHHHHHHhhhhhhhhhhhhhhh—

—Pause to again practice vocalizing—

The sounds of labor commonly make people around the laboring person uncomfortable. Drugs frequently get offered to laboring people to quiet them down or even shut them up. The hospital staff often tries to protect themselves as they offer "compassion" to the patient. I was once at a birth when the woman I was attending let out a tremendously strong, long, and hall-ringing kind of howling-moaning song. I thought she was doing great, and she was. But within moments of her contraction ending there was a knock at the door. It was the anesthesiologist, who said: "Hi, I just heard you and thought you must be ready for your epidural." I politely thanked him for checking in on us, while the laboring woman assured him she was fine. As it dawned on him that she wasn't interested, he got a perplexed and worried look on his face and ran out the door. The laboring woman and I had a good laugh at his nervousness and she got back to her work.

Over my years of teaching, I have heard many wonderful stories about how vocalizing has been useful to people during birth. One woman shared that if she could find the right pitch, then it would really help her cope. She said everything would vibrate and be loose and she felt like the sound was opening her up. She said that finding the right note at the start of each contraction took some work; she would start with a low note, then slowly, as she moved up and down her own musical scale, she would hunt for the note that worked best to really help her open. Another woman described that during her labor she felt so internally focused that she thought the vocalizations she made would help her partner know where to find her as she felt a little lost in her "labor-land." In my own vaginal birth, my vocalizations felt like a way to communicate to my husband *exactly* how big the contractions were.

One of my funniest vocalizing stories involves a giant, howling curse word. I was attending a birth with a couple along with the pregnant woman's mom. We were all at the hospital in the labor room with a nurse. The labor had been progressing beautifully all day, but the birthing woman was entering her transition and her posture and attitude were beginning to crumple. She was sitting, slumped over in a rocking chair, feeling sad and frustrated. I was thinking through what I might offer her next as a support technique when, all of a sudden, a sound started low and then grew and grew and grew as she released the biggest, loudest, howling-ist curse I had ever heard: "fffffffffffffffff-fUUUUUUUUUUUUUUUUUUUUUUuuuuuuuuuuucK!" What happened next was nothing short of amazing. She cracked herself up laughing! In fact, the entire energy of the room changed. I'm pretty sure her mom wet her pants she was laughing so hard, and her husband and I were also cracking up. Talk about a release of tension—wow! The nurse was pretty funny, too; she turned bright red and jumped across the room to close the door. That, of course, made us laugh even harder. Shortly after that massive "f-bomb" release, the birthing woman asked the nurse if she had one of those squat bars that go across the bed. The nurse put the squat bar in place, the mom climbed up on the bed, and she began to bear down with gusto. Her beautiful baby boy was born soon after. I will forever be humbled by the power of that gigantic curse.

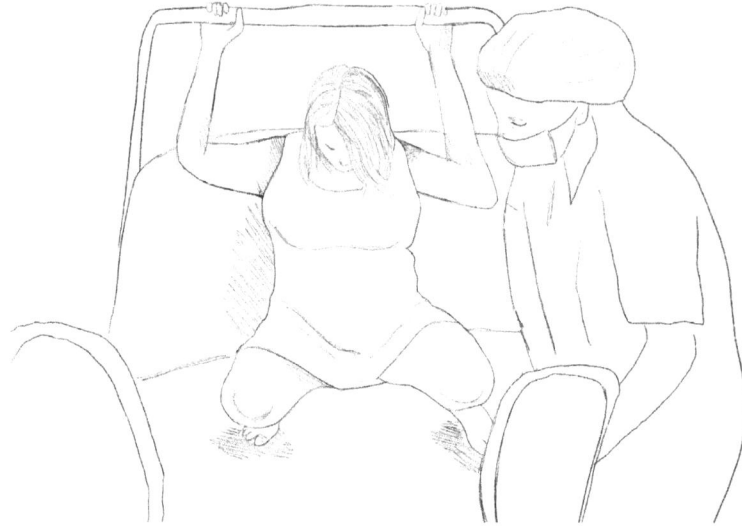

As I mentioned above, I have been teaching this vocalization technique (with or without curse words!) in class for as long as I have been teaching. And I almost always have a good percentage of people look at me sideways and comment that "vocalizing in labor may be good for some, but not for me!" Many people, maybe even you, think that they will be too shy, too internally focused, and much too quiet by nature to ever entertain a technique like this during birth. But then, time and time again, people come back to share their birth stories and report that vocalizing was not only something that they used, but it was one of the techniques they found most helpful. With this in mind, I encourage you to practice this technique so that you will have it readily available during birth. Work on getting used to the big sounds ahead of time. (Personally, I find this a satisfying technique for relieving all sorts of tension, like when I'm stressed and upset and I might otherwise yell at my kids or my husband. Instead, I sometimes go into a room and just release a gigantic, wailing howl and let my tension go—without hurting anyone else's feelings.)

In labor, if the support partner senses that the birthing person is resisting the work and holding their breath, the partner can initiate some vocalizations, too. The partner can start first by tuning into the person's breath pattern. Next, try to give a small sound to the truncated exhales they are currently making. Then, slowly elongate your sounds, which can help to encourage them to elongate their exhales. Allow your volume to grow as a gentle nudge for them to grow their volume too. Perhaps the birthing person will join you, or perhaps they'll tell you to shut up. If it's the latter, then you can go quiet. But if it helps, you'll be considered a genius!

The lip flap

I sometimes call this "horse lips" in my notes. I first learned this as a birth technique (along with several others) at a workshop led by Ina May Gaskin in the late 1990s. But, if I'm being completely honest, I really first learned this as "blowing raspberries" when I was a kid and then again as a young adult, usually on someone's belly. I'm betting you know this technique already, too! So let's do it together: Take a deep breath in and let your lips loosely flap together as you exhale through your mouth. Try again: Take another deep breath and relax your cheeks deeply as you let your lips flap from the air of your exhale. This technique helps to reduce tension in the cheeks and jaw. Plus, it's hilarious, and laughter is a great tension reliever.

By encouraging the mouth and jaw to relax you help to encourage your vagina to relax. This is, at its essence, a breathing technique that helps to elongate your exhalation, which reduces tension. A longer, fuller exhale will promote a deeper, fuller inhale. I find that the lip flap helps me to center myself. If you ever watch professional baseball games, for example, you can sometimes spot a pitcher, as he prepares to throw the ball, first take a centering lip flap exhalation as he discharges excess tension before he throws the pitch. In what other events might you see professionals using this technique? Practice the lip flap frequently so that it can become yours. Make this another coping technique in your repertoire. Like so many of the techniques and exercises presented in this book, if you don't practice it, then you may not think to try it during birth. Remember: your work of preparing is now; this will provide you with multiple coping mechanisms to tap during birth.

—Pause to practice the lip flap—

Acupressure and Shiatsu-style massage

Shiatsu (noun):
A form of healing massage in which the hands are used to apply pressure at acupuncture points on the body in order to stimulate and redistribute energy. Originating in Japan, it is used to treat various conditions such as back pain, migraine, insomnia, depression, and digestive problems.

Physical pressure at an acupuncture location can be an effective tool during pregnancy as well as birth. There are places on the body, along various energy routes, that can get blocked—meaning, the energy flow is reduced or stopped, which results in reduced function. Through shiatsu/acupressure these blockages can be released and good energy flow can be restored. The improved energy flow can not only improve the various functions listed in the dictionary definition above; shiatsu can also positively impact contraction strength and organization, fetal positioning, a reduction in maternal fear, deeper muscular release, and induction of labor. The potential benefits of shiatsu massage are plentiful and, beautifully, the risks are almost nonexistent.[334]

Acupressure points to support release can be found in the meaty area between thumb and index finger. Here the massager is crossing his own hands so that he can apply pressure to both of his partner's hands at once. These points, as I have learned from acupuncturists and experienced myself, can help one to release tension and can provide relief from headaches and constipation, and support the release of tears, and in labor the release of your baby.

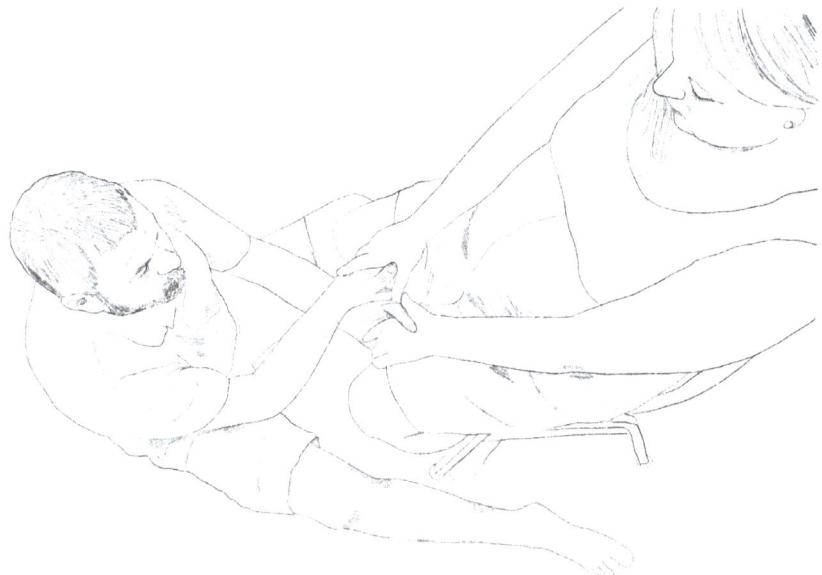

I say "almost" nonexistent because there is some risk involved when certain induction-coaxing release points are "worked." To "work" a pressure point is to apply a steady physical force for an extended duration of time combined with the mental intent of a particular outcome. For example, if you were to have someone try to induce your labor while you were still preterm, you could potentially start labor early, which you should never try to do. In my opinion, however, such a risk is connected to the *intent* of the person giving the massage along with the duration of time the points are held. When the person giving the massage has the intent to bring forth labor, the pressure points can be more effective. Therefore, it follows that when the partner has the intent to *not* bring about labor, and instead has the intent to open energy channels for love and calmness to flow through, and to help organize and optimize healthy function, then the pregnant person can feel confident to enjoy the benefits of shiatsu massage. Add to this the simple guideline to avoid "working" the two specific induction-related points and the risk will further decrease.

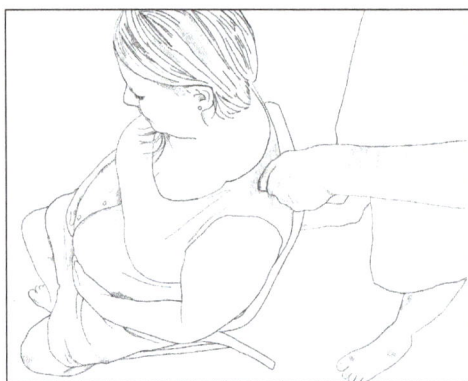

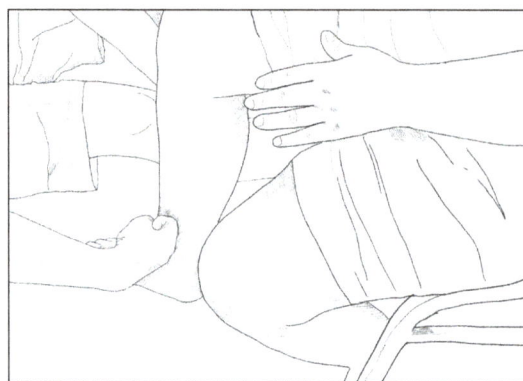

The two points to avoid until labor are 1) at the top of the shoulder, halfway between the base of the neck and the outer tip of the shoulder gridle just toward the back from the midline, in the meaty part of the top of the shoulder; and 2) on the inside of the ankle, four finger-widths distance up from the top of the protruding ankle bone (i.e., four of the pregnant person's own finger widths). I say all of this for informative purposes. While I caution you against putting any prolonged pressure on these two points preterm, don't be so cautious that you neglect to identify these points ahead of time. You can look for them on your own body and on a partner. You know you have found a pressure point when you find a spot near where you are looking and it feels more sensitive—usually more sore—than the surrounding area. If you can't find the "aha" spot, you may still activate some effect from applying pressure in the vicinity of the pressure point. Identifying these points now will help you to remember to use them in labor, when the time is right. So please explore. I'm simply saying that I don't want you to apply prolonged pressure and "work" these two specific points until labor actually begins or until you have evidence supporting the need for an induction.

—Pause to locate these acupressure points—

Shiatsu-style spinal massage

I will now teach you a massage technique that does not have any association with induction. This massage promotes calm and helps each person (giver and receiver) meditate on their own breath. Two points are worked at one time, one each on either side of the spinal column. This has a global calming effect on the nervous system.

To begin, the person receiving the massage should straddle an armless chair. Place one or two pillows across the back of the chair and allow the receiver to comfortably drape over the pillows. Encourage them to have their feet flat on the floor. Help them to get situated as comfortable as possible.

The massaging partner will start by first closing their eyes and taking a few deep, meditative breaths. This will help to focus their own energy and intention. They may also want to rub their hands together to generate some warmth before making contact. When they are ready, they can open their eyes and select the first two points high up on the spinal column. I was taught to start this massage at the base of the neck, gradually working down toward the sacrum in approximately two-to three-inch increments. Work each set of parallel points evenly for several moments to a few minutes each. The two points should not be on the spine; rather, each point is directly on either side of the spinal column, approximately two and a half to three inches horizontally apart from each other.

Once the starting points are selected, the massager can begin to apply a light but steady pressure by using either the middle knuckle of each index finger or the tips of the thumbs. Be mindful not to have the other parts of your hands making any contact with the pregnant person. You'll want the finger tips or knuckles to be the only points of contact between the two of you. Again, the massager will hold these two points for the duration of several full breaths (up to many minutes). The amount of pressure given in this massage should start out light. Just make contact. Then gradually increase the pressure as you feel any softening under your touch. As the massager listens with their hands, to feel the tissue soften, they can then gently sink in deeper with more pressure. The massager can verbally ask the receiver to think about softening at the points of contact, encouraging them to allow the pressure to sink in towards the center of their body. (Overall, however, words should be kept to a minimum throughout the massage.) The touch should be continuous and steady without any distraction. After several breaths (moments or minutes,

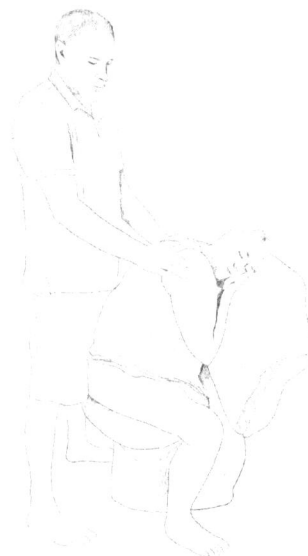

If you have access to a large ball you can try this position variation

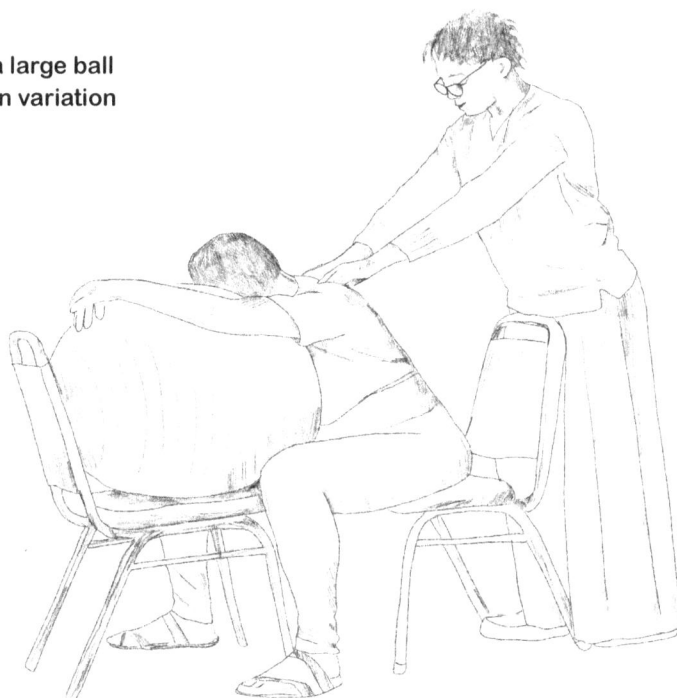

depending on your time frame), the massager will select two new points two to three inches farther down the spine, and repeat the sequence of starting out with a lighter pressure and gradually increasing. The massage is over when the massager has worked down the spine, stopping at or just above the pelvis. During labor someone may appreciate this massage in between contractions or during contractions.

Any massage can (and should) be thought of as a partnering breath exercise. The massaging partner should focus on their own internal posture and breath, as well as those of the receiver. Use your time to listen with your hands, your ears, and your heart. Invite your partner to yield under your touch.

The receiving person will want to focus their attention on following their own breath in and out, while trying to soften and yield into the points of contact. For the receiver, it will be interesting to experiment with focusing attention on different body parts as well. For example, try focusing sometimes on the body area being worked on and other times pull your attention to the outer reaches of your own body, away from where the massage is taking place. For example, try to relax the soles of your feet. It's also beneficial to sometimes just let your attention go, indulge your thoughts to go where they want to go. However, if your thoughts start to become uncomfortable or repetitive, bring yourself back to the present by directing your attention to your own breath. Feel and observe the action: I am breathing in... I am breathing out...

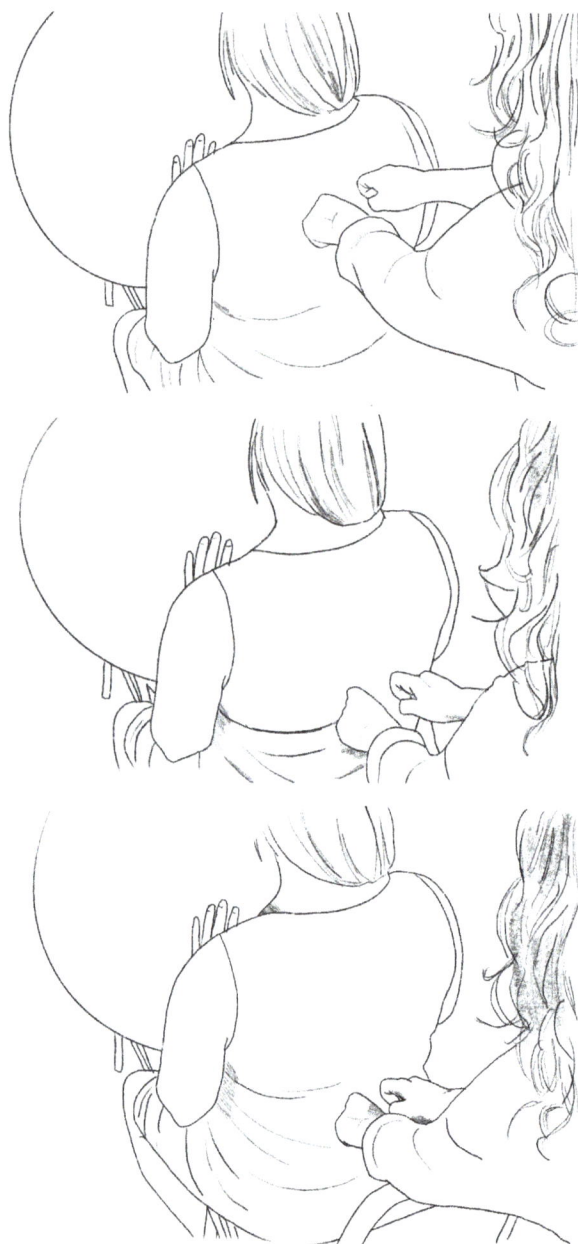

—Pause to try the shiatsu-style spinal massage—

Additional acupressure points useful during labor:

○ For pain: There are pressure points all long both sacroiliac joints. A partner can and should work two opposite points at a time. In early labor, start near the top of the sacrum. As the labor progresses, or if the points lose efficacy, find two new points farther down the sacrum. There are also points farther apart on the ilium, these may be most helpful in late first stage.

○ For fear: The bottom of the foot at the apex of the (smaller) arch, between the ball of the big toe and the ball of the littlest toe

Aromatherapy

Essential oils can be very comforting. They can help to reduce anxiety because our sense of smell works directly on our brain and "any odor you breathe in affects your limbic system, which governs emotional processing, motivation, fear, and pleasure."[335] The amount of pain a person feels is related to their tension levels, so things that are calming help to reduce one's perception of pain.[336]

There are several ways to utilize essential oils. A few drops can be mixed into a carrier oil such as grapeseed, sesame, or almond oil and then they can be massaged into the skin. Likewise, oils can be applied directly to a washcloth that is held near the face or put into a diffuser, which circulates the scents throughout the room. A midwife I have worked with recommends putting a drop of a calming essential oil on the palm of the hand. The person can then rub their hands together and then place their hands over their face to breathe in the scent. You may find this helpful in between the contractions, or during the contractions—either way can work. If the scent becomes unpleasant, then one can simply wash their hands. Alternatively, if you choose to place a few drops of oil onto a washcloth, then if the smell becomes distasteful it is easy enough to take the washcloth away.

Oils such as lavender, frankincense, and patchouli are three among many recommendations for calming and meditative scents. Lemon and peppermint oils can brighten a mood and lift up one's energy. Peppermint is excellent for improving mental clarity, which can really support a birthing person's ability to make decisions should the need arise.[337] Ideally the oils are produced from organic sources with no fillers added. In my community there are many midwives who recommend essential oils for aromatherapy during birth. Nevertheless, please do your own research and discuss these options with your providers before applying anything topically.

EXERCISE: SENSORY AWARENESS

I will now lead you through a sensory exploration. This is an adaptation of an exercise I learned first in a dance class and then again from the author Pam England.[338] If you are working with a partner, one of you can read aloud to the other. If you are working alone, then please read through once before closing your eyes and giving it a try.

"Settle into a comfortable, first-stage birthing position. Exhale and close your eyes. Focus your attention first on several breaths, flowing in and out. Allow these first breaths to help you arrive into this new position. Once settled please direct your attention to your sense of hearing. Listen through your ears, try to feel the sound waves going into and reverberating around your ears. What external sounds can you hear?"

—Reader pause—

"What internal sounds can you hear?"

—Reader pause—

"Please now focus your attention on your sense of touch. What can you feel? Are you wearing clothes? Can you feel the parts of you that are touching your clothes or the bed sheets or your partner? Can you feel the parts of you that are feeling the air? Notice the parts of you that are bearing weight or being supported."

—Reader pause—

"Please now focus your attention on your sense of smell. What can you smell? Where do you feel or sense smell? Can you smell your nostrils?"

—Reader pause—

"Now, with your eyes remaining closed, please bring your attention to your vision. What can you see inside your eyelids? With eyes remaining closed, explore your full range of eye movements and then let your eyes rest."

—Reader pause—

"Continuing to explore your vision, without moving your eyes or head, please now open your eyes. Allow your eyes to explore your total field of vision while leaving the head still. Explore your abilities to shift focus. Try to notice colors, textures, shapes, lines, lightness, and darkness."

—Reader pause—

"Allow your eyes to close and now please direct your attention to your sense of taste. What tastes can you detect in your mouth?"

—Reader pause—

"To conclude this exercise, in your own time and order, review and connect with each of your five senses: auditory, touch, taste, smell, and visual."

—Reader pause (long)—

"The exercise is now over. Please get comfortable to continue reading."

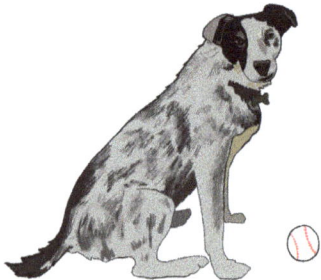

How was that? Were you able to follow along?

This sensory awareness technique is a kind of internal distraction technique and a potentially powerful birth tool. When you can conscientiously observe your own senses, you can use this ability to shift your focus during a birth contraction. The ability to shift your focus can help you to give yourself an attitude adjustment. When you feel a tremendous sensation, and maybe that sensation initially registers as pain, you can feel swallowed whole by the feeling. You can feel like pain is consuming you and allowing you only to be aware of it. But, if you can shift your focus, even just briefly, to an awareness of what you can *also* feel (the soles of your feet are strong on the ground, for example) or see (it's so sunny outside) or hear (my heart is beating) or taste (the last flavor was honey) or smell (the lavender oil on the nearby washcloth), then when your attention gets called back to your contraction, you have the experience of *returning*. The fact that you are returning to your strong birth sensations means that you were away from them for a bit. If you were away from these sensations, then labor hasn't swallowed you whole. You will live, you are safe. And you can return to the hard work with renewed strength and purpose. Labor is indeed hard. But it is also good for you and for the baby—and you can't be pregnant forever.

Visualizing your labor can aid your preparations

Imagine you are in your kitchen washing the dishes. All of a sudden you feel a strong cramp and then a trickle of water goes down your leg. Is it pee? You stand there, leaning on the counter for a moment, trying to process that 1) you didn't feel like you had to pee and 2) you had just had a good pee before you turned on the sink to wash the dishes. But if that wasn't pee... wait a minute... oh my gosh... maybe my water just broke?

And then, before you have time to get to the bathroom, a powerful sensation grips your lower abdomen. You feel a tightening squeeze that takes your breath away. It feels like a menstrual cramp on steroids and your whole abdomen is involved. You catch your breath and lean into the wall as you focus on a few good exhalations. Your belly relaxes and you continue on into the bathroom to get cleaned up. Your labor has started; a switch has been flipped.

That was six hours ago.

What are you doing now? Contractions are regular, coming about every five to seven minutes and lasting for a strong 45 to 60 seconds in duration. You have just had a whopper contraction. You currently can expect that you have between four and six minutes before the next contraction might arrive. Ask yourself the following questions:

- ○ What do you need/want to do right now?
- ○ How has it been going over the last six hours?
- ○ What have you been doing to cope?
- ○ How are you feeling about being in labor?
- ○ What do you think is coming next in terms of potential challenges?
- ○ Are you afraid? If so, of what?
- ○ Is there a coping technique you want to be sure to try?
- ○ Are there any techniques that you thought you would hate that now you might want to try? (Remember that sometimes the techniques we find repellent during pregnancy turn out to be very useful during birth.)
- ○ Where will you have your next contraction?
- ○ Can you rest?
- ○ Do you need to drink water and/or pee?
- ○ Would a massage feel good, or maybe a bath, or some fresh air, or kissing?

Reminder to the birthing partner: please don't ask questions mid contraction. Also, be mindful as the support partner not to ask too many questions throughout the process, as these can become burdensome.

In addition to the types of choices and decisions illuminated above, there are logistics during labor that need to be handled as well:

○ Are there any phone calls to be made?

○ If you are traveling for birth, do you have travel plans and arrangements made?

○ Are there things to pack?

○ Do you have cash or debit/credit cards or mobile payment options available? (I think it's always a good idea to have at least a little cash on hand when you are going to the hospital to have a baby. Or maybe I'm just old!)

○ If you are driving yourself, do you have gas in your car? (The mom in me is compelled to point out the obvious: no pregnant person should drive while in labor!)

○ Do you have a cell phone? Is it charged?

If possible, as soon as birth begins to demand your attention, you'll want to be able to tune into the singular focus of the loving-work of birth. So it's best to plan ahead and get all this practical and logistical stuff sorted out well in advance and then again very early in labor. Continuing a practice of visualizing possible labor scenarios can help you devise plans and utilize a variety of coping tactics. Early on in your pregnancy you should learn the locations of and directions to your area hospital(s). Better to know where they are and not need them, than to need them and not know where they are. It is also great to have extra hands around to handle any chores or logistics that need tending to, such as childcare (if you have older children), pet care, transportation, carrying bags, cleaning up, etc. A doula makes for a great set of extra hands! (More on doulas next week.)

Please take a moment to reflect on the visualization of your labor and write down or draw some notes here.

If I am planning a homebirth, when in labor should I contact the midwife?

Midwives generally want you to call them as soon as you become aware of any signs of labor. Midwives tend to stay in close communication with you as the labor progresses until you are ready for them to come to you. It is common for a midwife to describe what this care-juncture will look like as an embedded part of the homebirth/client communication early in your association. Always reach out when you want to. None of us can see the future and actually know what our own births will entail. I encourage you (those with homebirth plans) to read the following section on when to make a planned transfer to a hospital birth location just in case your plans should change. Everyone, please always seek immediate midwifery or medical attention should you have any concerns for yourself or your baby's wellbeing—during labor, now, or at any time in between.

If I am planning a hospital birth, when in labor should I go to the hospital?

The quick answer is: go to the hospital whenever you want to, get checked and then decide to stay or not based on how you feel after getting checked out (e.g., your blood pressure, the fetal heart tones, and possibly a vaginal exam). Short of an (even mildly) pressing desire to transport you'll want to consider a number of variables, such as how far do you need to travel and are there weather or traffic conditions or other obstacles that could influence the travel time. Also, what is the apparent furiousness—or lack thereof—of your labor progression and what's your provider's counsel, your intuition, and your preference. Short of any other compelling reasons or signs, if your goal is to get the majority of labor work done at home, and your travel time doesn't exceed 30 – 40 minutes, I generally counsel my clients to look for signs of transition (that unique phase at the end of first stage) to make their travel decision. Once you see any benchmarks of transition, which include self-doubting, being newly scared or newly easily angered, new feelings of being emotionally overwhelmed or a bit disoriented or uncertain, plus physically shaking, big temperature changes (sweating or freezing or both), new onset belching, flatulence or nausea, new onset vomiting, and contractions coming rapidly with noticeably shrinking recovery time between them, then it is probably time to go. (Review expressions of transition in Week 9.) If your travel time is one hour or longer it gets a little trickier to figure out. One way to mitigate that challenge would be to save up for a hotel room near the hospital. This can give you a private place close by to rest, should you want to go into the hospital for evaluation and have an easier option not to be admitted (yet) and not have to travel as far back as home. You will eventually come back again and you still won't know exactly when that will be.

Many providers rely on the timing of contractions for travel instructions for labor. (Review Week 6 for timing contractions.) Providers often instruct the 5-1-1 plan, which dictates that a pregnant person should go to the hospital when contractions are 5 minutes apart, each contraction is lasting for 1 minute, and this pattern has been occurring for at least 1 hour. Recently, some providers are now using the 4-1-1 plan: come in when the contractions are four minutes apart, lasting one minute each, and you're in that pattern for one hour. But tic tock, do you need the clock?

As I addressed in Week 6, how long the contractions are and how far apart they are is information that *can* add some clues as you try to understand something about how the birth is progressing. But this information is not a definitive, reliable way to know what is happening with your labor. In other words, the pattern of your contractions is not dependable as the sole source of decision making for when it's time to go to the hospital. Beware of making decisions in labor based solely on timing or other *singular* variables of assessment, such as cervical dilation.

That being said, a trusted midwife pal once told me that her experience has taught her that if labor begins with contractions that are 10 minutes or more apart, then there is a good chance that your labor will take a bit longer to progress. If contractions start off closer than 10 minutes apart, then there is a reasonable chance that your labor will progress a bit quicker.

As you think about what making this decision will be like in your birth, it is useful to understand something about your own birth values, and to have some loose goals or plans about how you hope the birth unfolds. Knowing your concerns around birth can help you with this decision, too. In my classes I point out that the less time physically in the hospital helps one avoid some routine interruptions and interventions, and this may be desirable.

I think it is useful to consider that the hospital staff are trained to do *things*, they have a long list of protocols to follow (i.e., things to do), and they assume that when you show up in labor you are ready for them to go through their lists and do their things that make up standard hospital practice. It follows then that, the less time you are physically there in labor, the less of those things get done. I don't mean to suggest that you not get the care you need or want. I just want you to be aware of what your hospital protocols are ahead of time so that you can make informed decisions. And sometimes making less decisions is preferable. Ideally you will have your provider's approval and support for your plan to labor at home, and also have (and use) access to them by phone throughout labor until you arrive at your location. Please, if at any point you want to go into the hospital (because you feel safer there), then go. If you want to stay at the hospital even if you sense that you are early in your process, then stay early. Your body will work best when and where you feel safest. But it is important to understand that more hours in the hospital means more opportunities for interruptions and interventions.

When you are deciding to go to your birth location, weigh the average of timings from a sample of recent contractions (noting how long they last and the time from the start of one contraction to the start of the next) while also considering the bigger picture of your experience: Have you recognized any of the emotional expressions of labor? Do you have intuition about where you are in that continuum of emotion? Consider the circumstances of your travel, including how and how far will you have to go to your birth location as well as any weather, traffic, or other obstacles. Evaluate your emotional reasons for why you want to go or why you are not ready to go. Do you have concerns? Does your provider have concerns? I repeat: you can and should go to your hospital anytime you want to. Your providers can only help you if they know what is going on and you need to follow your feelings. There should be no reason to stress going early because you don't have to stay and be admitted. If once you are observed by a maternity care provider, and all seems well but you appear to be still early in the process or your labor activity has slowed down with the tumult of the travel, then please do consider leaving until you get further into the process. Sometimes, as an intermediary step, it is useful first to go to your provider's office, if they are open. Based on your labor patterns and the results of your physical examination, you can then decide if it makes sense to stay and be admitted or to leave to get more work done under more private circumstances. Often being newly assured that all is going well can really help boost your progress in the birth. Of course, it would be wonderful to discuss this decision point well ahead of time with your provider.

For first-time parents, the tendency is to get to the hospital sooner rather than later. If you can anticipate this as possibly your situation, ask yourself how you can calm yourself down enough to get the bulk of your work done at home. Hiring a birth doula is one great way to build your confidence and add an additional support person. Hiring a maternity care provider who, in general, supports the plan to labor at home can also help you to find confidence.

Another action to consider around the time of moving to the hospital is calling the maternity floor directly as soon as you are ready to leave your home. In general, you don't need to do this because you will already have had a conversation with your practitioner, and once the decision to go into the hospital has been made, they will notify the maternity floor. Nevertheless, it's a good idea to have this number in hand well ahead of time, so that if you want to call you can. If you do call, you'll want to let the maternity floor know that you are on your way now and you can request a nurse who is knowledgeable about and supportive of natural pain relief techniques. This call also provides you with the chance to request a birthing ball, squat bar, birthing stool, birthing tub, etc., while giving the maternity floor advance time to ready this equipment and make the best nursing assignment.

Your intuition is an important safety alert system

I want you to cultivate trust in your instincts. To do that you have to give yourself permission to need and utilize support. If something doesn't seem right to you—if you have a hunch, an urge, an antsy feeling, an inclination, if you have questions, or just want to be checked because you are worried, or you express that, at any time, "something doesn't seem right," then you should contact your caregiver for attention. How can you relax into the experience and take care of yourself in labor (or pregnancy) if you're anxious? Open communication with your provider (and with yourself) is essential for good health. People are reliable reporters of their own well-being and the baby's, too; after all, the baby is a part of the gestating person.

I have lived through several stories of women who've had strong emotional reactions to seemingly normal symptoms, and once those instincts were followed they found out that their fears had been justified. One woman who comes to mind stayed after class one night to share her concerns with me. She described normal Braxton Hicks contractions; her symptoms were a general tightening around the abdomen, not too strong, but noticeable enough to stop what she was doing and take a deep breath. She said she had been getting them periodically throughout the day. Her description sounded exactly like any healthy Braxton Hicks contractions, but with one exception: they were making her unusually nervous. After she expressed her concern to me, I encouraged her to follow up with her provider. She told me that she had called earlier and spoken to a nurse that day, but that the nurse simply told her she was having Braxton Hicks contractions and that she shouldn't worry about it. I had known this woman for several weeks of intimate, in-person classes and she had not seemed to be particularly anxious or jittery. I knew her to be emotionally grounded and quite reasonable. Braxton Hicks contractions don't usually make a pregnant person overly nervous, especially when they're educated and know that practice contractions are a healthy part of pregnancy. Now, however, this woman was really upset by what she was feeling. It was her anxiety, therefore, that caught my attention. I pushed her to call her doctor's office back and to insist that she get checked out.

The next day she called me from the hospital. She had called the doctor after leaving class and insisted she needed attention. The doctor had her come into the hospital, where it was discovered that her baby was experiencing a cardiac complication. The doctor was then able to treat the baby by giving the mother medications. The medications allowed the baby to gestate several more weeks, reaching term. The baby was then born by cesarean section and was able to undergo medical care directly. This baby is now a big, strong child. That woman's caregivers were able to help her baby because her own early warning alert system—call it her intrinsic fetal monitoring—was good and she listened to it (and so did I). Please, trust your instincts. Health care providers can't help us if they don't know what's going on.

I had another client once call me in labor to ask when her contractions would get to five minutes apart and start to last one minute each. She was currently in labor and had been for 15 hours already. She told me that her labor had started with the contractions about three minutes apart, each lasting from 30 – 40 seconds. She reported that the contractions were still about three minutes apart, although some were closer to two minutes apart, and they were now lasting about 45 – 50 seconds each. She said they had gotten tougher to get through and she had been working hard, but that her labor pattern hadn't changed. She was starting to feel a lot of increased pressure on her rectum even between contractions. I said that it sounded like she might never see contractions that are five minutes apart and a minute long. In other words, she likely wouldn't fall into the 5-1-1 pattern. This surprised her because her doctor had been so clear and so specific. After hearing the woman on the phone through her next contraction, I suggested that if she and her partner thought they might be ready, they should make their move to the hospital. She was fully dilated when she arrived at the hospital and gave birth shortly after she got there. If she hadn't called someone to discuss her timing *in relation to everything else*, she might not have made it to the hospital before birth.

This client of mine was trying to be a good patient. She equated safe birth with following the "rules" and doing everything that the doctor said. This is a logical train of thought. Following your doctor's instructions is ostensibly one of the reasons you chose to work with them through your birth. I encourage you, however, to balance the information from your providers with what you are feeling during labor (or at any time during your birth experience). You must own part of the decision-making process. It needs to make sense to you; and it needs to go beyond just, "they told me this timing," or, "when I spoke to them this morning in my early labor, they said I should come to the hospital at 6pm tonight." If, for example, it doesn't make sense to come in at 6pm, because at 6pm you feel like you need to, want to, or can postpone going in, you can certainly decide to do so. Likewise, if you are nervous and want to go in earlier than 6pm to be checked, please advocate for that, and you can always just go to the hospital. Communicate with your caregivers, while knowing that the decision is ultimately up to you. Trusting your instincts is critical to making good choices.

Surprise! How to catch your baby

Were you planning a home birth but not at home when the baby is coming? Is your midwife delayed in getting to you? Are you planning to transport for birth? If you get caught by surprise in any of these kinds of scenarios, and the feeling to push has come on strong, then your support person should first visually check to see if the perineum is swollen with the baby's head. If it is, then birth is imminent and you should stay put, call emergency support (911), and prepare to catch the baby. You should not attempt to travel if the baby is coming *now*.

Chances are slim that you will find yourself in a situation where the baby is coming out and you aren't where you were expecting to be or with a professional birth attendant to assist you. But if your baby is coming and you are without a trained caregiver by your side, then you'll appreciate some assurance knowing that you have already had some guidance on how to catch your baby on your own. It's useful to gain some degree of emergency preparedness now, just in case. (Plus, even if it's not your baby that is making a surprise arrival, you never know when you might happen upon another person in need of emergency birth assistance.) The need to catch your baby can happen at home, if you don't have time to make it to the hospital, or even at the hospital—because, well, these things happen. One of my clients, while in the hospital, did exactly this. It was a busy night, and not even a nurse was there with her and her partner. But both had been well trained by the Bradley Method®, so they stayed calm and did remarkably well.

Imagine that you and your support partner are in the car, on your way to the hospital, when the baby decides she can't wait. While your partner is driving you turn to them and say, "Oh my gosh <grunt>, the baby is coming *now*!" The first thing that should happen is that your partner trusts that you know what you're talking about. The second thing that should happen is that your partner should check your surroundings and look for a safe place to stop the car. Stopping the car safely, well off the road, is the most important job in this moment—even if you can see the hospital in the distance. Please, don't try to speed up (run red lights or roll through stop signs) to get to the hospital; stop the car. In fact, drive with extra caution until you can pull over and safely stop the car. (Note that the hormones released during a stressful event can reduce your peripheral vision, so please act responsibly.[339]) A baby coming out is not an emergency in and of itself, but a motor vehicle accident would be. You are going to catch the baby. That is all. You'll all be okay.

Now, to the support partner's role: Once the car is safely off the road and stopped, put it in park but keep the motor running. Put your flashers on, turn up the heat, and then dial 911 for help. (If you don't have a phone, try *briefly* to get a passerby to call for help.) Assuming you have a phone and have reached 911, the first thing to do is to make sure that they have your location. Explain to them that you will keep the line open, but that you must put the phone down. You can't catch a baby with a cell phone in your hand. EMS dispatchers are well trained to keep you on the phone. You may think to put the phone on speaker mode, but you don't really need to hear the dispatcher.

What you'll want is the line open should you have any questions for them. Be brave—your baby is counting on you.

Remember and trust what you already know about birth and, in particular, second stage labor. Remember that people can and do birth their babies all by themselves. The job of support partners is to help make it easier by providing practical help and by keeping the laboring person calm, positive, and confident in their abilities. If the birthing person still has their bottoms on, you can help to get them off. You can remind the birthing person, and yourself, to breathe fully. Next, help them to get into the best position they can, given the situation. Perhaps getting on hands and knees in the back seat or in the passenger seat with the back reclining would be good. (If you own a vehicle consider exploring some potential positions ahead of time.) As the partner, please work hard to remain calm. (Remember that obstetric complications are generally surrounding times when the baby is not progressing down. So if the baby is already on its way out, then there is rarely a problem.) Encourage the birthing person to listen to their urges and instincts. If they can listen inwards, they will know when to squeeze down and when to relax. Encourage rest in between contractions. If you notice that there is some poop coming out of the birthing person before the baby, use some tissues or toilet paper or whatever you have on hand to wipe it away. Be sure to wipe any poop away from the vagina. (Keeping a good supply of tissues or toilet paper in the car is a good idea as you get closer to the actual birth. Additional recommended supplies to keep on hand follow further ahead, so keep reading.)

Now your job as the partner is pretty straightforward: try to stay calm (or fake calm, if you have to), love the birthing person, and catch. *Do not pull on the baby* or try to twist or turn the baby. Do not try to reach inside the birthing person. You want to "do no harm," and allow the birth process to unfold into your hands. Then... catch.

Once the baby is out, depending on what position the birthing person was in, you will either place the baby on the birthing person's belly (pull their shirt up for skin to skin contact, if they have a top on) or you may need to hold onto to the baby as you help direct them to sit or lie back. If they gave birth on their hands and knees you will need to hand them the baby through their legs so that they may sit back. Be careful not to put any traction on the umbilical cord, which is still attached to the placenta inside and also attached to the baby outside. The baby should be placed tummy down on the birth parent's abdomen or chest (depending on how long the cord reaches easily). If the birthing person has a bra on, help them to take that off as well. Next use a towel to dry the baby and wrap birth parent and baby together in a blanket or another towel or whatever you have access to for warmth (newspaper can work in a pinch). Be sure to keep the baby's face clear. *You want to keep the baby as warm as possible, which means you will want to dry the baby as quickly as possible. Again, wrap the baby and birthing person up together with a blanket, dry towel, or whatever else you have. Keeping birth parent and baby together with skin-to-skin contact will help the baby warm to the perfect temperature.*

Remember that the placenta may follow the baby within the first five minutes, or it may take up to 45 minutes after the birth. Because the baby will still be attached to the umbilical cord and the placenta is still inside attached to the uterus, this is a wonderful back up for the baby's transition to being an independent being. The cord and placenta will continue to supply some oxygenated blood to her, at least for a few more moments. If your baby is crying, then she is breathing. If she is quiet, then she may be breathing or she may need a bit of encouragement. Talk to your baby and massage her back with some vigor.

Again, do not pull on the umbilical cord at any time. There is no need to pull on the cord for any reason and you shouldn't do anything else with the cord (such as cutting it); soon enough help will arrive. But do feel free to touch the cord. Directly after the birth, you will be able to feel it pulsate for a few moments while any of the remaining blood from the placenta and cord at the moment of birth is delivered to the baby.

Once you have established that the baby is breathing, both you and the birthing parent should take a few deep breaths for yourselves. Smile! Your baby is here. The birth is over. And you did it! Continue to talk to and touch the baby. If you have some juice or water with you, offer the birth parent a sip.

It is likely that emergency medical help has arrived or is arriving at this moment; however, in the unlikely event that you are still on your own, you'll want to consider the tone of the uterus as your next step. Having effective post-birth contractions are critical to control blood loss and aid in delivery of the placenta. Stimulation of the breasts will encourage them to secrete oxytocin, which will contract the uterus to control the bleeding. If the baby will cooperate, nursing would be ideal. Even if the baby doesn't nurse, but only nuzzles at the breast, it will help to stimulate the gestational parent to secrete enough hormones to help contract the uterus. Encouraging a calm atmosphere will help, too. If there is any concern, the partner should massage the lower abdominal region, trying to identify the uterus, and the birthing parent or baby should tweak and roll the birthing parent's nipples. (The uterine massage will need to dig in kind of deep and it may not be very comfortable.) Breast stimulation should continue intermittently until you are under the care of a birth professional who can gauge the uterine tone and blood loss. Periodic checks of the uterine tone are important in preventing postpartum hemorrhage, although as a lay person that may remain elusive. Do the best you can but also calm yourself with your common sense; know that if the birth parent is feeling okay and their energy and skin color remain normal, then everything is working out well and as expected. Continued uterine massage may be necessary if they are not feeling or looking well, and in rare instances drugs such as Pitocin are beneficial to control blood loss.[340] (This is why you started by calling 911. Remember that they are on the line and you can get support as you need.)

If the placenta comes while you are still on the side of the road or otherwise unattended, keep the placenta connected to the baby. *Do not* cut the cord. Place only the placenta into a plastic bag or basin or wrap it up in a towel bundle. You will then have the baby in one bundle and the placenta, *still attached to the cord*, in another bundle. The cord can be cut whenever you are finally being cared for by birth professionals. In the meantime, continue to keep the baby warm, talk to her, allow her access to the gestational parent's breasts, and give her plenty of time to study your faces. The placenta should be examined by a healthcare professional as soon as possible. A birth professional will be able to assess the edges of the placenta and rule out the possibility that some section of the placenta has been retained in the uterus.[341] (This is a rare and very serious complication, requiring immediate medical attention.[342])

If help still hasn't arrived, then you will now want to proceed to a hospital. Go to the hospital you are closest to, even if it's not where you thought you were headed. When you get there, you'll need to go to the emergency department rather than straight to the maternity floor. They will do a rapid assessment and do what they can when they can to get you onto the maternity floor. Congratulations. You caught your baby!

Please note that the information provided above is in no way intended to replace seeking out proper care. Again, what I discussed above is solely intended as an emergency backup plan. If you do find yourself in the unexpected situation of an imminent birth, and you are not in a car, but at your home or elsewhere, then extrapolate the information you need from these plans and adapt accordingly.

Supplies to keep in your car (for vehicle owners), just in case

I recommend packing the following list into your car, as emergency supplies. Some of the following supplies can be useful for anytime that you may be in labor and in a car (so you may want to pack a car-bag if you don't have a car), while some are specifically in case of an unexpected birth.

O Blanket
    It is a good idea to always have a blanket in the car, especially if you live in a climate with cold winters.

O Towels (1 or 2, ideally kept clean in a separate bag)
    Towels will be used to dry the laboring person if their water breaks and/or to dry the baby after she's born.

- Good supply of (old) plastic grocery bags

  If you double bag them they work well for vomiting into. Then just tie the handles into a top knot and discard. These bags also work well for garbage collection or as a container to hold a placenta.

- Tissues or toilet paper

  If either the pregnant person or the support person is throwing up or crying, you will need tissues to blow noses and wipe eyes/mouth. If the baby is being caught, then these supplies can be used to wipe away any poop that may come out ahead of the baby.

- Mouthwash

  This is great to rinse out a mouth after vomiting, or if the support partner had some coffee, banana, garlic, peanut butter, or other smelly breath agent that might bother the birthing person as they labor.

- Water bottle, for drinking (filled with water)

- Flashlight, cell phone, and other typical first aid supplies are always a good safety practice.

- Gas in your gas tank or full electrical charge.

Tips on preparing older siblings for birth

I strongly encourage my clients to prepare their older children (even the youngest toddlers) as if they will be at the birth, regardless of the gestational parent's actual plans. Even if you're sure you *don't* want your older child(ren) at the birth, please consider that they might see some of it anyway. For example, what if gestational parent and older child are home alone when labor begins and it comes on strong. Or, what if labor begins in the middle of the night and there is no immediate need to leave the house or wake the child, but then the child wakes up and sees the action? I think that when a parent has prepared their child(ren) as best they can, then whatever parts of the labor they may see comes with some context to understand what is happening. And in the moment of labor, this can be a good comfort. Children are very accepting of natural things, but some prior education can help to reduce the parent's tension surrounding their child's well-being. A little bit of preparation goes a long way.

Showing children videos of real births of humans and animals can be one useful way to teach them about birth. It may be useful to show your children video clips of births being attended by other children. You can also practice labor positions and conscientious breathing in front of your children. Let your children see you working hard at the practice of birth preparation. Show them different labor positions in different rooms around your home. Let them see you practicing massage techniques. Let the kids know the work will be hard by practicing your loud vocalizations around them. You can welcome them to get loud with you! Kids find it funny and fun to get loud inside the home. Note that children may also find this work a bit daunting, too. It's a big deal that a baby is coming, and it's okay to have some fears. Let them see you grimace and grunt. Teach them that birth is hard work, but that you, the birthing person, are strong and safe.

Engage your children in some mock labor practice. During these practice times try not to pay too much attention to the older sibling(s). Give siblings ways to be involved; birth is not a spectator sport. Think now about how the siblings can be/feel useful during birth. Maybe if massaging the gestational parent is too much distraction for the laboring person, the child can give the support person a massage, or be a birth photographer, or get the other support person a drink of water, or wipe the support person's brow with a wash cloth. (It's hard work to care for someone in labor, too!) Or maybe an older child can participate by drawing a picture, or several, for the new baby. Be creative! Consider that birth is a family event; everyone can do something to help support the process.

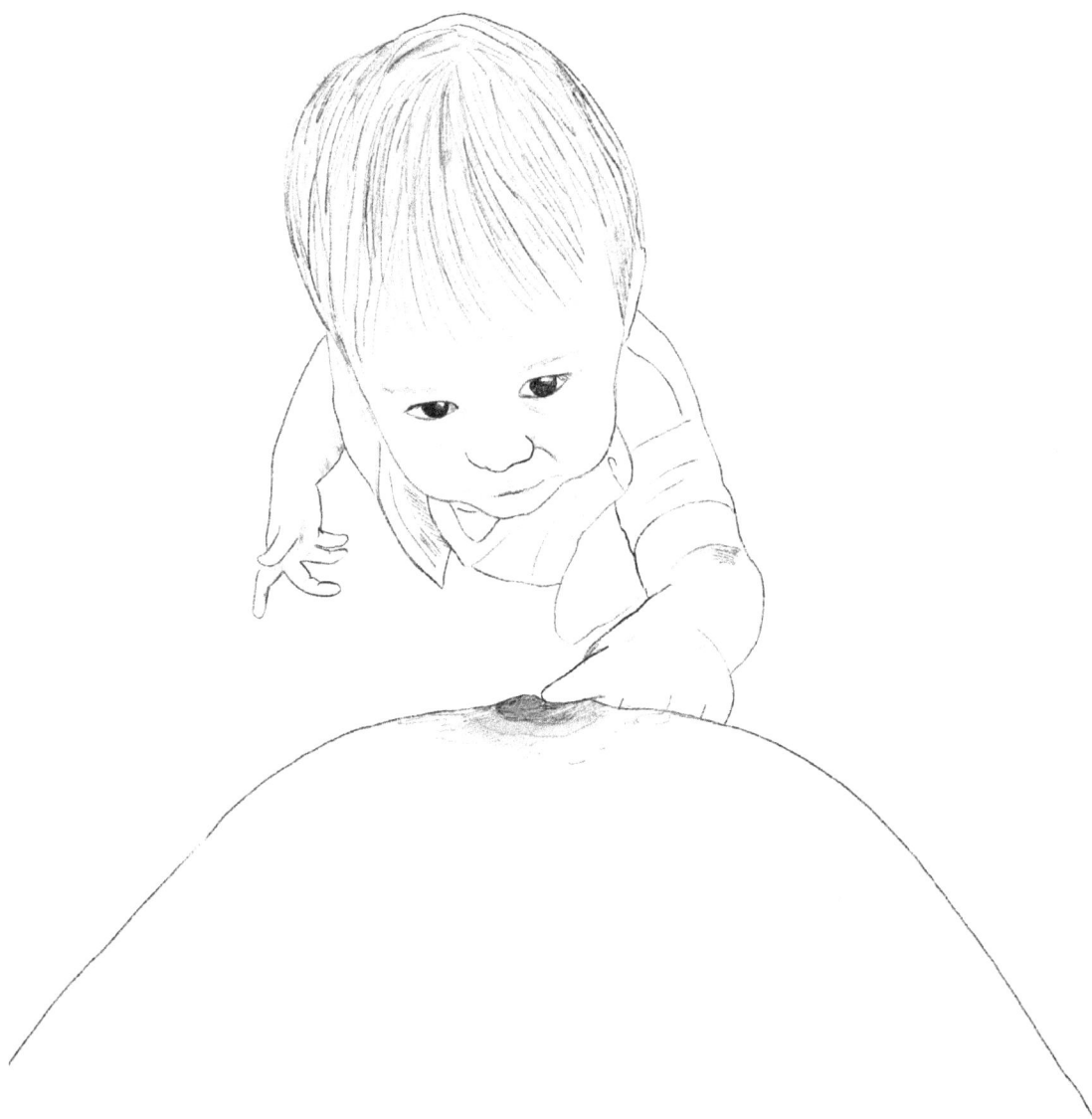

"Isn't my belly big? That's our baby growing in there!"

Some people believe having older children at birth decreases sibling rivalry. The thinking here is that when young children see that their new baby has come from their parent's body, then they understand more fully that this new person is a part of their parent, and therefore the family, which can in turn reduce rivalry. In my opinion, I think the most important thing to figure out is how the birthing person feels. Just like with so many other support techniques, the birthing person won't be able to know what really works best until labor has begun—and this includes the presence or absence of older children. Many people report to me that having their older children with them was a great source of comfort. Several parents have told me that it was calming for them, that they felt they could keep it together emotionally more easily when their older child was around. But I have also had parents tell me that everything was going along fine until they got to a place where they just *needed* their older child to leave; the presence of the older child had become a distraction. I don't think there is a right or a wrong here. I do think pregnancy is a great time for *everyone* to learn about birth.

Regardless of whether you want your older child(ren) to attend your birth or leave in the middle or whatever other scenario might emerge, you should be thinking about who can be a care provider for them during the birth and the immediate postpartum period. If you are planning a hospital birth, try to take your child to see the hospital in advance, so that they will understand where you go when you are away from them. And, finally, hold them close as often as possible. Their whole world is about to change drastically, too, resulting in all primary relationships shifting.

Fur babies

One of my former clients once commented: "When I reviewed labor positions at home, my dog was very unnerved and needed a lot of attention." I'm sure this is more common than not, so I would advise you to practice with your animals and to include some sound making, so that the pet(s) have a chance to get acclimated to what is to come. Of course, if you plan to birth at home, you can also separate any animals from the location of your birth. Likewise, talk to your veterinarian or animal trainer, as they are usually a good resource for suggestions on how to help a dog or other family pet adjust to the sights and sounds of labor and the new baby's arrival. Searching the internet may also afford some good suggestions (although be cautious of the rabbit holes—pun intended—you may find and evaluate the material to your comfort level). WebMD, for example, recommends to slowly acclimate your pets in advance of birth, and to realize that their lives are changing, too.[343] Finally, thinking ahead, if you can enlist some help for pet care during your birth and/or postpartum adjustment, please do!

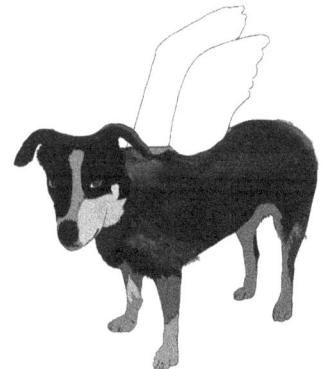

Congratulations on completing another week's lesson. You are a powerful and loving person, I am sure of it. This little being you are growing is so lucky to have found you. I am wishing you a wonderful week with a multitude of bright and light moments.

HOMEWORK:

A) Continue to build daily mindfulness routines

Practice relaxation techniques that you like, don't like, and are indifferent to. The more options you practice, the more you will have access to in labor. If you haven't been keeping up with a practice of using affirmations, consider revisiting those goals this week, too.

B) Continue to make practical plans

Discuss when to travel to the hospital with your providers or when to call your midwife to you. Make your plans for what you will wear, eat, drink, and transport, should that be or become a reality.

C) Practice mock labor sequences

Practice will build familiarity and make your tools more available. Include timing contractions, vocalizations, and a review of positions. Get the whole family involved, including older children and pets.

THIS SPACE IS FOR YOUR NOTES AND DRAWINGS

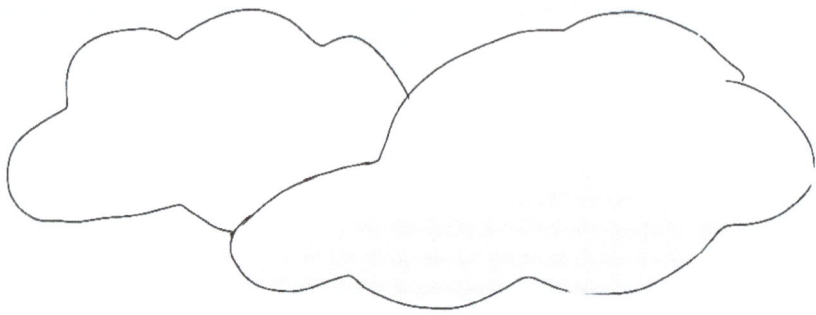

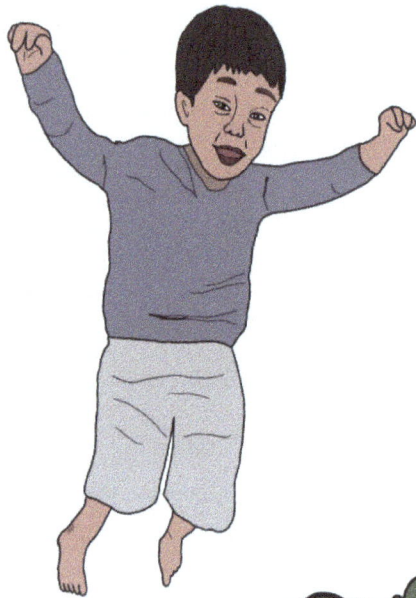

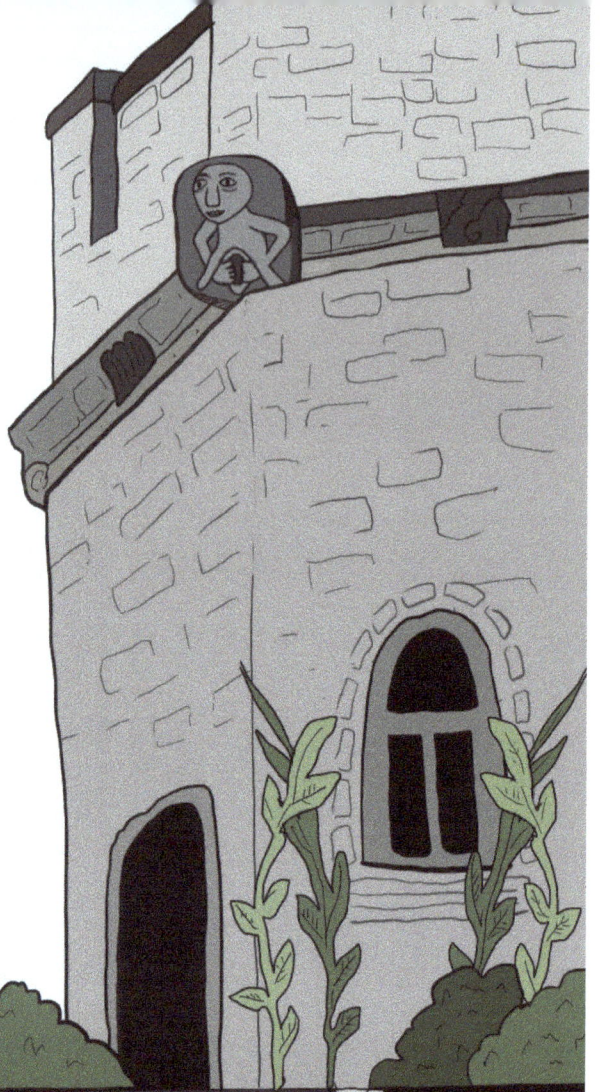

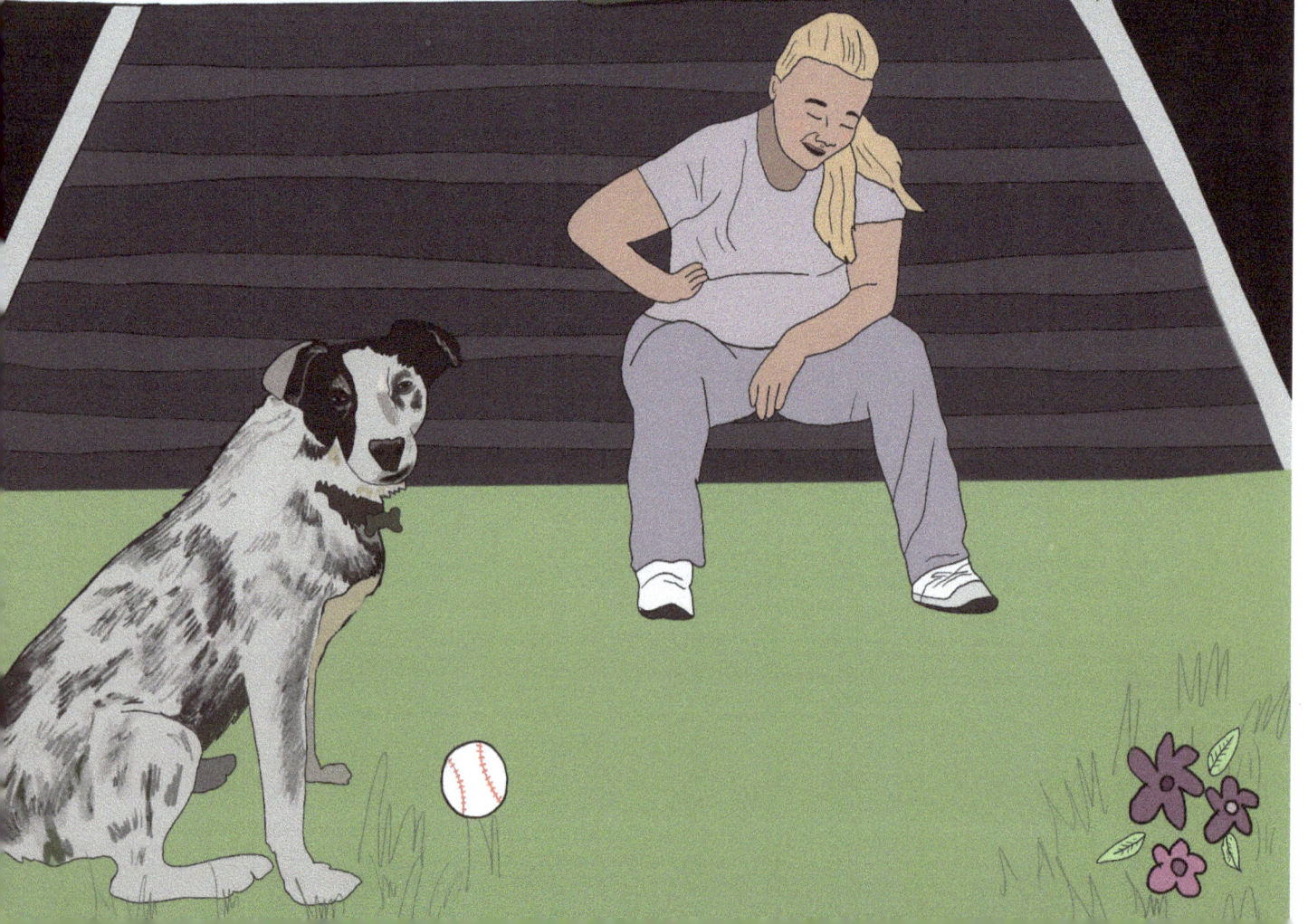

WEEK 15

Plan and Prepare

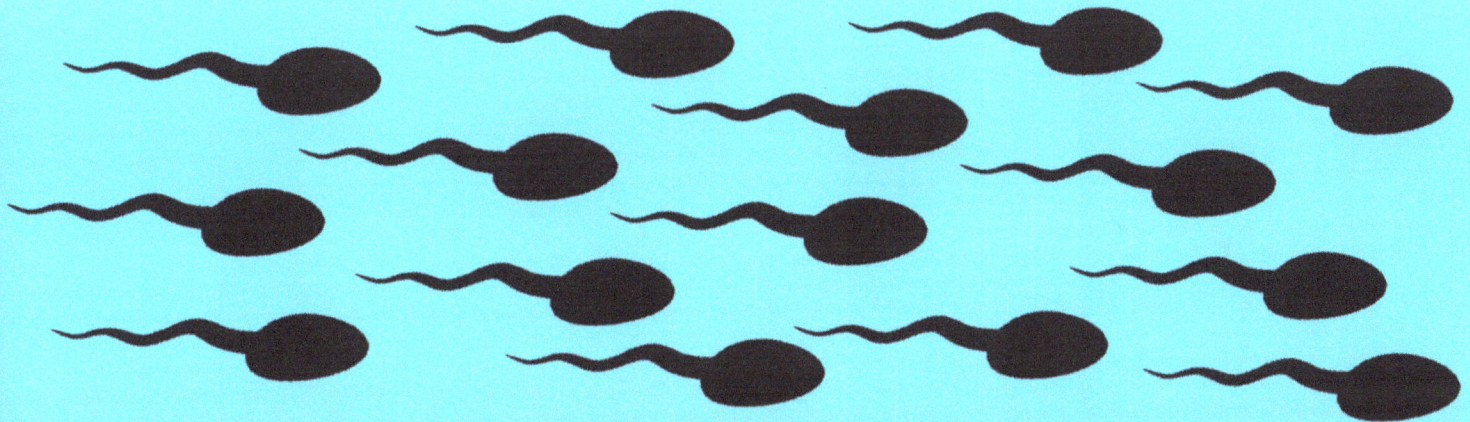

Chapter contents:

O *Doula care*

O *Postpartum planning*

THIS SPACE IS FOR YOUR NOTES AND DRAWINGS

Great to have you back for Week 15. You've already done so much wonderful work. I hope you're feeling strong and confident and excited to welcome your baby very soon! I also want to thank you for being you. Although we haven't met in person, this book serves as a conduit between us—between you, the beautiful and powerful birthing person, your support person(s), and me, your mentor and cheerleader. Because I have been cultivating my imagination through years of practicing and guiding visualization exercises, I imagine you are a nice, loving, and creative person. You care so much about being a great parent to your baby. You are a responsible, gentle, and thoughtful person, who wants to help make the world a more just and marvelous place. I said it last week and I deeply believe it is true and worth repeating: your baby is so lucky to have found you!

This week we will continue to discuss putting your best plans into place. As of today, where are you at with your healthcare decisions? Do you have a provider or an office from which you receive regular prenatal care? Did you have a prenatal appointment this past week? If so, how was it? Be it last week or an earlier date: how did you feel walking in the door, while you were there, and afterwards? Please write down some of your immediate thoughts below.

During one or more of your prenatal appointments, were you able to practice asking open-ended questions?

How do you feel about any answers you got?

I encourage you to respect your feelings. Do you feel a sense of relationship with any of the providers you've seen? Do you have options for alternative offices? If you have a choice, and you have made a choice, what are the reasons why? How do you feel about them?

If you haven't made any decisions yet, don't fret. Taking your time can be good, too; be thorough in your investigations. Should anything urgent happen before you commit to a provider, you can access urgent care or the emergency department at a hospital. While I fully support getting routine prenatal care from one practice, regardless of your plans to stay with them for care through your birth, sometimes you do need to end this relationship if the care you are receiving isn't good (your feelings about how you are treated count). Then you can begin with a new provider. Remember: even if you have decided and committed to a plan, plans are elusive—change is often possible during all phases of your pregnancy and birth.

Write down some additional notes now on any healthcare decisions you've made, or that you have been thinking about making. Make the category of "healthcare" as open to interpretation as you want as you think about any decisions you have had to make recently. (For example: moving might be a healthcare decision because where you live has a big impact on your health.)

Doula care

There are two kinds of doulas related to maternity care that I will address in this section: birth doulas and postpartum doulas. Birth doulas provide emotional support and continuity of care for the gestational parent and their partner through to the end of pregnancy and during birth. Postpartum doulas help the family recover from birth and adjust to life with a newborn. In addition, there are large differences in doula certification programs. Some birth doulas are trained, if not licensed, to perform vaginal exams in labor, monitor the fetal heart tones, and take the mother's blood pressure. Some doulas do not do any of these tests; they are there solely to provide emotional support, like reminding you of different labor positions to try, getting you food, parking the car, holding your hand, or cleaning up puke. Understanding the possibilities when it comes to doula care may help you to fine-tune your plans.

Doula care is a way to help make up for any gaps in extended family support. All people deserve to be cared for with knowledge, attention, and love. It's another sad commentary on our culture that many people need money to be able to afford what should be a birthright: to be nurtured through birth and postpartum adjustment. But don't despair. Maybe you can barter for services or find a doula-in-training that needs to attend births to complete their training, which can translate into working with you for free or at very low cost. Even if money is really, really tight, please do search for doula care anyway. Do not be shy to ask a doula to work out a payment plan. Many doulas work with sliding scale fees to accommodate different economic brackets. (And if you don't ask, you will never know.) I have never met a doula that was in this business to get rich. Consider what their hourly rate might drop down to if your labor lasts several days and you will start to understand that they have a calling to this work. Their skills are likely to be priceless to your experience, assuming you find a person who is a good fit.

A birth doula provides personalized emotional support from their point of hire in pregnancy and then through-out the birth. Birth doulas generally bring with them a wealth of labor coping techniques and an educated understanding of the healthy birth process. Birth doula's generally build their relationship with you through several prenatal visits, and then accompany you through labor. Birth doula services generally include several postpartum visits as well. The prenatal visits help to build a relationship of trust for the birth. Postpartum visits are beneficial for postpartum adjustment as they provide further continuity of care. Birth doulas are generally well informed on breastfeeding, infant care, and the wholistic needs of a postpartum family. Having a birth doula to process the emotional impact of the birth gives the gestational parent greater perspectives as they emotionally unpack the birth experience. Birth doulas are often good resources for community services and for what an expectant family may need. A good birth doula can provide support to a single parent or a couple, with the latter including a focus on the couple (or family) working well together.

Birth doulas generally follow a schedule of prenatal appointments that mimic a typical maternity care schedule. From the point-of-hire, the single parent or couple may meet with the birth doula monthly, then bimonthly, and then weekly at the end of the pregnancy. Birth doulas will usually make at least one home visit prior to labor. When labor arrives and you are ready for more support, they generally will come to your home and begin to care for you and your partner/family. If you are transporting to a hospital, they will travel with you, supporting you as you travel to your birth location. A birth doula typically doesn't leave your side until you're settled in and breastfeeding your baby. (Please be sure to discuss continuity of doula care during any interviews that you might have.)

Birth doulas attend hospital as well as home births. Doula care during labor and birth has been shown to reduce the need for medications and other interventions, such as cesarean sections.[344] Birth doulas increase a gestational person's satisfaction and lend great support to birth partners.[345] Doulas have been shown to provide a model of mothering behavior to new parents that supports excellent parent/infant bonding and breastfeeding. They help ward off postpartum adjustment problems and are usually good resources if additional postpartum care is needed.

A doula is *your* independent provider, charged with supporting you and your family. A doula does not make medical decisions. Their job is not to express their own opinions; a doula's job is to support you as you work through your process. A doula can remind you of what questions to ask to be able to make informed decisions. They can act as your sounding board as you process the choices before you. A birth doula should be awed by and respectful of the birth process and have a sizable degree of comfort with the sights and sounds of birth. A doula should have an assortment of (non-medication) pain relief techniques, and they should be knowledgeable and respectful of a person's choice to use pain medication. (Note: Just as you would ask your doctor about their approach to pain medication use, ask your birth doula the same question. This makes for a good topic of discussion and can help you to further determine if the doula is a good fit for you and your process. It is also useful to think back to the exercise in Week 6 describing physical, mental, and emotional support and look for any of those qualities you are hoping to boost with the help of a prospective hire.)

Once the baby is born and the primary nurturer and baby are settled in at home, postpartum doulas come to work. While postpartum doulas generally do not attend labor, you should ideally meet your postpartum doula prenatally, in order to establish a good relationship. Postpartum doulas frequently come for several hours a week over the first few weeks after baby is born and provide a range of basic breastfeeding support, emotional support, and household support. Your postpartum doula might hold the baby while you shower and then chat with you about your birth, or they might answer some of your breastfeeding questions while you feed the baby. As you nap with your baby, the postpartum doula might run to the market, swing by the post office for you, and then start cooking your dinner. You can awaken, feeling (at least a bit more) rested, clean, and calmer because the mail went out and dinner is well underway. Then maybe your tired partner will be home from work; your doula will leave and you can have dinner and enjoy some family time. All families deserve this kind of support from family, friend, and/or doula. Sadly, in my experience, most families go without.

The rewards that come from adequate support include reduced stress and workload on the whole family, plus more successful breastfeeding. These benefits are a great investment economically (formula is expensive, for example) and for the whole family's improved health. (Plus, the benefits of breastfeeding now include not having to worry about the formula shortages that have been plaguing the country since the Covid-19 pandemic.) I dream of a day when we have a healthcare system that includes both kinds of doula care available for all birthing families. Until that day, I urge you to research and then weigh your options carefully.

If you want to hire a birth and/or postpartum doula and you can't, fear not. There is an alternative! If you have a good friend or relative who is willing to commit the time to attend your birth and to learn about birth, then this person can often provide a high level of emotional support and continuity of care during birth or the postpartum period or both. Over my years of teaching Bradley® classes I have had several people bring a friend or relative along to class so their "novice doula" could prepare for their role in the upcoming birth. These people have all trained well and have been extremely successful at providing appropriate care. (Maybe reading this book can also help a novice doula gain skills and reduce fears?) One such woman recently called to thank me for that training, and then she shared that she had just made a life change: she was going to continue her training and become a professional doula! Birth is powerful. It can change the world, one person at a time.

Mary Beth, a Bradley® graduate, shares her daughter's birth story below and beautifully educates us on the ways her doula, Betsy, contributed to her birth. As you read her story, please look for the ways the doula directly reduced the birthing couple's workload and stress levels.

Betsy knew exactly what to do and where to go when we arrived at the hospital. Even though my husband and I had visited/toured the maternity ward and taken a waterbirth class, I certainly didn't think about the logistics of getting upstairs. Betsy got me a wheelchair and then had me kneel on it facing her as she pushed me down the hall to the elevator. My husband just left the car in front of the ER door—where it sat for hours I think before Betsy parked it in the garage for us.

We had brought the equipment required for waterbirth: a new hose and a skimmer bought at our local greenhouse and hardware supply. Betsy knew how to hook everything up to get the tub filled with water. When we arrived at the hospital, I was six centimeters dilated and completely effaced, but no one told me. I was glad not to know because I had learned in Bradley class that things could slow down or speed up at any time. It wouldn't do me any good to know the stats because the baby would come when she was ready.

As soon as I stepped foot in the tub, my entire body relaxed. The tub was big enough that I could float around with my legs limp. I stayed in the tub for quite a long time. Betsy or Greg [my partner] would give me sips of Recharge (an organic sports drink) periodically. I could easily shift positions due to the weightlessness of my body in the water. At some point I was shifting in a way that Betsy recognized was due to pressure on my rectum. I wasn't really conscious of this until she told me to go with the pressure. But I felt too hot in the tub and had to get out.

I tried different positions on the toilet and a birthing chair, leaning on Greg. I tried squatting, all fours. Finally, in the classic pushing position, I felt productive pulling tug-of-war with a sheet that Betsy had tied knots in at either end. But the baby still wasn't coming. The doctor came in to check on me again.

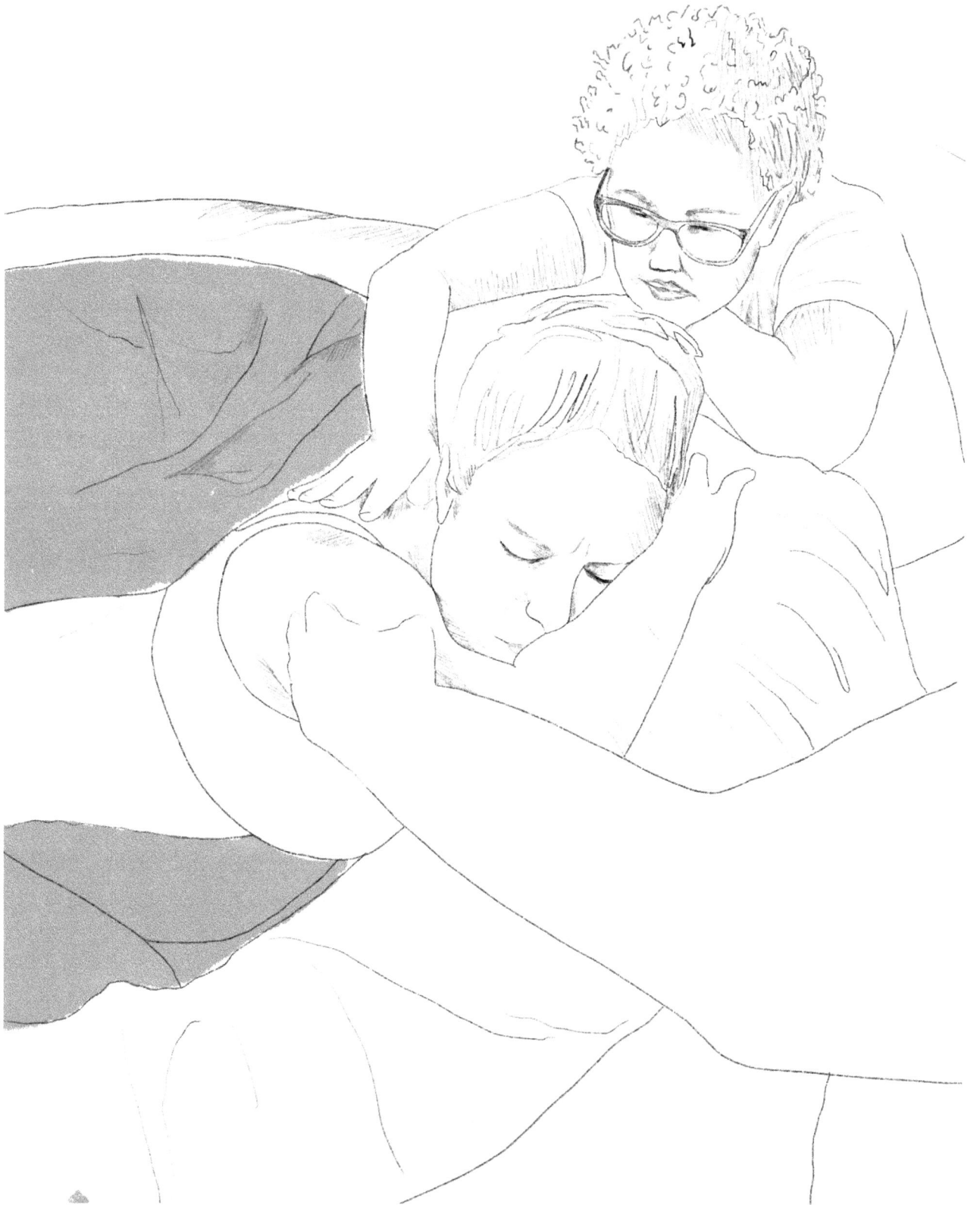

The contractions started to space out more. When it appeared that the baby needed some help, they gave me an oxygen mask over my mouth and nose. I could see the nurse wheel in some kind of liquid.

The conversation above me revealed that it was Pitocin. I ripped the oxygen mask off my face and said, "I don't want that." When the doctor suggested using vacuum suction to help the baby out, I asked him how much experience he had with that. While I don't remember the answer, Greg and I decided to go ahead and try the vacuum suction. The doctor attached the suction cup to the baby's head inside the birth canal [vagina]. This was more uncomfortable than anything up to this point. Betsy was encouraging me to keep pushing when the contractions came. I remember her saying, "Get mad." That's what pushed me harder. With the help of the vacuum suction to get the baby around my bone, I pushed the baby out after 4 hours [of pushing]. It was 8:53 PM. Greg cut the cord, the placenta passed without notice, and the doctor sewed up my episiotomy. I think the nurses weighed our new little girl before I held her. Because of Bradley class, we knew to request delay of a bath and eye ointment, which would have taken her away for a bit.

I held our little girl skin-to-skin. She migrated to one of my breasts and Betsy helped me to latch her on. I can't fully describe the feeling of holding this dark, curly-haired baby girl for the first time, but there was an immediate bond.[346]

Mary Beth's birth story illustrates the compassionate ways that doulas can work both before and during birth, as well as when complications occur. (Midwives have techniques that may have helped Mary Beth's baby find her way out without the suction. But when you have hired physicians, you rely on their techniques.) This mother felt supported in the choices she made and with the interventions that were used. The doula worked in concert with the partner, the obstetrician, and the nursing staff to create a team of support for the gestational parent and a welcoming environment for the new little babe.

For the sake of due diligence in your research, I encourage you, just as I encourage all of my clients, to investigate your local options for both birth and postpartum doula care. Again, if you are planning a hospital birth, the logistics of traveling in labor are vastly improved when you have the care of an attendant who travels with you. This care is invaluable to a single parent and allows a birthing couple to stay in their groove.

As you continue to plan out what your care will be like for the rest of your pregnancy and your birth, it is also wise to put real time into preparing for life after birth. This was the biggest transition I ever experienced and I have learned there is plenty that you can do to help smooth out the bumpy ride of adjusting to parenthood.

Postpartum planning

For starters: plan to write down your birth story, preferably in the first few days following your birth, when you likely won't feel like you have time or energy (because you won't!). But capturing these early memories and feelings can be very meaningful to you later on in life. It is easy to skip this wonderful gift to older you without a good plan.

Birthing your baby will be a profound experience, and yet as intense and important as it will be, it will only last a few hours or days. Once it is over, the baby will be here, and, spirits willing, stay with you for years and years to come. Pregnancy is, among other things, your job orientation for parenthood. So far in this book you have covered the basics of prenatal nutrition, exercise, relaxation skills, hiring your care providers, medical decision making, and getting through a well-supported birth. Now it is time to look ahead to your postpartum plans. What do you want your new family life to be like? Having some thought-out plans for this transition ahead of time can make a huge difference.

The first six weeks postpartum are a very unique time in your life. People all over the world have an array of different customs that help support the primary nurturer and the baby to bond and establish breastfeeding during this time. All gestational people also need to recover from the birth. Recovery takes time. A concept sometimes referred to as "cocooning" is desirable, when the primary nurturer and baby snuggle into a protected space—most commonly their home—free from the interruptions, responsibilities, news, and other stressors of the outside world. As you consider your postpartum plans please use six weeks as a loose time frame for your initial adjustment. Keep in mind, too, that you would be in good company if you get to six weeks and still feel unsettled. Many I have worked with, myself included, got to the six-week marker and thought, "What is different today? Everything still feels turned upside down." Nevertheless, as you are considering your postpartum plans realize that six weeks of special adjustment time is a reasonable goal.

How will you eat, get the dishes washed, have clean laundry, get to pediatrician appointments, have basic household chores done, and have emotional-social support in the weeks following your baby's arrival? Beyond your immediate postpartum adjustment, who will be the baby's primary caretaker? If you're in a relationship, is one of you more suited to care taking? Does one of you earn substantially more, have more job stability, or have more flexible hours? Are you planning on using daycare? Where? When? Do you know what it costs and how you might pay for it? Do you have older children? Can you enlist support to help with their care during your recovery and transition with the new baby? Do you have pets? Who will do pet care while you are tending to your new baby? These are some of the practical questions to consider. (Did you say yes to the idea of this pregnancy before actually thinking through all that it was going to mean to your life? I know I did!) Thinking about these questions (and more!) and their possible answers *before the baby arrives* can help you to make an easier transition to family life. Planning for your postpartum adjustment ahead of the birth of your baby leaves you free to focus on baby-care and self-care following the birth.

If you are feeling overwhelmed and some important information seems impossible to figure out, then take a deep breath and practice a conscientious breathing technique. Some focused relaxation can help you to think more clearly. When it comes to postpartum planning, start somewhere, anywhere, and give yourself positive encouragement along the way. Everything will work out—and what doesn't work out well can be changed. So much change is coming. Take a deep breath, and exhale slowly and fully.

It is important to understand that after your baby gets here it will be much more difficult to find the time and energy for self-care. Putting plans and practices in place now will help. So will acknowledging your thoughts and feelings. How do you feel right now when you remember that your baby is coming, and that she will be here to stay as your new constant companion and responsibility? You are likely feeling a range of emotions. Please describe briefly below how you feel at this moment. Jot down or draw some notes and say them out loud.

This is a big deal; you are having a baby! Your whole life is changing. Who you were before, and what you could get done in a day, is different than who you will be and what you will be able to accomplish in a postpartum day. It is no longer "business as usual." You will need to allow your priorities to shift. You will need time with your baby (which is time *not* doing other things) and you will need a lot of naps. If primary nurturer and baby are to make a healthy transition to family life, both should be nurtured and well supported by family and friends and/or a doula during this special time. The primary nurturer's goal should be to spend each and every postpartum day focused on baby and self-care, with a bit of extra energy squeezed out for any older children and partner (if you have one).

Again, you honor your transition to parenthood when you make plans for the details of life. The details are so important that it's worth repeating the questions over and again: What will be the food that you put in your mouth? Where will it come from? Who will prepare it? Who will wash the dish after you've eaten? Who will throw out the garbage? Wash the clothes? Fold the clothes? Buy the toilet paper? Etc. etc. etc. Good plans for basic care will help you to adjust and recuperate to your highest potential. Do you have freezer space? Can you cook and freeze some dinners? Can a friend or family member organize a meal train? Maybe ask your family for a meal subscription plan or a gift card for pizza delivery or the like in lieu of baby clothes and toys. (So many are compelled to buy the latter, but do you really need another cute baby outfit or soft toy? Perhaps not as much as you will need—and will welcome—a prepared dinner!)

By thinking through the daily chores needed for survival, you can start to evaluate where you need help and ways to receive support. The more support you can surround yourself with, the more time and energy you will have to tune into your baby and to yourself—and to each other together if you are coupled. The more you tune into your baby, the more joy you can find in parenting.

Learning the skills of planning for life's basic chores will also lay a foundation that will help you to live with less stress and improved health. For example, toddlers and teenagers alike will rely on you—their parent—to plan for nutritious meals, spaced out into even intervals throughout the day. Children thrive on the stability of good food, good sleep, good play and social interaction at regular intervals. Before I had my first child, it never really dawned on me that my new job as mother included 20 hours or more a week as Head Chef. I found that feeding my children well-balanced, home-cooked meals easily requires the workload of a second (or third, fourth, or fifth) part-time job.

With all of this in mind, I also want to encourage you to scale back your expectations of what you can get done during the first six weeks after birth. If you can seriously reduce your expectations as well as your actual workload, then you will emerge much stronger, more confident, and more cheerful when the time comes for you to resume additional work and responsibility. When primary nurturers can focus their energy on caring for their babies, napping, eating nutritious food, getting fresh air, and receiving emotional support, then the family starts off on their parenting journey with more solid ground underfoot and more joy in the heart.

I have seen many new parents who, by their own expectations, try to do too much too soon. They usually find themselves weepy, exhausted, and unhappy, with confidence lacking. Many new parents who have managed to make good plans for the first six weeks of cocooning, who really did reduce their postpartum responsibilities, have described to me that they *still* found themselves feeling tired, weepy and overwhelmed. Just imagine what those who try to steamroll through are up against. You truly can reduce postpartum stress with some planning.

Caring for a newborn is an emotionally consuming and physically demanding job. This cannot be repeated enough. Nurturing babies takes real time and energy. Babies need love and connection. Their neurological development is directly dependent on positive social interactions.[347] They need to be held, comforted, protected, and amused (don't we all?). And they need to sleep and eat and be cleaned. Plus, if you are going to breastfeed you will need extra energy, not just for baby-care, but for all of your increased metabolic work; your body has to make all that milk. When your baby arrives, you will find yourself nursing, nursing, nursing, and nursing some more. If you are bottle feeding, then you will have even more work to do with washing bottles and nipples, buying formula, testing temperatures, measuring mixes, etc. New parents must kick into survival mode.

Keep in mind: a postpartum breastfeeding parent is not a slacker! Realistically, you need to be able to cross things off your own to-do list and still be sure to get them done. Someone else (or, better yet, several other people) should help. Where can this extended support system provide you real relief? Ideally, this extra support comes from people other than your primary partner. They will certainly be working extra already, and they also need time to nap and snuggle with baby. If this is daunting to think about, take a deep breath, close your eyes, and look for your courage. Use your time now to plan for this wild transition.

To help you to visualize your plan, here's a glimpse into the future of a postpartum day—a day that is so full that you can absolutely not accomplish even one more thing:

- You will feed your baby. A newborn will feed every 2-3 hours, on average. When babies go through growth spurts then they can feed every hour or two. An average feeding can take 45 minutes or longer.

- You will change your baby's diapers. Babies should make at least 6 to 8 wet diapers in 24 hours and at least one poop diaper a day (but most infants poop more than that).

- You will need to change your baby's clothes at least once a day. Messy diaper explosions are common, regardless of diapering methods.

- You will need/want to coo, stare at, talk to, and otherwise interact with your baby. This takes time and energy. Nurturing is vital for human neuro development.[348]

- You will periodically need to clean your baby. You will initially give your baby sponge baths and then progress to full water baths once the cord stump dries up and falls off.

- You yourself will want/need to eat three good meals and maybe a couple of snacks per day. (Many breastfeeding parents describe being ravenous during breastfeeding.)

- You will need/want to drink plenty of water and other nourishing fluids, like juices and non-caffeinated teas. The output of fluid from breastfeeding demands attention to your hydration levels.

- You will need time to urinate and defecate. (Basic, I know, but these things take time. This is what I am talking about here: *survival mode*.)

- You will want to take a daily shower. Showering daily during the post-partum period is helpful because the birth parent may be funky from a lot of sweat as they excrete extra fluids leftover from pregnancy. Additionally, the shower is a great place to relax and/or cry. You can let the tears and the stress run down the drain. The water can soothe all your senses. And hopefully the shower coincides with a few moments of precious "off duty" time. The shower is also a good place to express some breast milk by hand, if you're feeling engorged when your milk first comes in. (If you don't have another helper to watch baby while you shower, consider placing baby in an infant carrier or even on a towel or blanket on the bathroom floor. It can calm you both to know you are in close proximity and ear shot, even if you can't physically tend to them in the next moment they want/need your attention.)

- When you get out of your shower you'll want/need to put on some clean pajamas or clothes.

- You must brush your teeth twice daily and floss once daily. (New parents and everyone else too!) Dental hygiene is crucial to good health. (And you will want to instill good habits; future dental bills—yours or your children's—are not what you want to look forward to. Children will do what you *do* more than what you say!)

○ The day should also include at least one nap (maybe after lunch) and ideally many naps throughout each day (maybe nap after breakfast and after dinner, too). Your sleep cycles will be knocked out of whack from adjusting to the needs of your newborn. The best rule of thumb is to sleep when your baby sleeps. This not only supports your physical and mental health; it helps if you are physically near each other during sleep so that the sleep cycles of you and your baby can regulate. If you can sleep when the baby sleeps, which takes discipline, you might get through this transition to family life without being continuously exhausted. Plus, you and your baby will be well on the way to a healthy sleep relationship. If I didn't nap during the day, during both of my postpartum periods, I was in tears by 4:00pm. This is not uncommon, so it is likely you will be, too.

○ You will also want/need to do some daily pelvic floor exercises, a few abdominal bracing exercises (review Week 3), and have a bit of fresh air and some gentle stretching, especially of the arms and upper torso. After the first few weeks, a short and easy walk outside will do wonders for your state of mind and it will help your body to return to your new normal.

And that is that. Those are my expectations—from personal and professional experience—for a very full post-partum day. Basic baby- and self-care will easily take up the entire day's efforts. In fact, I periodically get phone calls from teary new moms who ask me when they are actually supposed to find the time to floss, shower, or write down their birth story. Self-care is a huge challenge once the baby is born and yet, if you don't take care of yourself, there won't be much left of you to care for your family. The emotional recuperation embedded in self-care is essential to a primary nurturer's mental health. If a new parent is feeling down and overwhelmed, the solution often lies in helping them to get time for self-care for body, mind, and soul.

Please take note of what is *not* on a primary nurturer's list, given what was absent from the above example: No food shopping, cooking, or dish washing. No laundry, vacuuming, or pet care. No other household chores or errands. No email, texting, or social media. No sending out thank you notes for all the cute baby gifts. Plan to do nothing but the essentials. And take heart, because at the end of your postpartum period you will feel well-bonded to your baby, capable in your nurturing skills, and empowered to resume (most, if not all) of your prior responsibilities.

Now and throughout the rest of your pregnancy please check in with yourself using the following questions:

Will it be difficult for me to find or accept help from friends and family? If yes, how can I work through this?

Am I planning to breastfeed? Do I have any concerns about breastfeeding? How do my closest emotional support persons feel about breastfeeding?

Repeatedly asking yourself these questions can help you to create your postpartum plans as well as to help you identify challenges that you can begin working through now.

Time off from work is essential for postpartum adjustment. How much time off from work are you able/planning to take? If you are working in a professional role, are you planning to work right up until you go into labor? (It is best to remind your employers of the hard-to-plan nature of birth.) Most pregnant people I meet want to save up as much time as possible for after the birth, which is understandable. I want you to have that time with your baby, too. It saddens me that we don't honor new parents with more time for parenting. So again, what kind of time off from your professional life is possible? Check in with your employer and your partner. What, if any benefits are offered? Can you stack some of these benefits to create additional time, such as paid maternity leave (+ paid paternity leave?) + paid family leave + any paid sick days and/or vacation days and/or personal days you have accrued? Write down the information you gather below, simply to have it recorded somewhere for reference.

It is tricky to think about how much time will be needed for birth and immediately following birth. Most of us think that if the primary partner has one week off it will be one day for the birth and then 6 days off afterwards. That is what happens on TV; not so in real life. It is especially important to understand that a straightforward, healthy, natural birth process can easily chew up a week. Many people get little bits of labor work done over several days at the start of birth. Reading these signals and being responsive to the body's need for work and rest should be your priority. Many pregnant people find that they really need rest and support in the days leading up to birth. And, from my own observations, people clearly reap great benefits from taking time for self-care prior to birth. Remaining responsive to your feelings is paramount.

When thinking about your plans for the end of your pregnancy, it is imperative that you recognize the state of your own health. The signals your body sends you are more important than your ideas about how it is all "supposed" to go. If you were to develop a medical complication, for example, and your care providers were to prescribe bed rest, you would stop work immediately. If that can happen in such a dire situation, shouldn't it also be able to happen if it might *prevent* a dire situation? By reading this book and working through its lessons, doing the homework and practicing the offered exercises, you are already taking important steps to care for yourself and your baby, so why not continue this care in all possible ways? If you are too stressed and too tired at the end of your pregnancy or too distracted to focus on work or not feeling good for any reason—perhaps because you are trying to live a "business as usual" lifestyle—then your body may be giving you clear signals that you're doing too much. You may need to allow yourself to switch gears.

One of the single most important things you can do for the health of your baby and your birth process is to show up at your birth well-rested. Not only is it helpful to go into birth feeling good, learning to slow down before the baby arrives will help to ease you into parenthood. Having a bit of time before the baby arrives to really listen to and then yield to your own desires (e.g., do I want to take nap now or after my bath?) can make it much easier to put your baby's needs first when she arrives.

Lower your expectations for housework

What are your basic standards of housework, and can you relax them during your postpartum adjustment? For example, are there cleaning chores that can be reduced or modified for the first several months? What are your expectations about how clean and orderly your living space needs to be?

Each of us has different priorities for housework. There are some life chores we care more about than others. I have met a lot of people who have very specific ideas about how they want their laundry done, or they have needs for specific chores to *always* be kept up. What are your preferences for housework? Are there certain tasks that, if left undone, would drive you crazy and inhibit your ability to rest and to focus on your baby? Are there household needs that if they are not done, regardless of how you are feeling, you will get up and do them yourself? For myself, I don't care if I have a sink full of dirty dishes. (I have been known to leave them for days, eewww!). However, if the counters are messy when I walk into my kitchen, I get antsy and even a little stressed. I feel like this kitchen *has* to be cleaned! Yet I can easily imagine that, for someone else, the dishes in the sink would be the problem and they might care a lot less about the counter tops.

Figure out what you want/need done, prioritize your chores, and then go about planning for support. Maybe, if you feel like the vacuum cleaner must be run on a frequent schedule, you can enlist the help of a loved one or friend for that chore. (Think: six weeks of support = how many runs of a vacuum cleaner for you?) If there are certain quirks to the way you want a task done, why not have a planning party? Gather your support team together for a breakfast or a tea and go over any information that will help your team help you. It takes a village, after all.

Postpartum visitors

If you have family or friends coming from out of town for the birth or postpartum period, how does that feel? What are their expectations about how that time will be used? Are they expecting you to prepare food for them or to provide entertainment? What will their needs be? Will they want or expect to provide baby care? Take a moment to write or draw your immediate thoughts here.

New parents thrive on all kinds of support—except baby care. A new primary nurturer needs/wants to focus on the baby. It is everything else with which they need help. Do your family/friends have strong beliefs about the "best" way to care for your baby? They probably do have strong feelings; do you know what those feelings are? Will these people build your confidence or cause you to question your instincts?

My own mother, who is very supportive of breastfeeding, raised me with the information that mothers should breastfeed, that it is normal, and that it is incredibly satisfying for mother and baby. But even she once said to me, "Gee, you look so tired, do you want me to give the baby a bottle while you take a nap." This seemingly kind question left me wondering if she was correct. Was I wrong to commit to exclusive breastfeeding? What was I supposed to do? I was tired, which left me vulnerable to insecurity. This questioning caused even more exhaustion than the seemingly constant nursing and attention my baby required.

You'll want to focus your social time on the people that will be the most helpful and the most understanding. Evaluate your friends and family for their opinions on breastfeeding, for example. You'll want to surround yourself with people who won't undermine your confidence in your parenting choices. Remember that you will be learning to breastfeed; most of us don't learn at our best when we are being watched. This can be especially problematic if you have friends or family members watching and judging because they do not value breastfeeding and can't understand your decisions. This scenario is even more challenging when you and your baby must work hard at learning. When you have visitors there watching you, or distracting you from this work, it can easily exacerbate any exhaustion and stress already present.

As important as social support is, too many visitors and too much social time can also become a source of stress. You will likely feel super joyous and proud of your new baby and be genuinely happy and excited to show her off, but it is important to keep visits short. 15 minutes can be a long visit! Loved ones who come in bearing dinner, stop by your kitchen to wash a few dishes, and maybe pose for a few photos before they leave, are the kind of folks you'll want in the earliest weeks of your baby's life.

Learning to breastfeed requires a lot of breast exposure, too. It won't always require this, and you will likely be able to nurse quite discreetly, but initially full exposure is just easier. Ask yourself: if someone is watching you, are you really comfortable with them seeing your breasts? Are you comfortable with them seeing your attempts—possibly clumsy attempts—at breast feeding? It may become self-preserving to excuse yourself into a quiet bedroom for feedings. Will this create hard feelings with the visitors who just drove three hours to see you?

Who are the people in your life that you can anticipate wanting to come and visit? Do you have people who will want to come, but whenever they arrive they will let you know that they would "love a cup of coffee with cream and sugar, please?" If those people exist in your life (i.e., the ones that create more work than help), then think now about how you will handle them in your postpartum period. One of the tips in the Bradley® workbook suggests that you keep your bathrobe on and stay in bed when guests arrive. Even if you have been up with clothes on, when the doorbell rings, put your robe on and get in bed. Your guests will not stay as long if their expectations have been reduced around their visit. If you anticipate difficult family members or friends, strategize with your partner or a trusted friend; ask for help from someone who can act as a buffer. Talk, in advance of the birth, with your loved ones about what you are learning and preparing for. Be grateful for their love and connection to your baby, but also be clear about your boundaries. Once again, plan now for the rest and support that you feel will best help you through all your new adjustments. And be compassionate with yourself if/when your plans change.

It is always ok to blame the room emptying or house clearing on me. Blame it on this book and what you are learning from it: "My birth educator says I need to be in a quiet room when I am learning to nurse." If you don't want to use me as an excuse, and you still need one, blame your pediatrician or your midwife. Any perceived teacher or other type of authority figure will do!

I recently had a client ask, "What if the partner is the cause of all the company?" She is married to a person with a lot of local family, most of whom were expecting to descend upon the new family as soon as baby arrived. And she was worried about offending her partner's family. My answer, which you can adapt to your own needs, goes something like this:

> First, this is why we are talking about it now, before your birth. Our goal is to educate ourselves ahead of time so we can make plans, communicate effectively, and hopefully reduce conflicts later on. Let your family know that you are grateful for their support. Let them feel your love and gratitude. And then give your family a chance to understand what your needs and goals are for after the baby comes. Second, please try to appreciate and understand how awesome it is to have a huge family that wants to envelope you in love. It may ultimately feel fantastic to have everyone there loving you up, but when it's enough, it's enough. Talking about it now is a way to avoid hurt feelings later.

I want you to think about your parenting choices and how you are going to make your decisions. Are you going to feel secure enough to make mistakes as you fumble through, or will you feel in the shadow of the people around you who are there to "help?" Be honest with yourself. Evaluate the dynamics of the relationships you share with those who will be around you. Try to articulate your feelings about this in advance. Take "Aunt Martha" as a hypothetical example: she loves you and she wants to help. But sometimes she looks at you in disbelief when you state your preferences. Does this cause you to question your preferences? Did she breastfeed? Will she ultimately support your decisions? Or will she or somebody else subtly (or not so subtly) undermine your decisions and your confidence? Do you have positive role models? Are there people in your life that you can look up to for helpful information and genuine support? If you can identify them, name them out loud. If there are problems or communication struggles with friends or family now or on the horizon, try to engage in clear and kind boundary setting ahead of the birth.

Use this space below to help you identify any anticipated social stressors and to strategize possible coping methods.

Childcare plans

Try to put childcare plans in place during pregnancy so that you can use any maternity leave time you are taking for bonding and recovery. It really complicates the postpartum period if you need to use that time to figure out what comes next. At the same time, always keep in mind that any plans you make can be changed. If what you planned doesn't seem to be working, definitely take the time to figure out a new path. You can work to change whatever you need to whenever you need to. Ultimately, maternity leave is for you and baby to be together, however that can occur.

Picking a pediatrician

Ask everyone you know for references and be sure to inquire as to why someone is recommending a particular practice. Breastfeeding support groups are wonderful places to pick up resources. (In next week's lesson I recommend getting yourself to a breastfeeding support group while still pregnant.) Doula's can also be useful to identify supportive providers. I like to meet pediatricians who think of their job with new parents as being largely educational; their role is to guide and mentor new parents as they learn to care for their baby. With all this in mind, here are some questions to consider as you investigate and interview your options, before ultimately making your choice:

- Does this pediatrician have admitting privileges at the hospital you are planning to birth at? Or, is this pediatrician supportive of your decision to birth at home? When would they want you to come in for a newborn exam? If you're planning a hospital birth and your pediatrician does not have privileges at the hospital you birth at, then your baby will be cared for until discharged by a hospital staff pediatrician.

- Does this provider truly believe in and support breastfeeding? Do they offer breastfeeding support or education services? (Review Week 4 for information on interviewing providers.)

- Does this provider have special examination rooms for well babies? Some doctors will see well babies first thing in the morning, before regular visiting hours, in order to reduce the chance that your healthy baby picks up a bug while in the waiting room or exam room. Some providers have separate exam rooms for contagious kids and healthy kids, while some offices mix them all together.

- Who will you get on the phone when you call at 3:00am? (You will certainly have some late-night phone calls over the first few years.)

- Is this provider respectful of you?

As with any care provider, if you discover that the fit is not a good one after you have been working with them, it is wise to do the work to find someone new, if this is an option for you. Of course, this can be emotionally taxing, so again doing the homework upfront can help to alleviate work later on. With the baby coming there is always going to be so much work for later on. So do what you can now, right?

Pet care

From the moment you go into labor you'll want/need to be able to forget about your animals for a while. If you are walking out your door to go to the hospital, you have no idea when you will realistically be home. If you are having a home birth you will not want to be distracted by your animals' care needs or their reactions to your birthing energy. (Of course, some people find comfort during labor from the presence of their pets. So please take this into consideration, too.) If you end up needing to have a surgical birth, it will be at least three to five days at the hospital after the surgery. Who will be caring for your pets during this time? It should not be the primary partner, if at all possible. Your primary partner will want to be available to be with you and baby as much as possible. Can you arrange for your surrogate pet care folks to come to your home prior to your labor, in order to learn about how to care for your animals? Where is the food kept, how much do they get, and how often? Are they used to going for walks? Or having concentrated play time? If so when, how many/much, and for how far/long? Are there any medications that need to be given? As I've mentioned, it is also good to speak with a veterinarian or other related professional about helping your pets to acclimate to your new baby. The baby's safety should be urgently considered in a home with animals. Finding someone to help care for your pets during the birth and the first six weeks postpartum can bring great peace of mind. Is there someone to ask?

Reciprocity

As you start to digest your own postpartum needs, think too about ways that you can support the families currently around you. Do you know anyone with young children that you can help now? Reach out; reciprocity is a key factor in having good social support.

Maybe you can help with childcare or pet care? Or maybe, as another example among many more, you can pay it forward by organizing a dinner tree or meal train for another pregnant person in your community. Seek out a few people in their life who are willing to bring them a dinner after they give birth, during their postpartum period. Then make a list and a schedule and distribute it to the friends—and include any dietary concerns. Once the baby is born the new parent will call you to announce the baby's birth and to let you know when they would like their first meal. Thus begins the dinner tree. Once you bring their first meal, the next person on the list brings the second, then the third, etc. This can work automatically, as a preset schedule (there are apps for this!), or you can organize it as a phone tree, with each person on the list calling the next person on the list. You can organize the meals to arrive every day, every other day, once a week... whatever seems best based on your volunteers and the family's needs.

Expectations for meeting your baby

Oh my gosh! Your baby is really coming! What on earth is this going to be like?

What will this crazy new experience be like? Write your expectations below and then discuss them with yourself, your support partner, family, and friends. In other words, please examine your expectations for meeting your baby.

Meeting your baby

Wow. You did it! The baby is out. The pregnancy is over. Birth is over. Take a breath.

—Take a big, deep, world-changing breath—

Now it's time to recover. Drink some juice. (Orange juice is a Bradley Method® suggestion for a first fluid after birth.) The only need the birthing person and baby really have at this point is to be cared for as one. Their needs as a unit are to maximize skin-to-skin contact, be kept warm, chatted with, and observed. The birthing person needs to be closely watched for blood loss and uterine tone, as explained in Week 10.

While meeting your baby, let her hear your voice, look at her, and let her see your face. Touch, massage, and smell your baby, too. Your stimulation through voice and touch helps your baby to make her transition from your womb to your arms. Be compassionate with yourself when you first meet your baby (and thereafter, too). Try to accept however you feel as reasonable. Who can know what it will really be like until you're there?

I believe that you'll feel tremendous relief; the birth is over. The baby is out of your body! Then, at some point your focus will shift. The reality of the baby and her circumstances will impact your next set of emotions. You may feel euphoric and wild wonderment, mushy love, or perplexed—where did this baby come from? You may feel nervous and unsure or exhausted, self-occupied, and not quite ready to drink in your baby's arrival. You can't know the future. None of what you feel in this moment is the end-all of who you will grow into as a parent. My advice is: try to accept your feelings for what they are, your feelings *in the moment*. Later you will have other feelings, and you'll have still more after that. If we judge ourselves harshly when our feelings don't live up to our expectations, these judgments can create emotional hurdles that need to be overcome before we can move onto the next phase of feelings. What if you feel nervous or uneasy when you meet your baby, and then the next thought you have is "why didn't I feel overcome with love"? Does that mean you're not a good parent? No. All this questioning and judgment creates extra stuff for you to work through. By contrast, if you can look for acceptance of your feelings, if you can think, "this is so weird, I thought I would feel x, y or z," then you can follow up with, "and I guess that's okay for now." That response demonstrates compassion and acceptance and makes way for an open mind about what comes next. If you should face tough feelings, you can look for hope in knowing everything changes—likely with something good down the path.

You, your baby, and your providers will make initial evaluations of your baby's well-being and yours. Your judgements will be based on intuition and common sense. Your providers will use observation and rely on a tool called the "Apgar Test" to make their initial newborn assessment. The Apgar Test measures five attributes of newborn health:[349]

- ○ Respiratory effort
- ○ Heart rate
- ○ Muscle tone
- ○ Reflexes/grimace response
- ○ Skin color

Each attribute will be given an independent score of 0, 1, or 2, depending on what your provider observes. A total score of 7 or above means the baby seems healthy and doesn't need any medical support. A total score of 6 or under means the baby has need for medical care. Newborn needs can range from precautionary, supplemental oxygen (easily handled bedside) to large amounts of intervention provided in a neonatal intensive care unit (NICU). Babies almost never score a perfect 10 on the Apgar Test because, if nothing else, some blue color in the hands and feet is typically present.

The Apgar Test can be performed while your baby hangs out on your body. It is done at one minute postpartum, and again at five minutes postpartum. Think of the Apgar Test in the following way: the one-minute test gives some idea of how the baby tolerated the birth process and the five-minute score evaluates how well the baby is adjusting to life outside the womb.

Newborn characteristics

(note: see Addendum meconium 2 page 498)

Healthy newborn babies can be pretty weird looking.[350] Reality is vastly different than the advertised images of new babies that many of us have in mind. The following are all considered normal characteristics:

○ Cyanotic hands and feet. (Cyanotic means bluish in color, due to reduced circulation.)

○ Sometimes the head can seem quite dark purple(ish), but baby's color should even out quickly. If a baby's color is significantly off, supplemental oxygen may be appropriate.

○ Crossed eyes. These can be quite disconcerting to parents, but the muscles usually strengthen over time and the eyes straighten out. Dr. Sears says, "Don't panic if your infant's eyes appear to be crossed. It's normal for babies' eyes to be crossed in the early months of life and straighten out by the end of the first year."[351]

○ Swollen Genitals. This, too, is normal, and sometimes pretty funny. Enlarged genitals are a result of substantial amounts of hormones passed from gestational parent to baby. This will regulate over time.

○ Lanugo. This is baby fur or peach fuzz. Newborns can have "fur" (actually a type of hair) in lots of strange places on their bodies, such as the rim of the ears or the low back or arms. Again, this is normal and falls out over time.

○ Vernix caseosa. This is nature's protective skin cream, which covers baby in a creamy white substance made from the lipids protecting your baby's skin in the uterus. Lipids are fatty acids and non-water soluble, so they don't wash off in the amniotic fluid. Some babies have a lot of vernix still on them at birth; for others, it has already worn off. Vernix is good for their skin, so any that remains after birth can be rubbed in or ignored. It doesn't need to be washed off with soap. There are special antimicrobial qualities in the vernix that have helped the baby to fight off any potential bad bugs while inside the uterus or on the way out into the world.[352] In fact, lanugo and vernix work together:

> Lanugo plays an important role in binding the vernix caseosa to the skin of fetuses. Vernix caseosa is the viscous white covering on newborns that protects their skin, prevents water loss, plays an important role in thermoregulation, and contributes to innate immunity. It protects the fetus from damaging substances found in amniotic fluid, most notably urea and electrolytes.[353]

○ Milia. These are baby acne-like bumps on the face, commonly found across the bridge of the nose and on the cheeks. Please do not pick at them, just cleanse the baby normally and ignore. These, too, will go away in good time.

○ Fontanels. Your baby's head will have two "soft spots" where the bones of the skull have not yet fused together. This is a great evolutionary development, as it allows for the baby's skull plates to shift and mold during her decent through the vagina. Then, during the early days outside, the head regains its round shape and over time the skull plates will fuse. These fontanels will stay soft for months. They are called "soft spots," but they are not really that soft. It is ok to touch them. It is actually a good idea to touch the fontanels, gently of course, and get a feel for what seems normal. Knowing what they feel like normally can help you to determine whether or not your baby has any serious dehydration issues later on, should that question arise. Dehydration concerns are usually associated with illness or breastfeeding concerns. When a baby is dehydrated, the fontanels can start to become quite sunken.[354] This would be a clear indication that your baby needs medical attention.

As you continue to ponder what meeting your baby will be like and how you will tend to the details of your life postpartum, it's helpful to understand that many (most?) people encounter huge emotional upheaval during the transition to family life. Here again some advance processing can be protective.

Emotionally adjusting to your new role as parent

We hold stress in our bodies, which we then communicate to our babies. If your baby is picking up a lot of stress from you, then she may work it out by being fussy. This fussiness can in turn be disconcerting to you, which can cause more stress. This can be a tough cycle to break. We do best when we can look for healthy ways to utilize and release our negative stress.

Having a new baby is stressful no matter how happy (or not) you are about it. How will you perceive the stresses of having a baby? Stress can be positive or negative, depending on how you feel about it.[355] It's beneficial for coping later on to examine now what kinds of things create negative stress for you, not necessarily connected to your pregnancy process (but certainly including it). Please write examples of stressors with negative impacts down here.

Can you identify stressors that have positive outcomes?

What kinds of stressors can you anticipate once your baby arrives?

The adjustment to becoming a new parent is as big as an adjustment can get. It is therefore potentially as stressful as an adjustment can get, too. All of your primary relationships change and shift when a new baby enters the home. Add to this any potential challenges brought on by your post pregnancy body, as well as the inevitability of interrupted sleep, and this all creates a lot of new terrain to navigate. Babies are happy blessings, and yet happy things can cause stress, too.

It is important to acknowledge that the stress associated with this transition in your life is in no way a barometer for how much you love your baby or if you are a good parent or any such judgments. Stress acknowledges the reality of this huge change and marks the arrival of critical new responsibilities—likely more responsibility than you have ever felt or participated in before. The weight of this responsibility can be fatiguing in and of itself, not to mention the adjustment to disrupted sleep patterns. We need to sigh and cry, and to encourage ourselves to let some of the stress go. Mindful breathing, relaxation exercises, a shower, and a nap can all really help. A gentle walk outside can feel restorative, too.

Asking your loved ones for support remains a vital resource for help, even if this help is in the form of becoming a sounding board for your venting. A lot of new parents are afraid to express what is a fairly normal, occasional and generally temporary feeling of, "I feel miserable right now. What was I thinking? How could I have been so stupid as to think having a baby was a good idea? My whole life is over!" Parenting is such a big adjustment. These unhappy feelings (or some variation of them) are difficult to feel and may be very threatening for a partner to hear, especially if the partner is feeling responsible or is being somehow blamed. A weepy mom once shared the following with me:

> Before we had our baby, we [my partner and I] loved doing things together and being together. It seemed like the idea of having a baby was something that we would do together. But now that the baby is here, I am taking care of the baby and he has gone back to work, and it doesn't feel like we are doing it together.

The need to express these big feelings is palpable. Yet it's also understandable that a primary partner might feel too overwhelmed themselves to be a good listener for expressions of frustration such as these without becoming defensive or judgmental. Who will you be able to vent to? Realizing that we have a variety of social support needs that are best fulfilled by different people will be useful preparation, especially for the toughest days. Can you identify any specific friends or relatives that you can count on? Consider taking some notes here on who you can reach out to and what kind of support you can anticipate receiving from each special person.

While primary nurturers need their partners' support, they also really grow with the support of other primary nurturers. Your partners are working hard at adjusting, too. They have their own adjustment issues and challenges to cope with. Therefore, just as you should work to maintain a high level of intimacy with your partner, and to support each other's emotional needs, you should seek out other parents, as they can often help you to process or simply witness your negative or trying feelings. As primary nurturers, our perspectives are unique and experiential. Consequently, we can perhaps best learn nurturer-coping skills from other nurturers. Moreover, wouldn't it be wonderful if partners or other caregivers had the opportunity to connect with other partners or caregivers? Of course it would. I suggest, therefore, that whichever type of caregiver your partner may be, they try to set something up in advance of your birth that provides them a connection with people of the same experience.

Talking with other new parents can enable you to put things into perspective. Talking with more experienced parents can illuminate solutions to parenting challenges. Social connections will simultaneously combat the isolation that contributes to familial stress levels and help you to learn more deeply about this new responsibility. In other words, social support is its own kind of anti-stress medication. This is why I strongly recommend that, in addition to reading and working through this book, you also investigate taking an in-person birth class. This will provide another opportunity to make new connections and friendships with folks going through the same transformations. The stress is coming, along with some of the highest love-filled highs imaginable. Having a clue as to how you will cope with it all will help you through the rough spots.

Adjustment difficulties: Postpartum Depression, Anxiety, Post-Traumatic Stress Disorder (PTSD), and Postpartum Psychosis

Every new primary nurturer I have ever spoken to in the U.S. has had periods of weepy sadness, bouts of depression and anxious times. But for some people their chemistry is even more off balance and feelings can become quite magnified and distorted, and genuine mental illness can ensue. If you have suffered with mental health issues prior to pregnancy, then you will want to be extra vigilant. People who suffer with depression before pregnancy have a higher incidence of depression post baby.[356] If you have a history of mental illness, then it's helpful to alert your closest support people to be particularly mindful and attentive during the first year following your birth.

Typically, when we think of depression, it is common to think of it manifesting itself as someone who does not want to get out of bed, neglects social interactions, and exhibits sadness and lethargy.[357] For people who have just given birth, many adjustment disorders get lumped into the term "postpartum depression." Postpartum depression can certainly present with the above attributes, but you should also be on the lookout for increased anxiety, recurring intrusive thoughts (particularly any recurring thoughts or feelings of despondency, panic, fear of the baby, or fear of harming the baby,) and/or a lack of emotional connection to the baby. In practice there are a wide variety of symptoms to be alert for.[358] Sometimes adjustment disorders take on the form of anxiety. People who have reported being overly anxious have expressed fears about being alone with the baby, afraid they may hurt the baby, afraid of the baby, afraid of an intruder, or any number of other fears that can surface. Some people report symptoms that are more closely aligned with post-traumatic stress disorder (PTSD).[359] PTSD symptoms are more common when people have experienced trauma during their birth.[360] PTSD symptoms can include frequent nightmares, intrusive and disruptive thoughts, and flashbacks to the offending moments of the birth. And for a rare few their births can lead to experiences of psychosis, including delusions, hallucinations, and disorganized thinking.[361]

Unfortunately, mental illness still carries with it a negative stigma, which often prevents people from speaking up about their challenges. Mental health disease is not a weakness of character, it's not a moral failing, and it doesn't come from poor parenting or low IQ. Our mental health is an expression of our physical health. Blaming someone for mental health issues is like blaming someone for getting cancer. The only thing scarier than the way mental illness feels is not getting proper care. Adjustment disorders impact the health of the whole family, in fact the whole community. I believe it is incumbent upon all of us to speak up and help break the stigmas that prevent people from seeking care. If something seems off to you, about your feelings and your thinking, speak up and get the help you deserve.

Postpartum mental health issues are treatable and can often resolve with timely intervention. Treatments can include talk therapies, support groups, medications, exercise, diet changes, and getting more logistical support in the home. If the primary nurturer is unable to care for themself and/or the baby, or if the partner or a close family member or friend express concern about the primary nurturer's mental health, or if something just seems unusually off, then professional evaluation should be sought—without hesitation. Timely professional help may be lifesaving.

After my second child was born, I suffered with some postpartum anxiety. The day that I knew something was truly wrong was when Arlo was about one month old. Jasper, my older child, was six years old. One morning Julian came into the room to say goodbye; he was on his way to work. I was seated and nursing the baby. I experienced a wave of panic and asked with near hysteria, "How am I going to give everyone lunch? How can I get through this? What will we eat for lunch?!" Now, let's reflect for a moment: the baby is entirely breastfed and nursing was going well; Jasper could have easily made himself a peanut butter sandwich or grabbed a bowl of cereal; and he could even have prepared something for me to eat. So what was really going on? How could I be so terrified of lunch and of being left alone? Lunch was my excuse. What I was actually freaked out about was being left alone again with both the children. We were all adjusting to Julian's recent return to work. I was using lunch unconsciously as a fixation point. I was genuinely afraid and perplexed by how this was supposed to be ok. I couldn't understand how this was really going to work out all right for us. I was suffering under a tremendous amount of anxiety, which seemed to swell up out of thin air. Julian looked at me with much concern and disbelief. By his response, and the hugeness of my feelings, I knew something was off. I could tell that my fears didn't seem logical, and yet that didn't help to diffuse them. He knew for sure, and I was kind of sure, that I needed some help. I needed concrete, professional support or I might crack—whatever that meant. Thankfully I had the resources available to get help when I recognized these early symptoms.

Your first step toward being able to access resources for help is being aware that postpartum adjustment disorders are common, treatable, and *not your fault*. Please let the heavy stuff go. You're doing your homework *right now*. You're doing the hard work before the hard work! So keep at it. I recommend that you search for some postpartum counseling support during pregnancy, as an additional way to prepare. Remember, identifying your resources now and then not needing them is better than needing resources you haven't yet identified. Just like the information on loss from Week 13, this information and the resources you locate can be filed away in the deep crevices of your brain and written down in an accessible location. Trust that the information will be there should you need it.

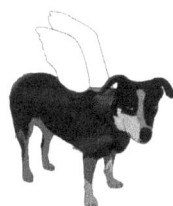

EXERCISE: DR. ANDREW WEIL'S "4,7,8" BREATHING PRACTICE[362]

Read this exercise through one time and then try it.

- ○ Breathe in for a count of 4.

- ○ Hold your breath for a count of 7.

- ○ Exhale for a count of 8.

- ○ Repeat 1 to 4 times in a row.

When Dr. Weil teaches this technique, he explains that the yogi he learned it from told him not to do it more than four times in a row. In my personal practice, as well as in the classes through which I lead my clients, we practice this exercise two or three times in a row. Immediately after the last exhale of the last sequence of 4,7,8 allow your breath to resume your regular pattern. Notice how the breath goes in and how it goes out. Keep your attention on your natural, comfortable breathing pattern for a few more breaths. Try to articulate something that you noticed as a result of this exercise. Then allow your attention to shift.

—Pause now to try this exercise—

How was that? Please continue to practice the 4,7,8 exercise in the coming week. Make it your own, as this will, in turn, make it more available to you during birth and in other times of stress.

Hello Baby!

We've been doing a lot of thinking around the logistics of postpartum planning. Before I close this chapter, I want to include some of the fun stuff, too. I think it is enchanting to think about who this new person—your baby—will be. What characteristics will they inherit and/or learn from you and the people who love them so much? We do pass down a part of ourselves when we raise a child, regardless of genetic connections. A child will "inherit" or learn about their sense of self and many other important personality traits from a biological as much as a non-biological parent.

To both the birthing person and the familial partner, please take a turn now for each one of you to read the following sentence out loud. Then write in your responses below.

(For the partner)
A quality I hope my baby gets from me is

A quality I hope our baby gets from my partner is

(For the gestational parent)
A quality I hope my baby gets from me is

A quality I hope our baby gets from my partner is

With those musings about who your baby is, I bid you farewell for the week. Congratulations on yet another chapter read (the second to last chapter in this book!). I trust you feel proud of how much you've been learning! I wish you a week of low stress, filled with fun and excellent selfcare.

HOMEWORK:

A) Contact a doula (or several!)

Ask birth doulas what their services include and what payment plans are available. Include questions about continuity of care and feelings about pain medications in labor. Also call postpartum doulas and ask about what their services include, as well as their breastfeeding education experience, payment plans, and scheduling.

B) Reflect on your housework issues

Make a list of the areas in your life, including specific chores, that you anticipate wanting/needing help with. Then figure out who will do what.

C) Consider your social support

Do you have positive helpers and role models? Who may be a challenge to your confidence and how can you protect yourselves? Who can you confide in when you need to vent?

D) Investigate pediatric care and postpartum mental healthcare options

Consider pediatricians or family practice doctors as well as professional mental health support, should you encounter postpartum adjustment disorders.

E) Pay it forward in support

Offer help to new families.

F) Keep up with your mindfulness skill development

Practice Dr. Andrew Weil's "4,7,8" breathing exercise. Be careful not to do it more than 4 times in a row.

THIS SPACE IS FOR YOUR NOTES AND DRAWINGS

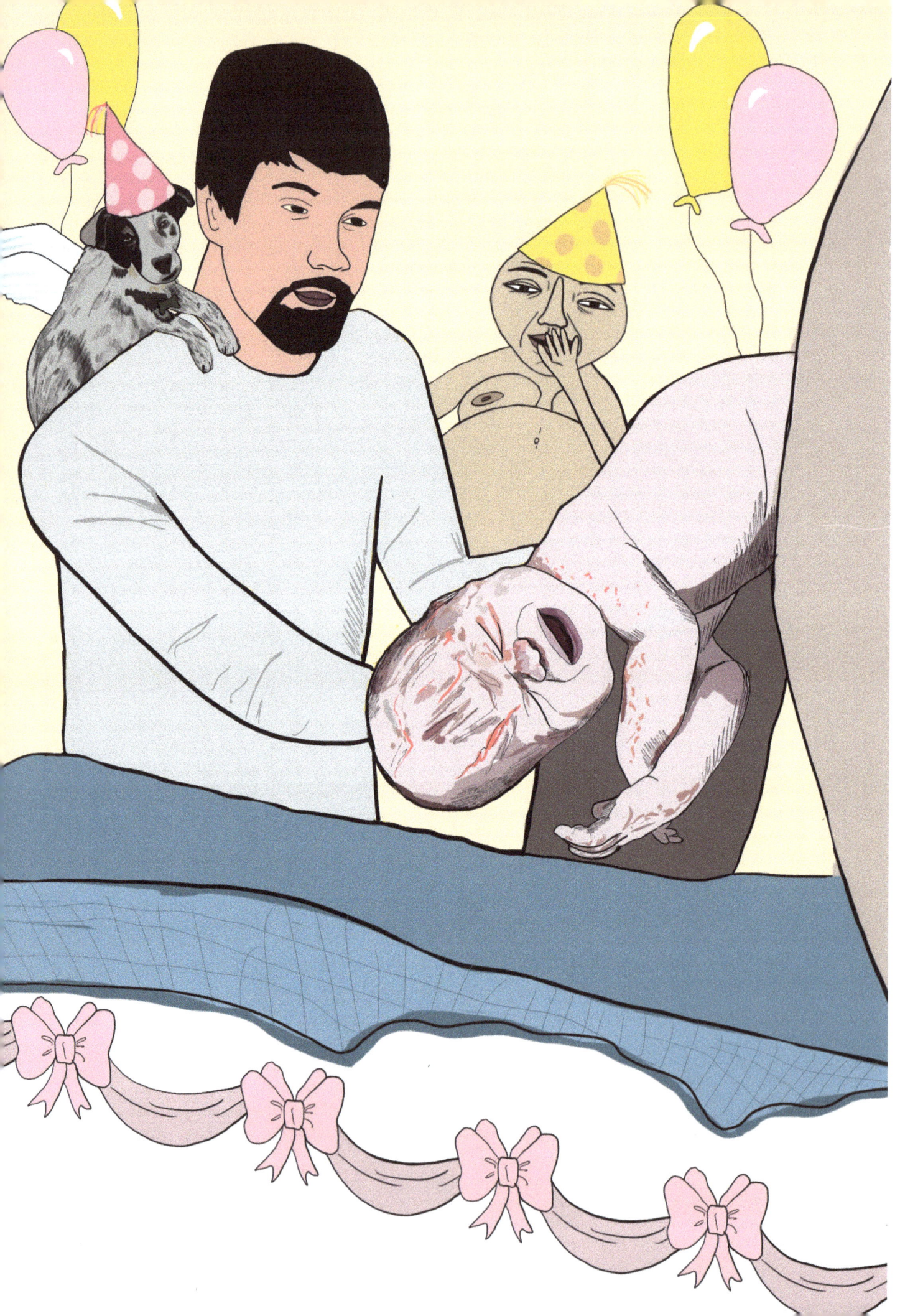

WEEK 16

Eat
Sleep
Repeat

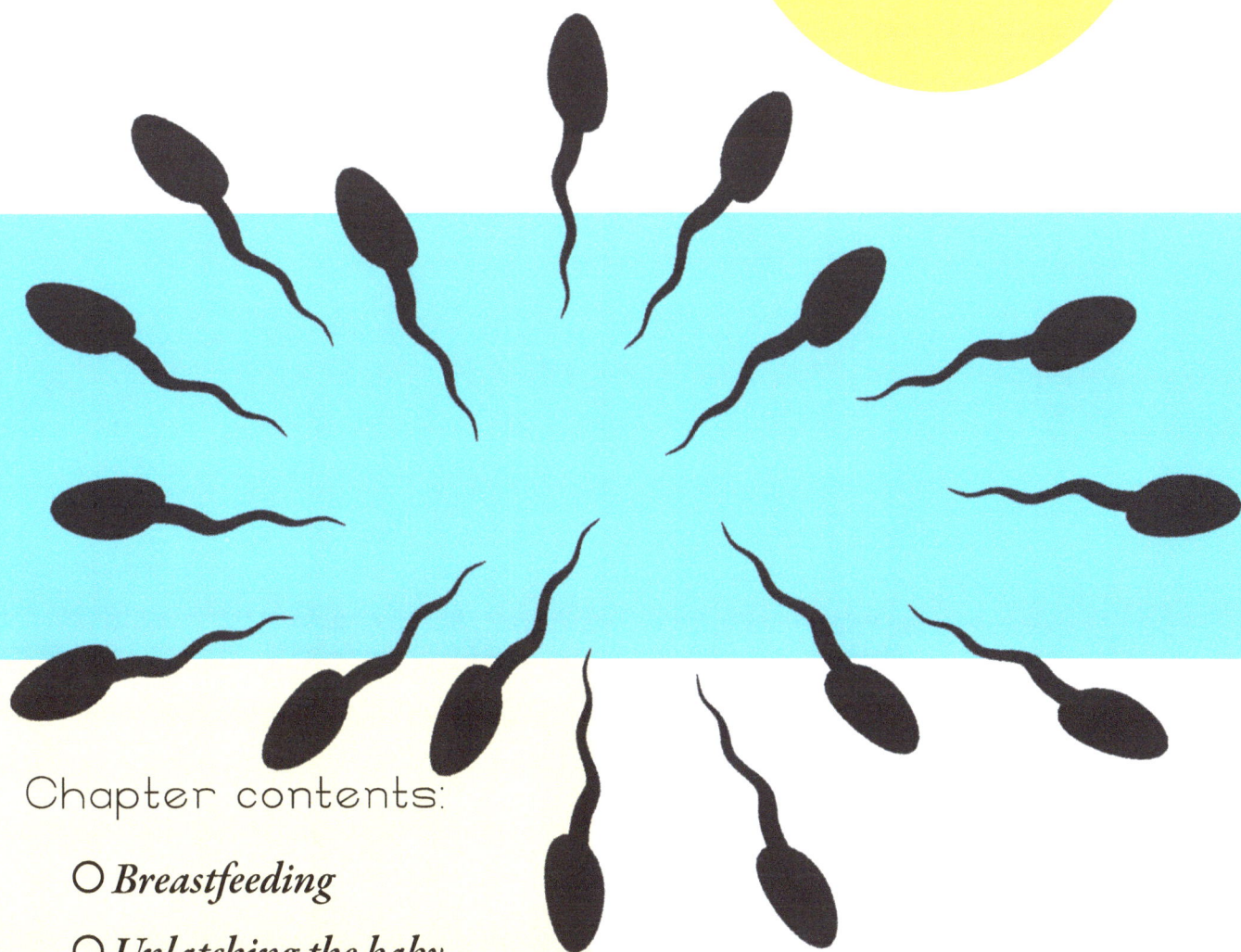

Chapter contents:

O *Breastfeeding*

O *Unlatching the baby*

O *Introducing Solid Food*

O *Sleep*

THIS SPACE IS FOR YOUR NOTES AND DRAWINGS

Welcome back. I hope your week was peaceful and productive. Did you try the "4,7,8" breathing exercise? If so, what did you notice? If not, what stopped you? How can you reset and try again? Did you contact any doulas or pediatricians? How are your postpartum plans shaping up? If you have not gotten "anything" done, try not to feel burdened by your list. Don't create a mountain out of a molehill. Small, simple steps will be stress-reducing and will yield great results. Being here in this moment, feeling this present breath is an admirable accomplishment. Rejoice in this moment.

From last week's lesson my hope was that you would gain some insight into the challenges that face new parents as they adjust as well as some ways to mitigate those challenges with advance preparation. In this final chapter I continue that conversation from the perspective of how that preparation benefits the baby, and, by extension, the world. When families can create the time and attention to tune into their little one we can improve public health. When you can ease into family life, you and your baby are more likely to emerge through your big transition with a deepened connection, with each of you developing a more grounded sense of self. This connection will make the coming work of family life healthier and infinitely more rewarding for you and your baby, and it can prove critical to creating family and global peace. What I mean by this is that without ample time or attention spent bonding with your new baby, the workload ahead will surely increase for you and for society as a whole:

> In a report published by Sutton Trust, a London-based institute that has published more than 140 research papers on education and social mobility, researchers from Princeton University, Columbia University, the London School of Economics and Political Science and the University of Bristol found that infants under the age of three who do not form strong bonds with their mothers or fathers are more likely to be aggressive, defiant and hyperactive as adults. These bonds, or secure attachments, are formed through early parental care, such as picking up a child when he or she cries or holding and reassuring a child.[363]

Responding to your baby's cues does require a lot of time and energy, and goes best with a well-built social support system. Every little bit of support helps you to have more energy and good will towards connecting—forming "secure attachments"—with your baby. If families are forced to take on too much too soon with too little support, then sadness, tears, fatigue, and stress adjustment issues can kick in. These challenges are not just experienced by the family; the ripple effects will be experienced by everyone your child will grow up to interact with in future relationships. Learning the skills to build trusting relationships begins at birth. The Sutton Trust report goes on to state:

> When helpless infants learn early that their cries will be responded to, they also learn that their needs will be met, and they are likely to form a secure attachment to their parents... However, when caregivers are overwhelmed because of their own difficulties, infants are more likely to learn that the world is not a safe place—leading them to become needy, frustrated, withdrawn or disorganized.[364]

You may have to take on more by necessity. Life is complicated, I understand. But, again, what can you plan for now, ahead of time? How much work can you (plan to) take off your plate? Who can you let into your life and your heart to help? It is often very difficult to ask for help and equally difficult to accept help. We think of ourselves as strong and capable and the idea that we need help with basic life tasks can be disconcerting. Nevertheless, it's valuable to give yourself the assignment to learn how not only to ask for help, but also to receive help. It's a skill set that will be an essential support through all your days of parenting. Learning to plan for your needs and learning to let people help you are important life skills that can make an immeasurable difference in how you bond with your baby and how you feel about your new job as a parent.

Unfortunately, with millions living under tremendous financial stress and uncertainty, coupled to woefully inadequate family-skills education across all economic levels, bonding with your baby is not a guaranteed part of childbearing. From research out of Princeton University comes the following deeply troubling finding:

> In a study of 14,000 U.S. children, 40 percent lack strong emotional bonds—what psychologists call "secure attachment"—with their parents that are crucial to success later in life. Researchers found that these children are more likely to face educational and behavioral problems.[365]

40%. That is a large number. Please take the advice offered throughout this book to heart and think now about how you will create the time to nurture and get to know your baby. What will it take for your baby to feel secure in her relationship with you?

Nurturing social relationships requires daily maintenance. Bonding and maintaining intimacy over time with your baby, older children, and your partner will take time and attention. Moreover, with babies this includes plenty of skin-to-skin time. The Cleveland Clinic website points out that "compared with babies who are swaddled or kept in a crib, skin-to-skin babies stay warmer and calmer, cry less and have better blood sugars."[366] Therefore, the easiest way to check off most of your postpartum goals is to spend most of your time mostly naked while home in bed with your baby. If only it were that easy...

Where you lack in resources, try to be extra compassionate with yourself and give yourself credit for trying the best that you can. Inadequate parental leave policies and economic inequalities clearly impact family bonding; we see the results in the abyss of social ills swirling around us. Faced with a culture that doesn't adequately support new families, you can only ask yourself to do the best that you can, given your particular circumstances. Scale back your workload where you can. Reduce anything unnecessary. For example, let the house get messy, don't waste time on social media or on electronic devices, tune out the news of the day. Regardless of your other responsibilities, try to keep your attention on supporting your own good health and on connecting with your baby. Do the best that you can and that will be plenty good enough.

Introduction to breastfeeding

Babies come hard-wired to breastfeed; it's our default setting as mammals. But breastfeeding isn't for everyone. Perhaps the gestational parent is not physically able to breastfeed, or is HIV positive, for example. (HIV can be transmitted through breastmilk.) Or maybe this parent is not emotionally equipped to breastfeed. Babies need love and physical connection in equal parts with nutrition, so if stress related to breastfeeding is causing you to avoid time with your baby, you may need to reconsider your options. Alarmingly, the U.S. has been plagued with infant formula shortages leading up to the publication of this book. My hope is that these supply issues are resolved quickly. To cope with these excruciatingly tough formula shortages, I suggest you consult potential pediatricians about what your best alternatives may be if you cannot or choose not to breastfeed. Please don't feel compelled to make any decisions now. If it works for you, plan to breastfeed and then adjust as needed.

For the best start at breastfeeding, the baby should go directly from birthing person's vagina to their naked belly for skin-to-skin contact. (Note: please don't fret any potential future complications if this ideal cannot be met. Many people overcome their circumstances and successfully breastfeed without having immediate skin-to-skin contact, myself included. And if need be, you can too.) With baby and gestational parent together, they can be cared for and observed as one by a provider. A blanket can be wrapped around them together if it is cool in the room. The baby will then, if given the opportunity, find her own way to the breast with a journey now called "the breast crawl" or "self-attachment." After unmedicated births, when baby and birthing person remain together, babies generally show a great deal of direction to the breast. They get there with the help of mouthing activity at their hands, which have smells from the amniotic fluid on them similar to the smells of the oils secreted by the breasts. In short, when baby and birthing parent are left undisturbed, the baby will exhibit just how preprogrammed to breastfeed we really are.

But as simple as the process can be, we do tend to complicate it, in large part because the United States does not have a breastfeeding culture.[367] If you are skeptical about this claim, then consider this: If we were a breastfeeding culture, we wouldn't bother to ask pregnant people if they were "intending to try" to breastfeed. If we were a breastfeeding culture, it would be assumed. We also wouldn't experience the taboo of breastfeeding in public. But there is good news. Regardless of our nationality, we *are* mammals, and mammals nurse their young quite well. So from now on, each time I make the point that primary nurturers, or breastfeeders, and babies must *learn* to breastfeed, I want you to remind yourself that you are a mammal. "I am a mammal and mammals can nurse. I will have to learn." Both claims are true.

Each primary nurturer and new baby will need to work out breastfeeding together as a couple. A baby must open her mouth wide, make good placement, and figure out how to suckle. A breastfeeder must learn how to help with offering and positioning. There is much cue-reading to learn for both participants. Learning to read each other's cues begins in the moments after birth and continues for years to come. (I find cue-reading is a skill all members of my family must work on continuously for harmony to exist).

We all make mistakes and go through varying levels of frustration while learning any new thing. For the first six weeks or so of your baby's life, their cues will largely be all about nursing, sleeping, and levels of energy for engagement. (Perhaps your baby will also want to tell you some funny jokes or about their memories *in utero*?) Primary nurturer and baby must build a foundation for communication and trust. This takes time together and a mutual willingness to learn, change, and adapt, each in relation to the other's needs. Additionally, the breast milk supply is established with a supply and demand feedback system. The more the baby nurses, the more milk the breastfeeder will make. Getting that system in sync takes time and, again, a mutual willingness to learn, change, and adapt, each in relation to the other's needs. (See the pattern?) We are mammals. We are supposed to breastfeed. But we have a lot to learn, especially when it comes to dodging the stressful obstacles that are commonly thrown in front of new breastfeeder/baby couples.

Hospital staff can sabotage breastfeeding—often inadvertently—with the use of supplemental bottles and pacifiers. Any time the baby is suckling on something that isn't the breast, there is important information the breastfeeder's body is denied about their baby's need to suck. This doesn't mean you can't occasionally offer your newborn a clean finger to suck on for a little extra soothing or to buy the primary nurturer a few extra minutes before feeding. It simply means the bond between baby and breastfeeder needs to be nurtured and tended to with as much opportunity as possible. Well-meaning nurses, some who may have lactation training and others who may not, can sometimes give conflicting information from one shift to the next, which can also cause uncertainty and stress. This, in turn, can impede milk production.

It is important to educate parents, for example, that counting the number of pee diapers in a day can show them if the baby is getting adequate amounts of breast milk. In between baby's medical weight checks, six to eight wet diapers a day and at least one poop per day has been the guideline for the last several decades for assessing if baby is getting enough milk. These guidelines have been a useful tool, but healthy babies do have more poops than that and so scientists continue to rethink these guidelines, investigating a combination of factors.[368] In the meantime, looking for those six to eight wet diapers and at least one poop remains a useful tool. Consider that when using traditional disposable diapers, it can be tricky to notice when baby is wet. If it's a small amount of pee and the diaper is super absorbent, you may need to hold it up to the light to check. Some diapers now have wetness indicators on them, and many types of new diapers are always coming on the market. Some may even alert your phone with a message about what type of waste your baby has released! (I am not sure I would have wanted that when my babies were babies, but you might find these advances helpful.)

Keep in mind that useful breastfeeding education is often scant. We mostly think of (or are more comfortable with) breasts being a way to sell cars or beer or to fondle during sex, rather than for feeding our babies. An important look at this cultural disconnect can be found in the book, *The Breastfeeding Café*, by Barbara Behrmann.[369] This book weaves a tapestry of stories about breastfeeding in America. One of the representative stories is of a breastfeeding mom who was asked to leave a Hooters® restaurant for nursing her baby. If you're unfamiliar, Hooters® is restaurant chain world-famous for featuring scantily clad waitresses with mostly large and largely revealed breasts. They bluntly market the female breast to sell beer and burgers. In fact, breasts (and butts) help to create the heterosexual male-oriented ambience of the so-called dining and drinking and sports-watching experience. Notice, then, the hypocritical stance of a restaurant that considers you inappropriate for feeding your baby at the breast while at the same time promoting an environment that depends almost completely on breasts to sell their products. This focus is literally written into their company name, as a pejorative! (Breastfeeding rights, including whether or not you can be asked to leave for nursing, vary by state.[370] See Appendix for information on checking your state's laws.)

Secondary to the marketing of breasts, we have developed a host of breast/body issues: our breasts are not perky enough, too small, too big, or just wrong. Many people with breasts have deeply internalized the complicated issues of sexual objectification, with tremendous obstacles to be overcome. Early history included experiential learning. Breastfeeding education once included that by the time a person gave birth to their own child, they would already have witnessed countless people nurse, and nurse frequently! They would have understood the work and support it requires through firsthand observation. In the here and now, all we typically see of breasts are beautiful models looking sexy in uncomfortable clothes trying to bring attention to various products and sexuality. Consequently, with little to no previous exposure to breastfeeding, but with lots of indoctrination to the idea that breasts are mostly for sex, and with an emphasis on the male gaze and marketing, breastfeeders come to the challenges of breastfeeding ill-equipped—embarrassed, even.

We typically spend the duration of our pregnancies absorbing the tag line "breast is best," but then we are also told plenty of stories about people "choosing" to breastfeed and then "failing." Most people go into their births with this information and this information alone: "Breastfeeding is the best thing for your baby, but you might not be able to do it." Strange that the best system that there is—breastfeeding—is frequently portrayed as not working. This conflicting messaging adds unnecessary anxiety to an already highly charged process. In other words, after the exhausting experience of birth, your exhaustion can be exacerbated by a variety of postpartum newborn procedures (such as injections, eye ointments, weighing, washing, etc.), resulting in birthing parents experiencing a delay in placing their babe to their breast and then just hoping for the best. The baby may or may not latch; the breastfeeding person may or may not get any useful help from the hospital staff; the baby may or may not get formula; and then the pair is sent home. With postpartum expectations built not on reality but on visions designed by advertising professionals, birthing people often face a rude awakening. They suddenly realize how little they have been taught about real parenthood. Add to this breast engorgement and fatigue, plus the baby's cries, and you likely have a much-stressed primary nurturer. ("Engorgement"[371] is the term we use for large swollen breasts that are super full, especially when the colostrum first transitions to milk. Also note that fatigue is often a direct result of fabricated sleep philosophies that frequently work against successful breastfeeding.[372] For more on engorgement and also on sleep keep reading.)

Once at home, people lacking support (and even many of us with support) can become consumed with conflict, fear, pain and guilt, all while sleep disrupted and with their hormones struggling to adjust to their new normal. The potential for breastfeeder and baby to both grow frustrated is high. When you have a primary nurturer who is still recovering physically from birth, compounded by sore breasts and exhaustion, plus a baby who is needy and hungry and can sense her parent's growing stress, you have the potential for a volatile situation to emerge.[373] Having this greater, even if a bit unnerving, understanding of the broader context within which you will be learning to nurse will help you to make better plans.

One woman I know got pregnant and had her first baby shortly after completing her training as a pediatrician. When her maternity leave was over she returned to work part time in a group pediatric practice. She was a new mom and a new doctor, which puts her low down on the power ladder. Breastfeeding had been difficult for her at the start and was continuing to be a challenge. She was stressed and without adequate support at home. She readily shared that her training as a pediatrician was useless in helping her to adjust to the demands of motherhood. She felt her training was particularly useless when it came to learning how to breastfeed. But even more poignant was the fact that as she was trying to balance the demands of working and caring for her baby, she was also realizing that she didn't have enough time to pump at her job. There she was, counseling parents that "breast is best" and yet when it came to breastfeeding her own baby she had no support from her colleagues. If pediatricians don't automatically support each other in breastfeeding, then how can they, the supposed "experts," truly support sustainable breastfeeding for their clients? With this in mind, use your interview skills to align yourselves with breastfeeding-friendly professionals. Also understand that your pediatrician is likely *not* an expert in breastfeeding. For locating expert support keep reading!

La Leche League: the breastfeeding experts

La Leche League started in 1956 as a small group of moms chatting about breastfeeding in Franklin Park, IL. These mothers quickly realized that there was a lot to share and learn so they decided to meet again (and again) for that purpose. Today, La Leche League is an international organization that promotes breastfeeding as well as breastfeeding education and support. They have become the breastfeeding authority the world over with hundreds of global and local leaders. They offer breastfeeding support in over 15 languages, are present in 89 countries to date, and both the American Medical Association and the World Health Organization look to La Leche League for breastfeeding information.

La Leche League is a great place for (many of) you to go for breastfeeding guidance and support, as well as to make new friends who share your values and dedication to breastfeeding. They run small, monthly meetings by region around the world, with leaders certified by La Leche League. Meetings are currently open to all *women* and their nursing babies. Hopefully one day soon this will change and all breastfeeders will be welcome. (That day could be today, so contact your local group and inquire!) It is free to go and check it out, but if you want to participate on a regular basis there is a nominal fee. La Leche League meetings are also usually a great place to get referrals for pediatricians, midwives, doulas, and other baby-friendly businesses and services in your area.

I strongly encourage all of you to get yourselves to a La Leche League meeting now, or some similar type of breastfeeding support group, before your baby arrives. Hospitals often run their own breastfeeding support groups and your provider may also be a good resource for other groups in your area. It is so much easier to get yourself out of the door now. You don't have to negotiate with your baby: stop first to feed, change, etc. You simply get the address and get yourself there. But it's not just physically easier to get yourself there now, before the baby comes; it's emotionally easier, too. Today, you will just be there to do research: to observe. You are curious but not in need. Once the baby arrives, you may well be feeling a bit needy. You might have questions and concerns about your baby's behaviors, or her bowels, or her sleep. You might need help with breast pain or information on building your milk supply or reducing engorgement.

Having a need, coupled with your changes in hormone levels and sleep (not to mention juggling your baby), can put you in a very vulnerable place. It is often hard to reach out and go someplace new and meet new people when you are feeling uncertain and insecure. Better to go now to meet the group leader and some other members. Then, once your baby arrives, you will already have people to reach out to. Plus, you will know where the meetings are, should you feel inclined to go there for support. Quite often my clients report that when they arrived at a breastfeeding support meeting pregnant, the members treated them like rock stars. They got them a chair or offered a snack; they were so proud of them for coming while still pregnant. They were impressed that pregnant people were being proactive about breastfeeding education. La Leche League is grass roots support (almost) at its best. They are all about mothers helping mothers and mother's teaching mothers. (I do hope one day they will more directly accommodate those that are gender diverse.) Please investigate all of your local breastfeeding support organizations to determine which one is the best fit for you.

Lactation consultants

Sometimes it's not group meetings or social support that you need for breastfeeding help. You might need help to get your baby's mouth properly on your breast, or someone to evaluate your baby's latch and suckling motions. A lactation consultant is a medical professional trained to do just that, and many are employed by hospitals for inpatient care.[374] Many make home visits, too (which is super helpful!). A lactation consultant watches you interact with your breastfeeding baby and then points out problems or redirects what is going on. If there are problems with the latch, or the baby's ability to suck, or with milk production, then they help you with appropriate solutions and referrals. For example, a lactation consultant can help screen for a tongue-tie (when the frenulum, the web of skin underneath the tongue that anchors the tongue's movements, is extra thick) and/or a lip-tie (when the top lip is more attached to the top gum than usual). These are two common, potentially complicating, congenital formations that your baby should be evaluated for whether by a lactation consultant, midwife, pediatric dentist, pediatric nurse, or even experienced other parents. This is an important evaluation if you are experiencing breastfeeding challenges; in particular nipple pain, especially when there appears to be a good latch but it still really hurts. Tongue- and lip-ties do not always cause a breastfeeding problem. But there is a simple surgical procedure to release a tie, which can be done on a newborn or later in life—really, at any point the anomaly proves to cause a problem.

Some breastfeeding challenges are not likely to develop or be noticed until the milk arrives, which is generally after the first few days when most people are already at home. You may need somebody who can take the baby's head and your breast and (clap of hands) help the two come together. A lactation consultant may need to touch and manipulate your breasts, with consent, and they should be comfortable to do so. (If they stand across the room when meeting with you, for example, then find a new consultant.) You want someone who can comfortably help guide your baby to the breast, and someone that you are comfortable with doing that. Per my usual recommendation, you should gather your list of resources now and put it someplace handy for after the baby comes.

If you birth in a hospital, you should ask to see a lactation consultant before your discharge. The hospital likely has one and they will come if you request them, but you will have to ask because this is not a routine service. (Note that the Affordable Care Act,[375] signed into law in 2010, mandates as of the publishing of this book, that health insurance companies must pay, at least in part, for lactation consultants.) By the same token, please understand that not all hospital lactation support is effective or adequate. Breastfeeding support groups, doulas, birth educators, and maternity care providers can all be possible resources for finding good, independent lactation consultants. (That is another reason to get to a breastfeeding support meeting while still pregnant; you can survey the attendants to learn names of consultants that have proven effective within your community.)

My first child had very little issue at the start, and we breastfed for a long time, until he weaned himself shortly after his third birthday. By the time my second child was born I was not only experienced with nursing my own, I had also been teaching breastfeeding and had successfully helped most of my clients. But when my second child arrived I did need the help and support of a lactation consultant. This was a different baby, I was a different mama, and I just didn't get what wasn't working. I had been teary the whole night, "Boo hoo! (real sobbing!) There is a problem and I can't fix it..." I'll never forget my dear husband asking, "What would you tell your clients to do?" In the morning, Julian made the phone call to a lactation consultant, who immediately asked when we next expected to feed. She was at our door in time for that next feeding. She evaluated my baby's suck and closely watched me try to nurse. She made one positioning adjustment and presto: happily nursing baby. The adjustment she recommended was that, for the cradle position I was using, I tilt the breast upwards—with my breast-supporting hand—as the baby was latching and aim to have my nipple contact the roof of the baby's mouth. This helps the baby create the suction that forms a good latch. (It's important to have the breast-supporting hand at or close to the chest wall and away from the areola tissue. You'll want the baby to have access to a large area of breast, including the area underneath the nipple and areola area for a big full mouthful of breast when they latch.) My lactation consultant was really supportive and I was a pretty quick study from my past experience, so in a couple of seconds she was able to guide me through that small adjustment and the problem was solved. It won't always be that easy, but the help is just that, real help—so pick up the phone! Later in the day this same lactation consultant called to see how my next feeding had gone, and then she checked in a few days later to make sure we were really all set. The support was wonderful and went well beyond the value of the dollars we had given her.

Breastfeeding benefits

The benefits of breastfeeding are so great they are almost incalculable for breastfeeder and baby. (If you are unable to breastfeed, this may be hard to read about, but I think it's important that the information be known. Regardless of your circumstances, I am confident that you are doing the best you can. And the best you can do is plenty good!) Many of the direct benefits, such as a decreased risk of breast or ovarian cancer, type 2 diabetes, high blood pressure, and osteoporosis for breastfeeder, and increased immunities and cognitive abilities for baby, are well documented. Breastfeeding also helps baby establish a healthy digestive tract and reduces the amount and severity of many ailments, such as ear infections, diarrhea, and food allergies. And I suspect there are many more benefits we are still to discover.

As I discussed earlier in this book, nursing immediately after birth (or even just skin-to-skin contact with nuzzling at or near the breast) helps a birth parent's body to secrete oxytocin, a hormone that contracts the uterus and controls postpartum bleeding. Over the first several postpartum weeks, additional uterine contractions brought on by nursing will work to help the uterus return to its pre-pregnant size.[376] Oxytocin and other love hormones flood the breastfeeder while they nurse, facilitating birth parent/baby bonding and helping to regulate birth parent's moods (fending off potential adjustment disorders). Nursing helps the parent and baby learn to read each other's cues and form a secure attachment.[377]

Breastfeeding requires great muscular effort from the baby. The hard work of suckling helps to develop the musculature of the head and neck.[378] It also helps to shape the baby's soft pallet, thus reducing the potential for problems associated with pallet shape later in life, such as snoring and sleep apnea.[379] This complex, physical, and regulatory work likewise helps to develop the baby's brainstem (where the brain meets the spinal column[380]) by continuously refining the suckling process.[381]

Other breastfeeding considerations

○ Finances: Formula (which, at the publication of this book, is hard to find in stores due to national shortages) will cost in the area of $1500 per year (as of 2023). By contrast, although breastfeeding is expensive in analogous ways when we calculate the economic value of the breastfeeder's time, you are likely to miss fewer work days due to caring for a sick baby/toddler/child and have fewer medical bills, which could then translate into better maintenance of your earning capacity. [382]

○ Happier family: Research is ongoing, but current evidence shows that breastfeeders are less likely to suffer with depression and breastfed babies tend to be less antisocial as adults.[383]

○ Sleep and night waking: Breastfed babies do wake more through the night, but when the breastfeeder is close by they get back to sleep faster. Night waking helps a baby regulate their sleep/wake cycles, which has been found to be protective to the baby.[384] Sudden Infant Death Syndrome (SIDS) is thought to occur in babies that have, amongst other risk factors (such as secondhand smoke exposure and prematurity), a malfunction of their sleep/wake regulation.[385] Breastfed babies are also found to have improved sleep from breastfeeding around the clock. This doesn't mean longer hours; it means more efficient sleep processes and better sleep/wake regulation. Moreover, the amounts of hormones and certain proteins in breastmilk, including melatonin and tryptophan, change over the course of 24 hours to be in sync with circadian rhythms. These variations in the breastmilk are associated with improved newborn sleep.[386]

○ Time: Breastfeeding is generally faster and easier than preparing bottles of formula. Hence, more time in bed with baby skin-to-skin and less time in the kitchen.

○ Lastly, some partners feel left out of the intimacy between breastfeeder and baby, but this can be remedied if the partner takes an active role in all other baby care, such as bathing, burping, diapering, dressing, and playing. Plus, soon enough your baby will eat solid foods, leaving toddler and the non-breastfeeding parent to go out together for a slice! (Yum, pizza!)

The first feeding

As I've already described, your baby, if given time, support, and access, will find her way to your breast when she's ready. Swedish researcher, Dr. Lennart Righard, studied and identified the Breast Crawl.[387] When birthing parent and baby are left undisturbed after an unmedicated birth, and the baby is left midline on their birthing parent's naked torso, the baby will crawl up to their breast, open her mouth wide, self-attach, and begin to suckle. You can encourage and support your baby to find your breast on her own by placing your hands so that they rest

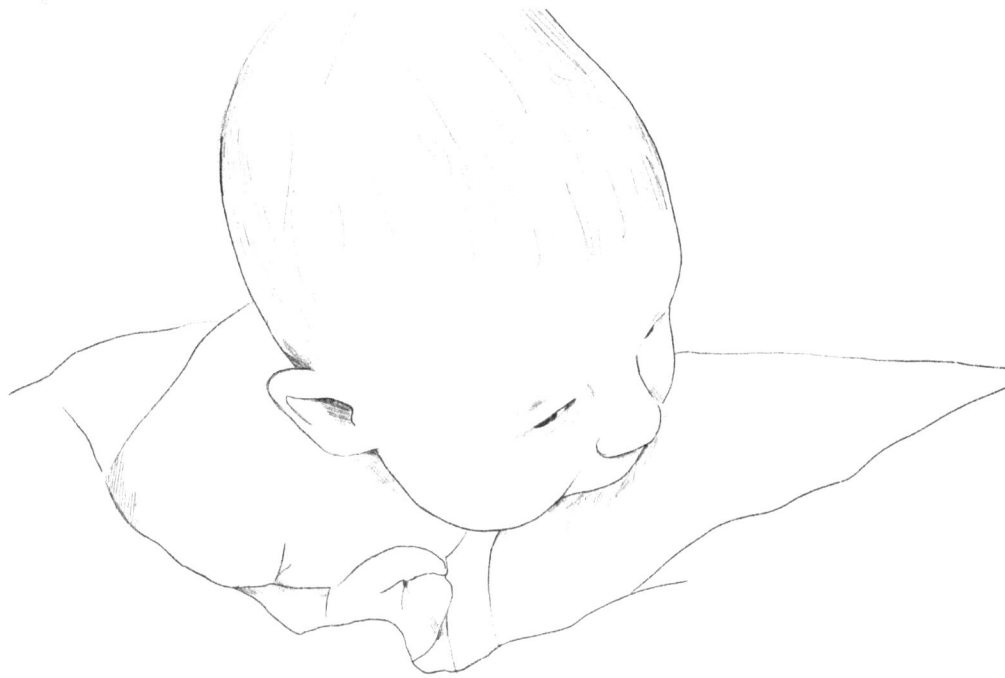

comfortably on your abdomen while at the same time touching the bottoms of the baby's feet. This gives the baby important support in her breast crawl.[388] Remember: any and all breast stimulation the baby causes will help to contract the birth person's uterus, reduce bleeding, and help to expel the placenta if it is still inside.

For the first feeding, and thereafter, work toward trusting and tuning into your baby's instincts. Importantly, try to relax fully into this new and wild experience. There is no rush. You and baby will figure this all out. Babies are well equipped to handle any glitches in the feeding process. I know of one extreme and upsetting story in which a baby had been abandoned after birth and was not found for six days—the baby survived, albeit hungry and I am sure freaked out.[389] Although this is a horrific story, it shows us that babies are resilient and well stocked to handle even the harshest transition from inside to out. Refer to it to gain assurance that a term-healthy newborn, cared for by attentive and loving parents, has what she needs if there are any delays in feeding once born. So, please, try to relax; know that you and your baby have time to learn. During the first hour or two of life babies are usually alert and interested in their parents' faces. The baby may appear super hungry or not at all hungry. It doesn't really matter. Go easy on yourself. Get to know each other, take your time, be gentle, talk to your baby and your loved ones, and be awed that the birth is finally over.

One major way that prenatal education supports family life is to reveal that if new parents can learn what to expect, then they can remain calmer in the face of some of nature's stranger moments—like meeting your newborn. Ask yourself, for example: what will your needs be after birth? Will you be hungry? Then eat something. One of my clients shared that she had used early labor to bake a chocolate cake that they brought with them to the hospital. Following birth, she reported that she ate six pieces! She then felt sick, of course. But she laughed as she told the story several weeks later and said she only regrets the last two pieces. And, if she has more babies, she will plan to bake another cake! Maybe you need physical help repositioning yourself with the baby in your arms? Ask for help. Perhaps you have questions? Speak up and ask them. Your care providers can hopefully answer your questions as you gently ease yourself into the first meeting and feeding. If your after-contractions are uncomfortable, exhale through them as you did during labor. The more you relax, the more your baby can relax. Babies are very intuitive and connected to the emotions of those around them, especially their gestational parent. Research published in 2019 finds evidence for what many gestational parents have already known:

Mothers' and babies' brains can work together as a 'mega-network' by synchronizing brain waves when they interact. The level of connectivity of the brain waves varies according to the mum's [sic] emotional state: when mothers express more positive emotions their brain becomes much more strongly connected with their baby's brain. This may help the baby to learn and its brain to develop.[390]

Note that actual evidence on birth education exists but has not been well studied.[391] Prenatal and postpartum education is based largely on observation and common sense.[392] In short, it's okay to rely on the experience, insight, and wisdom of mentors in the birth process (such as doulas and midwives) as well as those that have given birth before you!

Colostrum

Starting in late pregnancy and continuing through the first three to four days postpartum is the release of a fluid called "colostrum." This first liquid is the perfect food and drink for your baby. Colostrum contains all the nutrition and fluid your newborn needs until your breast milk develops, or "comes in." Generally, the colostrum changes over to milk in those three to four days after the birth, but this can take longer in cases of birth by cesarean section. Delayed skin-to-skin contact, stress from major abdominal surgery, and delayed initiation of breastfeeding all can impact the onset of milk production. Whenever your milk does come in you will notice the differences, the breasts tend to get very full and enlarged and the breastmilk looks more like cow's milk. The colostrum is yellowish in color and thicker than the breast milk.

I suspect that scientists will continue to learn amazing things about colostrum in the future. It is already known that in addition to nutrition and fluid, colostrum contains a power-packed dose of the gestational parent's immune system. This is true for all mammals. And because the newborn gut starts off quite porous, the colostrum acts like a protective sealant or coating. Additionally, colostrum contains leukocytes, which are cells beneficial to establish a healthy environment in the newborn gut.[393] With a newborn's tiny stomach, not much colostrum is needed. So what they do get is very important to their health.

As I mentioned above, pregnant people typically start to make colostrum during the last trimester of pregnancy (but some do make it earlier). During the seventh month of my first pregnancy, one hot summer night, I was sitting around playing Scrabble® with my husband and we were discussing that I might be making colostrum. Curious, I decided to give my breast a gentle, kneading squeeze. I milked my breast from the base of my chest out to the nipple and, sure enough, some thick, yellowish fluid came out. When I did this, I also learned that my nipple didn't contain just one hole for the fluid to come out, but several tiny little holes. Nipples are more like a shower head than a garden hose. "Holy cow!" I shrieked with excitement. "It's really there!" It was exciting, kind of sexy, and also so totally bizarre! There really was a baby coming, too! I tell you this fun anecdote because I hope that when your time comes you will appreciate your colostrum and what a precious gift it is for your baby.

After the initial meeting and feeding (on colostrum), the baby is usually ready for a nap. It has been a big deal to be born and to meet your loved ones. Now it is time for a rest. If newborn procedures, such as applying antibiotic eye ointment and/or a dose of vitamin K are to be administered, then waiting until after the first two hours of life is less disruptive to normal bonding than doing procedures during these first two hours. I can't write this enough: do your research now so that you can have confidence in your decisions once the baby is born. Having done your research ahead of time will allow you more energy to focus on getting to know your baby and resting. Remember to ask prospective care providers (maternity as well as pediatric) about what to expect following birth. What routines can you anticipate? By now you know that learning ahead of time about what to expect from your providers following birth will better enable you to make your best decisions and navigate care options for yourself and your baby with confidence.

Your first week postpartum

Once you are settled into your bed after a home birth, or returned home from the hospital after birth, please plan to spend at least one week in bed (i.e., a full seven days, if not longer). I do not mean a kind of glued-to-the-bed-afraid-to-get-up bed rest; I just mean to suggest that your bed is your home base—hang out in bed all day long if you can. If a friend comes over and you want to sit in another room for a small bit of time (15-20 minutes or so), please do so. If it is a beautiful day and you want to step outside for some fresh air, please do so! Connecting to nature can be a powerful restorative tool. Feel the sun on your skin, let the breeze blow your hair, but keep your activities brief and easy. Then return to your bed. Hopefully your partner, support team, and any older children can camp out on or near your bed.

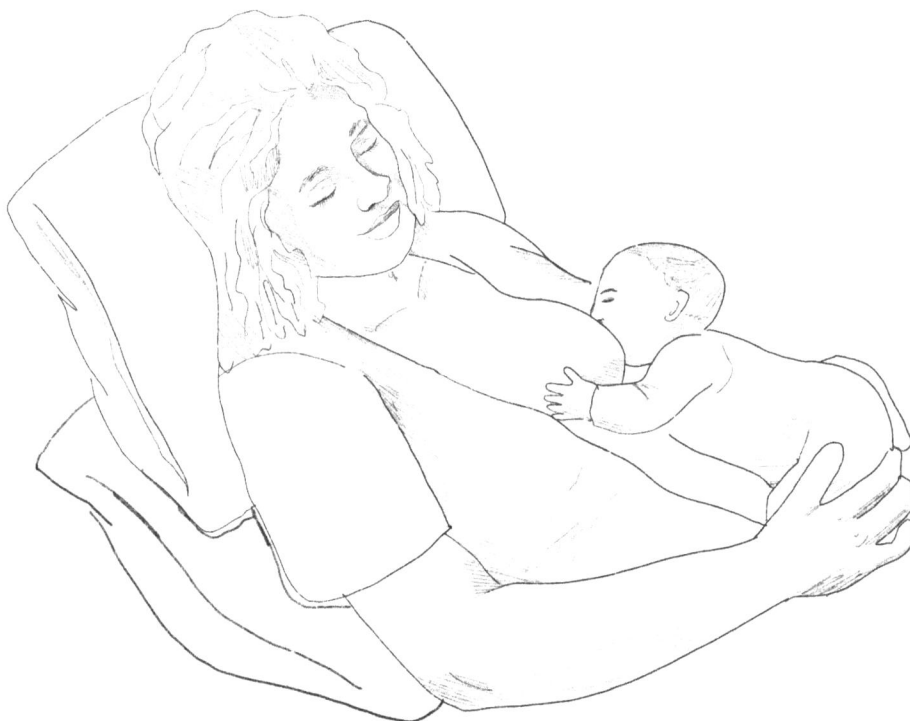

Giving yourself plenty of time in bed and near your bed gives you ample opportunity to heal, to learn about breastfeeding, and to bond with your baby. Remember: nurturing takes time, access, and energy. This is a special time to let go of the rest of the world. You need recovery and, again, you and your baby both benefit from skin-to-skin time. Staying in bed provides for these needs. Napping frequently is also a critical tool for your adjustment to family life. Sleep for a few hours to get through a few hours. I am sure this is a very different pattern than you were used to, but your whole life is changing now. When your baby falls asleep, lay down and close your eyes.

Lochia

Lochia is a menstrual-like blood flow that follows the birth. This flow can last up to six weeks, although many people's bleeding subsides sooner than that.[394] Your lochia is a helpful tool in gauging whether or not you are doing too much physical activity too soon after birth. Your lochia flow will start off bright red, looking very much like fresh blood, but within a few days the flow should start to look darker brown in color, resembling older blood. If you are overdoing your physical activities, this flow will return to a bright red. When this happens, you will have to get back into bed and take it easy. Think of the site where the placenta was attached almost like a big, open wound that needs to heal. So easy does it! (If you have any concerns or seem to be bleeding a lot, be sure to contact your provider right away. As I mentioned in Week 10, hemorrhage is a risk for the first 12 weeks postpartum.)

Postpartum care of your pelvic floor and vagina

After birth, your vagina and/or perineum may need some sutures or may have some swelling or bruising. If this is true for you, and with your provider's permission, apply ice packs. In the hospital they will likely have some cold pads for you to place on top of your pad that collects the lochia. If you are preparing for a home birth, you can make your own: Toward the end of your pregnancy buy some sterile gauze 4x4 pads and soak them in water. Then lay the gauze, folded in half, on a clean cookie sheet and freeze. Once they are frozen, place them in a freezer container and store until needed. After the birth, apply the frozen pads to the perineal area by placing them on top of your sanitary pad, in your underpants.

After my vaginal birth, when I asked my midwife how long I should continue to place the ice pads in my undies, she gave me a sly smile and said, "Oh, you'll know." Well, I had no real idea what she meant, but the relief that I felt from the iced pads was clear and immediate, so I didn't dwell on the question. A day later when I shrieked from the cold of the ice, I learned what she had meant. I quickly removed the ice pad. Initially following birth, the ice had felt amazingly good. Just two days later it felt like you would expect ice on your genitals to feel—shriek worthy! I knew at that point I was done with the need for ice.

One of the other soothing things that my midwife suggested immediately after the birth was to squirt warm water on my genitals as I peed. I was given a small, plastic squirt bottle and told to fill it with warm water prior to urinating. (Nurses call these squirt bottles "peri-bottles.") Without the warm water the urine would have stung my swollen and newly stitched perineum, but with the warm water spray I was fine. Being able to pee with minimal discomfort is important as that is also likely a brief respite from nursing. Uh oh, baby is hungry again!

And what about pelvic floor and vaginal toning exercises? Discuss with your provider first, but generally it is not only safe, but advantageous to begin toning your pelvic floor and vagina within a day or two of labor. Go gently and stop if you feel discomfort. You've been through a lot, and rebuilding muscular strength and integrity is important, but you will want to be wary of overdoing it. Once you determine the right level of practice for you, you might even do some toning exercises while you are nursing. This kind of multitasking is achievable, which is a good thing because, uh oh, baby is hungry again!

Newborn feeding cues

When you learn to read your baby's hunger cues you can respond to your baby's needs before she starts to get upset. Feeding her before she gets upset will help keep everyone's stress levels in check. There are different levels of feeding cues that babies give with increasing urgency.[395]

1. Mouthing activity; or, lots of opening and closing of the mouth. This activity may be subtle and can easily be missed if you're not looking for the cue.

2. If you missed the early mouthing cues, the baby will make her point with a little more emphasis by moving on to stick her hand—or whatever else she can get a hold of—into her mouth.

3. And if cues 1 and 2 were missed, cue 3 will be harder to miss: crying. Crying with hunger may start as some whimpers, but baby will surely progress to screams if you are still missing the cue or are otherwise delayed.

While learning to breastfeed it's really impossible to offer the breast too frequently. You can't over-nurse your baby. If she doesn't want to nurse, she won't. When she's older you won't ever have to offer the breast, she'll clearly communicate her needs. But for the first couple of months you should be offering the baby your breast at frequent intervals, at least every two to three hours throughout the day when she is awake. At the same time, you don't have to dwell on the clock; just tune into your baby. If your baby makes a funny face, offer her the breast. If she seems upset, offer her the breast. If she is squirmy, shares a memory, or tells you a joke (all in baby language of course), offer her the breast. This is how you both learn. Offer her the breast, because babies nurse for comfort as well as nutrition, and comfort is important too.

Take time out now for a stretch break.

EXERCISE: STRETCH
TO MAKE ROOM FOR YOUR BABY

You know the drill, read aloud or record. Tune into and follow your breath and be gentle with your body.

"Stand again with your feet about hips' width apart. Let your arms hang down by your side. Now take a nice deep breath in. As you do, soften your knees and reach your arms over your head. Look up at your arms. Feel a gentle back stretch. As you exhale, gently release your arms back down to your side and straighten your legs. Repeat at least 4 times."

—Reader pause—

"As you breathe in, reach up and look up. Exhale as you relax your arms back down by your side and return your head to a neutral position. Feel your long spine with the crown of your head reaching up to the sky and your heavy tailbone reaching down toward the ground."

—Reader pause—

"Reach up again as you inhale, this time focusing on one side of your body lengthening at a time. Allow one side to reach up really high, making room on that side. Imagine that you are opening up the spaces between your ribs and between your rib cage and your pelvis. Next, allow the first side to soften as you reach high up with the other side, opening yourself up equally on both sides. Repeat each side several times. Open up the sides of your body and feel the expansion. Babies take up a lot of room in our bodies. You can open yourself up to make more room through stretching. You'll feel better if you can make room for your baby."

—Pause here and give this exercise a try—

Positioning for breastfeeding

First and foremost, you need/want to be comfortable in your breastfeeding position. (You are going to be doing a lot of breastfeeding! Your comfort and care really matter!) The initial position from the first feeding—i.e., reclining back, skin-to-skin, with baby midline on your chest, is wonderful for all the breastfeeding to follow. But learning a variety of positions over the first few weeks, including side lying, cradle hold, and cross cradle hold, will help you to optimize the wonderful flexibility inherent in breastfeeding. Use pillows for support wherever needed, such as between your legs if you are lying down. For seated positions use lumbar support; you can roll up a towel and place it behind you in the curve of your lower back. Be mindful that your posture is not hunched over in seated positions (if it is, you will surely develop neck and back pain). While seated, use a foot rest to raise your lap and place pillows on your raised lap to help raise the baby up to breast level (instead of hunching over to bring breast to baby.) While in seated positions try using pillows or couch arms and the like to rest your elbows. The goal is for you to be as well supported and comfortable as possible. In seated positions it will be useful to use one hand (and not the one holding the baby) to support (hold) your breast. Support your breast from near the chest wall, making sure your hand is well away from the areola, especially on the underside of the breast. (Many of us, while trying to support our breast, unknowingly cover the underside of that breast close to or covering the areola with our hand, thus blocking the baby from getting enough breast in her mouth.) You can then use your hand to slightly tip the nipple up and aim it towards the roof of the baby's mouth, like my lactation consultant helped me to do.

Next, it's time to think about the baby's posture. A common and useful guideline is to think about you and the baby being "tummy to tummy." The baby's spine should be in good alignment, with their chin slightly tucked. Imagine how hard it would be to drink while your neck was extended or your head was cocked to one side.

The baby then needs to open their mouth wide, really wide, to get a whole big mouthful of breast, including a sizeable portion of the underside of your breast. If they are only open a little bit they will clamp down on the nipple. Not only will this be painful; it will not allow for the baby to get enough milk out. When they get a big mouthful of breast, they can use their tongue to massage the milk ducts, which helps them to extract ample amounts of milk (or colostrum).

Some babies are slow to grasp the importance of opening wide. Remember, they're learning too! We can help them. One way is to use your breast-supporting hand to gently brush your nipple up and down over the baby's lips, making sure to bring your nipple higher than the baby's mouth on the upswing. This nudges them to reach up for the breast, opening wide. Another trick that a lactation consultant taught me was that you can have a helper (simply because you don't have enough hands) apply gentle pressure on the baby's chin. This helps to direct their lower jaw down as they are opening

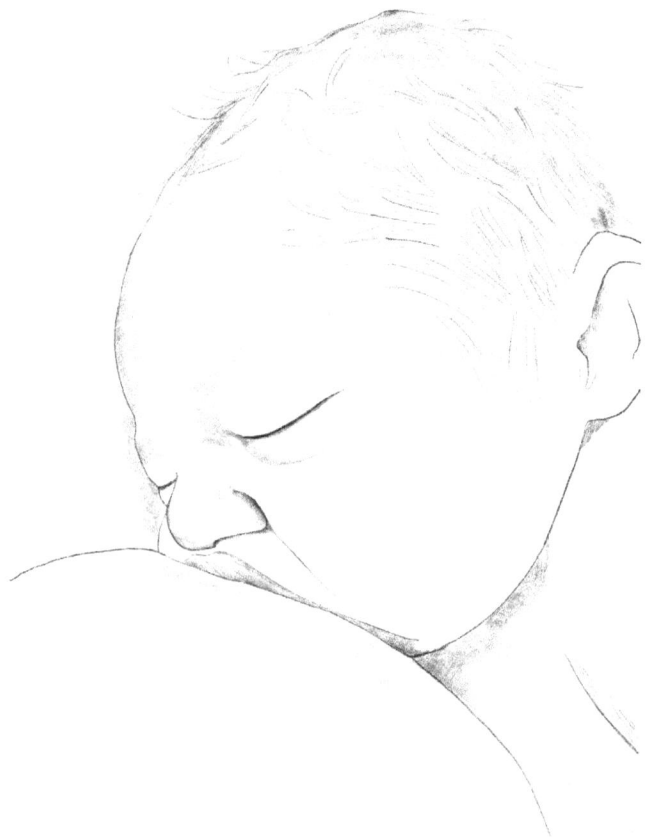

their mouth, thus helping them to open wider. When my eldest son was born, and we arrived home from the hospital, I realized by my sore nipples that my son wasn't opening wide enough at the start of feedings. We used the above tip, with my husband gently pulling our baby's lower jaw down as he was opening to latch. We did this for three feedings in a row and then by the fourth feeding he opened very wide at the start all on his own. He had learned, and your baby will too.

If your baby is latched on and it feels or looks wrong, you will want to take them off and try again, and again, and again. You may need to take them off and try again a lot of times to get it right. That is okay. You are both learning, and learning is really challenging sometimes. This can be frustrating for you and your baby, but it is important not to nurse with a poor latch. It is possible, if you allow the baby to nurse with an incorrect latch, to have so much pain from sore nipples later on that you can have a rough time distinguishing between a good or a poor latch. If you are struggling with your baby's latch, I urge you to contact a lactation consultant sooner rather than later. You'll want to keep any small stumbles from becoming larger issues, i.e., more discomfort and more ingrained poor nursing habits.

Once your baby is latched on properly, you will likely (but not necessarily) hear them gulping and swallowing. Although you may feel a lot of sensation, it shouldn't be painful. Take notice of how hard the musculature of the baby's jaw is working. Some babies are like little barracudas, they are furious eaters and can drain a breast with efficiency and steadfast determination. Other babies are more like philosophers, they may take a sip, contemplate the world's existence, and then eventually take another sip. These babies may take significantly longer to drain a breast. In general, it's beneficial to let a baby nurse as long as they want at one breast. There are important benefits for the baby to get the milk that comes later in a feeding at one breast. This hind milk contains more fat, and this fat is very beneficial to baby.[396] It is therefore important to allow the baby to nurse as long as they want to at the first breast before burping and switching to the other side.[397] But some babies can get really comfortable nursing and dozing with the nipple still in their mouth. As the breastfeeder, your comfort and intuition matter too! If you sense that the baby has really had a decent feed at that breast you can unlatch them, burp them, and then offer the other breast.

Unlatching the baby

Holy Moly! Your baby's latch, even an incorrect one, can be super strong! You can't just pull the baby off or you will surely cause yourself pain and possibly even damage your nipple tissue. (Think: Pitbull dangling from a tree branch!) To safely unlatch your baby, you first need to break the suction. You can do this by sliding your (clean) finger alongside your breast, down towards your nipple, and at the corner of the baby's mouth. You'll need to stick your finger all the way into the corner of their mouth, in between the two halves of their jaw. This will break the suction, allowing you to then slide the baby off. (Phew!) Now you can either try to re-latch if you need to help baby with a better latch, or, if you had a good latch and they have emptied the breast but are lingering in their happy place, you can unlatch them and declare that they are finished on that side. It's then likely time to burp the baby and offer the other breast.

Burping

Just as important as a proper latch, is helping your baby under four months of age to pass gas. You do this by burping them.[398] To help your baby burp, hold her upright, lean her against your chest, and gently pat her back. Positions such as resting her over your shoulder, across your forearm, or over your thigh can also place additional pressure on her gut and thus aid in the process. Try to burp your baby when she has finished the first breast, finished at the second breast, or anytime they seem fussy or cranky. Gas pains can range from super uncomfortable to extremely painful. If you have an available partner, burping can be their job. It's a great way to include the partner's involvement in feeding while you are exclusively breastfeeding.

Milk production and switching sides

Offer both breasts at each feeding. As I mentioned above, and as a general rule, you will want your baby to let you know when they are done at a particular breast so that they are sure to get your important hind milk. Remember: making milk is a supply and demand system. You supply some milk, baby demands more, your supply increases. When your baby nurses your body gets stimulated to make more milk. It's a system regulated by our hormones (our body's chemical messenger system). It is also impacted by emotions. You need to have reduced stress levels to make ample milk. Good nutrition and plenty of fluids are likewise key to your supply. Nursing at both breasts helps you to keep up with the baby's needs. Plus, if you only breastfed on one side, then that breast would get really big from making all the breast milk while your other side would stay small, resulting in some likely uncomfortably lopsided anatomy! I have seen imbalances arrive after just a few days of accidently ignoring one side. But the good news is that a breast production imbalance is usually rectified easily over the course of a few days.

Switching sides also provides good bilateral physical stimulation for the baby. If you do not breastfeed and are relying on bottle feeding, it is healthy for your baby if you mimic the skin-to-skin and bilateral contact (switching sides) of breastfeeding as you bottle feed. But sometimes babies have different opinions. I once had a client whose baby vehemently refused to nurse on one side of his mother. The mom tried everything, but she just couldn't get the baby to nurse on that one side. Frustrated and upset she sought care from a chiropractor who had good experience working with newborns. The chiropractor found that the baby had a cervical spinal subluxation (meaning, something in his spine was out of alignment), which, according to the chiropractor, likely occurred during the birth. Once the chiropractor adjusted the baby, he happily nursed on the side he had been refusing. The little guy had probably been quite uncomfortable on the side he was refusing, so once the pain subsided there was no more trouble.

Breast engorgement

Engorgement is when your breasts get super swollen with milk. You might become engorged when your milk first comes in, and thereafter whenever it's been too long a time since you've fed your baby. When your breast milk first changes from colostrum to milk, your body is not sure how much milk to make so it makes *a lot*. It's a bounty, but it can also be a pain. Engorged breasts are uncomfortable; I felt like I was going to pop. Engorged breasts can become so hard that they are difficult for the baby to latch onto. Thus, as you become aware of your breasts growing full with your new milk, somewhere between day 2 and day 5, the first course of action is to try to nurse, nurse, nurse! Hopefully your baby will cooperate and help you out by nursing like crazy. This is really what is best for both of you (although your nipples might complain a bit).

Your body is looking for information from your baby about what to do. Consequently, the more you nurse your baby the more your body will learn to make just the right amount. Use of a breast pump at this point is likely to increase your milk supply beyond what your baby needs, thus perpetuating the engorgement problem. The simplest solution for engorgement, when your baby will comply, is to nurse your way out of it. But if you can't get your baby to nurse, because the breast is too hard from engorgement, the baby is too sleepy, or she's just plain too full, then the next thing to try is hand expression of breast milk. As I mentioned, I like the shower for hand expressing (assuming there is no need to collect the milk) because the warm water helps to wash away some stress, too.

Begin to milk your breasts as if you were milking a cow: place both hands around the breast at the chest wall and gently kneed out toward the nipple with repetitive motions. Generally, all you really need to do is to get a few squirts out to help you feel better and to soften the breast enough to get baby latched on. Too much hand expressing, like pumping, can backfire by communicating to your brain that you need to make more milk. Once you get some relief, stop there. (If hand expressing, or any pumping for that matter, does not make you laugh, try mooing like a cow as you do it. If mooing makes you cry, stop, but realize that crying is a good release, too. We've all been there.) Many breastfeeders successfully use their hands to express some milk, but there is also a manual pump device called a Haakaa® that breastfeeders find helpful.[399] A Haakaa® is useful if there is a need/want to save the milk you extract. It's a small, hand-held and -operated silicone pump that creates some suction as you squeeze it.[400]

If you continue to be in a lot of pain from engorgement, another option is to apply ice compresses to help reduce inflammation. Or, follow the old wives' tale (now supported by scientific evidence): frozen cabbage leaves.[401] Applying frozen cabbage leaves will feel good, can decrease your discomfort, and can make the breast softer and easier to nurse. 20+ years ago I was taught that the effect of cabbage leaves would be so strong that it could be used to help suppress lactation, and so for treatment of engorgement the leaves should only be left on the breast until symptoms start to resolve. At the time I was taught this there wasn't any concrete evidence to support this practice. But I tried it and it worked! It's hilarious and fantastic: if you peel off a couple of cabbage leaves and place them in your freezer they will freeze into a bra-cup shape!

Again, it usually takes a solid six weeks for your milk supply to regulate to your baby's needs. Some people will feel comfortable breastfeeding after a couple of weeks, for others this can take longer. Many new breastfeeders tell me that it really takes several months to figure out breastfeeding, well beyond their expectations that in six weeks everything would be sorted out and life would feel "back to normal."

Take a moment now to check in with your feelings around nursing. Use the space below to jot down your reflections.

Is your baby getting enough milk?

If your baby seems alert when she is awake, has some calm periods, and if she seems interested in feeding, then chances are excellent that all is well. Well-baby visits and newborn weight checks will confirm this. By contrast, if you sense that your baby is lethargic, her lips seem dry, she is not peeing and pooping, her fontanels seem depressed more than usual, or she is constantly upset, then please seek attention from a breastfeeding-savvy healthcare provider. If your baby has any of those symptoms, then she should be evaluated for feeding issues, weight gain, and dehydration.

With any concerns about a need to boost milk production, it's important to evaluate the primary nurturer's nutrition, as well as sleep and stress levels. Is there a lack of support? Or perhaps there is an emotionally stressful reaction to parenthood that is affecting selfcare? Assuming that the breastfeeder is eating and drinking, my tried-and-true solution for boosting supply is skin-to-skin contact with baby coupled to bed rest. If breastfeeder and baby get into bed, mostly naked for a week or longer, then they typically emerge with a built-up milk supply and a more connected relationship.

Unfortunately, this solution is often unattainable for so many new parents because it relies on a lot of external support. It's shameful that in such a wealthy country, after the first two or three weeks, most breastfeeding parents cannot afford to spend enough time in bed with their baby—it becomes financially and logistically impossible. That's what I mean by "it takes a lot of external support for a person to breastfeed their baby." During this time, the breastfeeding couple (i.e., gestational parent and baby) will greatly benefit from extra love and emotional support. But breastfeeding parents have physical needs, too. They need practical help to have meals prepared, clothes cleaned for them and their baby, older children cared for by others, pet care handled by others, paying the bills handled by others, etc. That would be the kind of support that would allow a breastfeeding parent to stay in bed a week to ten days to boost their milk production. Stress and fatigue are huge inhibitors for lactation and maternal-infant bonding. As I have said numerous times, breastfeeding parents and baby need restful time together. When breastfeeding parents can reduce their focus to nothing but lounging and bonding with baby, and baby has continuous access to the breast with plenty of skin-to-skin time, breastmilk supply is boosted.[402]

I write of ideals here to help you plan, not to set up unattainable goals that leave you feeling down. Parents throughout time have survived horrors of cruelty and persevered. You are strong, and you will do the best you can and that will be good enough! As daunting as this workload is, you will be able to handle what comes your way. And when your baby snuggles in cozy and melts your heart you will understand that it is their love that gives us strength.

Bottle feeding and pacifiers

To best establish breastfeeding refrain from giving baby any supplemental sucking devices until her one-month birthday. As long as breastfeeding is well established, feel free to introduce a bottle and/or a pacifier after the first month.

How to introduce the bottle to your one-month-old

Step one, collect some breast milk. Get out the breast pump, clean it, and familiarize yourself with and figure out all its parts. Important note: when using electric pumps, be sure to check for the ability to control the force of the suction. Start with the lowest possible suction setting. You can then slowly increase the suction once you have the hang of it. But *please start slowly*. I have heard from several women who hurt themselves by starting with suction levels that were too strong.

Step two, introduce the bottle. For the first few introductions of the bottle you won't need more than an ounce or two of breastmilk. Initially, this process is just about getting your baby comfortable with the bottle because the bottle requires a very different action than actual breastfeeding. During breastfeeding the baby must use her tongue to massage the breast while simultaneously sucking very strongly. To bottle feed the baby must use her tongue to slow down the positive flow from the bottle. Your baby will need time and practice to figure out the difference.

Ideally, if breastfeeding is to be continued, it shouldn't be the breastfeeding parent who ever gives the baby a bottle. To reduce confusion, the breastfeeding parent should always be for breastfeeding and the other parent, or grandma, or friend or other caretaker should always be for bottle feeding.

Picking the right moment to introduce the bottle will help it go smoothly. Wait for a time when the baby isn't super hungry, exhausted, or over stimulated. A quiet, alert time is best. The first few bottle feedings should be viewed as experiments, not supplemental feeding. Over time baby and bottle can work up to replacement meals, but this should happen gradually.

Most babies at one-month-old take to the bottle without problem. Sometimes, however, families then put away the bottle, because the breastfeeding parent may not be returning to work for several more weeks, making the opportunity to breastfeed feel ever-present. The thinking usually is, "gee, this bottle feeding and pumping is a lot of work, and my baby took the bottle without hesitation, so let's leave this alone until I need to return to work." What can happen here is that an older baby, who hasn't been consistently given a bottle from 4 – 5 weeks of age on, becomes savvy of their own control; they may refuse the bottle, holding out for their parent's breast. (Smart babies! Who wouldn't prefer the real thing if you knew there was a choice?) The point here is that even when the baby takes the first bottle or two without issue, now the goal is to make it a daily routine. The non-breastfeeding parent or other caregiver should now give one bottle a day, even if the breastfeeding parent will still be home for a few more months, or longer. Not only does this help baby; it also gives the nursing parent a chance at a nap or shower. Simply put, it can provide a few glorious moments of being off duty.

If you are ultimately unable to use breastmilk to feed your baby, please do your research. Some families use goat's milk as a substitute for breastmilk or formulas based in soy or cow's milk. Fresh cow's milk should be avoided until the baby reaches at least one year of age. There are some large proteins in cow's milk that make it tough for young babies to digest. Commercial formula, as I have mentioned, might be hard to purchase, but if you can, it can be a reasonable substitute for many babies. However, the Cornucopia Institute (a nonprofit watchdog/consumer protection organization) presents research showing that many formula makers are adding Synthetic DHA and ARA oils solely for marketing purposes and some babies don't tolerate them well.[403] So again, do your research.

Solid foods

Scientists recommend that babies begin to learn about solid foods after their 6-month birthday. I believe that a baby should be able to independently sit up before you consider any solid foods. I also like the barometer of judging how guilty you feel eating in front of them! My boys would stare us down with funny baby indignation that they weren't getting any of our solid food. Two reasons to delay the introduction of solid foods is that they are super messy and will definitely amp up the amount of cleaning you need to do—from the baby and the floor to the poopy diapers! And whoa solid food poops really begin to stink like a big person's poop. Breastmilk diapers are benign in comparison. You have a wonderful lifetime ahead of eating and experimenting with solid foods with your children, so I wouldn't rush it if I were you.

Weaning

La Leche League teaches child-led weaning. I support this, too, and it worked out very well for us. After the first few months of life I never really offered the breast. I just followed my kids' lead. If they wanted to nurse, they could. Each baby, in his own time, stopped asking. Jasper weaned himself at three years of age and Arlo weaned himself at four. It was a beautiful process for us, and not without phases of increased clingy-ness leading to huge spikes in nursing frequency. These increases in frequency seemed to come around times of big developmental milestones, such as crawling, walking, and talking. It wasn't easy for me to always meet the increased demand joyfully, but I was brave and persevered. What I found was that if the child was extra clingy and nursing a lot, and if I could work to yield to his needs and give him the increased attention and time, then his requests would settle down rather quickly and we would get back on track. By contrast, if I would resist and pull away and feel resentful during these times, then the need would intensify and be prolonged. Both people matter in the nursing couple, and so I encourage you to dig into why it might be challenging to meet your baby's needs if/when such feelings arise. Consider, too, how brief a time in your parenting relationship this phase really is. And always remember: your feelings matter too; you can change what is working when or if you need to. If nursing is too stressful and keeping you from fully opening up to and connecting with your baby, it may be best to wean. Babies need love to flourish as well as nutrition.

Napping

Are you a good napper? When you are tired do you recognize the feeling and then lie down to rest with closed eyes (meaning, with no reading, no TV, radio, music, or other distractions)? Throughout my years of teaching, I continue to ask my clients if they are good nappers—most answer no. Then I ask them if they would like their babies to be good nappers and they *all* answer yes. Finally, the obvious question is asked: how will you teach your baby to be a good napper if you don't teach them by your own example? And, seriously, how tired will you be if you try to get through the childbearing year without naps? *Very, very tired,* and likely cranky and miserable. What will you/can you teach your family about sleep hygiene if you are walking around like a grumpy zombie? In fact, it's been found that in the United States many of us are already chronically under slept: "It is estimated that 50 to 70 million Americans chronically suffer from a disorder of sleep and wakefulness, hindering daily functioning and adversely affecting health and longevity."[404]

The good news is that you can build your napping skill set.[405] You will need to create time to practice. Try scheduling one nap on every day off between now and the baby's arrival. In your immediate postpartum period I guarantee you'll be in tears by 5:00pm if you haven't napped at all that day. Crying is good, crying isn't a bad thing, but being grumpy and sad from exhaustion sucks—for everyone. For new gestational parents during the postpartum period, the Bradley Method® recommends three one-hour naps per day. I think this is a good goal for partners, too!

As I have mentioned before *rest when your newborn rests.* Whether you like it or not, your baby is going to teach you a thing or two about your own sleep needs. I encourage you to embrace these lessons early on. Napping is a must to survive the postpartum adjustment period. Think about it: your baby isn't tired when she's awake, and when she is tired she goes to sleep. Babies sleep a lot when they are little. If you sleep when your baby sleeps, then you can get a lot of sleep, too. You can better transition through this time by having a good plan, and a good plan when you have a newborn is to sleep when the baby sleeps.

Directions for napping (they sound simple, but putting them into practice truly is a skill):

○ Make the room as dark and quiet as possible. (No phones or reading or music.)

○ Lay down and close your eyes.

○ Resist moving.

○ Try to relax your body and to quiet your mind by focusing on your breath.

- If you are tired, sleep will come.

- If sleep does not come, you will still reap restorative rewards from your rest.

- Sleep/rest for as long as your baby does! (Feel free to set a clock when practicing your napping skills before baby arrives.)

Baby's sleep

The current safe sleep guidelines from the American Academy of Pediatrics (AAP) indicate that your baby should sleep on her back, in a crib in your room, and with a pacifier in her mouth.[406] I am not telling you to disregard the AAP guidelines, but, as always, I encourage you to do further research. For example, both Dr. James A. McKenna[407] at Notre Dame University, who has done extensive research into mother/infant sleep sharing, and Dr. William Sears,[408] who is a pediatrician, author, and father of eight, both readily support the option of safe co-sleeping.

Understanding something about sleep cycles can help you make decisions as you negotiate with your newborn about sleep. Have you ever had the differing experiences when the alarm clock goes off and sometimes it's really hard to get up, even when you have had a pretty reasonable amount of sleep, while other times you're up easily, even when you haven't had an adequate number of hours? Whether you wake up easily or with more difficulty is usually attributed to where you are in your sleep cycle when the clock goes off. If you are in the deepest part of your cycle, then it is much harder to wake up. You and your baby can work toward aligning your cycles so that your night waking is less disruptive to your sleep needs.

For years I have been sharing the story of how my family learned to sleep well in a family bed. I do this not to convince anyone that they should make my same choices, but to encourage families to think outside the box. I want parents to understand that they are the experts of their family's needs and that with enough information parents can make their own best choices. Sleep is a critical element of family health. I encourage you to do whatever you need to do to reduce sleep struggles and cultivate sweet dreams for all.

The story of our family bed

During my first pregnancy I assumed that I would buy a crib and fix up the alcove we'd assigned as the new nursery. I knew I didn't know that much about parenting, yet I assumed that the one fact I did know was that babies sleep in cribs. So we bought a rocking chair and a foot stool to set beside the crib and a cute little mobile to hang over it. We were counseled to buy a drop-down crib and add bumpers to protect the baby from the edges. (Mobiles, drop down cribs, and padded bumpers are no longer considered safe. But in 1993 things were different.) It seemed to me that by purchasing these objects I would become a "mother." What I didn't know then was a lot, like cribs can present safety concerns, other mammals sleep with their young, and there is a strong, systemic belief in the U.S. that babies should be "independent sleepers." This idea of independent sleeping is a contemporary cultural construct and not an absolute truth about babies. I also didn't understand that being chronically tired meant I'd also be chronically unhappy. Nor did I know that when a baby first falls asleep, they go into a light sleep before shifting into a deeper sleep—and this is the opposite of adult sleep.[409] What this means is that when you try to transfer a baby that has just fallen asleep in your arms or elsewhere into a crib, they will usually wake up. Thus as I would rock and nurse and gentle my baby to sleep, and then try to put him down in his crib, he would wake up and start to fuss and want me to rock and nurse and gentle him back to sleep again (and again and again and again, in an unnerving cycle).

As both me and my baby grew more tired, we would both get more upset with the waking. When I did successfully get him to sleep in his crib (and this was not always a success), I would quickly retire to my own bed, exhausted. Just an hour or three later I would be woken up by my baby's early waking sounds—a grunt, a coo, a gurgle. I would pray to myself that he was merely shifting and that he would fall back asleep. He never did. Instead, he would continue his little grunts and coos and gurgles and then he would escalate quickly to screaming. To me, his first sounds translated to, *Hello. I am up, and I need you.* Then he would progress to an impatient, *Hey, where are you?! You're late!* And if I still wasn't there, he would explode in surging hysteria, something akin to *Oh my god, have you abandoned me completely and left me to be eaten by wolves, if I don't starve to death first?!* To which I'd respond in my head, "Alright. I get it, I am sorry. I thought you might just go back to sleep. I'm coming!" Then I would drag my sleepy butt out of bed and begin the cycle all over again:

○ Step 1: Pick him up and start to calm him down from his hysterical crying.

○ Step 2: Try to get the boob into the crying mouth.

○ Step 3: Settle into my rocking chair to nurse, rock, and gentle him back down.

○ Step 4: Try again to make the transfer back to the crib.

○ Step 4: Try again and again (and again and again).

There were many times when I tried just to pat his back to help him get back to sleep, without picking him up, but he never liked that and would only cry harder. I was exhausted nightly and daily, and I had growing stress about how I would be able to return to work on this kind of a sleep schedule.

One day, after a particularly tough night, with my return to work looming large, I called an older-than-me mother I had grown to trust, who also happened to be my own Bradley® instructor. I had reached out to her a few times before with questions and she had always been helpful and supportive. This time she asked me if I had ever brought my baby to bed. "What?! You can do that?!" I shouted. (I was clueless.) She explained that she had co-slept with all four of her children and that many breastfeeding mothers do, finding it more manageable. She said it was very important to consider safety, but once a few reasonable measures were taken, many families did it with great success. She outlined the dangers of suffocation from pillows, blankets, and any other objects that could cover the baby. She said we shouldn't bring the baby to bed if we slept on a waterbed, or if either of us were drunk or stoned or in any way altered in our awareness. And she said to be extremely mindful of the baby's proximity to the edge of the bed. She reminded me that even if my baby wasn't rolling over on his own today that could easily change by tomorrow. She had offered this information as something that I may want to consider, not as a directive. She went on to mention some resources on infant sleep and she offered support by saying that the best course of action would likely be the one that made the most sense for me. Finally, she encouraged me to discuss sleep concerns with my partner, and then we got off the phone. (See Appendix for infant sleep resources.)

It took me about a second to realize that I absolutely wanted to try it. I was desperate and wanted to try anything that might lead to more sleep. Bringing the baby into bed with us sounded logical and so much simpler. When Julian got home I discussed my plan and he was all in. He knew that being so tired all the time was making me sad and he was eager to try something like this if it meant we might all get a little more rest.

That same night we made our nest. The baby was between us with his own receiving blanket (a light-weight baby blanket). I had my own blanket and Julian had his, which ensured that neither of us would accidently pull our blanket over the baby. I then nursed the baby in bed until he fell asleep. I was so comfy all snuggled up near him that

I found myself dozing while nursing him. I woke up to him coming off my breast. He was sound asleep and, clearly, I had been, too. With us both in bed there was no need to stir him. I closed my eyes and was soon back asleep myself. A few hours later he made some gurgles alerting me to the fact that he was awake. I skootched over to him, pulled up my tee shirt and aided him as he latched on. Because I was right next to him, all he had to do was let me know he wanted to nurse with some little gurgles and coos. With no waiting time he had no reason to get upset; no crying! Because neither of us had to recover from his vigorous, wailing cries, this made it much quicker to get to the business of nursing and also much easier to get right back to sleep for both of us. He nursed a few more times before morning.

When we did get up in the morning Julian looked at me in disbelief and shock and said, "Oh my gosh, he slept through the night?!'

"No," I said. "But you did!"

To which Julian replied: "How many times did he get up? I can't believe I didn't hear him."

I couldn't answer him fully; the process—the whole night—had been so effortless. Was it two, three, or four times? I couldn't be sure. All I knew is that there was no crying; I didn't get out of bed; and I felt rested and happy for the first time in a long time. I was absolutely going to try this again.

Over the next couple of weeks of bed-sharing we were really finding our groove. There were still sleep disruptions but they were tolerable. We were enjoying the close proximity we had to each other as well as our own improved good cheer from the rest we were getting. Although I would still get up to change a diaper or to nurse, I had drastically reduced the impact of the night-wakings. More importantly, I was starting to feel the confidence build in my ability to parent. I started to see a glimmer of light towards a return to a place of stability and even began to think about work outside the house once again.

Then, as we were chugging comfortably along in our family bed, the slow dawn of a realization hit me: my baby was getting huge quickly! It seemed like my rapidly growing baby and my 6'4" husband were taking up the whole bed, leaving me to hover on the edge. I was getting anxious about my own lack of room to roll over coupled to the threat of my baby falling out of bed. Initially I was crest fallen, thinking that now we would have to go back to the crib and battle that battle all over again. I discussed these issues with Julian and we fielded different solutions. Suddenly, as Julian looked around our apartment, it was like a light bulb went off:

"Hey, let's get rid of our futon frame and put our mattress on the floor," he said. "That will take care of the worries about the baby falling out of bed. And then we can pull over that other futon, the one that we use folded up on the floor as an improvised couch, and we can put that mattress next to our existing one and we will have full sized areas to sleep on."

At first, I balked. Get rid of our furniture?! Convert our lovely multifunction studio apartment into one giant bedroom? How could we have guests over? Julian helped me to focus in on the immediate concern: we needed to improve our sleep. He reminded me to think outside the box. He reminded me that right then our only two priorities were safety and sleep. Okay. So out went the futon frame, and presto-change-o our studio apartment now looked like one giant futon-lined sleep area! I was a desperate momma willing to try anything that held the possibility of better sleep. And I was grateful to have a supportive partner by my side.

After the first night in our new set up I was sold for life. This appeared to be the ideal. There was ample and glorious room for each of us. Julian and I could have a whole futon to ourselves once the baby was asleep, and I could easily roll over to him if he woke up. Or, I could leave Julian and the baby on one futon and occasionally get the whole other futon to myself. Sheer bliss.

Not only did our sleep improve; we were deepening our connection to our baby. One morning I woke up to a grinning, happy husband and a jolly, smiling baby. Julian said, "I love having the baby in our bed. I feel like I get all these extra hours to cuddle." Our sleep cycles were getting in sync and sometimes I would even wake up moments before the baby, only to watch him open his eyes. It was magical and I couldn't believe how rested I was staying. I had completely believed that having a new baby would mean absolute exhaustion. Now I was finding out that this didn't have to be so. Our fears about the safety of bed sharing were calmed as we both experienced such an increased awareness of our son. I began to learn that sleeping with my child—for me—was not only happier and easier; it also felt safer. In fact, I felt that I was able to be vigilant even in my sleep because the close proximity felt protective rather than dangerous.

I called my Bradley® teacher back one day to report on how well things were going and to thank her for her generous support. I thanked her for not pushing ideas but rather for informing us of possibilities. As we were chatting, she shared some of her stories. She mentioned that she liked to wake her husband up if she ever had a bad dream or was frightened in the middle of the night. She would naturally turn to him for comfort and couldn't understand why that was okay for her to do, but a baby waking his momma up for comfort in the night was not. We discussed the strange cultural idea that babies must become independent sleepers.[410] Babies will and do become independent beings. But our sleep time together, for our family, helped to improve our intimacy and trust in all our interactions.

Meanwhile, the backlash we faced from some of our friends was astounding. One person said that having the baby in our bed was a sign that our marriage was in trouble. Another person assumed that this meant that we would be unable to have sex. And still another comment we received was that our baby would *never* be independent. I am sure all such comments were well-intentioned and meant to be informative, even supportive, but we were not amused. Once Julian responded, "Geez, if you only have sex in your bed I feel sorry for you! If the baby is in our bed, then we still have the kitchen, the bathroom, the living room, the hallway… you name it!" (I blushed with embarrassment in the moment, but we laughed hysterically about it later.)

On that note, our only chance of having any energy for sexual intimacy was if we were getting enough rest. And having the baby in bed with us was bringing us closer together as a family, not tearing us apart. There is no single approach or solution that fits every family, but we knew that, for our family, this was the best change we could make. Parenting a baby is hard work, damn hard work. So if what we were doing seemed to be working out well, we were going to keep doing it. Our baby was cheerful and good humored, and we were starting to feel that way, too.

We continued with the family bed for as long as our children needed it. I believe that when children have developmental needs and they are met, then they mature out of them as soon as they are ready. Each boy eventually had his own bed. When Arlo was born, Jasper had already been sleeping in his own room for some time. And both boys were happily independent enough to go to grandma's house for the weekend by age three.

The new challenge, with two boys, was how to lie down and read bedtime stories with Jasper while also nursing and caring for baby Arlo. Empowered by Julian's earlier problem solving and parenting brilliance, we decided to move our recently acquired king size mattress onto the floor in baby Arlo's room. Then Jasper and I started to sleep with the baby, in the baby's room, on the king mattress on the floor. Nirvana again. I could lie down and nurse the baby while reading bedtime stories with Jasper. We could all snuggle and sleep bond. Julian was free to come and join us or he could sleep in another bed we set up in our own room. Eventually I weaned myself out of the baby's room and the two brothers slept together for several years.

Then one day 6-year-old Arlo kicked 12-year-old Jasper out of his bed: "Get out and sleep in your own room! Your feet and your farts stink and you steal the blankets!" Jasper was a bit shocked, but he was also ready to become a teenager in his own space.

And with that, you, dear reader, are ready too! You have taken in a tremendous amount of practical information, and you are now ready for your birth journey from pregnancy to childbirth to postpartum and beyond! I hope you have enjoyed yourselves throughout our time together and that you have gained greater and greater confidence in the birth process and your own abilities. Thank you for taking this time to prepare for your family life. I trust that you are now more equipped to make your own best family healthcare choices; well motivated to continue practicing conscientious breath and labor coping techniques; and empowered to define your own journey. Eat well, rest well, exercise, and love fiercely. Continue to evaluate and communicate with care providers, partners, family, and friends. Investigate your options for birth classes and breastfeeding support groups. Practice reciprocity with other new families and look to build support for your postpartum adjustment. Together, we will go forth and do our work for a just and peaceful world.

I wish you and your family a love-filled and productive life. With admiration and joy I wish you a final congratulations—you made it to the end of this pregnancy guide! I know it took a conscientious effort. I bet your biceps have gotten so strong from repeatedly lifting this heavy content! Know that you can return to any part of this book anytime you need it. I am confident your baby will appreciate your new strengths. I wish you good health, happiness and courage. I would be thrilled to hear how you're doing or to receive any feedback you have on this course. You can reach me through my website: www.ConscientiousBirth.com. Now I say goodbye with one final image to help you realize your amazing potential to open wide. Behold the Sheela Na Gig:

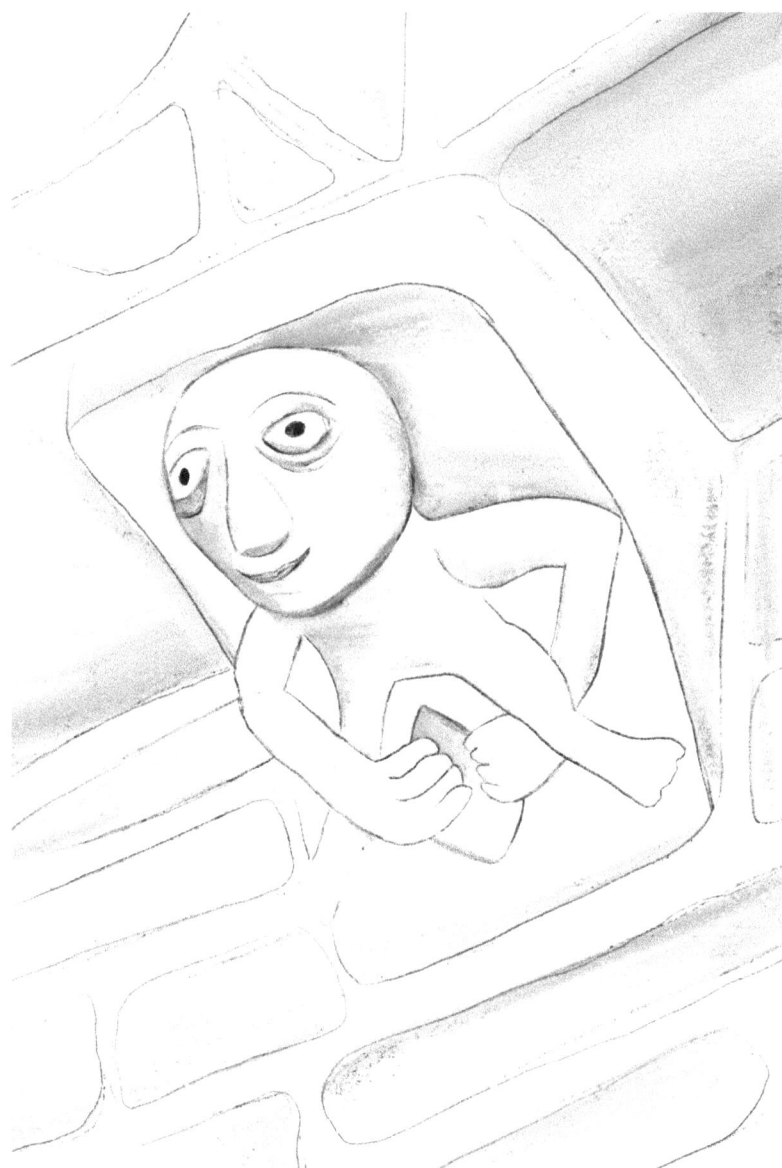

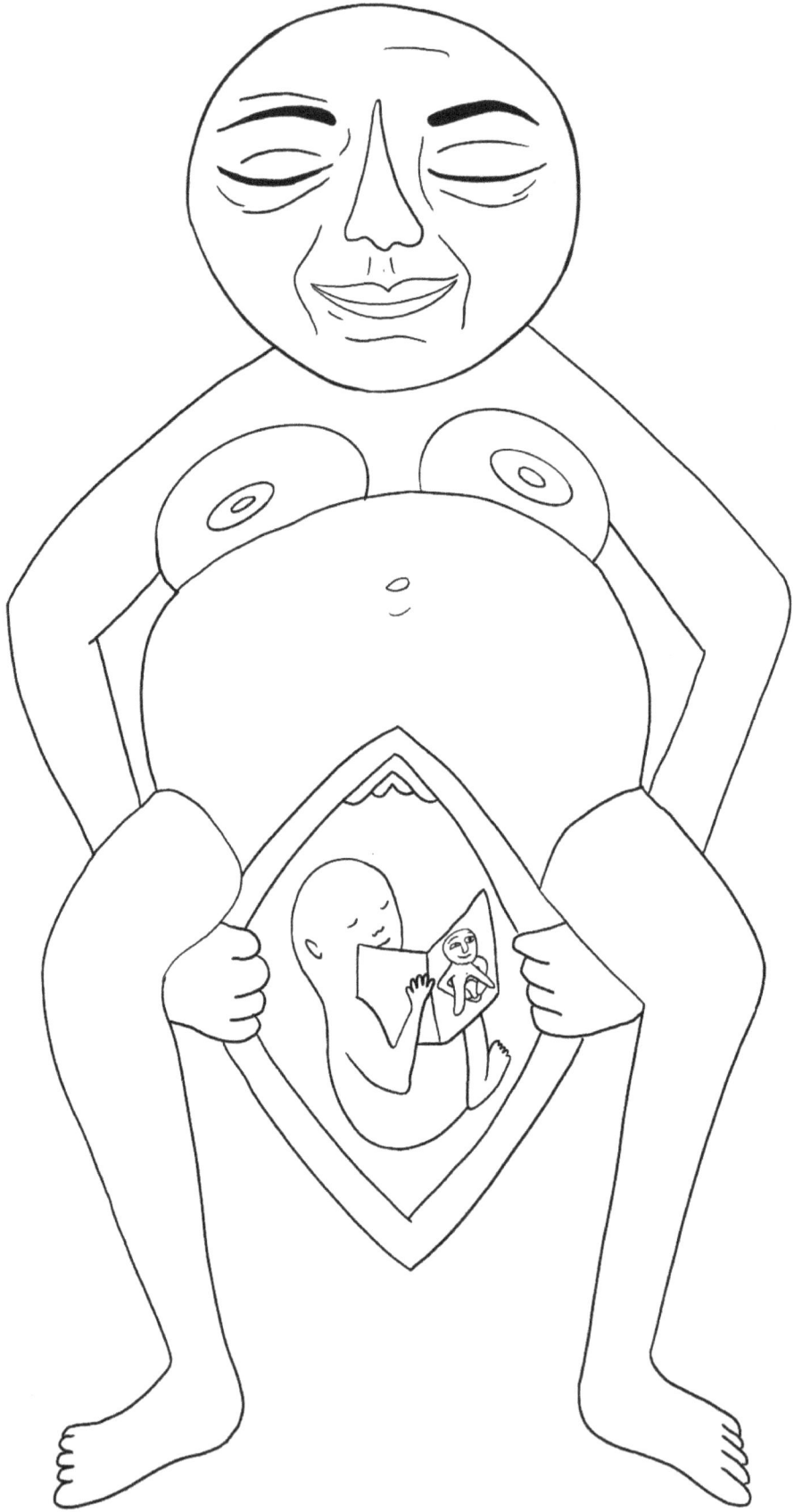

Acknowledgements

A very special thank you to my editor—my book-midwife—Janelle A. Schwartz, she expertly and compassionately guided me to find my voice and make it readable. She was a steadfast support through the hardest parts of birthing my author-self. I also want to thank the outstanding humans that generously shaped my birth education: Tisha Graham, Betsy Mercogliano, Heidi Ricks, Carrie Kimball, Lisa Preller, Vicki Nolan Marnin, K. Michelle Doyle, and Sandy Jamrog. To Shennan Jarboe and Rebeca Torres, I am grateful beyond measure for your willingness to share your experiences, thank you. I am equally grateful for my time with Luca and Jackson, I visualize their spirits playing at various ages. Anni Rudegeair, Arden McCrossan, Dan McCrossan, Sydney Klugman, Bobbi, Sherman, and Jerry Sherman, thank you! And a giant thanks to Anna Schupack: your courage, your skill, and your ability to read my mind as we brought Sheela to life made working with you a joyful and often hilarious experience. Thank you to Karen Schupack for your continued technical assistance, and for growing magnificent Anna! And a special debt of gratitude to the countless other providers, families, and individuals that have taught me, encouraged me, contributed their stories, and allowed me into their lives through their most intimate transformations to family life. Thank you also to Rachel Gartner, your friendship is my oxygen. And finally, a very special thank you to my true love, Julian Marynczak who said, "Em, you really must write a book!" I am overwhelmed with gratitude and deeply indebted to you all. Without your honesty, support, patience, and love, this book would never have come through its own protracted, and empowering, trying, birth process.

REFERENCES

Preface and introduction

1   John Harding, "Sheela Na Gig," in *Britannica*, June 6, 2016, https://www.britannica.com/art/Sheela-Na-Gig.

2   Dana-Ain Davis, *Reproductive Injustice: Racism, Pregnancy, and Premature Birth* (NYU Press, 2019), https://nyupress.org/9781479853571/reproductive-injustice/.

3   Judith Lothian, "Safe, Healthy Birth: What Every Pregnant Woman Needs to Know," *Journal of Perinatal Education* 18, no. 3 (2009): 48–54, https://doi.org/105812409X461225.

4   Marsden Wagner, *Born in the USA: How a Broken Maternity System Must Be Fixed to Put Women and Children First* (University of California Press, 2006), https://www.amazon.com/Born-USA-Broken-Maternity-Children/dp/0520256336.

5   Roosa Tikkanen et al., "Maternal Mortality and Maternity Care in the United States Compared to 10 Other Developed Countries," Common Wealth Fund, November 18, 2020, https://www.commonwealthfund.org/publications/issue-briefs/2020/nov/maternal-mortality-maternity-care-us-compared-10-countries.

Week 1

6   Wayne State University Physician Group, "Alpha-Fetoprotein Screening," Wayne State University Physician Group, 2020, http://www.wsupgdocs.org/family-medicine/WayneStateContentPage.aspx?nd=1727.

7   Mayo Clinic, "Mayo Clinic Laboratories," Mayo Clinic Laboratories, 2020, https://www.mayocliniclabs.com/test-catalog/Clinical+and+Interpretive/113382.

8   The Fetal Medicine Center, "Harmony Test," The Fetal Medicine Center, 2020, https://fetalmedicine.com/harmony-test.

9   Mayo Clinic Staff, "Amniocentesis," Amniocentesis, March 8, 2019, http://www.mayoclinic.com/health/amniocentesis/MY00155/DSECTION=risks.

10 Julia Belluz, "We Finally Have a New US Maternal Mortality Estimate. It's Still Terrible.," *Vox*, January 30, 2020, https://www.sciencedaily.com/releases/2013/01/130130101839.htm.

11 Wayne State University Physician Group, "Alpha-Fetoprotein Screening."

12 Sarah Buckley, "Executive Summary of Hormonal Physiology of Childbearing: Evidence and Implications for Women, Babies, and Maternity Care," *Journal of Perinatal Education* 24, no. 3 (2015): 145–53, https://doi.org/10.1891/1058-1243.24.3.145.

13 "Your Baby in the Birth Canal," MedlinePlus, 2020, https://medlineplus.gov/ency/article/002060.htm.

14 CDC, "Rates of Cesarean Delivery," MMWR Weekly, 1993, https://www.cdc.gov/mmwr/preview/mmwrhtml/00036845.htm.

15 Centers for Disease Control and Prevention, "Method of Delivery," CDC.gov, February 7, 2022, https://www.cdc.gov/nchs/fastats/delivery.htm.

16 James Nestor, *Breath, The New Science of a Lost Art* (Penguin Random House UK, 2020).

17 Saleem Reshamwala and Dan Harris, "Welcome to the Dread Project," 10 Percent Happier/More Than A Feeling, n.d., 2022, https://www.tenpercent.com/mtaf-podcast-episodes/welcome-to-the-dread-project.

Week 2

18 Annie Murphy Paul, "How the First Nine Months Shape the Rest of Your Life: Cancer. Heart Disease. Obesity. Depression. The New Science of Fetal Origins Traces Adult Health to Our Experiences in the Womb," *Time Magazine*, September 20, 2010.

19 Murphy Paul.

20 M Magley, "Eclampsia," Stat Pearls, January 2022, Magley M, Hinson MR. Eclampsia. [Updated 2022 Feb 16]. In: StatPearls [Internet]. Treasure Island (FL): StatPearls Publishing; 2022 Jan-. Available from: https://www.ncbi.nlm.nih.gov/books/NBK554392/.

21 Lily Nichols RDN, CDC, *Real Food for Pregnancy, The Science and Wisdom of Optimal Prenatal Nutritionisbn*, 2018.

22 R. Elango and RO Ball, "Protein and Amino Acid Requirements during Pregnancy.," *Pub Med Central*, July 15, 2016, https://doi.org/10.3945/an.115.011817.

23 Gail Sforza Brewer and Thomas Brewer, *What Every Pregnant Woman Should Know: The Truth about Diet and Drugs in Pregnancy* (Penguin Books, 1985).

24 Kris Gunnars, "Why Are Eggs Good for You?," *Healthline*, April 26, 2018, https://www.healthline.com/nutrition/why-are-eggs-good-for-you.

25 Sforza Brewer and Brewer, *What Every Pregnant Woman Should Know: The Truth about Diet and Drugs in Pregnancy*.

26 "Floradix," Flora, accessed June 15, 2020, https://www.florahealth.com/us/floradix/.

27 Staff Cleveland Clinic, "Can You Have a Safe Vegetarian Pregnacny? Planning and Variety Are 2 Keys to Success," Medical, Cleveland Clinic.org, July 8, 2020, https://health.clevelandclinic.org/can-you-safely-have-a-vegetarian-pregnancy/.

28 Staff Drugs and Lactation Database, "Vitamin B12.," *LactMed Internet. National Library of Medicine (US)*, October 18, 2021, https://www.ncbi.nlm.nih.gov/books/NBK534419/.

29 Alina Petre, "7 Supplements You Need on a Vegan Diet," *Healthline*, October 15, 2019, https://www.healthline.com/nutrition/7-supplements-for-vegans.

30 R. Raghavan et al., "Maternal Multivitamin Intake, Plasma Folate and Vitamin B 12Levels and Autism Spectrum Disorder Risk in Offspring," *Paediatr Perinat Epidemiol*, January 3, 2017, https://doi.org/10.1111/ppe.12414.

31 Ashley Marcin and Kay Carolyn, "Is It Safe to Consume Soy Products While Pregnant?," *Healthline*, March 30, 2021, https://www.healthline.com/health/pregnancy/soy-pregnancy.

32 Reed Mangels, *The Everything Vegan Pregnancy BookThe Everything Vegan Pregnancy Book* (Adams Media, 2011).

33 Ram Chandyo et al., "The Effects of Vitamin B12 Supplementation in Pregnancy and Postpartum on Growth and Neurodevelopment in Early Childhood: Study Protocol for a Randomized Placebo Controlled Trial," *BMJ* 7, no. 8 (2017), https://doi.org/10.1136/bmjopen-2017-016434. "The Effects of Vitamin B12 Supplementation in Pregnancy and Postpartum on Growth and Neurodevelopment in Early Childhood: Study Protocol for a Randomized Placebo Controlled Trial."

34 Chandyo et al.

35 "Vitamin B12," Centers for Disease Control and Prevention, December 14, 2019, https://www.cdc.gov/breastfeeding/breastfeeding-special-circumstances/diet-and-micronutrients/vitamin-b12.html.

36 Inaki Lete and Jose Allue, "The Effectiveness of Ginger in the Prevention of Nausea and Vomiting during Pregnancy and Chemotherapy," *US National Library of Medicine*, 2016, 11–17, https://doi.org/10.4137/IMI.S36273.

37 Louis Aronne, "Food Order Has Significant Impact on Glucose and Insulin Levels," *Weill Cornell Medicine*, June 23, 2015, https://news.weill.cornell.edu/news/2015/06/food-order-has-significant-impact-on-glucose-and-insulin-levels-louis-aronne.

38 S. Kobylewski and MF Jacobson, "Toxicology of Food Dyes.," *Int J Occup Environ Health.*, 2012, https://doi.org/10.1179/1077352512Z.00000000034.

39 F Hytten, "Blood Volume Changes in Normal Pregnancy," *PubMed* 14, no. 3 (October 1985): 601–12.

40 M Magley, "Eclampsia."

41 Camille Powe, Richard Levine, and S. Ananth Karumanchi, "Preeclampsia, a Disease of the Maternal Endothelium," *Circulation*, June 21, 2011, 2856–69, https://doi.org/10.1161/CIRCULATIONAHA.109.853127.

42 Sforza Brewer and Brewer, *What Every Pregnant Woman Should Know: The Truth about Diet and Drugs in Pregnancy*.

43 Jennifer Crowley, PhD, Lauren Ball, PhD, and Prof Gerrit Jan Hiddink, PhD, "Nutrition in Medical Education: A Systematic Review," *The Lancet* 3, no. 9 (September 1, 2019), https://www.thelancet.com/journals/lanplh/article/PIIS2542-5196(19)30171-8/fulltext.

44 Mayo Clinic Staff, "Preeclampsia," Mayo Clinic, 2020, https://news.weill.cornell.edu/news/2015/06/food-order-has-significant-impact-on-glucose-and-insulin-levels-louis-aronne.

45 Mayo Clinic Staff.

46   Jennifer Savage, Jennifer Orlet Fisher, and Leann Birch, "Parental Influence on Eating Behavior Conception to Adolescence," *US National Library of Medicine* 35, no. 1 (2007): 22–34, https://doi.org/10.1111/j.1748-720X.2007.00111.x.

47   World Health Organization, *Promoting Optimal Fetal Development* (World Health Organization), accessed July 28, 2015, https://www.who.int/nutrition/publications/fetomaternal/9241594004/en/.

48   Robert Schneider et al., "Stress Reduction in the Secondary Prevention of Cardiovascular Disease," *Circulation: Cardiovascular Quality and Outcomes* 5, no. 6 (n.d.): 750–58, https://doi.org/10.1161/CIRCOUTCOMES.112.967406.

49   Sara Bernard, "Neuroplasticity: Learning Physically Changes the Brain," October 1, 2010, https://www.edutopia.org/neuroscience-brain-based-learning-neuroplasticity.

50   Thich Nhat Hanh, *Happiness, Essential Mindfulness PracticesNhat Hanh, Thich. Happiness (EasyRead Comfort Edition). N.p., ReadHowYouWant.Com.* (Read How You Want.com, 2009).

51   Nhat Hanh.

52   Ina May Gaskin, *Ina May's Guide to Childbirth* (Bantam Books, 2003).

53   Gaskin.

Week 3

54   Serena Solomon, "Using Sports Psychology for Childbirth," *The New York Times*, January 15, 2019, https://www.nytimes.com/2019/01/15/well/family/using-sports-psychology-for-childbirth.html?auth=login-facebook&searchResultPosition=2.

55   Linda Szyamski and Andrew Satin, "Exercise During Pregnancy: Fetal Responses to Current Public Health Guidelines," *US National Library of Medicine* 119, no. 3 (2012): 603–10, https://doi.org/10.1097/AOG.0b013e31824760b5.

56   Roger Hammer, Jan Perkins, and Richard Parr, "Exercise During the Childbearing Year," *The Journal of Perinatal Education* 9, no. 1 (2000): 1–14, https://doi.org/10.1624/105812400X87455.

57   Board of Trustees of the University of Alabama, "Recommendations for Exercise In Pregnancy and Postpartum," NCHPAD Building Healthy Inclusive Communities, 2020, https://www.nchpad.org/17/104/Exercise~During~Pregnancy.

58   Cleveland Clinic, "Rated Perceived Exertion (RPE) Scale," Cleveland Clinic, February 25, 2019, https://my.clevelandclinic.org/health/articles/17450-rated-perceived-exertion-rpe-scale.

59   Cleveland Clinic.

60   American Academy of Family Physicians, "Sleep and Pregnancy," familydoctor.org, 2020, https://familydoctor.org/getting-enough-sleep-pregnancy/.

61   "Exercise and Depression," WebMD, 2020, https://www.webmd.com/depression/guide/exercise-depression#1.

62   Louise Barrett, "Cognition and the Modular Brain," in *Human Evolutionary Psychology* (Princeton University Press, 2002), 289, https://books.google.com/books?id=tVVtDwAAQBAJ&pg=PA289&lpg=PA289&dq=feelings+are+inextricably+bound+to+our+endocrine&source=bl&ots=4cIZPI18-Q&sig=ACfU3U2MncGQqUNe7KPOJNA0GoMo3ECb_A&hl=en&sa=X&ved=2ahUKEwiomvKTxKPqAhW0mHIEHShuANIQ6AEwAHoECAkQAQ#v=onepage&q=feelings%20are%20inextricably%20bound%20to%20our%20endocrine&f=false.

63   "Hormones," Prospec Protein Specialists, 2020, https://www.prospecbio.com/hormones.

64   Society for Endocrinology, "Relaxin," You and your hormones, March 2018, https://www.yourhormones.info/hormones/relaxin/.

65   The Johns Hopkins University, "Nutrition During Pregnancy," Johns Hopkins Medicine, 2020, https://www.hopkinsmedicine.org/health/wellness-and-prevention/nutrition-during-pregnancy.

66   Mother and Child Health and Education Trust, "Malnutrition," Mother and Child Nutrition, 2020, https://motherchildnutrition.org/malnutrition/about-malnutrition/impact-of-malnutrition.html.

67   "NICHD Research Weighs in on Weight Gain during Pregnancy," NIH, September 28, 2013, https://www.nichd.nih.gov/newsroom/resources/spotlight/082813-pregnancy-weight.

68   Mayo Clinic Mayo Clinic Staff, "Friendships: Enrich Your Life and Improve Your Health," Heatlhy Lifestyle, Adult Health, MayoClinic.org, July 1, 2022, https://www.mayoclinic.org/healthy-lifestyle/adult-health/in-depth/friendships/art-20044860.

69   Sanna Lignell et al., "Environmental Organic Pollutants in Human Milk before and after Weight Loss," *Chemosphere* 159 (2016): 96–102, https://doi.org/10.1016/j.chemosphere.2016.05.077.

70   "Maternal Diet," Centers for Disease Control and Prevention, February 10, 2020, https://www.cdc.gov/breastfeeding/breastfeeding-special-circumstances/diet-and-micronutrients/maternal-diet.html.

71   Mayo Clinic Staff, "Labor and Delivery, Postpartum Care," Mayo Clinic, 2020, https://www.mayoclinic.org/healthy-lifestyle/labor-and-delivery/in-depth/weight-loss-after-pregnancy/art-20047813.

72   UCLA Health, "Pelvic Floor Disorders," Center for Women's Pelvic Health at UCLA, accessed June 30, 2020, https://www.uclahealth.org/womens-pelvic-health/pelvic-floor-disorders.

73   "Vaginal Lubrication," ScienceDirect, 2020, cite https://www.sciencedirect.com/topics/medicine-and-dentistry/vaginal-lubrication.

74   Serena Ng, "As Births Slow, P&G Turns to Adult Diapers," *The Wall Street Journal*, July 16, 2014, https://www.wsj.com/articles/as-births-slow-p-g-turns-to-adult-diapers-1405554364.

75   Debra Pascali-Bonaro, *Orgasmic Birth* (Orgasmic Birth), accessed June 17, 2020, https://www.orgasmicbirth.com/products/films-soundtrack/#content.

76   "Kim Anami," 2020, https://kimanami.com/. http://kimanami.com/vaginal-kung-fu/.

77   Kim Anami, "Kim Anami," KimAnami.com, 2020, https://kimanami.com/.

78   *Aligned and Well Down There For Women*, 2012, https://www.youtube.com/watch?v=WR7C-fQkkOY.

79   "Your Baby in the Birth Canal," MedlinePlus, 2020, https://medlineplus.gov/ency/article/002060.htm.

80   Joseph McArdle, Les Michelson, and Albert D'Alonzo, "Action Potentials in Fast- and Slow-Twitch Mammalian Muscles during Reinnervation and Development," *Journal of General Physiology* 75, no. 6 (June 1, 1980): 655–72, https://doi.org/10.1085/jgp.75.6.655.

81   Florence Williams, *Breasts: A Natural and Unnatural History* (W. W. Norton & Company, Inc, 2012), https://www.amazon.com/Breasts-Natural-Unnatural-Florence-Williams/dp/0393345076.

82   Debbi Goodman, "Pilates and Pregnancy: Safe Ab Exercises," Pilates Pro The Pulse of the Industry, 2008, https://pilates-pro.com/pilates-pro/2008/8/18/pilates-and-pregnancy-safe-ab-exercises.html.

Week 4

83   Dominic Polcino, "The Canine Mutiny," *The Simpsons* (Fox, April 13, 1997), https://en.wikipedia.org/wiki/The_Canine_Mutiny.

84   Healthline Editorial Team, "Labor and Delivery: Types of Midwives," healthline Parenthood, 2016, https://www.healthline.com/health/pregnancy/intrapartum-care-midwife#types-of-midwives.

85   "Medicaid Benefits: Nurse Midwife Services," State Health Facts, 2018, https://www.kff.org/medicaid/state-indicator/nurse-midwife-services/?currentTimeframe=0&sortModel=%7B%22colId%22:%22Location%22,%22sort%22:%22asc%22%7D.

86   "OB Guideline 15: Assessment and Monitoring in Labor and Delivery," crico, 2017, https://www.rmf.harvard.edu/Clinician-Resources/Guidelines-Algorithms/2017/OB-Guideline-Files/Guideline15-Assessment-and-Monitoring-in-Labor-and-Delivery.

87   March of Dimes, "Placental Abruption," March of Dimes, accessed March 2, 2022, https://www.marchofdimes.org/mission/march-of-dimes-leadership.aspx.

88   Rachel Naomi Remen, *Kitchen Table Wisdom: Stories That Heal* (The Berkley Publishing Group Penguin Group, 1994), http://www.rachelremen.com/books/kitchen-table-wisdom/.

89   Remen.

90   Kerasidou, Angeliki, and Ruth Horn., "'Making Space for Empathy: Supporting Doctors in the Emotional Labour of Clinical Care.' BMC Medical Ethics Vol. 17 8. 27 Jan. 2016, Doi:10.1186/S12910-016-0091-7," *BMC Medical Ethics* 17 8 (January 27, 2016).

91   Meghan Bohren et al., "Continuous Support for Women During Childbirth," *US National Library of Medicine* 7, no. 7 (2017), https://doi.org/10.1002/14651858.CD003766.pub6.

92   American College of Nurse-Midwives, "Our Philosophy of Care," American College of Nurse-Midwives, accessed July 15, 2020, https://www.midwife.org/Our-Philosophy-of-care.

93   Wagner, *Born in the USA: How a Broken Maternity System Must Be Fixed to Put Women and Children First* (University of California Press, 2006), https://www.amazon.com/Born-USA-Broken-Maternity-Children/dp/0520256336.

94   "La Leche Leauge International," 2020, https://www.llli.org/.

95   Paul Anderson, "Paul's Submission," 2009.

96   James Madison, "United States Constitution," August 18, 1787.

97   Staff Guttmacher Institute, "Substance Abuse During Pregnancy," Guttmacher Institute, 2022, https://www.guttmacher.org/state-policy/explore/substance-use-during-pregnancy.

98   Staff Centers for Disease Control and Prevention, "Data and Statistics on Birth Defects," Centers for Disease Control and Prevention, 2020, https://www.cdc.gov/ncbddd/birthdefects/data.html.

99   M.R. Torloni et al., "Safety of Ultrasonography in Pregnancy: WHO Systematic Review of the Literature and Meta-Analysis," *Wiley InterScience Online*, March 17, 2009, https://obgyn.onlinelibrary.wiley.com/doi/pdf/10.1002/uog.6328.

100   Kaelin A. Agten et al., "Routine Ultrasound for Fetal Assessment before 24 Weeks' Gestation.," *Cochrane Database of Systematic Reviews*, no. 8 (2021), https://doi.org/10.1002/14651858.CD014698.

101   Vanessa Burrows, FDA Historian, "Why X-Rays in Shoe Stores Were a Really Bad Idea," Medical Design & Outsourcing, May 23, 2017, https://www.medicaldesignandoutsourcing.com/radiating-shoe-sales/.

102   Shankar Shankar, Paul S. Pagel, and David S. Warner, "Potential Adverse Ultrasound-Related Biological Effects: A Critical Review," *Anesthesiology* 115:1109–1124 (2011), https://doi.org/10.1097/ALN.0b013e31822fd1f1.

103   Julia Milner and Jane Arezina, "The Accuracy of Ultrasound Estimation of Fetal Weight in Comparison to Birth Weight: A Systematic Review.," *Ultrasound (Leeds, England)* 26,1 (2018): 32-41. doi:10.1177/1742271X17732807 (February 7, 2018), https://www.ncbi.nlm.nih.gov/pmc/articles/PMC5810856/.

104   Rebecca Dekker, "What Is the Evidence for Induction for Low Fluid at Term in a Healthy Pregnancy?," Evidence Based Birth, August 30, 2012, https://evidencebasedbirth.com/what-is-the-evidence-for-induction-for-low-fluid-at-term-in-a-healthy-pregnancy/.

105   "What Is Relaxin?," Hormone Health Network, 2020, https://www.hormone.org/your-health-and-hormones/glands-and-hormones-a-to-z/hormones/relaxin.

106   The Editors of Encyclopaedia Britannica, "Corpus Luteum," Encyclopaedia Britannica, 2020, https://www.britannica.com/science/corpus-luteum.

107   Gloria Lemay, "Pelvises I Have Known and Loved," *Midwifery Today*, 1999, https://midwiferytoday.com/mt-articles/pelvises-known-loved/.

108   R. Bowen, "Placental Hormones," August 6, 2000, http://www.vivo.colostate.edu/hbooks/pathphys/reprod/placenta/endocrine.html.

109   The Editors of Encyclopaedia Britannica, "The Uterus and the Development of the Placenta," Encyclopaedia Britannica, 2020, https://www.britannica.com/science/pregnancy/The-uterus-and-the-development-of-the-placenta.

110   Kelly Young, "CDC Warns Against Consumption of Dried Placenta Capsules," *New England Journal of Medicine Journal Watch*, June 30, 2017, https://www.jwatch.org/fw113049/2017/06/30/cdc-warns-against-consumption-dried-placenta-capsules.

111   Patricia Guthrie, Cox News Service, "MANY CULTURES REVERE PLACENTA, BYPRODUCT OF CHILDBIRTH," *Chicago Tribune*, July 7, 1999, https://www.chicagotribune.com/news/ct-xpm-1999-07-07-9907070031-story.html.

112   *Amazing Talents of the Newborn*, DVD Video (Johnson & Johnson, 2011), https://www.worldcat.org/title/amazing-talents-of-the-newborn/oclc/857504358.

113   March of Dimes, "Health Topic: Stillbirth," March of Dimes, n.d., https://www.marchofdimes.org/complications/stillbirth.aspx.

114   Committee Opinion ACOG, "Delayed Umbilical Cord Clamping After Birth," American College of Obstetrics and Gynocologists Committee on obstetric practice, December 2020, https://www.acog.org/clinical/clinical-guidance/committee-opinion/articles/2020/12/delayed-umbilical-cord-clamping-after-birth.

115   Cari Nierenberg, "What Makes an Innie an Innie? And More Belly Button Mysteries," News, May 16, 2011, https://www.nbcnews.com/healthmain/what-makes-innie-innie-more-belly-button-mysteries-1C6437359.

116 Staff Cleveland Clinic, "Fundal Height," Patient Education, Cleveland Clinic, 2022, https://my.clevelandclinic.org/health/diagnostics/22294-fundal-height.

117 Gaskin, *Ina May's Guide to Childbirth* (Bantam Books, 2003).

118 Morgan Craig, Sneha Sudanagunta, and Megan Billow, "Anatomy, Abdomen and Pelvis, Broad Ligaments," *Statpearls*, 2020, https://www.ncbi.nlm.nih.gov/books/NBK499943/.

119 *Counting Breaths Meditation' - For Meditation Dreamers and Dropouts!*, 2021, https://www.youtube.com/watch?v=7Q_90_856RU&t=1320s.

120 "Yes, Pregnancy Affects Your Digestion," Gastrointestinal Specialists, 2022, https://www.gastrova.com/article/pregnancy-and-your-digestion/.

Week 5

121 "Changes in the Gastrointestinal System in Pregnancy," Moodle, 2014, https://moodle.digital-campus.org/mod/page/view.php?id=17796.

122 "Postpartum Hemorrhoids and Other Pains in the Butt," MamaMend, 2019, https://www.mamamend.com/postpartum-health/postpartum-hemorrhoids.

123 "The Consequences of Stress during Pregnancy," American Psychological Association, 2018, https://www.apa.org/monitor/2018/06/stress-pregnancy.

124 "Pica Cravings During Pregnancy," American Pregnancy Association, 2019, https://americanpregnancy.org/is-it-safe/unusual-cravings-pica/.

125 "Stress," Anxiety and Depression Association of America, 2018, https://adaa.org/understanding-anxiety/related-illnesses/stress.

126 "Are Congestion and Nosebleeds Normal during the Second Trimeseter of Pregnancy?," Grow by WebMD, 2018, https://www.webmd.com/baby/qa/are-congestion-and-nosebleeds-normal-during-the-second-trimester-of-pregnancy.

127 Judith Orloff, "The Healing Power of Tears," Judith Orloff M.D., 2020, https://drjudithorloff.com/the-healing-power-of-tears/.

128 Staff Johns Hopkins, "Labor," Medical, Johns Hopkins Medicine, 2022, https://www.hopkinsmedicine.org/health/wellness-and-prevention/labor.

129 Andrew McCarthy and Bill Hunter, *Obstetrics and Gynaecology* (Peking University Medical Press, 2003), https://www.worldcat.org/title/obstetrics-and-gynaecology-a-core-text-with-self-assessment/oclc/308641988.

130 McCarthy and Hunter.

131 McCarthy and Hunter.

132 Alan DeCherney et al., *Current Diagnosis & Treatment Obstetrics & Gynecology*, 12th ed. (McGraw Hill, 2019), https://www.amazon.com/Diagnosis-Treatment-Obstetrics-Gynecology-Gynecologic/dp/0071833900.

133 Mayo Clinic Staff, "Labor and Delivery, Postpartum Care," Mayo Clinic, 2020, https://www.mayoclinic.org/healthy-lifestyle/labor-and-delivery/in-depth/weight-loss-after-pregnancy/art-20047813.

134 "Muscle Fiber Contraction and Relaxation," ER Services, accessed July 1, 2020, http://cnx.org/contents/14fb4ad7-39a1-4eee-ab6e-3ef2482e3e22@7.1@7.1.

135 "Labor Contractions," Sutter Health, 2020, citehttps://www.sutterhealth.org/health/labor-delivery/labor-contractions.

136 Sandbox & Co, "First Stage of Labor," familyeducation, accessed July 1, 2020, https://www.familyeducation.com/pregnancy/dilation-effacement/first-stage-labor.

137 April Ronca et al., "Effects of Labor Contractions on Catecholamine Release and Breathing Frequency in Newborn Rats," *US National Library of Medicine* 120, no. 6 (2006): 1308–14, https://doi.org/10.1037/0735-7044.120.6.1308.

138 Barbara Hotelling, "From Psychoprophylactic to Orgasmic Birth," *Journal of Perinatal Education* 18, no. 4 (Fall 2009): 45–48, https://doi.org/10.1624/105812409X474708.

Week 6

139 Gaskin, *Ina May's Guide to Childbirth* (Bantam Books, 2003).

140 Amy Cuddy, *Your Body Language Shapes Who You Are* (TEDGLOBAL, 2012), http://www.ted.com/talks/amy_cuddy_your_body_language_shapes_who_you_are?language=en.

141 Cuddy.

142 Daniel Miller, "Try Getting Past This Lot! Elephants Huddle Round Female to Protect Her from Prowling Hyenas While She Gives Birth," News, Daily Mail, February 29, 2012, https://www.dailymail.co.uk/news/article-2108183/Herd-elephants-huddles-round-female-gives-birth.html.

143 Zawn Villines and Holly Ernst, "Can Dehydration Affect Pregnancy?," Medical News Today, June 22, 2018, https://www.medical-newstoday.com/articles/322230.

144 Jill Seladi-Schulman, Ph.D and Alana Biggers M.D. MPH, "Can Dehydration Affect Your Blood Pressure?," Healthline News, January 15, 2020, https://www.healthline.com/health/dehydration-and-blood-pressure.

145 Anisha Nair, "Is Vomiting During Labor Helpful?," firstcry parenting, 2018, https://parenting.firstcry.com/articles/is-vomiting-during-labour-helpful/.

Week 7

146 Sara Kassabian et al., "Building a Global Policy Agenda to Prioritize Preterm Birth: A Qualitative Analysis on Factors Shaping Global Health Policymaking," *Pub Med Central* 4:65 (June 22, 2020), https://www.ncbi.nlm.nih.gov/pmc/articles/PMC7578407/.

147 Olivia Campbell, "Here's What Happened When Reagan Went after Healthcare Programs. It's Not Good.," Timeline, September 13, 2017, https://timeline.com/reagan-trump-healthcare-cuts-8cf64aa242eb.

148 RE Behrman and AS Butler, "Preterm Birth: Causes, Consequences, and Prevention," *National Academies Press (US)*, 2007, https://www.ncbi.nlm.nih.gov/books/NBK11385/.

149 Dana-Ain Davis, *Reproductive Injustice: Racism, Pregnancy, and Premature Birth* (NYU Press, 2019), https://nyupress.org/9781479853571/reproductive-injustice/.

150 Ann Jefferies, "Kangaroo Care for the Preterm Infant and Family," *US National Library of Medicine* 17, no. 3 (2012): 141–43, https://doi.org/10.1093/pch/17.3.141.

151 Keith Moore, "How Accurate Are 'Due Dates'?," *BBC News*, 2015, https://www.bbc.com/news/magazine-31046144.

152 Moore.

153 Justin Wolter, "The Process of Implantation of Embryos in Primates," The Embryo Project Encyclopedia, 2013, https://embryo.asu.edu/pages/process-implantation-embryos-primates.

154 "Signs Labor Has Begun," News Medical Life Sciences, 2019, https://www.news-medical.net/health/Signs-Labor-Has-Begun.aspx.

155 Robin Elise Weiss, "Fetal Postitions for Labor and Birth," verywellfamily, 2019, https://www.verywellfamily.com/fetal-positions-for-labor-and-birth-2759020.

156 Janie McCoy King, *Back Labor No More!!: What Every Woman Should Know Before Labor*, second (Plenary Systems, Inc., 2008).

Week 9

157 Alan DeCherney et al., *Current Diagnosis & Treatment Obstetrics & Gynecology*, 12th ed. (McGraw Hill, 2019), https://www.amazon.com/Diagnosis-Treatment-Obstetrics-Gynecology-Gynecologic/dp/0071833900.

158 "Newborn Head Modling," in *Medline Plus* (US National Library of Medicine, 2022), https://medlineplus.gov/ency/article/002270.htm.

159 Pavilion for Women, "Changes During Pregnancy: What's Normal and What's Not?," Texas Children's Hospital, 2020, https://women.texaschildrens.org/blog/2019/05/changes-during-pregnancy-what's-normal-and-what's-not.

160   Pavilion for Women.

161   Your.MD, "Sexual Arousal in Women," Your.MD, 2020, https://www.your.md/condition/goodsex-sexualarousalinwomen.

162   Kazem Azadzoi and Mike Siroky, "Neurologic Factors in Female Sexual Function and Dysfunction," *Korean Journal of Urology* 51, no. 7 (2010): 443–49, https://doi.org/10.4111/kju.2010.51.7.443.

163   Cindy Cockeram, "Putting Your Knees Together Can Help Push Your Baby Out!," Lamaze.org, January 10, 2020, https://www.lamaze.org/Giving-Birth-with-Confidence/GBWC-Post/TitleLink/Putting-Your-Knees-Together-Can-Help-Push-Your-Baby-Out.

164   Christina Marie Tussey et al., "Reducing Length of Labor and Cesarean Surgery Rate Using a Peanut Ball for Women Laboring with and Epidural," *The Journal of Perinatal Education* 24, no. 1 (2015): 16–24, https://doi.org/10.1891/1058-1243.24.1.16.

165   Dekker, "The Evidence on: Birthing Positions," Evidence Based Birth, 2018, https://evidencebasedbirth.com/evidence-birthing-positions/.

166   Andrew Kotaska, "Informed Consent and Refusal in Obstetrics: A Practical Ethical Guide," *Birth Issues in Perinatal Care*, 2017, https://doi.org/10.1111/birt.12281.

167   Paul Moyer, "Less Pelvic Floor Damage Associated With Unchoached Than Coached Pushing During Labor," *Medscape Medical News*, August 2, 2004, https://www.medscape.com/viewarticle/484738.

168   L Reveiz, HG Gaitan, and L Cuervo, "Enemas during Labour," Cochrane, 2013, https://www.cochrane.org/CD000330/PREG_enemas-during-labour.

169   Natalia Hailes and Ash Spivak, "The Uterus: Oh How It Grows (and Shrinks!)," in *Why Did No ONe Tell Me This?: The Doulas' (Honest) Guide for Expectant Parents* (Singapore: Hachette Book Group, 2020), https://www.amazon.com/Why-Did-One-Tell-This/dp/0762495669/ref=sr_1_1?dchild=1&keywords=9780762495672&linkCode=qs&qid=1593794673&s=books&sr=1-1.

170   George Osol and Maurizio Mandala, "Maternal Uterine Vascular Remodeling During Pregnancy," *Physiology (Bethesda)*, 2009, 58–71, https://doi.org/10.1152/physiol.00033.2008.

171   John Smith and Ronald Ramus, "Postpartum Hemorrhage," *Medscape*, June 27, 2018, https://emedicine.medscape.com/article/275038-overview#a0103.

172   "Postpartum Hemorrhage," March of Dimes, 2020, https://www.marchofdimes.org/pregnancy/postpartum-hemorrhage.aspx.

173   John Smith, "Management of the Third Stage of Labor," Medscape, 2015, https://emedicine.medscape.com/article/275304-overview.

174   Ann Evensen, Janice Anderson, and Patricia Fontaine, "Postpartum Hemorrhage: Prevention and Treatment," *American Family Physician* 95, no. 7 (2017): 443–49.

175   Austin McEvoy and Maggie Tetrokalashvili, "Physiology, Pregnancy Contractions," StatPearls, 2018, https://www.ncbi.nlm.nih.gov/books/NBK532927/.

176   Sarah Buckley, "Synthetic Oxytocin (Pitocin, Syntocinon): Unpacking the Myths and Side-Effects," Dr. Sarah Buckley, 2019, https://sarahbuckley.com/pitocin-side-effects-part1/.

177   K. Bischoff, M. Nothacker, and C. LeHane, "Lack of Controlled Studies Investigating the Risk of Postpartum Haemorrhage in Cesarean Delivery after Prior Use of Oxytocin: A Scoping Review.," *BMC Pregnancy and Childbirth*, November 29, 2017, https://doi.org/10.1186/s12884-017-1584-1.

178   Marsha Walker, "Influence of the Maternal Anatomy and Physiology on Lactation," in *Breastfeeding Management For The Clinician: Using The Evidence*, 1st ed. (Jones and Bartlett Publishers, Massachusetts), https://books.google.com/books?id=nuRf-YXawAcC&pg=PA66&lpg=PA66&dq=stress+impedes+release+of+oxytocin+and+prolactin&source=bl&ots=DR7Kd4vkB2&sig=ACfU-3U3nXpYUMvBsTdwmXdjJq0RnzAWhlg&hl=en&sa=X&ved=2ahUKEwiPos3Ts63qAhUCmXIEHZHaAhEQ6AEwDXoECAwQAQ#v=onepage&q=stress%20impedes%20release%20of%20oxytocin%20and%20prolactin&f=false.

179   Walker.

180   Janice Anderson and Duncan Etches, "Prevention and Management of Postpartum Hemorrhage," *American Family Physician* 75, no. 6 (March 15, 2007): 875–82.

181 Monika Thakur and Angesh Thakur, "Uterine Inversion," StatPearls, 2020, https://www.ncbi.nlm.nih.gov/books/NBK525971/.

182 CM Begley et al., "Delivering the Placenta in the Third Stage of Labour," Cochrane, 2019, https://www.cochrane.org/CD007412/PREG_delivering-placenta-third-stage-labour.

183 Smith and Ramus, "Postpartum Hemorrhage."

184 "Prevalence of Anemia among Pregnant Women," The World Bank, 2020, https://data.worldbank.org/indicator/SH.PRG.ANEM.

185 Allison Fisher and Elizabeta Nemeth, "Iron Homeostasis during Pregnancy," *The American Journal of Clinical Nutrition*, 2017, 1567–74, https://doi.org/10.3945/ajcn.117.155812.

186 "Vitamin K," 2020, https://www.health.ny.gov/professionals/hospital_administrator/letters/2020/docs/dal_20-03_vitamin_k.pdf?fbclid=IwAR2qXY91j0tpcnN1YP1xfgb_Y0L_kR9zdzC8h65O5LS5lm8VKH8q7iDHbLQ.

187 F.Z. Karimi et al., "The Effect of Mother-Infant Skin to Skin Contact after Birth on Third Stage of Labor: A Systematic Review and Meta-Analysis," *Pub Med, Iranian Journal of Public Health* 48, no. 4 (2019), https://www.ncbi.nlm.nih.gov/pmc/articles/PMC6500522/.

188 Karimi et al.

189 "WHO Recommendation on the Use of Uterine Massage for the Treatment of Postpartum Haemorrhage," The Reproductive Health Library, 2018, https://extranet.who.int/rhl/topics/preconception-pregnancy-childbirth-and-postpartum-care/postpartum-care/postpartum-haemorrhage/who-recommendation-use-uterine-massage-treatment-postpartum-haemorrhage.

190 Sarah Buckley, *Gentle Birth, Gentle Mothering* (California: Celestial Arts, 2009), https://sarahbuckley.com/gentle-birth-gentle-mothering/.

191 Jo Lewin, "How to Get More Iron from the Diet," MedicalNewsToday, 2020, https://www.medicalnewstoday.com/articles/322272.

192 Saraswathi Vedam et al., "The Giving Voice to Mothers Study: Inequity and Mistreatment during Pregnancy and Childbirth in the United States," BMC Reproductive Health, 2019, https://reproductive-health-journal.biomedcentral.com/articles/10.1186/s12978-019-0729-2.

Week 10

193 Colette Bouchez, "Exercise for Energyy: Workouts That Work," JUMPSTART by WebMD, 2020, https://www.webmd.com/fitness-exercise/features/exercise-for-energy-workouts-that-work#1.

194 Alice Park, "The Case for the 1-Minute Workout Is Getting Stronger," *Time Magazine*, April 28, 2016, https://time.com/4311373/interval-training-benefits/.

195 Christina Gregory, "The Five Stages of Grief," PSYCOM, 2020, https://www.psycom.net/depression.central.grief.html.

196 Jeanne Faulkner, "Uncontrollable Shaking During Labor and Pregnancy Hormones," yahoo!life, 2019, https://www.yahoo.com/lifestyle/uncontrollable-shaking-during-labor-pregnancy-185956124.html.

197 Antonia Whyatt and Ariel Brewster, "Involution: How to Deal with Postpartum Afterpains," Today's Parent, 2017, https://www.todaysparent.com/pregnancy/giving-birth/involution-how-to-deal-with-birth-afterpains/.

198 "Physical Examination," healthline Parenthood, 2020, https://www.healthline.com/health/pregnancy/evaluation-physician#End-of-Visit.

199 Maria Pyanov, "Small Pelvis? Big Baby? Here's The Truth About CPD," bellybelly, 2020, https://www.bellybelly.com.au/birth/small-pelvis-big-baby-cpd/.

200 Alan DeCherney et al., *Current Diagnosis & Treatment Obstetrics & Gynecology*, 12th ed. (McGraw Hill, 2019), https://www.amazon.com/Diagnosis-Treatment-Obstetrics-Gynecology-Gynecologic/dp/0071833900.

201 Mayo Clinic Staff, "Labor Induction," Mayo Clinic, 2020, https://www.mayoclinic.org/tests-procedures/labor-induction/about/pac-20385141.

202 Rebecca Dekker, "The Evidence on Membrane Sweeping," Evidence Based Birth, 2017, https://evidencebasedbirth.com/evidence-on-membrane-sweeping/.

203   M. Czosnykowska-Łukacka et al., "Milk Immunoglobulin Profile During Prolonged Lactation," *Frontiers in Pediatrics* 8:428 (August 7, 2020), https://www.ncbi.nlm.nih.gov/pmc/articles/PMC7426452/.

204   Rachel Reed, "The Anterior Cervical Lip: How to Ruin a Perfectly Good Birth," MidwifeThinking, June 15, 2016, https://midwifethinking.com/2016/06/15/the-anterior-cervical-lip-how-to-ruin-a-perfectly-good-birth/.

Week 11

205   Colleen de Bellefonds, "Fetal Development: Baby's Nervous System and Brain," what to expect, 2019, https://www.whattoexpect.com/pregnancy/fetal-development/fetal-brain-nervous-system/.

206   The American Cancer Society medical and Editorial content team, "What Is Informed Consent?," American Cancer Society, 2020, https://www.cancer.org/treatment/finding-and-paying-for-treatment/understanding-financial-and-legal-matters/informed-consent/what-is-informed-consent.html.

207   "2018 Annual Report," America's Health Rankings, 2020, https://www.americashealthrankings.org/learn/reports/2018-annual-report/findings-international-comparison.

208   "Patients' Rights," The Free Dictionary, 2008, https://legal-dictionary.thefreedictionary.com/Patients%27+Rights.

209   Travis Peeler, "What Is Assault and Battery?," LegalMatch, 2020, https://www.legalmatch.com/law-library/article/assault-and-battery---victim.html.

210   Ruth Faden, Tom Beauchamp, and Nancy King, *A History and Theory of Informed Consent* (Oxford University Press, 1986), https://www.amazon.com/History-Theory-Informed-Consent/dp/0195036867.

211   Lone Storgaard and Niels Uldbjerg, "The Use of Amniotomy to Shorten Spontaneous Labour. A Survey of a Cohrane Review" 171, no. 47 (November 16, 2009): 3438–40.

212   Brad N. Greenwood et al., "Physician–Patient Racial Concordance and Disparities in Birthing Mortality for Newborns," *Proceedings of the National Academy of Sciences*, August 13, 2020, 201913405, https://doi.org/10.1073/pnas.1913405117.

213   Pam England and Rob Horowitz, *Birthing from Within: An Extra-Ordinary Guide to Childbirth Preparation*, 1st ed. (New Mexico: Paratera Press, 1998), https://www.amazon.com/Birthing-Within-Extra-Ordinary-Childbirth-Preparation/dp/0965987302.

214   NYU Langone Health, "Obstetric Anesthesia," NYU Langone Health, accessed June 24, 2020, https://med.nyu.edu/anes/subspecialties/obstetric-anesthesia.

215   NYU Langone Health.

216   Janice A. Sabin, "How We Fail Black Patients in Pain," Association of American Medical Colleges, January 6, 2020, https://www.aamc.org/news-insights/how-we-fail-black-patients-pain.

217   Rebecca Dekker, "Evidence on: IV Fluids During Labor," Evidence Based Birth, May 31, 2017, https://evidencebasedbirth.com/iv-fluids-during-labor/.

218   "IVs" (Phoenix Children's Hospital, 2015), https://www.phoenixchildrens.org/files/inline-files/IVs-107.pdf.

219   American Society of Anesthesiologists, "Most Healthy Women Would Benefit from Light Meal during Labor," Press release, November 6, 2015, https://www.asahq.org/about-asa/newsroom/news-releases/2015/11/eating-a-light-meal-during-labor.

220   Dekker, "Evidence on: IV Fluids During Labor."

221   Edmund Funai and Errol Norwitz, "Management of Normal Labor and Delivery," *UpToDate*, 2017, http://enjoypregnancyclub.com/wp-content/uploads/2017/05/Management%20of%20normal%20labor%20and%20delivery.pdf.

222   Donna Murray, "Weight Loss in the Breastfed Baby," verywellfamily, 2020, https://www.verywellfamily.com/weight-loss-in-the-breastfed-infant-431641.

223   Joy Noel-Weiss, Genevieve Courant, and A Kirsten Woodend, "Physiological Weight Loss in the Breastfed Neonate: A Systemic Review," *Open Medicine* 2, no. 4 (2008): e99–110.

224   Rebecca Dekker, "Evidence for the Saline Lock during Labor," Evidence Based Birth, 2012, https://evidencebasedbirth.com/the-saline-lock-during-labor/.

225 Frank A. Maffei, "Intraosseous Cannulation," Medical, Medscape, April 11, 2019, https://emedicine.medscape.com/article/908610-overview.

226 Z. Alfirevic et al., "Continuous Cardiotocography (CTG) as a Form of Electronic Fetal Monitoring (EFM) for Fetal Assessment during Labour. Cochrane Database Syst Rev.," *Pub Med Central*, February 3, 2017, https://www.ncbi.nlm.nih.gov/pmc/articles/PMC6464257/.

227 Rebecca Dekker, "The Evidence on: Fetal Monitoring," Medical, Evidenced Based Birth, May 21, 2018, https://evidencebasedbirth.com/fetal-monitoring/.

228 Dekker.

229 Dekker.

230 HL Brown, "Does the Use of Diagnostic Technology Reduce Fetal Mortality?," *Pub Med Central*, April 2019, https://doi.org/10.1111/1475-6773.13103..

231 Ellen Blix et al., "Intermittent Auscultation Fetal Monitoring during Labour: A Systematic Scoping Review to Identify Methods, Effects, and Accuracy," *US National Library of Medicine* 14, no. 7 (2019), https://doi.org/10.1371/journal.pone.0219573.

232 Dekker, "The Evidence on: Fetal Monitoring."

233 Dekker.

234 Dekker.

Week 12

235 The Cleveland Clinic, "Labor without Medication: Coping Skills," Cleveland Clinic, 2020, https://my.clevelandclinic.org/health/articles/15586-labor-without-medication-coping-skills.

236 Floyd Bloom, "Analgesic," Encyclopaedia Britannica, 2017, https://www.britannica.com/science/analgesic.

237 Yvette Terrie, "An Overview of Opioids," Pharmacy Times, 2011, https://www.pharmacytimes.com/publications/issue/2011/June2011/An-Overview-of-Opioids.

238 Toshiharu Kasaba et al., "Epidural Fentanyl Improves the Onset and Spread of Epidural Mepivacaine Analgesia," 1996, 1211–15.

239 Alan William Cuthbert, "Anesthetic," Encyclopaedia Britannica, 2018, https://www.britannica.com/science/anesthetic.

240 NHS, "Epidurals and Spinals: Information about Their Operation for Anyone Who May Benefit from an Epidural or Spinal," *Royal Berkshire*, 2020, https://www.royalberkshire.nhs.uk/patient-information-leaflets/Anaesthetics/Anaesthetics%20epiduraandspinalsls.htm.

241 Matrix Anesthesia, "What Is the Difference between an Epidural and Spinal Block?," MatrixAnesthesia, 2019, http://www.matrixanesthesia.com/faqs/obstetrics/what-is-the-difference-between-an-epidural-and-spinal-block.

242 Katherine Arendt and Scott Segal, "Why Epidurals Do Not Always Work," *Obstetrics and Gynecology* 1, no. 2 (2008): 49–55.

243 WebMd Staff, "Fentanyl Patch, Transdermal 72 Hours - Uses, Side Effects, and More," WebMD, accessed October 6, 2022, http://www.webmd.com/pain-management/fentanyl.

244 "Stadol Solution Side Effects by Likelihood and Severity," WebMD, 2020, https://www.webmd.com/drugs/2/drug-982/stadol-injection/details/list-sideeffects.

245 Waknine, "FDA Safety Labeling Changes: Nubain and Zocor."

246 Devin Larsen and Christopher V. Maani, "Nalbuphine," *National Center for Biotechnology Information*, May 8, 2022, https://www.ncbi.nlm.nih.gov/books/NBK534283/.

247 "Demerol," RxList, September 19, 2018, https://www.rxlist.com/demerol-drug.htm#description.

248 Drugs.com, "Bupivacaine Pregnancy and Breastfeeding Warnings," Drugs.com, April 13, 2020, https://www.drugs.com/pregnancy/bupivacaine.html.

249 Laura Goetzl et al., "Maternal Epidural Analgesia and Rates of Maternal Antibiotic Treatment in a Low-Risk Nulliparous Population," *Journal of Perinatology*, 2003, 457–61.

250   Segal, "Labor Epidural Analgesia and Maternal Fever."

251   Marcos Silva and Stephen Halpern, "Epidural Analgesia for Labor: Current Techniques," *Dovepress*, 2010, 143–53, https://doi.org/10.2147/LRA.S10237.

252   Gilbert Grant, "Adverse Effects of Neuraxial Analgesia and Anesthesia for Obstetrics," *UpToDate*, May 2020, https://www.uptodate.com/contents/adverse-effects-of-neuraxial-analgesia-and-anesthesia-for-obstetrics.

253   "All About Epidurals: A Safe Pain Management Option During Labor," MU, 2020, https://www.muhealth.org/our-stories/all-about-epidurals-safe-pain-management-option-during-labor.

254   Waknine, "FDA Safety Labeling Changes: Nubain and Zocor."

255   Manuel C. Vallejo and Mark I. Zakowski, "Pro-Con Debate: Nitrous Oxide for Labor Analgesia.," *BioMed Research International* 2019: 4618798. (August 20, 2019), https://doi.org/10.1155/2019/4618798.

256   Rebecca Dekker, "Nitrous Oxide During Labor," Evidence Based Birth, March 2018, https://evidencebasedbirth.com/nitrous-oxide-during-labor/.

257   Vallejo and Zakowski, "Pro-Con Debate: Nitrous Oxide for Labor Analgesia."

258   Cleveland Clinic Staff, "Homocysteine," Health Education, Cleveland Clinic.org, accessed October 7, 2022, https://my.clevelandclinic.org/health/articles/21527-homocysteine.

259   Vallejo and Zakowski, "Pro-Con Debate: Nitrous Oxide for Labor Analgesia."

260   Vallejo and Zakowski.

261   Vallejo and Zakowski.

262   Ob/Gyn Nursing, "Allnurses," allnurses, 2020, https://allnurses.com/ob-gyn-c24/.

263   F. Khan, G. Kabiraj, and et al, "A Systematic Review of the Link Between Autism Spectrum Disorder and Acetaminophen: A Mystery to Resolve.," *Cureus* 14, no. 7 (July 18, 2022), https://doi.org/10.7759/cureus.26995.

264   P. Good, "Evidence the U.S. Autism Epidemic Initiated by Acetaminophen (Tylenol) Is Aggravated by Oral Antibiotic Amoxicillin/Clavulanate (Augmentin) and Now Exponentially by Herbicide Glyphosate (Roundup).," *PubMed*, February 23, 2018, https://doi.org/10.1016/j.clnesp.2017.10.005.

265   Media Relations CDC staff, "1 in 3 Adults Don't Get Enough Sleep, Centers for Disease Control and Prevention," Press release, February 18, 2016, https://www.cdc.gov/media/releases/2016/p0215-enough-sleep.html.

266   A.M. Jukic et al., "Length of Human Pregnancy and Contributors to Its Natural Variation," *Human Reproduction Oxford Journals* 28, no. 10 (2013): 2848–55, https://doi.org/10.1093/humrep/det297.

267   "39 Weeks Infographic," March of Dimes, 2020, https://www.marchofdimes.org/pregnancy/39-weeks-infographic.aspx.

268   Alison Abbott, "Neuroscience: The Brain, Interrupted," *Nature* 518, no. 7537 (February 3, 2015), https://www.nature.com/news/neuroscience-the-brain-interrupted-1.16831.

269   Allen Wilcox, David Dunson, and Donna Day Baird, "The Timing of the 'Fertile Window' in the Menstrual Cycle: Day Specific Estimates from a Prospective Study," *BMJ* 321, no. 7271 (November 18, 2000): 1259–62, https://doi.org/10.1136/bmj.321.7271.1259.

270   Otto Umana and Marco Siccardi, "Prenatal Non-Stress Test," StatPearls, 2020, https://www.ncbi.nlm.nih.gov/books/NBK537123/.

271   Mayo Clinic Staff, "Biophysical Profile," Mayo Clinic, 2020, https://www.mayoclinic.org/tests-procedures/biophysical-profile/about/pac-20393061.

272   Rebecca Dekker, "Evidence on: Induction or Cesarean for a Big Baby," Evidence Based Birth, August 21, 2019, https://evidence-basedbirth.com/evidence-for-induction-or-c-section-for-big-baby/.

273   Julia Milner and Jane Arezina, "The Accuracy of Ultrasound Estimation of Fetal Weight in Comparison to Birth Weight: A Systematic Review. (Leeds, England) Vol. 26,1 (2018): 32-41. Doi:10.1177/1742271X17732807," *Ultrasound* 26,1 (2018), https://www.ncbi.nlm.nih.gov/pmc/articles/PMC5810856/.

274   "Fractured Clavicle in the Newborn," Medical Encyclopedia, MedlinePlus, May 2, 2020, https://medlineplus.gov/ency/article/001588.htm.

275 Jennifer Holzman, Ivica Zalud, and Marguerite Lisa Bartholomew, "Ultrasound of the Placenta," *Donald School Journal of Ultrasound in Obstetrics and Gynecology* 1, no. 4 (2007): 47–60.

276 Deborah Wing, "Protocol 49: Induction of Labor," Wiley Online Library, 2015, https://onlinelibrary.wiley.com/doi/abs/10.1002/9781119001256.ch49.

277 Rebecca Dekker, "The Evidence on: Due Dates," Evidence Based Birth, 2019, https://evidencebasedbirth.com/evidence-on-due-dates/.

278 Philippa Middleton et al., "Induction of Labour at or beyond 37 Weeks' Gestation," *Cochrane Database of Systematic Reviews*, no. 7 (July 15, 2020), https://www.cochranelibrary.com/cdsr/doi/10.1002/14651858.CD004945.pub5/full.

279 Eugene Declercq, Candice Belanoff, and Ronald Iverson, "Maternal Perceptions of the Experience of Attempted Labor Induction and Medically Elective Inductions: Analysis of Survey Results from Listening to Mothers in California," *BMC Pregnancy and Childbirth* 20, Article 458 (2020), https://bmcpregnancychildbirth.biomedcentral.com/articles/10.1186/s12884-020-03137-x#citeas.

280 Wing, "Protocol 49: Induction of Labor."

281 Wagner Marsden, *Born in the USA: How a Broken Maternity System Must Be Fixed to Put Women and Children First* (University of California Press, 2006), https://www.amazon.com/Born-USA-Broken-Maternity-Children/dp/0520256336.

282 "Misoprostol- Oral, Cytotec," MedicineNet, 2013, https://www.medicinenet.com/misoprostol-oral/article.htm.

283 Becky Little, "The Science Behind the 'Abortion Pill,'" Smithsonian Magazine, 2017, https://www.smithsonianmag.com/health-medicine/science-behind-abortion-pill-180963762/.

284 Rebecca Allen and Barbara O'Brien, "Uses of Misoprostol in Obstetrics and Gynecology," *Obstetrics and Gynecology* 2, no. 3 (2009): 159–68.

285 Wagner, *Born in the USA: How a Broken Maternity System Must Be Fixed to Put Women and Children First.*

286 Austin McEvoy and Maggie Tetrokalashvili, "Physiology, Pregnancy Contractions," StatPearls, 2018, https://www.ncbi.nlm.nih.gov/books/NBK532927/.

287 Sarah Buckley, "Synthetic Oxytocin (Pitocin, Syntocinon): Unpacking the Myths and Side-Effects," Dr. Sarah Buckley, 2019, https://sarahbuckley.com/pitocin-side-effects-part1/.

288 SW Kim, D. Nasioudis, and LD. Levine, "Role of Early Amniotomy with Induced Labor: A Systematic Review of Literature and Meta-Analysis.," *Am J Obstet Gynecol MFM*, November 2019, https://pubmed.ncbi.nlm.nih.gov/33345842/.

289 Ganesh Acharya and Vasilis Sitras, "Oxygen Uptake of the Human Fetus at Term," *Acta Obstetricia et Gynecologica*, 2009, 104–9.

290 Acharya and Sitras.

291 G. Torres, M. Mourad, and JR Leheste, "Perspectives of Pitocin Administration on Behavioral Outcomes in the Pediatric Population: Recent Insights and Future Implications.," *Heliyon* 29;6(5) (May 2020), https://www.ncbi.nlm.nih.gov/pmc/articles/PMC7264063/.

292 Ashik Siddique, "Pitocin May Have Adverse Effects On Newborn Babies," Medical Daily, 2013, https://www.medicaldaily.com/pitocin-may-have-adverse-effects-newborn-babies-245641.

293 Mayo Clinic Staff, "Labor Induction," Mayo Clinic, 2020, https://www.mayoclinic.org/tests-procedures/labor-induction/about/pac-20385141.

294 Homa K. Ahmadzia, Chad A. Grotegut, and Andra H. James, "A National Update on Rates of Postpartum Haemorrhage and Related Interventions," *Blood Transfusion* 18,4 (2020), https://www.ncbi.nlm.nih.gov/pmc/articles/PMC7375891/.

295 Mark Curran, "Bishop Score Calculator," perinatology, 2020, http://perinatology.com/calculators/Bishop%20Score%20Calculator.htm.

296 Kaori Takahata et al., "Effects of Breast Stimulation for Spontaneous Onset of Labor on Salivary Oxytocin Levels in Low-Risk Pregnant Women: A Feasibility Study," *PLoS One* 13, no. 2 (2018), https://doi.org/10.1371/journal.pone.0192757.

297 Rebecca Dekker, "Natural Labor Induction Series: Breast Stimulation," Evidence Based Birth, 2017, https://evidencebasedbirth.com/evidence-using-breast-stimulation-to-naturally-induce-labor/.

298 "Can Labor Be Induced Naturally?," Grow by WebMD, 2020, https://www.webmd.com/baby/inducing-labor-naturally-can-it-be-done#1.

299 Jukic et al., "Length of Human Pregnancy and Contributors to Its Natural Variation."

Week 13

300 Deborah Siegel-Acevedo, "Writing Can Help Us Heal from Trauma," *Harvard Business Review*, July 1, 2021, https://hbr.org/2021/07/writing-can-help-us-heal-from-trauma.

301 Crystal Raypole, "How to Use Drawing as a Coping Tool for Anxiety," *Healthline*, January 28, 2021, https://www.healthline.com/health/mental-health/anxiety-drawing.

302 Audre Lorde, "The Transformation of Silence into Language & Action," *Sinister Wisdom* 6 (1978).

303 Carolyn Ross, "Are You Stressed Out and Exhausted?," Psychology Today, 2016, https://www.psychologytoday.com/us/blog/real-healing/201605/are-you-stressed-out-and-exhausted.

304 Carol Burke and Roma Allen, "Complications of Cesarean Birth," *American Journal of Maternal/Child Nursing* 45, no. 2 (2020): 92–99.

305 Frances Anderson-Bagga and Angelica Sze, "Placenta Previa," StatPearls, 2019, https://www.ncbi.nlm.nih.gov/books/NBK539818/.

306 Anderson-Bagga and Sze.

307 Mayo Clinic Staff, "Placental Abruption," Mayo Clinic, 2020, https://www.mayoclinic.org/diseases-conditions/placental-abruption/symptoms-causes/syc-20376458.

308 "External Cephalic Version (Version) for Breech Position," Michigan Medicine, 2020, https://www.uofmhealth.org/health-library/hw180146.

309 "Using the Rebozo to Turn Breech, Transverse and Oblique Babies," Magicalbirth, 2015, https://magicalbirth.wordpress.com/2015/12/24/using-the-rebozo-to-turn-breech-transverse-and-oblique-babies/.

310 "Sideways/Transverse," Spinning Babies, 2020, https://spinningbabies.com/learn-more/baby-positions/other-fetal-positions/sidewaystransverse/.

311 Melissa Teresa Chu Lam and Elizabeth Dierking, "Intensive Care Unit Issues in Eclampsia and HELLP Syndrome," *International Journal of Critical Illness & Injury Science* 7, no. 3 (2017): 136–41, https://doi.org/10.4103/IJCIIS.IJCIIS_33_17.

312 Rebecca Dekker, "Evidence on: Prolonged Second Stage of Labor," Evidence Based Birth, 2017, https://evidencebasedbirth.com/prolonged-second-stage-of-labor/.

313 E. Bornstein et al., "Implementation of a Standardized Post-Cesarean Delivery Order Set with Multimodal Combination Analgesia Reduces Inpatient Opioid Usage.," *Journal of Clinical Medicine* 10, no. 7 (January 2021), https://www.ncbi.nlm.nih.gov/pmc/articles/PMC7793107/.

314 Susan Donaldson James, "Placenta Accreta: Multiple C-Sections Can Kill Mother," News, ABC News, April 18, 2011, https://abcnews.go.com/Health/caesarian-rates-placenta-accreta-contributing-rise-maternal-death/story?id=13399308.

315 Society for Maternal-Fetal Medicine American College or Obstetricans and Gynocologists, "Placenta Accreta Spectrum," *ACOG Consensus Paper* 7 (2021), https://www.acog.org/clinical/clinical-guidance/obstetric-care-consensus/articles/2018/12/placenta-accreta-spectrum.

316 American College or Obstetricans and Gynocologists.

317 Mayo Clinic, "C-Section," Mayo Clinic, 2020, https://www.mayoclinic.org/tests-procedures/c-section/about/pac-20393655.

318 OE Keag, JE Norman, and SJ Stock, "Long-Term Risks and Benefits Associated with Cesarean Delivery for Mother, Baby, and Subsequent Pregnancies: Systematic Review and Meta-Analysis.," *PLoS Med* 15, no. 1 (2018), https://www.ncbi.nlm.nih.gov/pmc/articles/PMC5779640/.

319 The American College of Obstetricians and Gynecologists, "Vaginal Seeding," ACOG, 2017, https://www.acog.org/clinical/clinical-guidance/committee-opinion/articles/2017/11/vaginal-seeding.

320　Yao Yao et al., "The Role of Microbiota in Infant Health: From Early Life to Adulthood," *Frontiers In Immunology*, October 7, 2021, https://www.frontiersin.org/articles/10.3389/fimmu.2021.708472/full.

321　The American College of Obstetricians and Gynecologists, "Vaginal Seeding."

322　Sutapa Bandyopadhyay Neogi et al., "Risk Factors for Stillbirths: How Much Can a Responsive Health System Prevent?," *BMC Pregnancy and Childbirth* 18, no. 1 (January 18, 2018): 33, https://doi.org/10.1186/s12884-018-1660-1.

323　Duaa Eldeib, "Her Child Was Stillborn at 39 Weeks. She Blames a System That Doesn't Always Listen to Mothers.," *ProPublica*, November 13, 2022, https://www.propublica.org/article/stillbirths-prevention-infant-mortality.

324　Eldeib.

325　ACOG staff, "Management of Stillbirth," *Obstetric Care Consensus* 10 (March 2020), https://www.acog.org/clinical/clinical-guidance/obstetric-care-consensus/articles/2020/03/management-of-stillbirth.

326　Staff American Pregnancy Association, "Stillbirth: Surviving Emotionally," American Pregnancy Association, 2021, https://americanpregnancy.org/pregnancy-loss/stillborn-surviving-emotionally/.

327　Joan Didion, *The Year of Magical Thinking* (Vintage Books, 2005), https://www.goodreads.com/book/show/7815.The_Year_of_Magical_Thinking.

328　Yasemin Saplakoglu, "Why Does a Mother's Body Keep Some of Her Baby's Cells After Birth?," *Live Science*, February 22, 2022, https://www.livescience.com/62930-why-mom-keeps-baby-cells.html.

329　"The Role of Hormones in Childbirth," childbirth connection, 2020, http://www.childbirthconnection.org/maternity-care/role-of-hormones/.

330　"The Cascade of Intervention," childbirth connection, 2020, http://www.childbirthconnection.org/maternity-care/cascade-of-intervention/.

331　Liz Gibbons, "The Global Numbers and Costs of Additionally Needed and Unnecessary Caesarean Sections Performed per Year: Overuse as a Barrier to Universal Coverage," *ResearchGate*, January 2010, file:///Users/sydneyklugman/Downloads/The_Global_Numbers_and_Costs_of_Additionally_Neede.pdf.

332　Ferris Jabr, "Why Your Brain Needs More Downtime," *Scientific American*, October 15, 2013, https://www.scientificamerican.com/article/mental-downtime/.

Week 14

333　Mayo Clinic Staff, "Stress Management," Mayo Clinic, 2020, https://www.mayoclinic.org/healthy-lifestyle/stress-management/in-depth/social-support/art-20044445.

334　Rebecca Dekker, "Acupuncture or Acupressure for Pain Relief during Labor," Evidence Based Birth, 2018, https://evidencebasedbirth.com/acupuncture-and-acupressure-for-pain-relief-during-labor/.

335　"The Limbic System," Queensland Brain Institute, 2019, https://qbi.uq.edu.au/brain/brain-anatomy/limbic-system.

336　Ariana Ayu, "Can You Smell Your Way to a Better Brain? Science Says Yes.," *Ayutopia International*, accessed July 6, 2020, https://www.inc.com/ariana-ayu/can-you-smell-your-way-to-a-better-brain-science-says-yes.html.

337　Ayu.

338　Pam England and Rob Horowitz, *Birthing from Within: An Extra-Ordinary Guide to Childbirth Preparation*, 1st ed. (New Mexico: Paratera Press, 1998), https://www.amazon.com/Birthing-Within-Extra-Ordinary-Childbirth-Preparation/dp/0965987302.

339　Victoria Tennant, "The Powerful Impact of Stress," *Scribd*, n.d., 19.

340　Kathy Alden, "Nursing Care of the Family During the Postpartum Period," in *Studyguide for Maternity Adn Women's Health Care* (Cram101, 2016), 216, https://www.amazon.com/Studyguide-Maternity-Womens-Health-9780323293686/dp/1538832860/ref=sr_1_1?dchild=1&keywords=9780323293686&linkCode=qs&qid=1594084400&s=books&sr=1-1.

341　"Placenta Examination after Birth- Practice Guideline" (NHS Foundation Trust, 2018), https://www.royalberkshire.nhs.uk/Downloads/GPs/GP%20protocols%20and%20guidelines/Maternity%20Guidelines%20and%20Policies/Intrapartum/Placenta_examination_guideline_V3.0_GL886_NOV18.pdf.

342   Robin Elise Weiss, "Placental Exam After Birth of the Baby," verywellfamily, 2019, https://www.verywellfamily.com/placental-exam-2758770.

343   "Prepping Your Pet for Your New Baby," Fetch by WebMD, accessed July 31, 2020, https://pets.webmd.com/features/pets-and-new-baby#2.

Week 15

344   MA Bohren et al., "Continuous Support for Women during Childbirth," Cochrane, July 6, 2017, https://www.cochrane.org/CD003766/PREG_continuous-support-women-during-childbirth.

345   Jacqueline Fortier, "Doula Support Compared with Standard Care," *US National Library of Medicine* 61, no. 6 (2015): e284–92.

346   Mary Beth Bobish, "Mary Beth's Birth Story," 2009.

347   J. Ronald Lally and Peter L Mangione, "Caring Relationships: The Heart of Early Brain Development," naeyc, 2017, https://www.naeyc.org/resources/pubs/yc/may2017/caring-relationships-heart-early-brain-development.

348   CDC staff, "Child Development, Early Brain Development," Centers for Disease and Control and Prevention, March 25, 2022, https://www.cdc.gov/ncbddd/childdevelopment/early-brain-development.html.

349   US National Library of Medicine, "Apgar Score," MedlinePlus, 2020, https://medlineplus.gov/ency/article/003402.htm.

350   Mayo Clinic Staff, "What a Newborn Really Looks Like," Mayo Clinic, 2020, https://www.mayoclinic.org/healthy-lifestyle/infant-and-toddler-health/multimedia/newborn/sls-20076309?s=4.

351   Jennifer Matlack and Virginia Sole-Smith, "Common Vision Problems: Is The World Blurry for Your Kid?," *Parents*, 2020, http://www.parenting.com/article/ask-dr-sears-concerned-about-crossed-eyes.

352   Maria Tollin et al., "Vernix Caseosa as a Multi-Component Defence System Based on Polypeptides, Lipids, and Their Interactions," *US National Library of Medicine* 62, no. 19–20 (2005): 2390–99, https://doi.org/10.1007/s00018-005-5260-7.

353   Brendon Verhave, Ali Nassereddin, and Sarah Lappin, "Embryology, Lanugo," StatPearls, 2020, https://www.ncbi.nlm.nih.gov/books/NBK526092/.

354   Aaron Kandola, "Sunken Fontanel: Everything You Need to Know," MedicalNewsToday, 2018, https://www.medicalnewstoday.com/articles/323912#causes.

355   Angela Grippo, "Why Stress Is Both Good and Bad," Psychology Today, 2016, https://www.psychologytoday.com/us/blog/the-wide-wide-world-psychology/201601/why-stress-is-both-good-and-bad.

356   "Depression During Pregnancy & Postpartum," Postpartum Support International, 2020, https://www.postpartum.net/learn-more/depression-during-pregnancy-postpartum/.

357   "What Is Depression?," American Psychiatric Association, 2017, https://www.psychiatry.org/patients-families/depression/what-is-depression.

358   "Symptoms Postnatal Depression," NHS, 2018, https://www.nhs.uk/conditions/post-natal-depression/symptoms/.

359   "Postpartum Post-Traumatic Stress Disorder," Postpartum Support International, 2020, https://www.postpartum.net/learn-more/postpartum-post-traumatic-stress-disorder/.

360   Ilana Strauss, "The Mothers Who Can't Escape the Trauma of Childbirth," The Atlantic, 2015, https://www.theatlantic.com/health/archive/2015/10/the-mothers-who-cant-escape-the-trauma-of-childbirth/408589/.

361   "What Is Postpartum Psychosis?," Action on Postpartum Psychosis, accessed July 15, 2020, https://www.app-network.org/what-is-pp/.

362   Andrew Weil, *Breathing Exercises: 4-7-8 Breath* (Weil, 2020), https://www.drweil.com/videos-features/videos/breathing-exercises-4-7-8-breath/.

Week 16

363   B. Rose Huber, "Four in 10 Infants Lack Strong Parental Aattachments," *Woodrow Wilson School of Public and International Affairs*, March 27, 2014, https://www.princeton.edu/news/2014/03/27/four-10-infants-lack-strong-parental-attachments?section=topstories.

364   Sophie Moullin, Jane Waldfogel, and Elizabeth Washbrook, "Baby Bonds," *Sutton Trust*, March 2014, https://www.suttontrust.com/wp-content/uploads/2020/01/baby-bonds-final.pdf.

365   Huber, "Four in 10 Infants Lack Strong Parental Attachments."

366   Marie Gerecke, "Breastfeeding: How to Establish a Good Milk Supply," Cleveland Clinic, 2020, https://health.clevelandclinic.org/breastfeeding-how-to-establish-a-good-milk-supply-infographic/.

367   "Breastfeeding Report Card," Centers for Disease Control and Prevention, 2018, https://www.cdc.gov/breastfeeding/data/report-card.htm.

368   Nancy Mohrbacker, "Diaper Output and Milk Intake in the Early Weeks," Breastfeeding USA, 2020, https://breastfeedingusa.org/content/article/diaper-output-and-milk-intake-early-weeks.

369   Barbara Behrmann, *The Breastfeeding Cafe: Mothers Share the Joys, Challenges, and Secrets of Nursing* (Ann Arbor Michigan: The University of Michigan Press, 2005), https://www.amazon.com/Breastfeeding-Caf%C3%A9-Mothers-Challenges-Secrets/dp/047206875X.

370   U.S. Department of Agriculture, "Your Breastfeeding Rights," WIC Breastfeeding Support, accessed July 8, 2020, https://wicbreastfeeding.fns.usda.gov/your-breastfeeding-rights.

371   Regents of the University of Michigan, "Breast Engorgement," Michigan Medicine, 2020, https://www.uofmhealth.org/health-library/hw133953.

372   James McKenna, "Night Waking among Breastfeeding Mothers and Infants Conflict, Congruence, or Both?," *Evolution, Medicine, & Public Health*, 2014, 40–47, https://doi.org/10.1093/emph/eou006.

373   La Leche League International, "Sleep-Training... or Not," la leche league international, 2020, https://www.llli.org/breastfeeding-info/sleep-training-or-not/.

374   "Breastfeeding Your Baby," March for Babies, 2019, https://www.marchofdimes.org/baby/breastfeeding-your-baby.aspx.

375   U.S. Centers for Medicare and Medicaid Services, "Patient Protection and Affordable Care Act," HealthCare.gov, accessed June 27, 2020, https://www.healthcare.gov/glossary/patient-protection-and-affordable-care-act/#:~:text=Get%20Answers-,Patient%20Protection%20and%20Affordable%20Care%20Act,amended%20version%20of%20the%20law.

376   Parvin Abedi et al., "Breastfeeding or Nipple Stimulation for Reducing Postpartum Haemorrhage in the Third Stage of Labor," Cochrane Database Syst Rev, 2016, https://www.ncbi.nlm.nih.gov/pmc/articles/PMC6718231/.

377   Hilary Flower, "The Nature of Breastfeeding Contractions," kellymom, 2020, https://kellymom.com/tandem-faq/03bfcontractions/.

378   Brian Palmer, "Snoring and Sleep Apnea: How It Can Be Prevented in Childhood," *Das Schlafmagazin* 3 (2005): 22–23.

379   Dana Festila et al., "Suckling and Non-Nutritive Sucking Habit: What Should We Know?," *Clujul Medical* 87, no. 1 (2014): 11–14, https://doi.org/10.15386/cjm.2014.8872.871.df1mg2.

380   Catherine Watson Genna and Lisa Sandora, "Breastfeeding: Normal Sucking and Swallowing" (Jones & Bartlett Learning), accessed July 8, 2020, http://samples.jbpub.com/9781284093919/9781284093919_CH01_GennaSample.pdf.

381   "Functions of the Brain Stem," Medicine LibreTexts, 2020, https://med.libretexts.org/Bookshelves/Anatomy_and_Physiology/Book%3A_Anatomy_and_Physiology_(Boundless)/11%3A_Central_Nervous_System/11.4%3A_The_Brain_Stem/11.4A%3A_Functions_of_the_Brain_Stem.

382   Kaitlin Bell Barnett, "My Mommy Tax: Six Months of Nursing Cost More than a Year of Formula," The Guardian, 2016, https://www.theguardian.com/commentisfree/2016/feb/02/my-mommy-tax-six-months-of-nursing-cost-more-than-a-year-of-formula.

383   Kathleen Kroi and Tobias Grossmann, "Psychological Effects of Breastfeeding on Children and Mothers," *Bundesgesundheitsblatt Gesundheitsforschung* 61, no. 8 (2018), https://doi.org/10.1007/s00103-018-2769-0.

384   La Leche League International, "Infant Sleep," la leche league international, 2018, https://www.llli.org/infant-sleep/.

385   Mayo Clinic Staff, "Sudden Infant Death Syndrome (SIDS)," Health Information, Mayo Clinic.org, 2022, https://www.mayoclinic.org/diseases-conditions/sudden-infant-death-syndrome/symptoms-causes/syc-20352800.

386   J. Cubero et al., "The Circadian Rhythm of Tryptophan in Breast Milk Affects the Rhythms of 6-Sulfatoxymelatonin and Sleep in Newborn.," *Neuro Endricronology Letters* 6, no. 657–61 (2005), https://pubmed.ncbi.nlm.nih.gov/16380706/.

387   *Delivery Self-Attachment* (Geddes Productions, 1990), https://www.geddesproduction.com/product/delivery-self-attachment/.

388   *Natural Breastfeeding for An Easier Start* (Natural Breastfeeding, 2020), https://www.naturalbreastfeeding.com/.

389   Anna Patty, "Newborn in Drain: How a Baby Can Survive for Six Days without Food or Water," The Sydney Morning Herald, 2014, https://www.smh.com.au/national/nsw/newborn-in-drain-how-a-baby-can-survive-for-six-days-without-food-or-water-20141124-11sg2a.html.

390   "Mothers' and Babies' Brains 'more in Tune' When Mother Is Happy," ScienceDaily, 2019, https://www.sciencedaily.com/releases/2019/12/191217105210.htm.

391   "Examining the Effects of Prenatal Education" (McMaster Forum, 2019), https://www.sciencedaily.com/releases/2019/12/191217105210.htm.

392   Judith Lothian, "Does Childbirth Education Make a Difference?," *The Journal of Perinatal Education* 25, no. 3 (2016): 139–41, https://doi.org/10.1891/1058-1243.25.3.139.

393   "La Leche Leauge International," 2020, https://www.llli.org/.

394   "Pregnancy: Physical Changes After Delivery," Cleveland Clinic, 2020, https://my.clevelandclinic.org/health/articles/9682-pregnancy-physical-changes-after-delivery.

395   Kelly Bonyata, "Hunger Cues- When Do I Feed Baby?," kellymom, 2020, https://kellymom.com/bf/normal/hunger-cues/.

396   La Leche League International, "Foremilk and Hindmilk," la leche league international, 2020, https://www.llli.org/breastfeeding-info/foremilk-and-hindmilk/.

397   Kelly Bonyata, "Foremilk and Hindmilk- What Does This Mean?," kellymom, 2020, https://kellymom.com/bf/got-milk/basics/foremilk-hindmilk/.

398   Taylor Norris, "Illustrated Guide for Burping Your Sleeping Baby," healthline Parenthood, 2018, https://www.healthline.com/health/how-to-burp-a-sleeping-baby#why-burping-matters.

399   "The Holy Haakaa," Work & Mother, 2019, https://www.workandmother.com/the-holy-haakaa/.

400   Rachel The Analytical Mommy, "Everything You Need to Know About Haakaa Silicone Breast Pumps!," The Analytical Mommy, accessed August 3, 2020, https://www.theanalyticalmommy.com/haakaa-silicone-breast-pump-review/.

401   Boh Boi, Serena Koh, and Desley Gail, "The Effectiveness of Cabbage Leaf Application (Treatment)," *National Library of Medicine* 10, no. 20 (2012): 1185–1213, https://doi.org/10.11124/01938924-201210200-00001.

402   unicef, "Skin-to-Skin Contact," unicef United Kingdom, 2019, https://www.unicef.org.uk/babyfriendly/baby-friendly-resources/implementing-standards-resources/skin-to-skin-contact/.

403   Cornucopia Institute, "Infant Formula Report," The Cornucopia Institute, December 19, 2019, http://www.cornucopia.org/2008/01/replacing-mother-infant-formula-report/.

404   HR Colten and BM Altevogt, eds., "Extent and Health COnsequences of Chronic Sleep Loss and Sleep Disorders," in *Sleep Disorders Adn Sleep Deprication: An Unmet Public Health Problem* (Washington DC: National Academies Press (US), 2006), https://www.ncbi.nlm.nih.gov/books/NBK19961/.

405   "Napping," SleepFoundation.org, 2020, https://www.sleepfoundation.org/articles/napping.

406   "Safe Sleep: Recommendations," American Academy of Pediatrics, 2020, https://www.aap.org/en-us/advocacy-and-policy/aap-health-initiatives/safe-sleep/Pages/Safe-Sleep-Recommendations.aspx.

407   James J. McKenna, *Safe Infant Sleep, Expert Answers to Your Cosleeping Questions*, First (Plotypus Media, 2020).

408   William Sears, *Nighttime Parenting: How to Get Your Baby and Child to Sleep* (Penguin Group, 1985), https://www.amazon.com/Nighttime-Parenting-Your-Child-Sleep/dp/0452281482.

409   *Amazing Talents of the Newborn*, DVD Video (Johnson & Johnson, 2011), https://www.worldcat.org/title/amazing-talents-of-the-newborn/oclc/857504358.

410   Mina Shimizu, Heejung Park, and Patricia Greenfield, "Infant Sleeping Arrangements and Cultural Values among Contemporary Japanese Mothers," *Frontiers in Psychology*, 2014, https://doi.org/10.3389/fpsyg.2014.00718.

APPENDIX

Week 3

(Note that some of the following films are available on online, and others may be harder to track down but would be worth your efforts.)

Birth films:

- ○ Everyday Miracles: A Celebration of Birth, Injoy videos, Julie Perry (2002)
  - ○ (YouTube: MothersAdvocate) https://www.youtube.com/watch?v=eE67bO8uEvk
- ○ Birth in the Squatting Position, Poly Morph Films (1979)
  - ○ (YouTube: Konstantin Varik) https://www.youtube.com/watch?v=aAF5n3GBkPA
- ○ The Business of Being Born, Abby Epstein (2008)
- ○ Orgasmic Birth: The Best-Kept Secret, Pascali-Bonaro (2008)
- ○ Born in the USA, Marcia Jarmel and Ken Schneider (2000)
- ○ Birth Into Being, Tatyana Sargunas (1999)

Pelvic floor videos:

- ○ The Pelvic Floor Demystified (YouTube: Nutritious Movement)
  - ○ https://www.youtube.com/watch?v=IOoTC9DpB3k
- ○ Squats for Improved Pelvic Floor function (YouTube: Lisa Gillispie)
  - ○ https://www.youtube.com/watch?v=z7j0UFiV3Z8

Week 4

How to file a medical complaint against a doctor or physician assistant

- ○ To file a medical complaint against a doctor, contact your state medical board.
  - ○ Find your state's medical board: https://www.fsmb.org/contact-a-state-medical-board/
  - ○ Federation of State Medical Boards: https://www.fsmb.org
  - ○ https://www.legalzoom.com/articles/how-to-file-a-complaint-against-a-doctor
  - ○ https://www.verywellhealth.com/complain-about-a-doctor-or-other-healthcare-provider-2614928

For complaints against midwives

- ○ American Midwifery Certification Board: https://www.amcbmidwife.org/about-amcb

Week 7

Information on fetal positioning

- ○ Spinning Babies, https://www.spinningbabies.com
- ○ The Miles Circuit, http://www.milescircuit.com
- ○ The Webster Technique, https://icpa4kids.com/training/webster-certification/webster-technique/

Week 16

Breastfeeding laws by state
- ○ Breastfeeding laws by state, National Conference of State Legislatures (NCSL)
  - ○ https://www.ncsl.org/research/health/breastfeeding-state-laws.aspx
- ○ Your Breastfeeding Rights, WIC (Women infant and children), U.S. Department of Agriculture
  - ○ https://wicbreastfeeding.fns.usda.gov/your-breastfeeding-rights.

Breastfeeding Videos:
- ○ Natural Breastfeeding for an Easier Start
  - ○ https://www.naturalbreastfeeding.com
- ○ Attaching Your Baby at the Breast
  - ○ https://globalhealthmedia.org/videos/attaching-your-baby-at-the-breast/
- ○ Delivery Self Attachment
  - ○ https://www.medicalvideos.com/video/10543/breast-crawl-self-attachment

ADDITIONAL READING AND WEBSITE SUGGESTIONS

Books:

Family Life

- ○ Cortes, Ricardo & Adam Mansbach. *Go the F**k to Sleep.* New York: Akashic Books, 2011. (Also take a listen to the talented Samuel L. Jackson read the book on YouTube: https://www.youtube.com/watch?v=SDCqgHLX8Ys)

- ○ Faber, Adele & Elaine Mazlish. *Siblings Without Rivalry: How to Help Your Children Live Together So You Can Live Too.* New York: W.W. Norton & Company, 1987.

- ○ Faber, Adele & Elaine Mazlish. *How to Talk So Kids Will Listen, And Listen So Kids Will Talk.* New York: Scribner, 1989.

- ○ Gwande, Atul. *Being Mortal: Medicine and What Matters in the End.* New York: Metropolitan Books, 2014.

- ○ Hanh, Thich Nhat. *Happiness: Essential Mindfulness Practices.* Berkeley: Parallax Press, 2009.

- ○ McKenna, James J. *Safe Infant Sleep: Expert Answers to Your Cosleeping Questions.* Washington, D.C.: Platypus Media, 2020.

- ○ Nestor, James. *Breath: The New Science of a Lost Art.* New York: Riverhead Books, 2020.

- ○ Payne, Kim John. *Simplicity Parenting: Using the Extraordinary Power of Less to Raise Calmer, Happier, and More Secure Kids.* New York: Ballantine Books, 2010.

Pregnancy/Birth

- ○ Nichols, Lily. *Real Food for Pregnancy*: *The Science and Wisdom of Optimal Prenatal Nutrition.* Lily Nichols, 2018.

- ○ Simkin, Penny and Phyllis Klaus. *When Survivors Give Birth: Understanding and Healing the Effects of Early Sexual Abuse on Childbearing Women.* Seattle: Classic Day Publishing, 2004.

- ○ Stanger-Ross, Iliana. *A is for Advice (The Reassuring Kind): Wisdom For Pregnancy.* New York: Harper Collins, 2019.

Pregnancy Loss

- ○ Burgess, Mary. *Mending Invisible Wings: Healing From the Loss of Your Baby.* Palm of Her Hand, 2009.

- ○ Davis, Deborah L. *Empty Cradle, Broken Heart: Surviving the Death of Your Baby.* Golden: Fulcrum Publishing, 2016.

- ○ Ilse, Sherokee. *Empty Arms: Coping with Miscarriage, Stillbirth and Infant Death.* Maple Plain, Wintergreen Press, Inc., 2015.

Postpartum

- ○ Lim, Robin. *After the Baby's Birth... A Woman's Way to Wellness: A Complete Guide for Postpartum Women,* Celestial Arts, 2001.

- ○ Wiessenger, Diane and Diana West. *The Womanly Art of Breastfeeding: Completely Revised and Updated 8th Edition.* New York: Ballantine Books, 2010.

Websites:

- O Black Mothers' Breastfeeding Association, https://blackmothersbreastfeeding.org/

- O Black doula project, https://blackdoulaproject.com

- O Black doulas, https://blackdoulas.org"

- O Bradley Method of Childbirth Education®, https://bradleybirth.com/

- O Breastfeeding USA, https://breastfeedingusa.org/

- O Centering Pregnancy, https://centeringhealthcare.org

- O Childbirth Connection, http://www.childbirthconnection.org/maternity-care/

- O DONA International (Doulas of North America), https://www.dona.org

- O Evidence Based Birth, https://evidencebasedbirth.com

- O Jason Headley, *F*ck That: An Honest Meditation*, https://www.youtube.com/watch?v=92i5m3tV5XY

- O Kelly Mom, https://kellymom.com/category/about/

- O La Leche League, https://www.llli.org/

- O Postpartum Support International, https://www.postpartum.net

- O United States Lactation Consultant Association, https://uslca.org/resources/find-a-lactation-consul-tant-map#!directory/map

- O WIC Breastfeeding Support, https://wicbreastfeeding.fns.usda.gov/

ADDENDUMS

Meconium (Fetal poop) Addendum 1

Babies don't generally poop while still inside, but they can if they are stressed. If your amniotic sac ruptures and you are not with your care providers you should contact them and let them know. It will be important to first try and evaluate the amniotic fluid yourself. Try to catch some in a container, look in the toilet, or check the area where you leaked such as your underpants or the bed. If the fluid looks clear, or slightly opaque with a tinge of white or pink color, those are all assuring variations. You will however now want to take extra precautions to avoid infection. Refrain from inserting anything into the vagina. (Vaginal exams should be carefully considered before consenting always, and especially once your membranes have ruptured. And if your fluid is clear, you might not want to run into the hospital right away if you are not in active labor as there are typically many more germs there than in your home.) If you do see any meconium in the amniotic fluid such as pale green or brown, thin, stringy debris, or darkly colored thick gloppy dense debris, that is a sign that your baby has pooped inside the uterus. Thick and dark meconium is a sign that your baby has just recently pooped and could be currently stressed. If this is the case please seek medical attention immediately. The other way meconium can present, thin and pale, indicates that at some point in the past the baby experienced stress and pooped. Older meconium warrants a prompt conversation with your provider too, but may not require immediate physical attention. Any meconium present will indicate medical attention at birth. If the baby has potentially inhaled any meconium the concern is that it could clog and infect the lungs. If after birth your baby shows no signs of distress, it's likely that no medical action is required. When symptoms of distress do present, providers will try to suction out any debris from the lungs. They may need to move the baby to a neonatal intensive care unit (NICU) to mechanically keep their lungs open for several days until any persistent meconium can be reabsorbed. In this case antibiotics will also be prescribed. Most babies who experience meconium aspiration and have access to care, recover with no long-term effects.

Meconium Addendum 2

Meconium is your baby's first fecal material. Your baby should pass a meconium poop within the first 48 hours of after birth. The meconium is usually dark green to black in color and it's sticky sticky sticky like tar. To clean meconium off you or your baby's skin try olive oil, we found that to be much more efficient than using baby wipes or soap.

INDEX

ABOUT THE AUTHOR

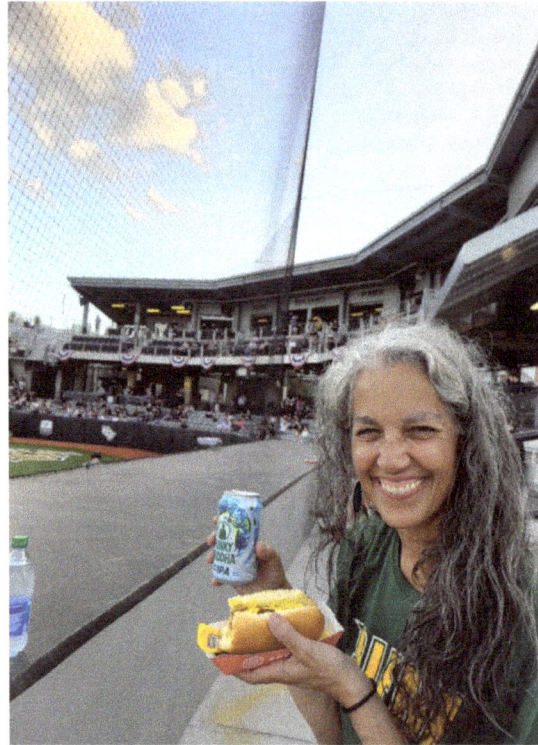

Emily Marynczak, birth educator, doula, activist, artist, and mother. Born in 1962 in Nyack, New York. In 1967 her family moved to New York City, where Emily experienced the activism and artistic energy of the 1960s and 70s. In 1980, Emily attended Antioch College in Yellow Springs, Ohio where she earned a B.A. in dance and documentary arts. Emily then went on to earn an advanced degree from the National Theater School of The Netherlands in their school of modern dance in Amsterdam. After grad school she returned to NY and worked a variety of jobs including as a company dancer with Yoshiko Chuma and the School of Hard Knocks, a nursery school teacher, and as script supervisor in the motion picture industry. On one special film job: the indie-classic Swoon, by Tom Kalin, Emily meet Julian. In 1993 baby number one arrived and Emily and Julian moved to Albany NY where she embraced her life as a mother, and became a childbirth educator. Emily is seen here in this photo at a very happy moment indeed; watching her youngest kid play baseball and celebrating 30 years of marriage. In all aspects of her life Emily strives to continuously chip away at unjust and oppressive power structures. Emily loves writing, walking long distances, and eating ice cream.

www.ingramcontent.com/pod-product-compliance
Lightning Source LLC
Chambersburg PA
CBHW042337030426
42335CB00030B/3375